INSTRUMENTAL METHODS OF ANALYSIS

DR. SUPRIYA S. MAHAJAN

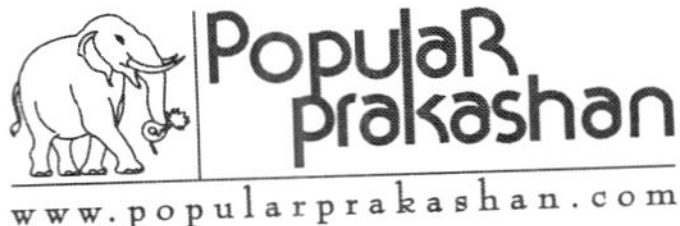

Published by
Asmita Mohite for
POPULAR PRAKASHAN PVT. LTD.
301, Mahalaxmi Chambers
22, Bhulabhai Desai Road
Mumbai - 400 026
info@popularprakashan.com

First Edition 2010
Reprint September 2010
Reprint December 2010
Reprint October 2018
Reprint July 2024

(4325)
ISBN 978-81-7991-577-6

Cover Design: Mahendra Ghanekar
Typesetting: Jyoti Nagap

Printed by
by Trinity Academy For Corporate Training Ltd.
Pune

Dedicated

to

My Dear Parents

to

Whom I Owe

Everything...

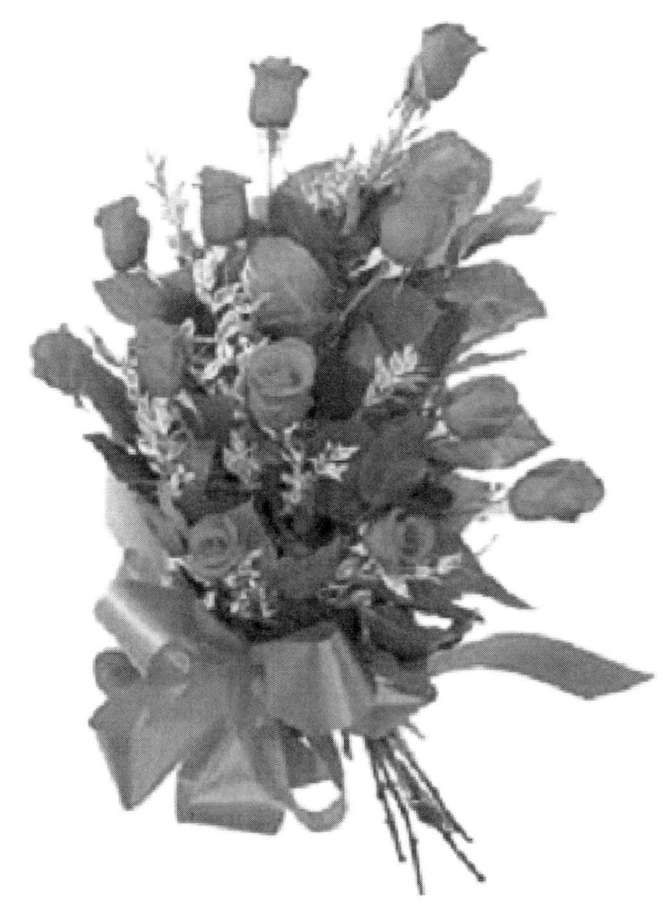

Foreword

Analytical chemistry has come a long way from its past obscurity to its present-day status of an independent science, encompassing many physico-chemical disciplines. The instrumental part of analytical chemistry is like mathematics. It expresses the result in numbers - like in mathematics, and yet unlike in mathematics, it does not assume numbers. Its results are final and can be reproduced again and again, and yet it hasn't got the status of a basic science. Instrumental methods of analysis are important tools used by many scientists working in different fields to prove or advance their theories.

The stepmotherly treatment given to analytical chemistry, and along with it, to instrumental methods of analysis, has unfortunately been prevalent for a long time. The Nobel Prize in Medicine for the discovery of the structure of DNA molecule went to James Watson, Francis Crick and Maurice Wilkins, but Rosalind Franklin, who did the spectacular work of X-ray diffraction on DNA, was all but forgotten. Nuclear magnetic resonance was first described by Isidor Rabi in 1938. Eight years later, in 1946, Felix Bloch and Edward Mills Purcell refined the technique for use on liquids and solids, for which they shared the Nobel Prize in Physics, much later in 1952, only after the application of NMR was found to be very good in many sciences. As recently as in 2002, the coveted Nobel Prize in Chemistry was shared by John Fenn, a scientist from USA and Koichi Tanaka, a scientist from Japan, for application of mass spectrometry in biological sciences.

I still remember the day when the Beckman spectrophotometer arrived in UDCT in 1950, where I was a post-graduate research student. The whole institute was filled with enthusiasm as if some VIP has arrived! Later on it was housed in a glass cabinet and was literally worshiped like a god!! No one was allowed to touch it except for a few people who were trained and trusted. We, the juniors, were only to submit our samples and wait for a day or two to get the results. The excitement petered out after a year or so, when the double beam instrument came along and the 'Beckman' lost its charm. With the advent of digital technology, electronics and entry of computers in the field of analysis, the whole scenario changed rapidly and a new generation of researchers came along, who knew only how to push the buttons on the instrument and get the results. They were totally unaware of what is meant by 'dark current,' 'slit adjustment,' or the 'aperture of the window,' because it was all done automatically by the "super-intelligent" instrument. In all this progress, the fundamental knowledge of the instrument and its application was lost. The instruments became a mere tool for mining of data - like what is said about computers - 'garbage in, garbage out.'

This book by my brilliant former student and colleague, Dr. Supriya Mahajan, has come out at the right time for this gadget-crazy generation. The book will tell them what is hidden behind the instrument and what it is capable of doing, besides neatly producing sheets of data. The basic fundamentals of instruments, which have been lost, as I said earlier, are revived in this book. The book has done an excellent job in reviewing these fundamentals of instruments.

Speaking of today's vast ocean of information, it is often said:

'Where is the knowledge that we lost in information?

Where is the wisdom that we lost in vast collection of knowledge?'

Let us not forget that we ultimately have to gain knowledge and through knowledge gain wisdom, both in science as well as in life.

This book will fill that gap between data - information - knowledge - and wisdom. I am confident that it will be appreciated both by students of analytical sciences as well as by their teachers.

Dr. H.P.Tipnis
M. Sc. (Tech), M.S., Ph.D.(USA)
Corporate Advisor - Pharmacy
Former Principal,
Bombay College of Pharmacy

Mumbai
March 2010

Preface

The growing need for the accurate and quantitative estimation of compounds has increased the demand for advanced analytical techniques with sophisticated instrumentation and user-friendly software. With this in mind, I have endeavoured to broadly cover the most widely-used instrumental analytical techniques.

The objective of this book is to create a basic understanding of the most popular analytical methods, instrumentation and applications. Wherever required, the concepts are lucidly explained with the help of simplified diagrams.

With the advent of computer software and with the development of high throughput screening, the process of drug design and development has been accelerated. The isolation of compounds using separation techniques is of great importance. The tremendous power of various chromatographic techniques for the isolation and estimation of compounds has created a special place for them in the field of qualitative as well as quantitative analysis. I have dealt with liquid chromatography and gas chromatography intensively. A variety of techniques such as exclusion chromatography, affinity chromatography, ion–pair chromatography, chiral chromatography, etc. are also discussed.

Hyphenated techniques using the combination of two analytical methods like LC/MS, GC/MS, TG/MS, DSC/MS, etc. have gained lot of popularity in the field of analysis due to increase in the speed of generating data and accuracy in the measurements. The technique of mass spectrometry is discussed in-depth with representative fragmentation processes. The electrochemical methods of analysis such as conductimetry, polarography and amperometry, which still continue to play role in the field of analysis, as also fluorimetry, ultraviolet spectrometry, infrared (IR) spectrometry, ^{1}H-NMR spectrometry, atomic spectrometry and X-ray diffraction spectrometry, have been discussed in great detail.

I have included several problems based on Beer-Lambert law, Fieser Woodward rules, IR, ^{1}H-NMR and mass spectrometry, as also mixed problems. In addition, there are plenty of problems for practice with the information and data required for solving them.

Lastly, I have given a few hints for the upkeep of the instruments to help prevent the equipment from going out of order, and to gain optimum efficiency from the instruments for many years.

I take this opportunity to thank my past and present students, whose inspiration and motivation made the arduous task of writing the book an easy one.

My heartfelt thanks to Dr. S. D. Bhandarkar, former Prof essor and Head of Department of Endocrinology and Associate in Clinical Pharmacology, Seth G. S. Medical College and K. E. M. Hospital and one of the authors of the iconic book, 'Pharmacology and Pharmacotherapeutics'. He edited this book critically and provided immeasurable guidance. His immense experience and vast knowledge helped me give a proper structure to this book. He has offered such a valuable help throughout the preparation of this book that words are inadequate to express my thanks.

I am deeply honoured to have the Foreword written by my teacher, mentor and the former Principal of Bombay College of Pharmacy, Dr. H.P.Tipnis, whom I respect very much. A accomplished author himself, he gave me the right dose of perception and intuition essential to the preparation of this book. I express my deep gratitude towards him.

It is a pleasure to acknowledge M/s Perkin Elmer, for providing the photographs for the cover page of this book.

It would be highly remiss if I do not use this platform to truly and fully appreciate the love, belief and support of my husband, Sudhakar. To my son, Akshay, sister, Supriya Dani and her husband, Shirish Dani, many thanks for being a constant source of love.

Thanks are due to Mr. Harsha Bhatkal of Popular Prakashan, and the staff, especially Mrs. Jyoti Nagap for their help.

I welcome suggestions and constructive criticism from my readers, so that I can make the next edition of the book even more useful.

Dr. Supriya Mahajan

About the Book

This book comes from the desk of Dr. (Mrs.) Supriya S. Mahajan, M.Sc. (Tech) from University Institute of Chemical Technology and Ph. D. (Tech) from Bombay College of Pharmacy, who has taught Pharmaceutical Chemistry, Pharmaceutical Analysis and Modern Analytical Techniques for the last 27 years, first in Bombay College of Pharmacy, Mumbai, and then in C. U. Shah College of Pharmacy, Mumbai. She is now Professor of Pharmaceutical Chemistry in the latter institute. She has been a member of several academic committees, and a recipient of many honors and awards. She has published scientific papers widely. The book is the culmination of her wide and long experience in teaching, writing and research in her subject.

The book covers a wide range of advanced analytical instruments, their internal structure, working, uses, and the details of how to use them effectively. It is well-planned and follows a uniform pattern in all chapters. Each chapter covers one topic, and is divided into sections and sub-sections to make it easy to understand. The language is simple and flows smoothly from section to section. There are many detailed diagrams of the instruments, graphs and summary tables.

Books on this subject, especially of this range and depth of treatment of the topics, are hard to come by, and this book will be a boon to everyone who needs this kind of information. That includes graduate and postgraduate students, as well as teachers, in any branch of pharmacy, chemistry; and those who run clinical and analytical laboratories of any description, both in hospitals and private practice.

I was privileged to read the book from an early stage of its preparation; and I have been educated by it and more than enjoyed it. To quote a cliché, "For the novice, it is the Bible (or the Geeta, if you will); and for the expert, it is a source of a quick reference". I recommend it to anyone who has to even remotely anything to do with any branch of pharmacy or chemistry.

Dr. S. D. Bhandarkar
Former Professor and HOD of Endocrinology and
Associate in Clinical Pharmacology,
Seth G. S. Medical College and K. E. M. Hospital

March 2010

About the Author

Dr. Supriya Mahajan is a professor of Pharmaceutical Chemistry at C.U.Shah College of Pharmacy in Mumbai and has over 27 years of teaching experience. Dr. Mahajan has done her M.Sc. (Tech) from the University Institute of Chemical Technology and Ph.D. (Tech) from the Bombay College of Pharmacy. Her research papers have appeared in several reputed national and international journals. She has also presented her research work at conferences in India and abroad.

She is a member of a panel that reviews research articles published in national and international journals. She is the resource person for a few colleges and seminars and delivers lectures on Modern Analytical Techniques and their Applications.

A guide for post-graduate and doctoral students of pharmacy, Dr. Mahajan is on the editorial board of *Indian Drugs*, the publication brought out by the Indian Drug Manufacturers' Association.

Important Physical Constants

1. Avogadro number (N) = 6.022137×10^{23} particles mol^{-1}
2. Boltzmann constant (k) = $1.38066 \times 10\text{-}^{23}$ JK^{-1} = 1.38066×10^{-16} erg deg^{-1}
3. Faraday constant (F) = 96,485 C mol^{-1} of electrons
4. Gas constant (R) = 8.31451 $JK^{-1}mol^{-1}$ = $0.0820578 \times 10\text{-}^{23}$ L atm K^{-1} mol^{-1}
5. Modified Planck constant ($\hbar$) = h/2ð = 1.05511×10^{-34} J sec
6. Planck constant (h) = 6.62608×10^{-34} J sec
7. Speed of light (c) in vacuum = 2.99792×10^{8} m sec^{-1}

Symbols Used

1. α : Alpha
2. β : Beta
3. γ : Gamma : Magnetogyric ratio
4. δ : Delta : (i) The chemical shift in NMR spectrum and (ii) the path difference between two beams (Michelson interferometer)
5. ε : Epsilon : Molar absorptivity
6. ζ : Zeta : Zeta potential
7. η : Eta : Viscosity
8. θ : Theta : Angle
9. κ : Kappa : Specific conductance or conductivity
10. λ : Lambda : Waevelength
11. Λ : Capital lambda : Equivalent conductance
12. $\overline{\Lambda}$: Capital lambda bar : Molar conductance
13. Λ° : Conductivity of a solution at infinite dilution
14. μ : Mu : Magnetic dipole moment
15. ν : Nu : Frequency of radiation
16. π : Pi
17. ρ : Rho : (i) Specific resistance or resistivity of a solution (ii) density
18. σ : Sigma :Shielding constant or a screening constant
19. τ: Tau : Chemical shift
20. Ω : Capital Omega : Ohms : Unit of resistance
21. A : Absorbance
22. a : Absorptivity
23. B : Magnetic field
24. C : Capacitance
25. D : Diffusion coefficient
26. d : diameter, grating spacing, thickness of dielectric layer
27. E : Energy
28. e : Electron
29. G : Conductance
30. H : Enthalpy
31. I : Intensity
32. i : Current
33. J : Joules
34. K : Equilibrium constant, Partition coefficient, Distribution coefficient
35. M : Molarity
36. Normality
37. n : Refractive index, number of equivalents, spectral order, number of electrons participating in the electrode reaction
38. P : Power of radiation
39. R : Resistance, Gas constant
40. s : Standard deviation N :
41. S/N : Signal to noise ratio
42. T : Transmittance, temperature
43. t : Time
44. V : Voltage
45. v : Velocity

Contents

CHAPTER 1

ELECTROMAGNETIC RADIATION

Electromagnetic radiation (EMR) is a type of energy that is transmitted through space at enormous velocities . The concept of wave-particle duality is applicable to EMR. Sometimes, EMR is considered as waves and sometimes, it is considered as particles or corpuscles.

Wave model is useful in explaining phenomena like reflection, refraction, diffraction, interference and so on. Corpuscular nature of EMR is useful in understanding interaction between radiation and matter, such as absorption or emission of energy by the matter. In the corpuscular model, EMR is treated as packets of energy, called *photons* or *quanta*. The wave model fails to account for the phenomena associated with the absorption or emission of the radiant energy. For these processes, it is necessary to view EMR as a stream of discrete particles of energy called photons.

1.1. WAVE PROPERTIES OF RADIATION

Wave properties are described by a number of parameters. Some of them are:

1) Wavelength (λ, Lambda, Gr. = Greek)

The distance between the two consecutive crests or two consecutive troughs (i.e. one cycle) of a wave is called wavelength (**Fig. 1.1**). It can be expressed in centimeters, nanometers or angstrom units (A°). These are interrelated as follows:

Wavelength Units:

$1A^\circ = 10^{-8}\,cm = 10^{-10}\,m$

$1nm = 10A^\circ = 10^{-7}\,cm = 10^{-9}\,m$

$1\mu m = 10^{3} nm = 10^{-4} cm = 10^{-6}\,m$

Note: In the earlier literature, the micrometer (μm) was called as micron (μ) and nanometer (nm) was called as millimicron (mμ).

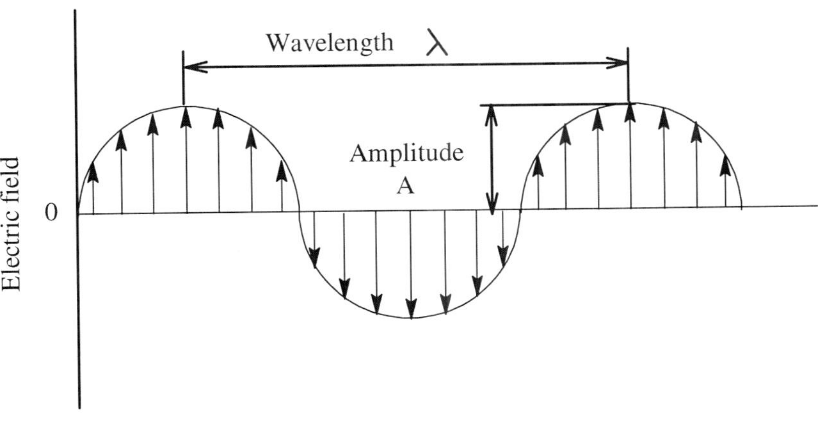

Fig. 1.1: Wave parameters

2) Amplitude (A)

The amplitude of the wave is the length of the electric vector at a maximum in the wave.

3) Frequency (ν, Nu, Gr.)

The frequency of radiation is the number of waves passing through a point in one second. The common unit of frequency is *hertz* (Hz). Frequency of 1 hertz corresponds to one cycle or one wave per second. Frequency is related to wavelength by the following equation-

$$\nu = c/\lambda \; \dots \; (1.1)$$

where 'c' is the velocity of light in vacuum.

$c = 2.99 \times 10^{8}$ m/s $= 3.00 \times 10^{10}$ cm/s

4) Wavenumber ($\bar{\nu}$, Nu bar)

The reciprocal of the wavelength in centimeters is called wavenumber. It is the number of complete waves or cycles in 1 cm. Its units are cm^{-1}. The relation between the wavenumber and the frequency is expressed by the following equation:

$$\bar{\nu} = \frac{1}{\lambda} = \frac{\nu}{c} \dots (1.2)$$

1.2. ELECTROMAGNETIC SPECTRUM

Electromagnetic spectrum of radiation is described in terms of its energy, wavelength, wavenumber or wave frequency. Based on these values, EMR is classified into different regions. The full range of wavelengths or energies of EMR is called an *electromagnetic spectrum.* In this spectrum, the human eye is perceptive to a very small portion. **Table 1.1** shows the wavelengths (λ) for different regions of the EMR.

Table 1.1: Wavelengths (λ) in different regions of the electromagnetic spectrum

γ-rays	X-rays	Far UV	UV	Visible	Near IR	Middle IR	Far IR	Micro waves	Radio waves
0.1-10 nm	10-100 nm	100-200 nm	200-400 nm	400-800 nm	0.8-2.5 μm	2.5-50 μm	50-1000 μm	0.1-100 cm	100-1000 cm

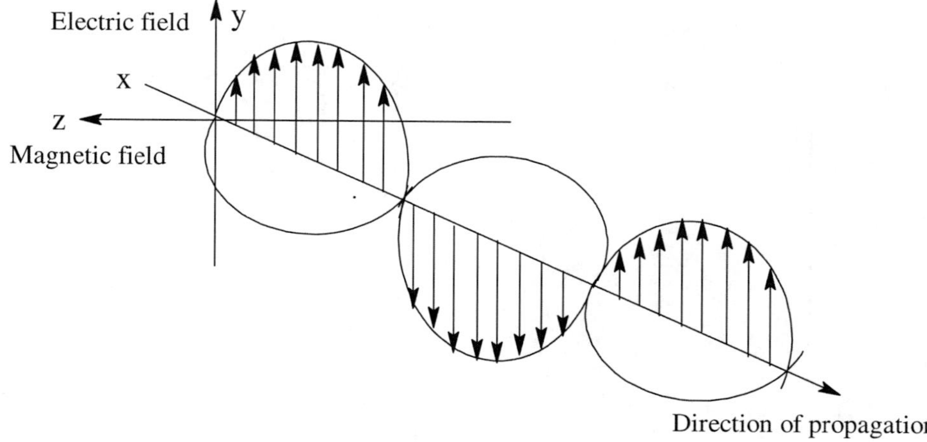

Fig.1.2: Electric and magnetic fields associated with the EMR

1.3. INTERACTION OF EMR WITH MATTER

Figure 1.2 shows the electric and magnetic fields associated with the EMR. These two fields are perpendicular to each other and to the direction of propagation of EMR.

In any medium containing matter, the electromagnetic field of the radiation interacts with the bound electrons in the atoms or molecules present. The radiant frequency always remains fixed and is determined by the source. Hence, as the radiation passes from a less dense medium to a denser medium, its wavelength decreases and vice versa. This is shown in **Fig. 1.3**.

The nature of the interaction of the matter with electromagnetic field of the radiation depends on the properties of the matter through which radiation passes and may lead to transmission, absorption or scattering of the radiation.

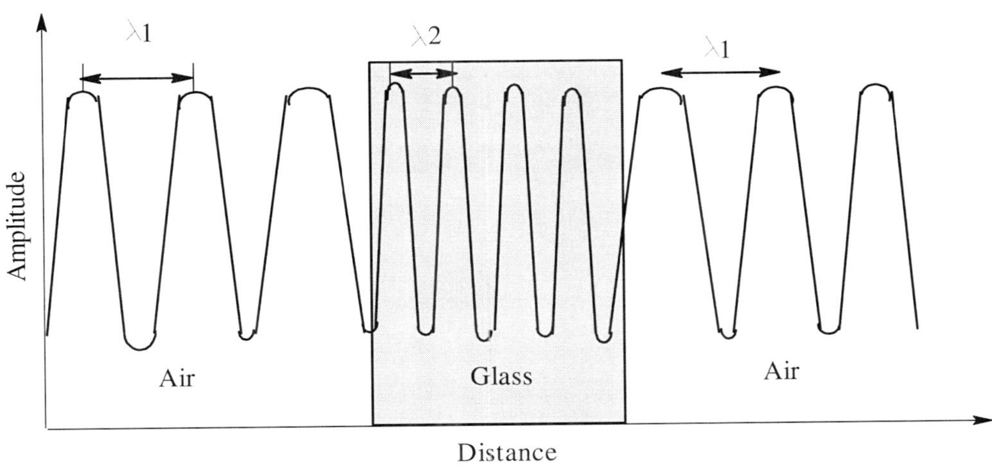

Fig.1.3: Interaction of matter with electromagnetic field of radiation

1.4. ABSORPTION SPECTROMETRY

Spectrometry is the spectroscopic technique used to assess the concentration or amount of a given species; and, a spectrometer is the instrument used for this purpose.

When radiation passes through a sample, the electromagnetic energy is transferred to the atoms or molecules constituting the sample. As a result, the latter are transformed from a lower energy state to a higher energy state. At room temperature, most of the substances are in their lowest energy state or ground state. Hence, the absorption of energy usually results in the transition from ground state to higher energy states. Ultraviolet radiation and visible radiation are sufficiently energetic to cause the transition of the outermost or the bonding electrons only, but X-radiation, being much more energetic, can interact with electrons closest to the nuclei. Depending on the region of wavelengths involved, absorption spectrometry can be classified as ultraviolet spectrometry, X- ray spectrometry and so on. Similarly, depending upon the nature of matter involved, spectrometry can also be classified as:

1.4.1. Atomic absorption spectrometry
1.4.2. Molecular absorption spectrometry

In the first case, atomic sample interacts with the radiation whereas in the second case molecular sample interacts.

1.4.1. Atomic Absorption Spectrometry

When a beam of polychromatic ultraviolet or visible radiation passes through a mono-atomic sample, such as vapor of mercury or sodium, only a few well defined frequencies are absorbed. This is because atoms possess only electronic energy levels. Vibrational and rotational energy levels are not present in atoms. The absorption of energy by atoms thus results in the transition of an electron from one electronic state to the other. Absorption to each higher energy level results in the production of a line in the spectrum. The intensity of each line depends on the number of electrons involved in a particular transition. If an atom contains four electronic states such as E_o, E_1, E_2 and E_3, as shown in **Fig. 1.4**, then the transition of an electron can be brought about from the ground state (E_o) to E_1, E_2 and E_3 electronic states.

The wavelength λ_1 having energy ΔE_1 can bring about transition of electrons from E_o to E_1. A still shorter wavelength λ_2, associated with higher amount of energy ΔE_2, can bring about transition of electrons from E_o to E_2. A wavelength λ_3, even shorter than λ_2, and associated with energy ΔE_3, higher than ΔE_2, can bring about transition of electrons from E_o to E_3. Absorption of these three energies can produce three lines, L_1, L_2 and L_3, in a spectrum at different values of wavelengths or frequencies. This is illustrated in **Fig. 1.4**. The intensity of each line depends on the number of atoms or electrons that are excited from the ground electronic state to the higher electronic state. Because of limited number of electronic states in an atom, very few lines appear in the atomic spectrum. Hence, an atomic spectrum is a *line spectrum* and is very simple in nature.

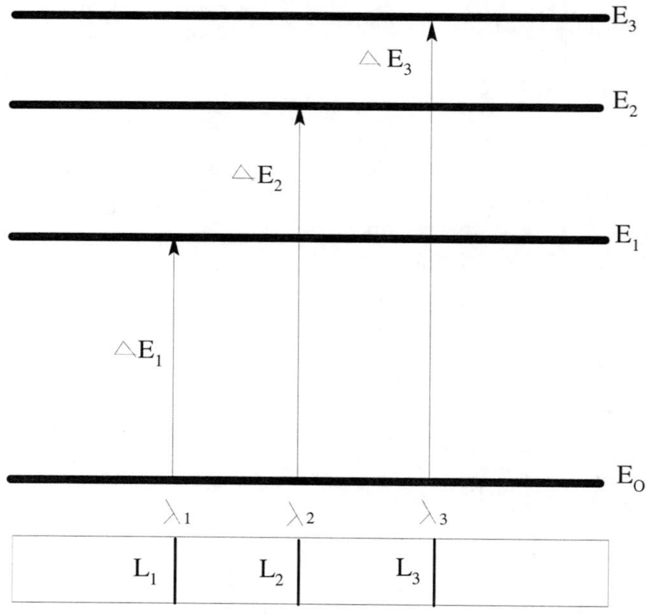

Fig. 1.4: A line (L) spectrum of an atom

1.4.2. Molecular Absorption Spectrometry

When a beam of polychromatic radiation, containing a broad range (> 50 nm) of wavelengths, passes through a multi-atomic molecular sample, several frequencies are absorbed. This is because unlike atoms, molecules possess electronic, vibrational and rotational energy levels. As shown in **Fig. 1.5**, each electronic state consists of a number of vibrational energy levels and each vibrational energy level in turn, consists of several rotational energy levels.

In **Fig. 1.5**, E_o, E_1 and E_2 are the ground, first and second electronic states, respectively. The vibrational energy levels are denoted by v_o, v_1, v_2 and v_3. The rotational energy levels are denoted by r_o, r_1, r_2, and so on.

The total energy of a molecule is the sum of its electronic energy ($E_{electronic}$), vibrational energy ($E_{vibrational}$) and rotational energy ($E_{rotational}$).

$$E = (E_{electronic}) + (E_{vibrational}) + (E_{rotational})$$

The absorption of energy by a molecule thus results in the transition of electrons from the ground state to the higher rotational, vibrational or electronic energy levels, depending on the amount of energy available.

The transition of electrons from one rotational energy level to another requires less energy and correspondingly a longer wavelength for excitation. The transition of electrons from one

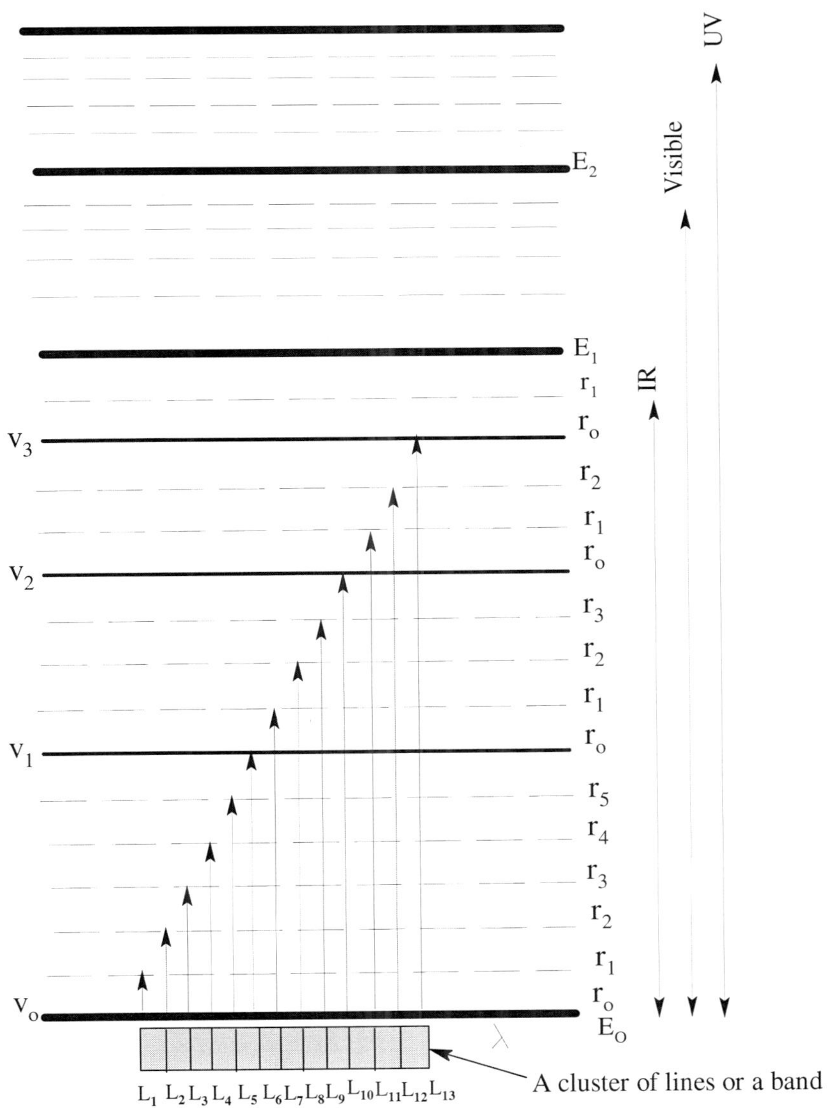

Fig. 1.5: A band spectrum of a molecule

vibrational energy level to another requires a little more energy than that required for the rotational transition, and a comparatively shorter wavelength can excite the electron. The transition from one electronic state to another requires still larger amount of energy and correspondingly a still shorter wavelength is required for the excitation. With a polychromatic beam, wherein a number of wavelengths are available for excitation, a molecule can undergo all the three types of transition. This results in the absorption of a number of frequencies. Since each absorption produces one line (L) in the spectrum, the absorption of a number of frequencies which are very close to each other, produces a cluster of lines which appears as a band in the spectrum (**Fig. 1.5**). Hence, a molecular spectrum is a *band spectrum* and is complex in nature.

For imagining the formation of a band from the cluster of closely spaced lines, let us consider the rotational and vibrational energy levels between the electronic states E_0 and E_1. Each transition, from say r_0 to r_1, r_0 to r_2, r_0 to r_3 and so on, would produce single line each (L_1, L_2, L_3, respectively). All these lines would be very close to each other because there is very little difference in the amount of energy required for the successive transitions. Correspondingly, there is very little difference in the frequencies of radiation, which are absorbed by the molecule. Since, in the spectrum, these lines are produced very close to each other they appear as a band in a low resolution instrument. The resolution of the band in the individual lines is possible only with a high resolution spectrometer.

Electromagnetic radiation of different energies brings about transitions to various energy levels of a molecule. These are shown in **Fig. 1.5**. Infrared radiation is less energetic than visible radiation and ultraviolet radiation and can bring about transition of electrons among the vibrational or rotational energy levels of the ground state (E_0). Visible radiation being more energetic than infrared radiation, causes excitation of electrons from E_0 to any of the vibrational or rotational energy levels associated with E_1. Ultraviolet radiation is more energetic than visible radiation and causes excitation of electrons from E_0 to any of the vibrational or rotational energy levels associated with E_2 or higher.

1.5. EMISSION SPECTROMETRY

In absorption spectrometry, the sample is exposed to some radiation of power P_0. The radiation interacts with the sample and transfers a part of its energy to the sample. This interaction results in the reduction of power of the radiation from P_0 to P. Measurement of incident power P_0 and the transmitted power P provides the information about the amount of energy transmitted, (P_0-P), from radiation to the sample. As a result of absorption of energy, the sample gets excited from ground state to higher energy levels.

In emission spectrometry, the sample is excited to higher energy level by using number of means such as bombardment with electrons or other elementary particles, exposure to high potential alternating current or absorption of EMR. The excited sample with higher energy is always less stable. To achieve more stability, the sample tries to come back to its original state by emitting out the excess energy. When this energy is given out in the form of radiation containing relatively few specific wavelengths, the resulting emission spectrum is discontinuous and is a line spectrum. It can be used for identification and determination of emitting species. Sometimes, the atoms in a solid or a liquid are so closely packed that the individual wavelengths are very closely spaced and the resolution is not feasible by ordinary means. This results in a continuous or a band spectrum.

Thus, in emission spectrometry, the power of the radiation which is produced by the excited sample while returning back to the ground state is measured.

1.6. SELECTION OF ABSORPTION OR EMISSION SPECTROMETRY

The difference between absorption spectrometry and emission spectrometry is explained diagrammatically in **Fig. 1.6**. In absorption spectrometry, the amount of energy absorbed by a compound is required to be determined. The amount of energy absorbed by a compound is (P_o-P). Hence, measurement of P_o as well as P should be accurate. These quantities can be measured accurately only if their magnitudes are sufficiently high. The power of the incident beam (P_o) is sufficiently high and can be measured accurately. The power of the transmitted beam (P) is sufficiently high only if incident radiation interacts with fewer molecules in the sample.

In emission spectrometry, the amount of energy emitted by an excited molecule while coming back to the ground state is measured. If the power or intensity of emitted radiation is to be measured accurately, a larger number of molecules should come back from an excited state to the ground state. Hence, emission spectrometry is used when a large number of molecules interact with incident radiation and get excited to higher energy level.

Thus, absorption spectrometry is selected when fewer molecules interact with incident radiation and get excited from the ground state to the excited state, whereas emission spectrometry is selected when a large number of molecules interact with incident radiation and get excited from the ground state to the excited state.

1.7. OPTICAL INSTRUMENTS

Common **optical instruments** are described below.

1) A **spectroscope** is an optical instrument used for visual identification of emission lines, which are produced as a result of emission of light from the excited sample.
2) A **spectrograph** is a record of emission lines on a photographic plate or a film.
3) A **photometer** is an instrument used to measure intensity of radiation. It is used for the measurement of absorption in the ultraviolet, visible and infrared regions. It is also used for the measurement of emission and fluorescence in the ultraviolet and visible regions. A photometer designed for fluorescence measurement is called **fluorimeter**. A photometer makes use of a source, filter and a photoelectric detector. The use of a filter for isolation of wavelengths from the source provides a *broad range* (25-50 nm) of wavelengths for the excitation of a sample.
4) A photometer used in the visible range of radiation is referred to as a **colorimeter**. A **colorimeter** is an instrument used for the absorption measurements of wavelengths, which are detected by human eyes.

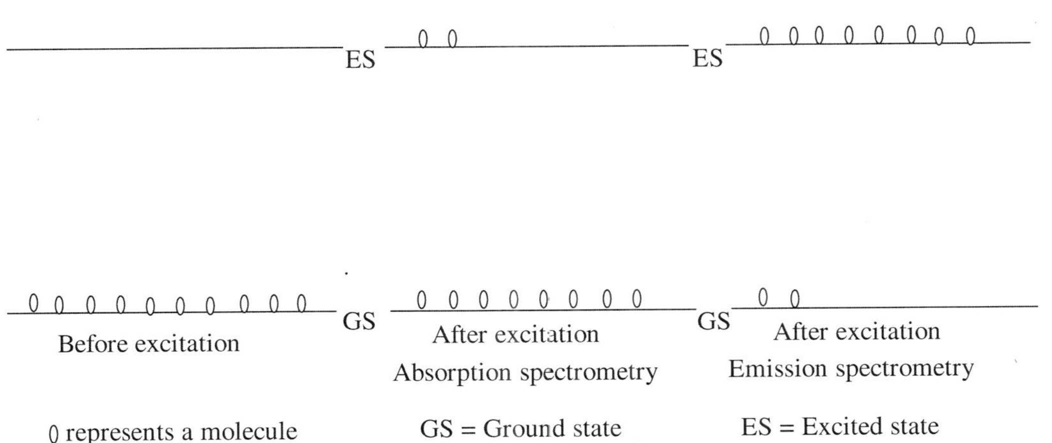

Fig. 1.6: A schematic presentation showing difference between the absorption and the emission spectrometry

5) A **spectrometer (a spectrograph or a spectroscope)** is an optical instrument used to measure properties of radiation over a specific portion of the electromagnetic spectrum, typically used in spectroscopic analysis to identify materials. A **spectrometer** is an instrument which makes use of a monochromator for isolation of wavelengths from the source. Use of a monochromator for the isolation of wavelengths from the source, makes available a *narrow range* (5-15 nm) of wavelengths for the excitation of a sample.
6) A **spectrophotometer** is a photometer that can measure intensity as a function of the color, or more specifically, the wavelength of radiation. A **spectrophotometer** makes use of a monochromator as a wavelength selector and a photoelectric detector. In case of a spectrometer and a spectrophotometer, each element of the spectrum is viewed serially. A spectrophotometer is used for measurements of absorbance in the ultraviolet, visible and infrared regions. It is also used for the measurements of fluorescence in the ultraviolet and visible regions. A spectrometer used for the measurement of fluorescence is termed as **spectrofluorimeter**.

CHAPTER 2

ULTRAVIOLET-VISIBLE ABSORPTION SPECTROMETRY

Absorption studies in the range of ultraviolet-visible (UV-visible) radiation are mainly carried out for quantitative estimation of compounds. Electromagnetic radiation (EMR) in the range of 200–400 nm constitutes ultraviolet (UV) range, whereas the EMR in the range of 400–800 nm constitutes the range for visible radiation.

2.1. COMMON TERMS USED IN ABSORPTION SPECTROMETRY

The following terms are commonly used in the absorption spectrometry.

1) Radiant power (P) or intensity (I)

The power (P) of the radiation is the energy of the beam reaching a given area per second, whereas the intensity (I) is the power per unit solid angle. Power and intensity are often used interchangeably though it is not correct to do so.

2) Transmittance (T)

When the radiation of power P_o is incident on the sample solution, the interaction between the photons of radiation and absorbing particles of the sample occurs. As a result, the power of the beam is attenuated from P_o to P as shown in **Fig. 2.1**.

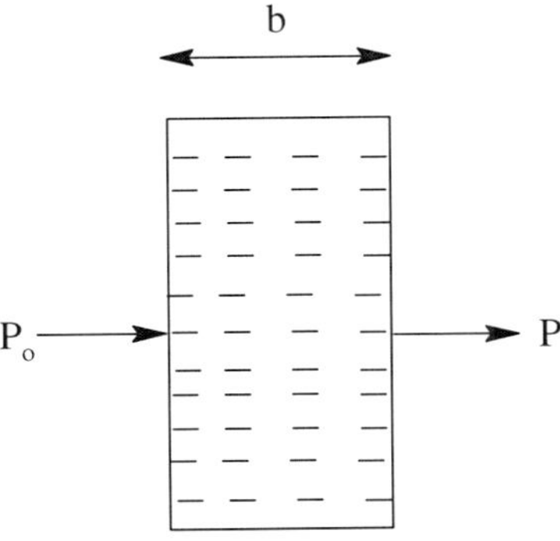

Fig. 2.1: Attenuation of power of radiation due to absorbing solution

The transmittance (T) of the solution is then defined as the fraction of incident radiation transmitted by the solution.

$$T = \frac{P}{P_o} \quad ...(2.1)$$

Usually, the term percent transmittance (% T), instead of transmittance is used.

$$\% T = \frac{P}{P_o} \times 100 \quad ...(2.2)$$

3) Absorbance (A)

When the power of the incident beam is P_o and the power of the transmitted beam is P, let the transmittance of the solution be T. The absorbance (A) of a solution is then defined as the negative logarithm of transmittance and is expressed as -

$$A = -\log_{10} T$$

$$= -\log_{10} \frac{P}{P_o} = +\log_{10} \frac{P_o}{P} \quad \cdots (2.3)$$

If the attenuation of the beam is more, the transmittance of the solution is less and the absorbance is more.

4) Absorptivity (a) and molar absorptivity (ε)

The absorbance (A) of a solution increases with the increase in the number of absorbing particles. When the thickness of the solution increases, the number of particles in the path of radiation also increases. Similarly, as the concentration of the solution increases, the number of particles interacting with the radiation also increases. Hence, absorbance increases with the increase in the thickness (b) and the concentration (c) of the solution. Thus, absorbance is directly proportional to the thickness of the solution ($A \propto b$) and also to the concentration ($A \propto c$) of a substance in the solution.

$$\therefore A \propto b \ \& \ A \propto c$$

$$\text{or } A = a.\ b.\ c \ ... \ (2.4)$$

where, 'a' is a proportionality constant called *absorptivity*.

a = absorptivity and has units of L g^{-1} cm^{-1}, when 'b' is in centimeters and concentration is in grams per liter.

a = ε (Epsilon, Gr.) = molar absorptivity and has units of L mol^{-1} cm^{-1}, when 'b' is in centimeters and concentration is in moles per liter. Molar absorptivity was formerly referred to as molar extinction coefficient.

a = $A^{1\%}_{1\,cm}$ = specific absorbance of an analyte, i.e. absorbance of a solution when 'b' is 1 centimeter and the concentration is in grams per 100 ml.

The magnitude of absorptivity indicates the ease of excitation of a molecule. The higher the absorptivity, the higher is the ease of excitation of a molecule. Its value changes with the change in the wavelength used for excitation.

5) Scanning

Scanning of a molecule in a particular range of radiation means exposing the molecule to the whole range of radiation in that region. For example, if a molecule is scanned in the UV range, it is exposed to the radiation in the range of 200-400 nm and the energy absorbed by it is recorded at each wavelength. Scanning is done in order to find the wavelength of maximum absorption (λ_{max}).

6) Wavelength of maximum absorption (λ_{max})

When a molecule is scanned using a range of wavelengths, it starts absorbing energy at a particular wavelength. Absorption increases with the increase in the wavelength, achieves maximum at a particular wavelength and then starts decreasing. The wavelength at which a substance absorbs maximum energy is called the wavelength of maximum absorption (λ_{max}).

2.2. QUANTITATIVE ASPECTS OF ABSORPTION SPECTROMETRY

We have seen that -

$$A \propto b$$

$$\propto c$$

Absorbance is quantitatively related to the thickness (b) of the solution and its concentration (c) by two separate laws. The relation between the absorbance and the thickness of the solution is governed by **Lambert's law**, whereas the relation between the absorbance and the concentration of the solution is governed by

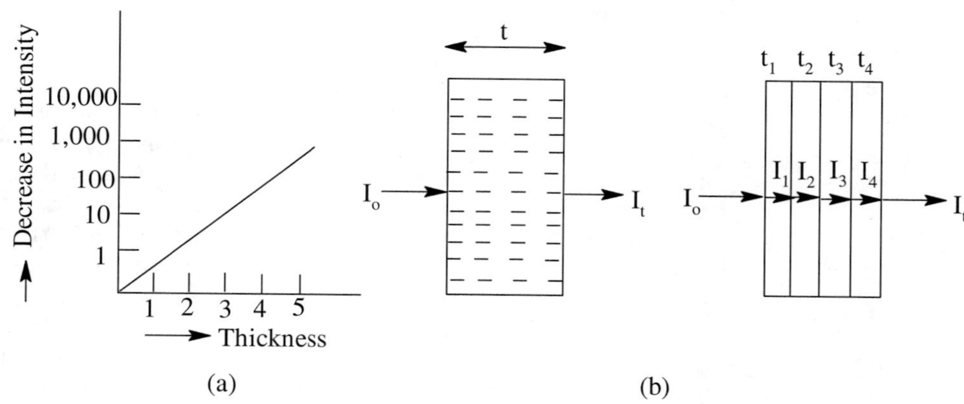

Fig. 2.2: (a) Exponential decrease in the intensity with arithmetic increase in the thickness of a solution (b) Decrease in the intensity of radiation with the increase in the thickness of a solution

Beer's law.

2.2.1. Lambert's Law

Statement

The intensity of a beam of a monochromatic* radiation decreases exponentially with the increase in the thickness of the absorbing species arithmetically. This is shown in **Fig. 2.2(a).**

OR

When a beam of light is allowed to pass through a transparent medium, the rate of decrease of intensity with the increase in the thickness of the medium is directly proportional to the intensity of the incident light (I). This is shown in **Fig. 2.2(b).**

According to Lambert's law –

$$-\frac{dI}{dt} \propto I$$

$$\text{or } -\frac{dI}{dt} = kI \cdots (2.5)$$

where, t = thickness of the solution,
k = a proportionality constant, and
I = intensity of an incident radiation
The negative sign in **equation (2.5)** indicates the decrease in the intensity (dI) with the increase in the thickness (dt) of the solution.
Rearranging and integrating **equation (2.5)**, we get -

$$+\ln\frac{I_0}{It} = k\,N$$

where, I_o = intensity of radiation at thickness, t = 0, and

$$-\ln\frac{I_t}{I_o} = k\,t \text{ OR } I_t = I_o\,e^{-kt}$$

$$\therefore +\ln\frac{I_o}{I_t} = k\,t$$

$$\therefore 2.303 \times \ln\frac{I_o}{I_t} = 2.303 \times k\,t$$

I_t = intensity of radiation at thickness, t = t
By replacing the product of two constants, (2.303 x k), by another constant, K, we get **equation (2.6).**

$$\log_{10}\frac{I_o}{I_t} = K\,t \cdots (2.6)$$

In **equation (2.6)**, K is the *absorption coefficient.*
According to **equation (2.3)**,

$$\text{Absorbance} = A = \log_{10}\frac{P_o}{P} = \log_{10}\frac{I_o}{I_t}$$

Hence, **equation (2.6)** can be written as -

$$A = Kt \ldots (2.7)$$

Thus, according to Lambert's law, absorbance is directly proportional to the thickness of the solution ($A \propto t$).
If I_o = 10 and I_t = 1, then by substituting these values in **equation (2.6)**, we get -

$$A = \log_{10}\frac{10}{1} = K\,t$$

Since $\log_{10} 10 = 1$, A = 1 = Kt
Hence, K = 1/t ... (2.8)

The absorption coefficient (K) is thus defined as the reciprocal of the thickness which is required to reduce the intensity of the transmitted radiation (I_t) to 1/10th of the intensity of the incident radiation (I_o).

2.2.2. Beer's Law

Statement

The intensity of a beam of a monochromatic radiation decreases exponentially with the increase

* A monochromatic beam, strictly speaking, is a beam containing a single isolated wavelength, which is very difficult to obtain even with the help of the most efficient monochromator. Hence, in practice, a beam containing a narrow range of wavelengths (approximately, 5-10 nm on either side of λ_{max}) is considered as a monochromatic beam.

in the concentration of the absorbing substance arithmetically.

OR

The successive increments in the number of identical absorbing molecules in the path of a beam of a monochromatic radiation absorb equal fractions of the radiant energy passing through them.

Mathematically, it can be expressed as –

$$-\frac{dI}{dn} \propto I$$

$$\text{or } -\frac{dI}{dn} = kI \cdots (2.9)$$

where, I = intensity of the radiant beam, and k = a proportionality constant

The negative sign in **equation (2.9)** indicates the decrease in the intensity (dI) with the increase in the number of particles (dn) of the absorbing species.

Rearranging and integrating **equation (2.9)**, we get –

$$-\int_{I=I_o}^{I=I_t} \frac{dI}{I} = k \int_{n=0}^{n=N} dn$$

where, I_o = intensity of the incident radiation when the number of interacting molecules, n = 0, I_t = intensity of the transmitted radiation when the number of interacting molecules, n = N, and N = total number of molecules in the path of radiation over the thickness (t) of a solution.

$$-\ln\frac{I_t}{I_o} = kN \text{ OR } I_t = I_o e^{-kN}$$

$$+\ln\frac{I_o}{I_t} = kN$$

$$2.303 \text{ x } \ln\frac{I_o}{I_t} = 2.303 \text{ x } kN$$

By replacing the product of two constants, (2.303 x k), by another constant, K, we get **equation (2.10)**.

$$\log_{10}\frac{I_o}{I_t} = KN \cdots (2.10)$$

According to **equation (2.3)**,

$$\text{Absorbance} = A = \log_{10}\frac{P_o}{P} = \log_{10}\frac{I_o}{I_t}$$

$$\text{Hence, } A = \log_{10}\frac{I_o}{I_t} = KN$$

$$\therefore A = K \text{ x } N \ldots (2.11)$$

Thus, according to Beer's law, the absorbance is directly proportional to the number of particles of an analyte in its solution.

A more convenient measure of the number of particles (N) effective in absorbing radiation is the product of concentration (c) of an analyte and the length of the path (t or b) of the radiation inside the solution. Thus, N = b x c. By replacing the term N, in **equation (2.11)**, by the product of path length (b) and the concentration (c) of a solution, and also by replacing a constant 'K' by another constant 'a', we get **equation (2.12)**.

A = a x b x c ... (2.12)

Equation (2.12) expresses Beer and Lambert law together because in this equation -

$A \propto b$ - (as per Lambert's law)

and $A \propto c$- (as per Beer's law)

2.2.3. Deviation from Beer's Law

Variation in the absorbance of a solution can be because of the variation in the path length (**Fig. 2.3**) or because of the variation in the concentration of a solution (**Fig. 2.4**). There is no exception for the linear relationship between the absorbance and the path length (b or t) at a fixed concentration (c_1) of an analyte but a deviation from linearity between the measured absorbance and the concentration, at a fixed path length, is observed many a times.

Different causes for deviation from Beer's law are given below.

2.2.3.1. Real Limitations to Beer's Law

Beer's law is applicable to only dilute solutions. It is not applicable to very dilute solutions or to concentrated solutions. This is because of the change in the molar absorptivity (ε)

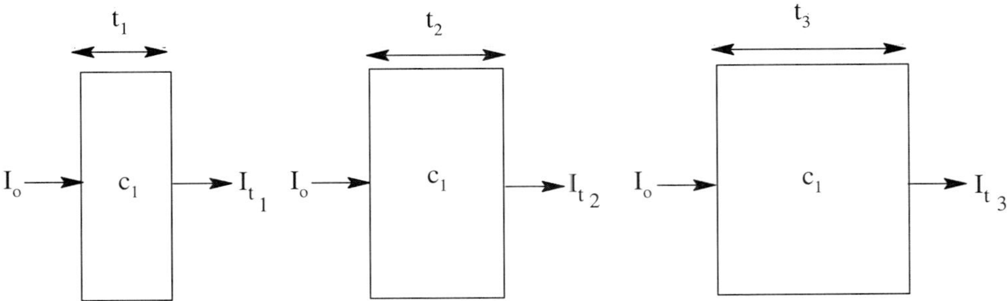

Fig. 2.3: Variation in the absorbance of a solution with path length (t) at a fixed concentration

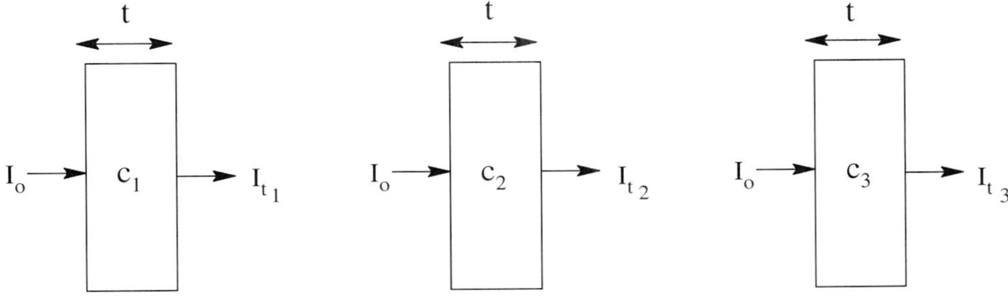

Fig. 2.4: Variation in the absorbance of a solution with concentration at a fixed path length

of an analyte, i.e. the ease of excitation of an analyte, with dilution, for most of the compounds. The change in the molar absorptivity with the change in the concentration is explained below.

At high concentrations (more than 0.01 M) of absorbing species, the molecules of an analyte are very close to each other. Hence, the average distance between the analyte molecules (intermolecular distance) is diminished. Two neighboring molecules start interacting and affect the charge distribution of each other. This in turn can alter their ability to absorb radiation of a particular wavelength. Thus, molar absorptivity of an analyte is changed.

Figure 2.5 shows interaction between the neighboring molecules of an amine as an absorber. In the absence of any interaction between the neighboring molecules, energy is required only for the excitation of non-bonding electrons on the nitrogen atom of an amine. When an intermolecular distance decreases (i.e. when the concentration of an absorber increases), an electron pair on the nitrogen atom of one molecule of an amine forms hydrogen bond with the hydrogen atom of another molecule of an amine. During the formation of a

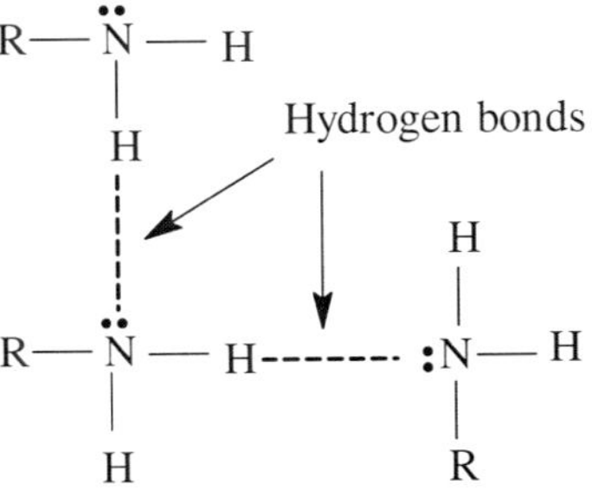

Fig. 2.5: Interaction between the neighboring molecules of an amine

hydrogen bond, some energy is released. This makes the system containing amine molecules more stable. In the presence of hydrogen bonding, excitation of the non-bonding electrons takes place, only after breaking of the hydrogen bond, which requires additional energy. The energy required to break the hydrogen bond between the two molecules is exactly equal to the energy released during its formation. Thus, excitation of amines, in the presence of hydrogen bonding requires larger amount of energy as compared to the energy required in the absence of hydrogen bonding. Correspondingly, the excitation of an amine is brought about at a longer wavelength (smaller energy) in the absence of hydrogen bonding and at a shorter wavelength (higher energy) in the presence of hydrogen bonding. This change in the absorption wavelength (λ_{max}) with the change in the concentration of an absorber results in the change in the absorptivity (ε) of an absorber, consequently resulting in the deviation from Beer's law.

At a low concentration of an amine as the absorbing species, the molecules are far apart and the solvent molecules (like ethanol) occupy the space between the two molecules of an amine. The interaction of the absorbing species with ethanol is shown in **Fig. 2.6**. This interaction changes the charge distribution in an absorber, which results in the change of λ_{max} and the molar absorptivity of an absorber, ultimately leading to the deviation from Beer's law.

$$R-\ddot{N}(H)-H \cdots :O(C_2H_5)-H \cdots :N(H)(R)-H$$

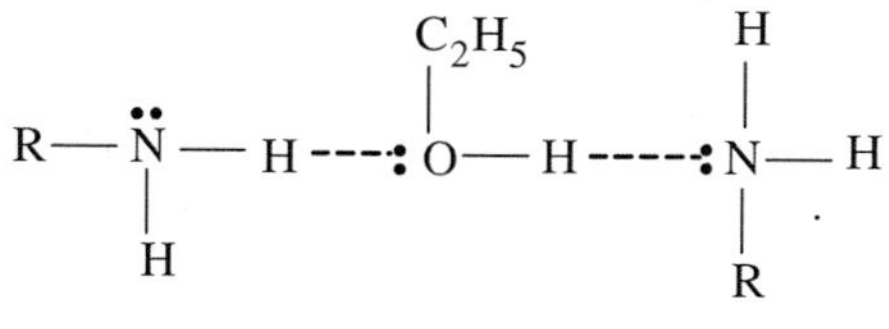

Fig. 2.6: Interaction of an absorber with ethanol

2.2.3.2. Apparent Chemical Deviation

The apparent chemical deviations from Beer's law are commonly observed in case of molecules which are able to undergo either association or dissociation or some chemical reaction with the solvent. For example, four molecules of benzyl alcohol associate in chloroform or carbon tetrachloride to form a polymer, as shown in **Fig. 2.7**. A monomer absorbs at a wavelength of 275 nm, whereas a polymer absorbs at a wavelength of 300 nm. The monomer is in equilibrium with the polymer. Deviation from Beer's law is observed when the shift in this equilibrium takes place with the dilution of the solution, i.e. with the change in the concentration of the monomer in its solution.

$$4\ C_6H_5CH_2OH \rightleftharpoons (C_6H_5CH_2OH)_4$$

Monomer (λ_{max} = 275 nm) Polymer (λ_{max} = 300 nm)

Fig. 2.7: Association of benzyl alcohol molecules

When the concentration of benzyl alcohol is less, the extent of association of its molecules is also less. Hence, the solution contains mainly the monomeric form of benzyl alcohol. Thus, at lower concentrations of benzyl alcohol, a straight line (B) is obtained for an absorbance vs. concentration plot (**Fig. 2.8**) at λ= 275 nm, which is the wavelength of maximum absorption (λ_{max}) of the monomer. As the concentration of benzyl alcohol is increased, four molecules associate with each other to form the polymer and equilibrium shifts towards the formation of the polymer. Because of this association, very little or negligible amount of the monomer remains in solution. Hence, sufficient increase in the absorbance is not observed at λ= 275 nm with the corresponding increase in the concentration of the monomer. This leads to the *negative deviation* with respect to line B (curve D, **Fig. 2.8**). Since more of polymer is present in the solution at higher concentration of the monomer, a greater absorbance is observed (curve E, **Fig. 2.8**) with respect to line B at λ=300 nm, which is the wavelength of maximum absorption (λ_{max}) of the polymer. Thus, a *positive deviation* is observed for a concentrated solution if the absorbance is measured at 300 nm.

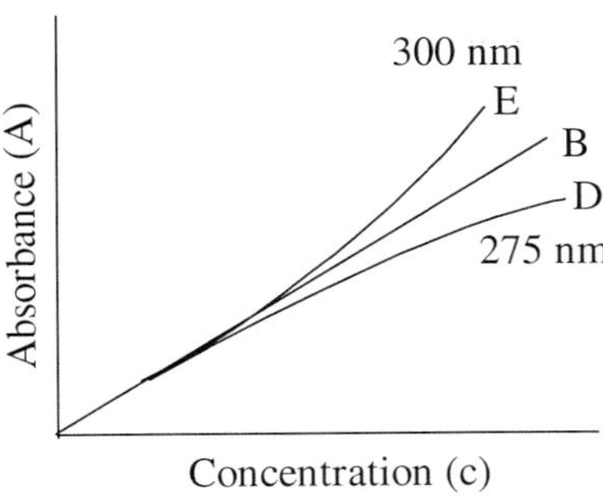

Fig. 2.8: The positive and the negative deviations in benzyl alcohol

Apparent deviation due to association of molecules can be corrected or predicted if equilibrium constant for the association is taken into consideration.

Another example of apparent deviation is the deviation from linearity between absorbance and total concentration of chromium because of change in color of unbuffered dichromate solution on dilution. **Table 2.1** shows wavelengths associated with various colors and **Fig. 2.9** shows pairs of complimentary colors.

An orange colored dichromate is converted gradually to a yellow colored chromate when water is added to it. The reaction of dichromate ions with water is shown below.

$$Cr_2O_7^{-2} + H_2O \rightleftharpoons 2\,HCrO_4^{-1} \rightleftharpoons 2\,CrO_4^{-2} + 2\,H^+$$

Orange (λ_{max} = 550 nm) Yellow (λ_{max} = 450 nm)

A dichromate solution appears orange because a radiation corresponding to an orange color is not absorbed by it but is transmitted out. This transmitted radiation reaches our eyes and gives the perception of an orange appearance to the dichromate solution. The radiation corresponding to its complimentary color (blue) is absorbed maximum by an orange colored solution. Thus, an orange colored solution of dichromate ions absorbs radiation of λ = 550 nm, whereas a yellow colored solution of chromate ions absorbs radiation of its complimentary color (violet) of λ = 450 nm.

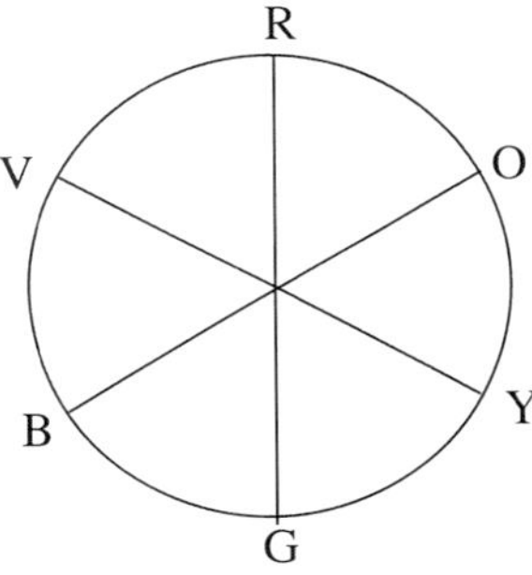

Fig. 2.9: A color wheel showing pairs of complimentary colors

Table 2.1: Wavelengths associated with various colors

Color	**Red**	**Orange**	**Yellow**	**Green**	**Blue**	**Violet blue**	**Violet**
Average wavelength (nm)	750	700	650	600	550	500	450
Range of wavelengths (nm)	720-780	680-720	620-680	580-620	520-580	480-520	420-480

At most wavelengths, the molar absorptivities of the dichromate and the chromate ions are quite different. The total absorbance of any solution depends upon the concentration ratio of dichromate to chromate. The ratio, however, changes markedly with dilution.

As concentration of dichromate ions is increased in solution, slowly its conversion to chromate ions is reduced, since the same amount of water is available for the hydrolysis of the increasing quantities of dichromate ions. If absorption of this solution is measured at $\lambda = 550$ nm, *positive deviation* from the linearity between the absorbance and the total concentration of chromium is seen. The same measurements at $\lambda = 450$ nm result in *negative deviation* from the linearity. This is shown in **Fig. 2.10**.

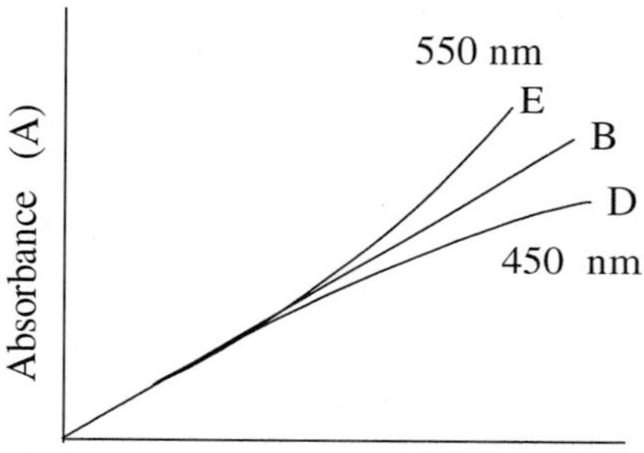

Fig. 2.10: Apparent deviation from linearity between absorbance and total concentration of chromium

Chromium (VI) exists as dichromate alone in an acidic solution and chromate alone in an alkaline solution. Deviations of this system from Beer's law are more apparent than real because one can correct these deviations if equilibrium constant for the conversion of dichromate to chromate and vice versa and also the molar absorptivities of chromate and dichromate ions at two wavelengths are known.

2.2.3.3. Apparent Instrumental Deviation from Polychromatic Radiation

Let the molar absorptivity of a substance exposed to a monochromatic radiation of wavelength λ_1 be ε_1. The absorbance A_1 is then given by the equation -

$$A_1 = \varepsilon_1 . b . c$$

The value of molar absorptivity for any compound varies with the wavelength of radiation. In practice, even an effective monochromator is not able to isolate one single wavelength from a polychromatic beam (a beam containing radiation of different wavelengths). What is considered as a monochromatic beam is an isolation of a narrow range of wavelengths from a polychromatic beam. If a substance is exposed to such a monochromatic beam, which is a mixture of few wavelengths, then separate equations for absorbances at different wavelengths can be written. For simplicity, let us consider that a monochromatic beam contains three wavelengths λ_1, λ_2 and λ_3. At these wavelengths, let the absorptivity values for a compound be ε_1, ε_2, and ε_3. Three equations for absorbances A_1, A_2 and A_3 at the wavelengths λ_1, λ_2 and λ_3, respectively, can be written as follows.

At λ_1	$A_1 = \varepsilon_1 . b . c$
At λ_2	$A_2 = \varepsilon_2 . b . c$
At λ_3	$A_3 = \varepsilon_3 . b . c$

Practically, the absorbance (A) recorded by the instrument is the sum of all these three absorbances.

$$A = A_1 + A_2 + A_3$$

Beer's law is obeyed if $\varepsilon_1 = \varepsilon_2 = \varepsilon_3$, i.e. if all the three molar absorptivities are same. If three molar absorptivities differ, then the relation between the absorbance and the concentration is no longer linear. Moreover, the greater the difference between the absorptivity values, the greater is the departure from the linearity. Thus, Beer's law is obeyed only when the radiation is truly monochromatic.

Usually, deviation from Beer's law due to the use of a polychromatic beam is not appreciable if the absorber does not show large changes in absorbance as a function of wavelength.

2.2.3.4. Apparent Instrumental Deviation in Presence of Stray Radiation

Stray radiation consists of a mixture of wavelengths which differ greatly from that of the principal radiation. Stray radiation is produced due to reflection from various internal surfaces of the instrument. Multiple reflections bring about loss in energy of radiation and correspondingly a change in their wavelengths. They cause deviation from Beer's law due to the reason similar to that for the deviation due to a polychromatic beam.

2.3. MOLECULAR STRUCTURE AND ELECTRONIC SPECTRA

Whether a molecule absorbs UV radiation or not and if it absorbs, then at what wavelength and to what extent it absorbs radiation, depends on the structure of a molecule or the type of electrons in the molecule. Usually, UV-visible radiation excites bonding electrons of a molecule and therefore, types of bonds in a species can be found out from the wavelength of absorption.

2.3.1. Different Types of Electronic Transitions

An organic molecule contains three types of electrons, viz., sigma (σ, Gr.), pi (π, Gr.) and non-bonding (n) electrons. All the saturated compounds like ethane, methane, etc. contain only σ bonds and therefore, only σ electrons. The unsaturated compounds like alkynes, alkenes or aldehydes, containing a triple or a double bond, possess π and σ bonds and therefore, they have π as well as σ electrons in their structures. Molecules having electronegative element such as nitrogen, oxygen, sulphur, halogen, etc. possess non-bonding electrons. For example, a molecule of acetaldehyde, shown in **Fig. 2.11**, possesses all the three types of electrons.

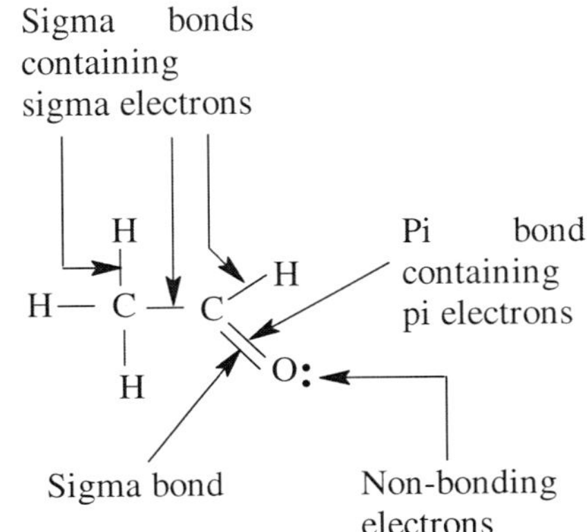

Fig. 2.11: Three types of electrons in the molecule of acetaldehyde

Sigma electrons are present in σ molecular orbitals. When these electrons absorb energy, they get excited to the corresponding σ* (sigma star) antibonding molecular orbital. When π electrons present in the π molecular orbital absorb energy, they get excited to π* (pi star) antibonding molecular orbital. Non-bonding electrons on the electronegative elements occupy either σ* or π* antibonding molecular orbital after excitation. Usually, the energy level of the non-bonding electrons lies between π and π* orbitals or between σ and π orbitals. Different energy levels of various molecular orbitals are shown in **Fig. 2.12**.

When a substance interacts with UV radiation, a few electrons in the molecule get excited to higher energy levels. Whether σ electrons are excited or π or n electrons, depends upon the energy or the wavelength of radiation interacting with the substance. Four different types of electronic transitions are possible when a substance interacts with UV radiation. These transitions are as follows.

1) σ - σ* Transition
2) n - σ* Transition
3) n - π * Transition
4) π - π * Transition

1) σ - σ* Transition

This transition is seen in molecules having σ electrons or σ bonds. For example, a molecule of methane contains only σ bonds and hence involves only a σ - σ* transition when exposed to energetic radiation. When a σ electron is excited, it enters σ* antibonding molecular orbital and the molecule is said to be in σσ* excited state. As seen in **Fig. 2.12**, it is obvious that relative to other possible transitions, the energy required to induce

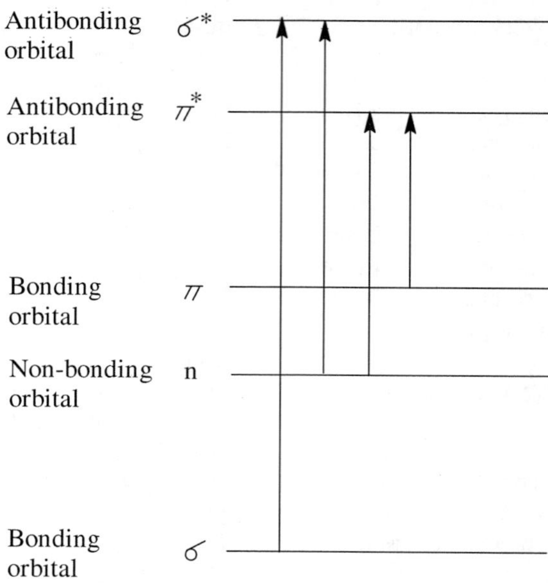

Fig. 2.12: Different energy levels of various molecular orbitals

σ - σ* transition is large. This energy can be provided to a substance if a substance is exposed to the radiation of wavelength in the region of 100 – 200 nm, usually < 185 nm ($E = hn = hc/\lambda$). Waves in this region being shorter, provide larger amount of energy required for σ - σ* transition. These waves are so energetic that some of the atmospheric components like N_2, O_2, etc. also absorb in this region. Hence, if the absorption is to be measured selectively for a substance which is to be analyzed, it is essential to remove these atmospheric components from the UV spectrometer by applying vacuum. Hence, UV spectrometry carried out by using vacuum, while working in the region of 100 - 200 nm, is referred to as *vacuum UV spectrometry*. This results into two major drawbacks. An analytical technique using vacuum adds up to the cost of analysis. Secondly, the absorption of a large amount of energy provided by the energetic radiation in this range results in breaking up of a σ bond in a molecule. Therefore, this range is not used ordinarily for day to day analysis. Thus, absorption maxima due to σ - σ* transition are never observed in the *ordinarily or readily accessible UV region* (Described later).

2) n - σ* Transition

Saturated compounds such as C_2H_5OH or CH_3-CH_2-NH_2, as shown in **Fig. 2.13**, containing non-bonding electrons or an unshared electron pair, can show n - σ* transition because they have only σ* antibonding molecular orbital available after excitation. The energy required for n - σ* transition is lesser than that required for σ - σ* transition. Hence, this transition occurs at a little longer wavelength of radiation, i.e. in the region of 150 - 250 nm, but most of the absorption peaks appear below 200 nm. The molar absorptivity (ε), i.e. the ease of excitation of electrons associated with this type of absorption, is intermediate in magnitude and usually ranges between 100-3000 L $mol^{-1} cm^{-1}$.

$C_2H_5\ddot{O}H$ (with two lone pairs on O) — Ethanol

$CH_3\,CH_2\,\ddot{N}H_2$ — Ethylamine

Fig. 2.13: Saturated compounds containing non-bonding electrons

In the presence of a polar solvent such as water or ethanol, the non-bonding electron pair of an analyte interacts with the electropositive atom of the solvent. For example, an electron pair on the nitrogen atom of an analyte (R-NH_2) interacts with the hydrogen atom of the solvent (ethanol), as shown in **Fig. 2.14**. This interaction results in the formation of a hydrogen bond.

H-bond between an amine and ethanol

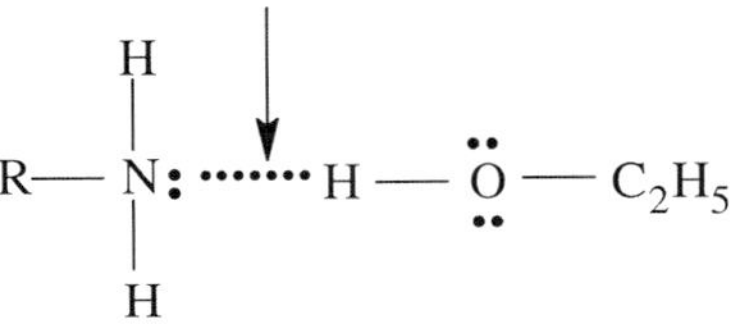

Fig. 2.14: Interaction between a solute containing a lone pair of electrons and a polar solvent (ethanol)

When a hydrogen bond is formed, some energy (E) is released and therefore, system becomes more stable, i.e. a ground state energy level of non-bonding (n) electrons goes down. When an n - σ* transition of one of the electrons from the pair occurs, the remaining single non-bonding (n) electron cannot maintain the hydrogen bond. Thus, energy of nσ* excited state is not affected by this type of solvent interaction.

From **Fig. 2.15**, it is clear that E is the amount of energy released in the formation of a hydrogen bond. Thus, in the presence of hydrogen bonding, the non-bonding electrons would require higher amount of energy for their excitation to σ* antibonding molecular orbital. Hence, in a polar solvent, non-bonding electrons require more energetic or shorter waves for their excitation or the absorption maximum shifts towards shorter wavelengths, as shown in **Fig. 2.16**. This shift is more if the polarity of a solvent is more. This shift in the absorption maximum

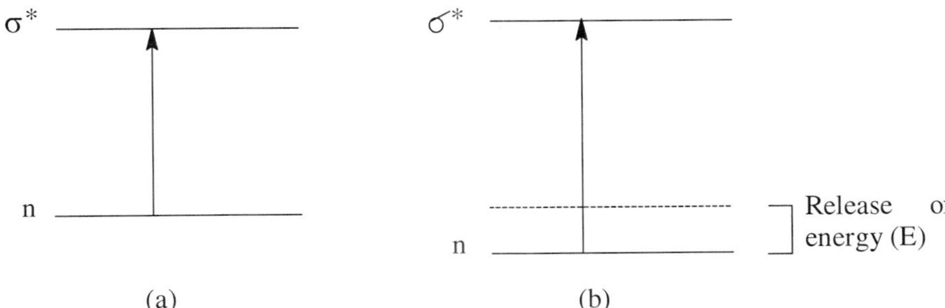

Energy required for excitation of non-bonding electrons (a) in the absence of hydrogen bonding and (b) in the presence of hydrogen bonding

Fig. 2.15: Release of energy (E) after hydrogen bond formation

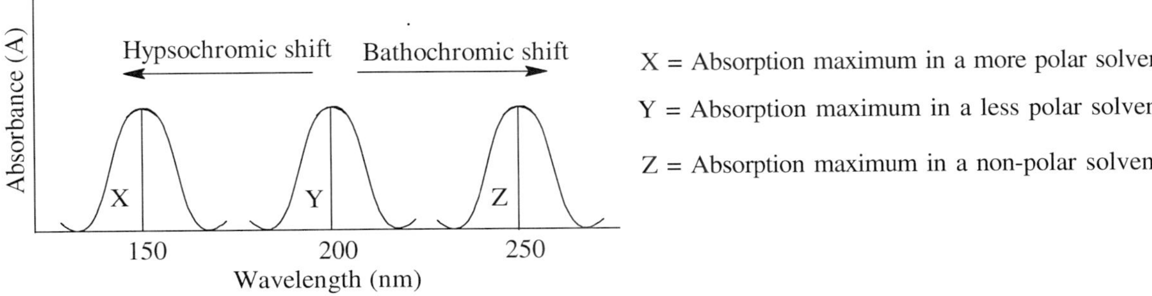

Fig. 2.16: Hypsochromic and bathochromic shifts

towards a shorter wavelength or towards the blue color is called a *hypsochromic shift* or a *blue shift*. A hypsochromic shift in a polar solvent is a characteristic of n - σ* transition. The number of organic functional groups with n - σ* peaks in the readily accessible UV region is relatively small.

3) and 4) n - π* and π - π* Transitions

These transitions are seen in unsaturated molecules having π* antibonding molecular orbitals. Molecules possessing unsaturation (either a triple or a double bond) as well as an electronegative element (oxygen, nitrogen, sulphur) in their structure, show n - π* transition. For example, 1,3-butadiene can show only π - π* transition because of the presence of a double bond, whereas acetaldehyde can show n - π* as well as π - π* transitions because of the presence of non-bonding electrons as well as a double bond. Structures of these molecules are shown in **Fig. 2.17**. These transitions require relatively smaller amount of energy than that required for other transitions. Thus, these transitions can occur at longer wavelengths, usually between 200 - 400 nm.

The compounds from the class of alkynes, alkenes, etc. involve π - π* transition and compounds from the class of aldehydes, ketones, amides, azo, nitro or nitroso, involve n - π* transition. The functional groups in such compounds absorb radiation easily because they require less energy for their excitation and are called *real chromophores*. Thus, chromophores are the functional groups, which require a small amount of energy for their excitation. Ultraviolet-visible spectrometry is mainly applicable to these chromophores.

The n - π* and π - π* transitions can be distinguished in two ways.

(i) The molar absorptivity (ε) for n - π* transition is in the range of 10-100 L mol $^{-1}$cm^{-1} and for π - π* transition it is in the range of 1000-10,000 L mol^{-1}cm^{-1}. Thus, ease of π - π* transition is more than that for n - π* transition and hence, π - π* transition is more intense than n - π* transition.

(ii) Another characteristic difference between the two types of transitions is the effect exerted by the solvent on the wavelength of absorption. In case of molecules containing non-bonding electrons or involving n - π* transition, the interaction of the non-bonding electrons with polar solvents is observed. The extent of interaction depends on the polarity of solvents. In the presence of non-polar solvents, the interaction of the non-bonding electrons with solvents does not occur. With polar solvents, the non-bonding electrons form hydrogen bond. The strength of this hydrogen bond increases with the increase in the polarity of solvents. Since the electrons which are to be excited are involved in the formation of a

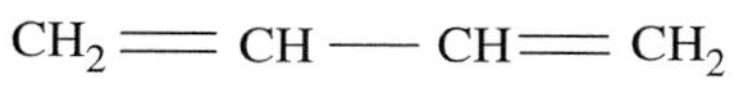

$CH_2{=}CH{-}CH{=}CH_2$

1,3-Butadiene

$H_3C{-}CH{=}\ddot{O}{:}$ (H–C(H)(H)–C(H)=O:)

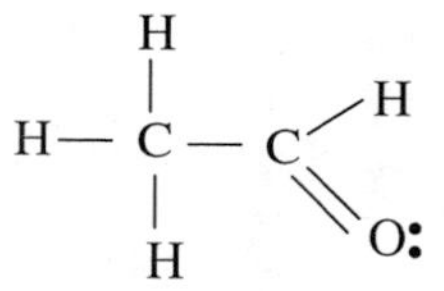

Acetaldehyde

Fig. 2.17: Molecules involving transitions to π* antibonding molecular orbital

The commonly used solvents such as methanol or ethanol do not absorb any radiation beyond 215 - 220 nm. The wavelength of radiation, beyond which a solvent does not show any absorption, is called the *cut off point* or the *cut off wavelength* of that solvent. There is no interference of any atmospheric components as well, in the region between 220 and 380 nm. Thus, beyond 220 nm and up to about 380 nm, the radiation interacts selectively with an analyte and therefore, this region is very widely used for accurate quantitative analysis of many substances. Hence, this region is known as *experimentally convenient spectral region* or *readily accessible UV region*.

hydrogen bond, the additional energy is required to be supplied to the molecule to break the hydrogen bond formed by it with the solvent. This additional energy corresponds exactly to the amount of energy released during the formation of a hydrogen bond. In order to supply this additional energy, more energetic or shorter radiation is required. Thus, in the presence of polar solvents, the peaks associated with n - π* transition are generally shifted to shorter wavelengths, i.e. this transition exhibits a *hypsochromic shift* or a *blue shift*. This hypsochromic shift is to the extent of 30 nm depending on the polarity of the solvent.

In case of both, n - π* and π - π* transitions, usually a *bathochromic shift* or a *red shift*, i.e. a shift in the absorption maximum towards the longer wavelengths is also observed (**Fig.2.16**). This can be explained as follows. When an alkene (C=C) or an unsaturated compound having electronegative element (C≡O or C≡N) is dissolved in a polar solvent, the electrons in the double bond or the electrons on the electronegative element are dragged away from them towards the electropositive atom of the solvent, as shown in **Fig. 2.18**. Because of dragging of electrons from a π bond towards a polar solvent, there is less electron density in the common overlapping region of orbitals of the two atoms which are bound by a π bond. This reduces the bond energy or the bond strength of a π bond. Since the bond becomes weaker, the energy of the π* antibonding molecular orbital is reduced, as shown in **Fig. 2.19(b)**. Thus, lesser energy is now required to excite π or n electrons to π* antibonding molecular orbital in the presence of a polar solvent. Therefore, in the presence of a polar solvent, π - π* transition or n - π* transition can be brought about by using longer wavelengths. This is known as a *bathochromic shift*. This is seen only to the extent of 5 nm. As seen from **Fig. 2.19(a)**, in compounds involving n - π* transition, the hypsochromic shift is more predominant as compared to the bathochromic shift, since the lowering of the energy (E_1) of the non-bonding orbital is more as compared to the lowering of the energy (E_2) of the π* antibonding molecular orbital. In **Fig. 2.19**, dotted lines indicate energy in the presence of a polar solvent and solid lines indicate energy in the absence of a polar solvent.

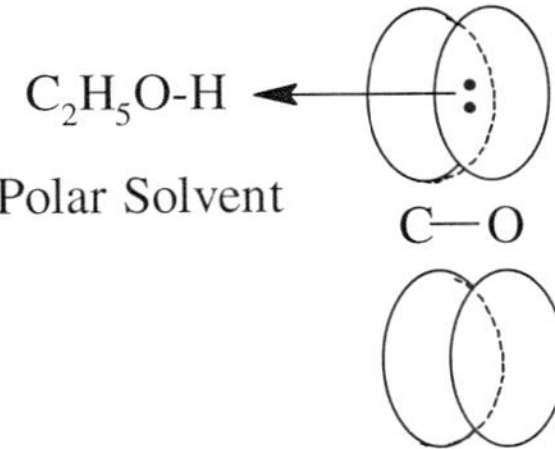

Fig. 2.18: Dragging of electrons from a double bond towards a polar solvent

2.3.2. Effect of Conjugation of Chromophores

Apart from the solvent effect, another factor that can bring about shift in absorption maxima is conjugation of chromophores attached to the doubly bonded atoms.

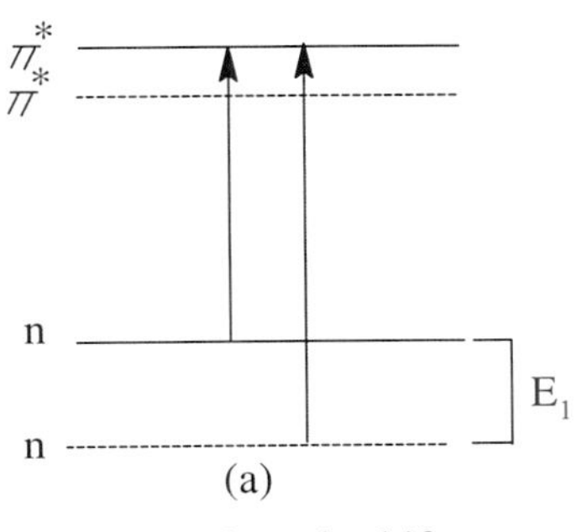

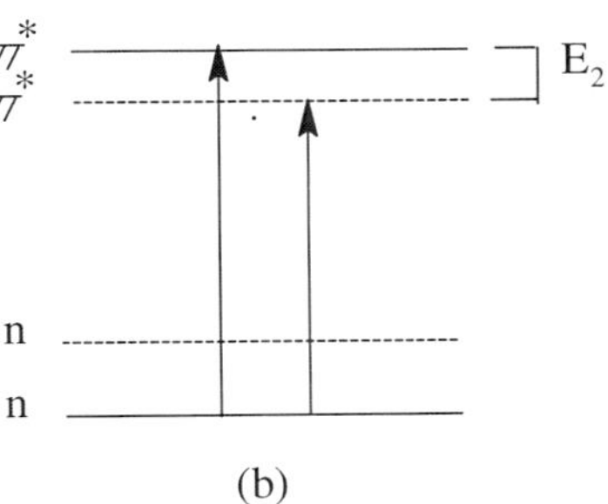

Fig. 2.19: The effect of solvent polarity on energy levels of orbitals

Consider a molecule of 1, 3- butadiene having the structure as CH_2=CH-CH=CH_2. As shown in **Fig. 2.20(a)**, the formation of double bonds in this molecule is by the sidewise overlapping of p-orbitals. Since the double bonds are conjugated, there is a possibility of delocalization of electrons in p-orbitals of all the four consecutive carbon atoms [**Fig. 2.20(b)**]. Under this situation, π electron can be excited to π* antibonding molecular orbital, easily. Because of the presence of four atomic centers and the

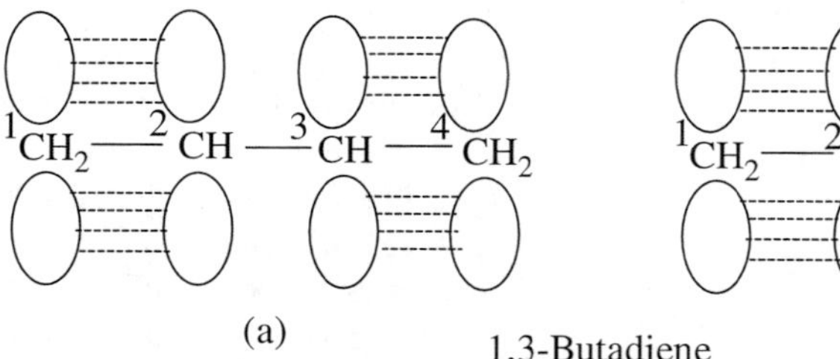

Fig. 2.20: (a) Formation of a double bond between C_1 and C_2 (b) Delocalization of electrons in p-orbitals of all the carbon atoms

conjugation of double bonds in 1,3-butadiene, the excited electron can enter or delocalize in any of the antibonding molecular orbitals, as shown in **Fig. 2.20(b)**. This lowers the energy of antibonding molecular orbital (π*) and gives less antibonding character to it. Since the energy gap between π and π* orbitals is reduced, lesser energy, i.e. a longer wavelength is required for the excitation of π electrons to π* energy level. This results in shifting the absorption maximum to the longer wavelength causing the bathochromic or the red shift in a conjugated system.

In 1,3- butadiene, a shift of 20 nm towards a longer wavelength, is observed as compared to the corresponding peak for an unconjugated diene. A similar bathochromic shift is observed when a doubly bonded oxygen (in aldehydes, ketones and carboxylic acids) and an olefinic double bond are in conjugation (-C=C-C=O). Analogous effects are also observed when two carbonyl or carboxylate groups are conjugated with one another. If there are many chromophores and if these chromophores are separated from one another by more than one single bond, then the absorption of multi-chromophores in a single organic molecule is additive.

2.3.3. Absorption by Aromatic Systems

All the aromatic hydrocarbons produce three sets of bands in the UV region. These three bands originate from π - π* transitions. For example, benzene has a strong absorption peak at 184 nm ($\varepsilon_{max} \approx$ 60,000), a weaker band, called the E_2 band, at 204 nm ($\varepsilon_{max} \approx$ 7900) and a still weaker band, called the B band, at 256 nm ($\varepsilon_{max} \approx$ 200). The position of all the three peaks of benzene is affected by the substituents present on the ring.

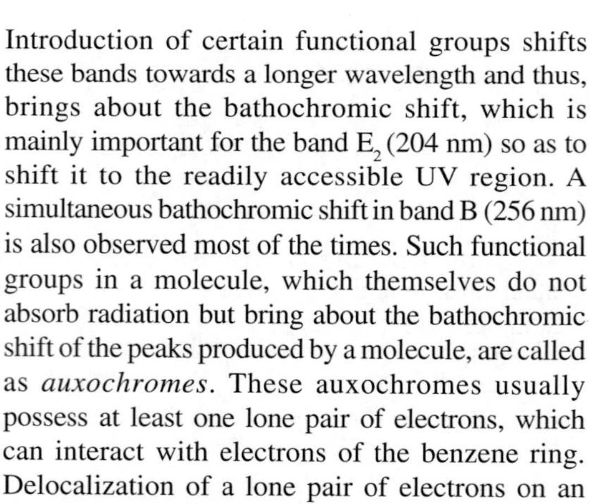

Introduction of certain functional groups shifts these bands towards a longer wavelength and thus, brings about the bathochromic shift, which is mainly important for the band E_2 (204 nm) so as to shift it to the readily accessible UV region. A simultaneous bathochromic shift in band B (256 nm) is also observed most of the times. Such functional groups in a molecule, which themselves do not absorb radiation but bring about the bathochromic shift of the peaks produced by a molecule, are called as *auxochromes*. These auxochromes usually possess at least one lone pair of electrons, which can interact with electrons of the benzene ring. Delocalization of a lone pair of electrons on an auxochrome in benzene ring, stabilizes the π* state, thereby lowering its energy. This is responsible for the bathochromic shift by an auxochrome and is referred to as an *auxochromic effect.*

Hydroxy (OH) and amino (NH_2) groups exert an auxochromic effect on the benzene chromophore, particularly with respect to the B band. The explanation for this goes as follows. In phenol, the oxygen atom of the hydroxy group has two lone pairs of electrons. If phenol is converted to the phenolate anion by dissolving it in sodium hydroxide, then a more pronounced auxochromic effect is observed. This is because in a phenolate anion, three electron pairs are available for delocalization in the ring. This is shown in **Fig. 2.21**.

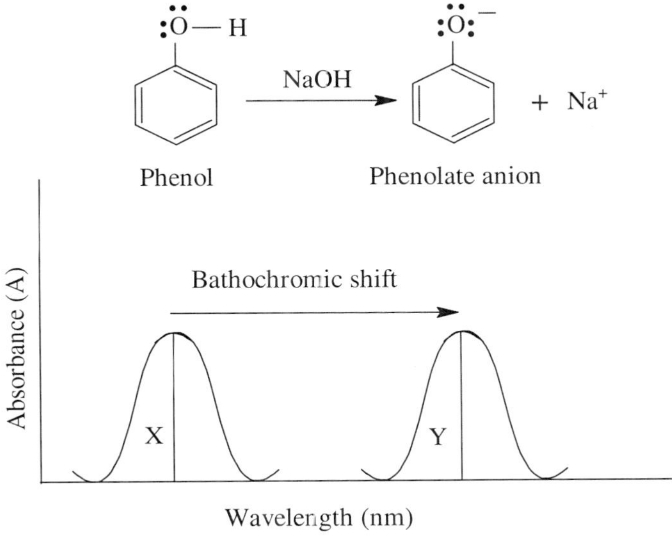

Fig. 2.21: An auxochromic effect in phenol in alkaline medium

In case of aniline also, an auxochromic effect is more pronounced in the alkaline medium. In the acidic medium, as shown in **Fig. 2.22**, its auxochromic effect vanishes since the lone pair of electrons gets involved in the formation of an anilinium ion and is not available for delocalization in the ring.

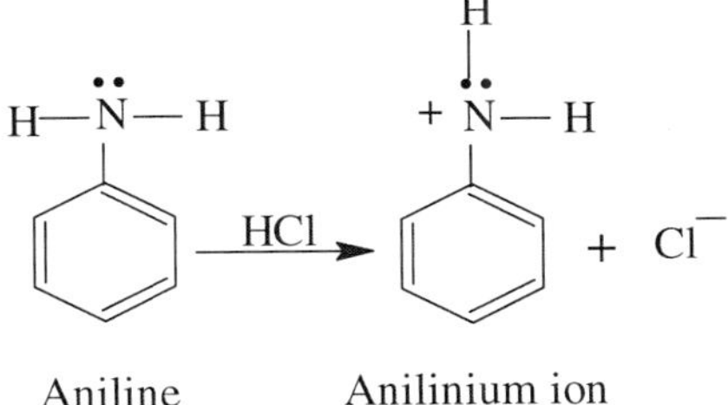

Fig. 2.22: Formation of an anilinium ion in the acidic medium

The auxochromic effect is similar to the bathochromic effect but in the auxochromic effect, an auxochrome does not show any absorption in the UV region and in the bathochromic effect, a chromophore does show absorption in the UV region.

2.4. INSTRUMENTATION IN THE UV-VISIBLE SPECTROMETRY

Components of a typical spectrometer

Typical spectrometers possess the following six components.

2.4.1. A Source of Radiation

A source produces radiation required for the excitation of an analyte. The source should be selected in such a way so as to get radiation suitable for a particular analytical technique, e.g. a source should make available radiation of wavelengths in the range of 400 - 800 nm for the visible spectrometry or for colorimetry. Similarly, a source should provide radiation of wavelengths in the range of 200 - 400 nm for the UV spectrometry.

2.4.2. A Wavelength Selector

A wavelength selector is a device that isolates a limited range of wavelengths from the mixture of wavelengths produced by the source. This device can be a filter or a monochromator.

2.4.3. A Sample Holder

A sample holder of a suitable material and size is required for holding the sample to be analyzed.

2.4.4. A Detector

A detector detects the presence of an anlayte in the path of radiation by converting radiant energy, usually to an electrical signal. It is also able to detect the amount of an analyte present in the sample and produce signal accordingly.

2.4.5. A Recorder

A signal produced by the detector is recorded by a recorder.

2.4.6. A Printer

The recorded signal can be printed on a piece of paper using a printer.

2.4.1. Sources of Radiation

The radiation in the UV-visible range is obtained by using hydrogen, deuterium, xenon and mercury lamps.

2.4.1.1. Hydrogen (H_2) Lamp

As shown in **Fig. 2.23**, in this source, hydrogen gas is filled under pressure into an evacuated tube. The tube has two electrodes embedded in its sides. When c urrent is passed through the gas, the electrons provided by this current collide with the hydrogen gas in the tube. Because of the collisions, the electrons in the hydrogen gas get excited to the electronic, vibrational and rotational energy levels. These excited electrons, while coming back to the ground state, give out energy and produce a continuous spectrum or a band spectrum, characteristic of molecules. The energy given out by the hydrogen gas corresponds to the radiation of different wavelengths. These wavelengths are made available for the excitation of an analyte.

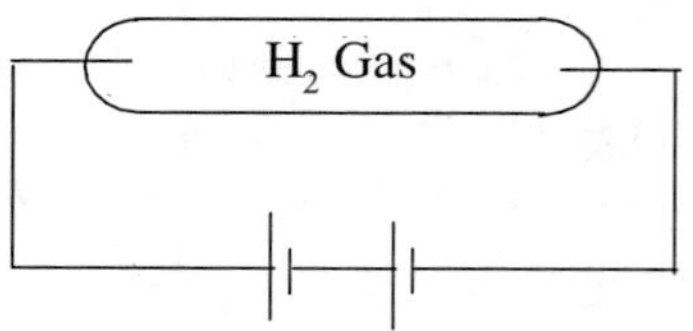

Fig. 2.23: Hydrogen lamp

It is observed that a band spectrum is produced when the hydrogen gas is under high pressure. Hence, under high pressure, the hydrogen lamp provides a continuous spectrum of all the wavelengths in the range of 120-350 nm (UV region). When the pressure of the gas is low, a line spectrum is obtained and hence, only few wavelengths are available for the excitation of a sample.

Advantages

(i) Hydrogen lamp is stable, robust and cheaper compared to a deuterium lamp.

(ii) It also provides quite intense radiation.

Hence, this source is widely used.

2.4.1.2. Deuterium (D_2) Lamp

Deuterium lamp contains deuterium (D_2) gas in place of the hydrogen gas in an evacuated tube. Like hydrogen gas, deuterium also produces a band spectrum under high pressure and a line spectrum under low pressure. It also produces a continuous spectrum in the region of 120 – 350 nm.

Advantage

Deuterium lamp produces 3-5 times more intense radiation than the hydrogen lamp. Hence, it is used when high intensity radiation is required.

Disadvantage

Deuterium lamp is more expensive than the hydrogen lamp.

2.4.1.3. Mercury (Hg) Arc Lamp

In this case, mercury vapor under pressure is filled into an evacuated tube. Mercury atoms in the tube are excited by an electric discharge. Being an atomic source, it produces an atomic spectrum, i.e. sharp lines are seen in its spectrum. The most intense lines are produced at 254, 366, 405, 436, 546, 577, 691 and 773 nm. Because it does not give a continuous spectrum, it is not suitable for the continuous spectral studies. Hence, it cannot be used for scanning of a substance, where a substance is required to be exposed to all the wavelengths in a particular spectral region.

2.4.1.4. Tungsten (W) Lamp

When an electric current is passed through a tungsten wire, it becomes red hot and emits radiation in the visible and IR range (350 – 2500 nm).

2.4.1.5. Xenon-arc (Xe) Lamp

This lamp contains xenon (Xe) gas in place of a hydrogen gas in an evacuated tube. The passage of current through xenon gas, results in the emission of intense radiation in the range of 250 – 600 nm.

2.4.2. Wavelength Selectors

A wavelength selector is used to convert a polychromatic beam to a monochromatic one. Ordinarily, it is not possible to isolate one single wavelength from the mixture of wavelengths emitted by the source but one can isolate few wavelengths from a polychromatic beam. As shown in **Fig. 2.24**, an effective wavelength selector can isolate a narrow range of wavelengths (say 5 - 10 wavelengths out of 100) from the source, whereas a less effective wavelength selector separates a broad range of wavelengths (say 25 - 50 wavelengths out of 100) from the source. A narrow bandwidth enhances the sensitivity of the absorbance measurement.

Wavelength selectors are of two types:
2.4.2.1. Filters
2.4.2.2. Monochromators

2.4.2.1. Filters

A filter is a device that allows radiation of the required wavelength to pass through it but absorbs radiation of other wavelengths, wholly or partially. Thus, one filter can be used for a specific analysis only. If a large number of species is to be analyzed, the corresponding number of filters has to be used. This is the major drawback of filters.

Filters are of two types.
1) Absorption filters
2) Interference filters

1) Absorption filters

Absorption filters absorb unwanted wavelengths and allow passing through them a wavelength or a band of wavelengths of interest. These filters are used for the analysis of compounds in the visible region, i.e. for colorimetry.

Construction

An absorption filter is a colored glass plate that has been colored either by dissolving or by dispersing a pigment in the glass. It can also be prepared by sandwiching a colored gelatin strip between two glass plates.

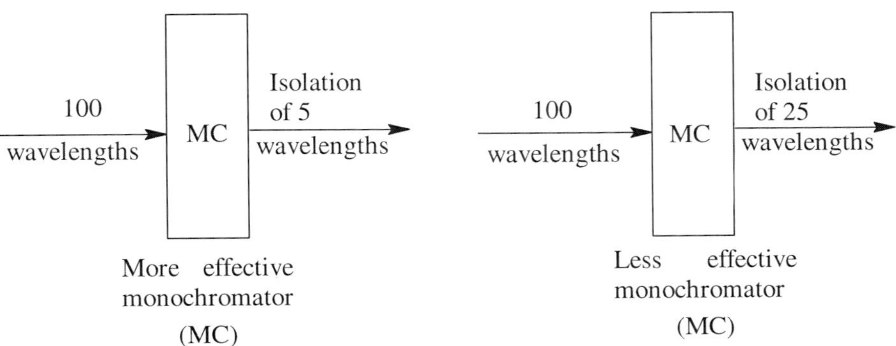

Fig. 2.24: Simple understanding of effectiveness of a monochromator

Principle

For a solution of a particular color, a filter of a specific color is used. Selection of a filter can be done from a color wheel as shown in **Fig. 2.9**. For a compound having some color, the filter having its complimentary color is chosen. For example, as shown in **Fig. 2.25**, a red object appears red because a wavelength corresponding to the red color enters our eyes, i.e. a red object does not absorb wavelength of red radiation, but it absorbs radiation of its complimentary color (Green) the maximum. If we arrange the wavelengths in the visible range, which starts from approximately 400 nm and ends approximately at 800 nm, in a circular form, we get a *color wheel*. The colors opposite to each other are the pairs of complimentary colors. The complimentary color of red is green. Hence, if a substance to be analyzed is red in color, it transmits red wavelengths the maximum and absorbs green the maximum. In order to supply green radiation to this red analyte, a green filter, which transmits wavelengths of green radiation, the maximum, should be used. Similarly, for an orange compound, a blue filter is chosen. Thus, a color wheel helps to select a filter for the analysis of colored compounds.

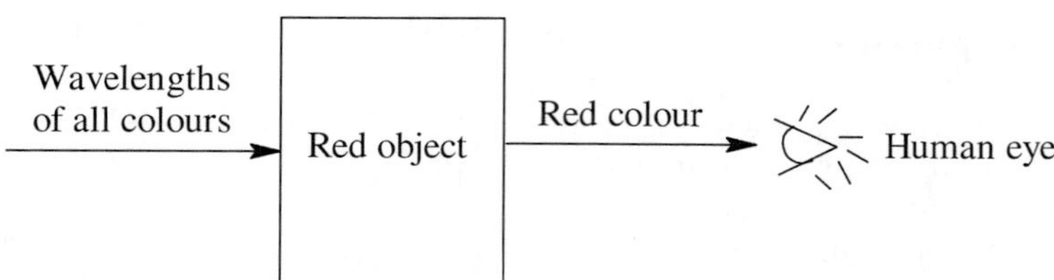

Fig. 2.25: Transmission of red wavelength by red object

Advantage

Absorption filters are simple to fabricate, cheaply available and their performance is adequate for reasonably accurate calculations.

Drawbacks

(i) These filters separate a broad range of wavelengths from the radiation given out by a source. In order to get a narrow range of wavelengths, a combination of filters can be used, but combination usually reduces the intensity of radiation.

(ii) Absorption filters find their use mainly in the visible region.

2) Interference filters

Interference filters are used for obtaining narrow band of wavelengths.

Principle

The principle involved in the separation of certain wavelengths from the mixture of wavelengths using interference filters is of interference of light. The desired wavelength undergoes a *constructive interference* whereas the unwanted wavelengths undergo *destructive interference*.

In the constructive interference, crest of one wave overlaps with the crest of another wave. Similarly, trough of one wave overlaps with the trough of another wave. The constructive interference of two waves, indicated by solid and dotted lines, is shown in **Fig. 2.26**. This adds up the energy of two waves and results in a bright

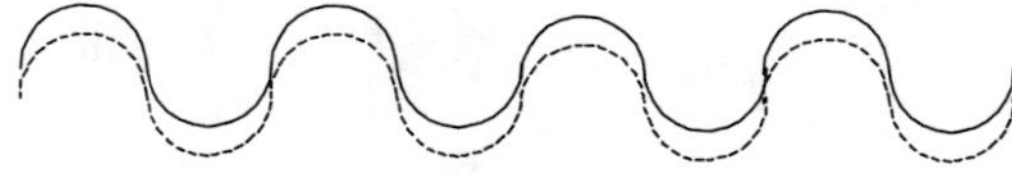

Fig. 2.26: Constructive interference of two waves

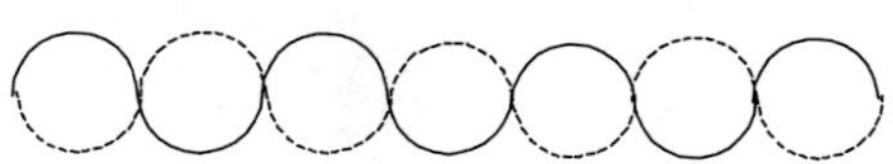

Fig. 2.27: Destructive interference of two waves

band. In the destructive interference, as shown in **Fig. 2.27**, crest of one wave overlaps with the trough of another wave and the energies of the two waves are nullified resulting in a dark band. These waves are therefore, not allowed to pass through the filter.

Construction

Interference filters can be prepared by using glass plates and metal plates. A glass plate is coated with a semitransparent metal layer, which in turn is coated with a thin layer of a dielectric material like magnesium fluoride (MgF_2). This is again coated by a thin film of a metal and finally this metal layer is coated with another glass plate. The construction of interference filters is shown in **Fig. 2.28**.

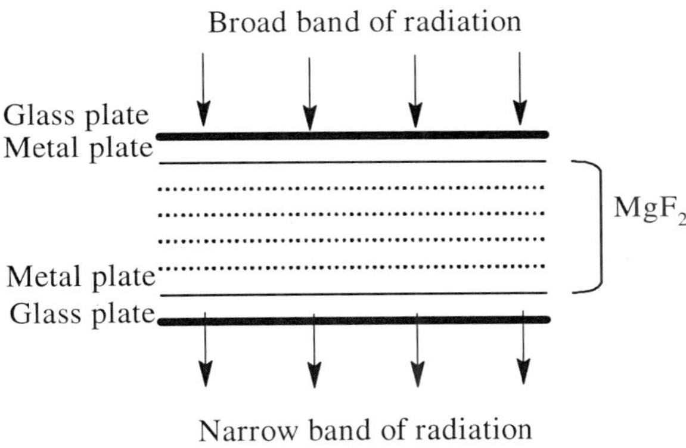

Fig. 2.28: An interference filter

Working

The working of an interference filter can be explained with the help of **Fig. 2.29**. When a ray of light is incident upon an interference filter at point 1 at an angle θ, a part of the light reflects back and part of the light is transmitted to point 2. The remaining light is again reflected back and transmitted out from point 2. The same process is repeated at points 3, 4 and also at the subsequent corresponding points in the filter. Several outgoing rays undergo constructive interference for those wavelengths which are exactly even multiples of the thickness of a dielectric material in the filter. If 'd' is the thickness of the dielectric material, then the constructive interference for the wavelengths would occur only if it satisfies the condition as expressed by the **equation (2.13)**.

$$2d = n\lambda/\cos\theta \quad \ldots (2.13)$$

where, 'n' is an integer indicating order of the spectrum and π is the wavelength of the radiation inside the material. Most of the times, θ = 0 because incident rays are exactly perpendicular to the surface of the filter, as shown in **Fig. 2.28**. Hence, cos θ = 1. Therefore, **equation (2.13)** takes the form of **equation (2.14)**.

$$2d = n\lambda \ldots (2.14)$$

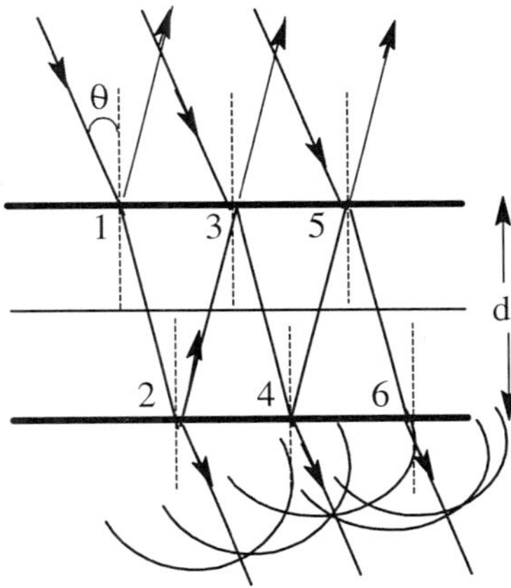

Fig. 2.29: Constructive interference by the interference filter

If λ_1 is the corresponding wavelength in air, then λ and λ_1 are related by the equation, $\lambda = \lambda_1 n_1$, where, n_1 is the refractive index of the dielectric material.

For isolating a wavelength λ_2 from a mixture of wavelengths from the source, a different thickness (d_2) of the dielectric layer is required. Thus, λ_2 undergoes constructive interference, if it satisfies the condition, $2d_2 = n\lambda_2$.

Thus, thickness of the dielectric layer is carefully controlled in order to isolate the wavelength of interest.

Advantages

(i) The interference filters can be used to isolate a narrow band of wavelengths.

(ii) These are useful in the UV, visible and IR regions.

Drawback

The interference filters produce higher order spectra, which correspond to n = 1, n = 2, n = 4, etc. in **equation (2.14)**. In this equation, let the product '2d' on the left hand side be equal to 800. The right hand side of the equation, i.e. në, can then be written as-

$$n\lambda = 800 = 1 \times 800$$
$$800 = 2 \times 400$$
$$800 = 4 \times 200$$
$$800 = 8 \times 100$$

Thus, waves of 100, 200, 400 and 800 nm can undergo constructive interference at this distance 2d. Hence, an interference filter separates a first order spectrum (n = 1) of 800 nm or a second order spectrum (n = 2) of 400 nm, a fourth order spectrum (n = 4) of 200 nm or an eighth order spectrum (n = 8) of 100 nm. Since the unwanted radiation can be easily removed by using a combination of filters, it is not considered as a serious drawback.

2.4.2.2. Monochromators

Each monochromator necessarily contains three elements which are as follows.

(i) An entrance slit

(ii) A dispersing element

(iii) An exit slit

An *entrance slit* allows a sharply defined beam of heterochromatic radiation to pass through it. A *dispersing element* disperses the polychromatic beam into its individual component wavelengths and thus makes possible isolation of different wavelengths for different analytical techniques or for different samples. An *exit slit* allows the wavelengths on either side of wavelength of interest to pass through it, which ultimately interacts with the sample to be analyzed.

The dispersing elements used are -

1) Prism or
2) Grating

These dispersing elements are costly. Because of the monochromator, a spectrometer becomes more expensive.

1) Prisms as monochromators

In less expensive monochromators, the dispersing element is prism. The prisms are generally made of glass, quartz or fused silica. The advantage of using glass is that it possesses highest resolving power but it absorbs very strongly in the region of 200-300 nm and hence, is not transparent in this region.

A widely used prism material for the entire UV range is either quartz or fused silica because they are transparent throughout the entire UV range. Fused silica prisms are preferred to quartz prisms, especially in the region of short wavelengths, because they are absolutely transparent in this region. Fused silica prisms are used only when very intense radiation is required.

Material used for fabricating prisms of a monochromator must transmit radiation in the frequency range of interest. Ideally, the transmittance should approach 100 %. The refractive index of the material used in the construction of prisms should be low in order to reduce reflective losses. At the same time, the material of construction should be such that its refractive index changes sufficiently with the change in the wavelength so that the dispersion and hence, the separation of wavelengths is more. This is responsible for determining spectral purity.

For UV, visible and near IR regions, a quartz prism is often employed. In order to cover the entire IR region, however, prisms of different materials like sodium chloride, potassium bromide or cesium bromide are required.

Two types of prisms are used as dispersing elements.

A) A Cornu prism

B) A Littrow prism

A) A Cornu prism

(i) As shown in **Fig. 2.30**, a Cornu prism is a 60 degree prism because the prism angle (α) is 60 degree.

(ii) It is made up of either racemic quartz or crystalline quartz, which is dextrorotatory and levorotatory in nature.

If a racemic mixture of two optically active forms - dextrorotatory and levorotatory - is used, then the prism is fabricated as a single block prism. If crystalline quartz is used to fabricate the prism, then two 30 degree prisms are joined together.

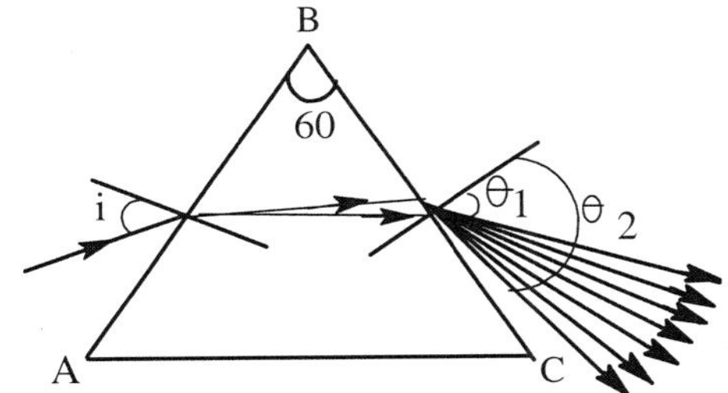

Fig. 2.30: A Cornu prism

One 30 degree prism is fabricated using a levorotatory form of quartz and another 30 degree prism is fabricated using a dextrorotatory form of quartz. This is in order to get a non-polarized beam which is more intense than a polarized beam because a polarized light has only one component of radiation whereas a non-polarized light possesses components in all directions, as shown in **Fig. 2.31**. Polarization caused by dextrorotatory quartz is reversed by levorotatory quartz and thus, radiation remains in the non-polarized form.

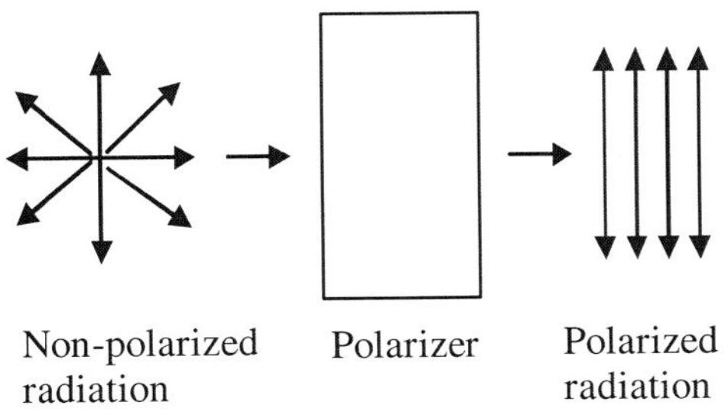

Fig. 2.31: Non-polarized and polarized radiation

In a Cornu prism, a beam of radiation is incident on one surface (AB) at an angle of incidence (i). This beam gets refracted twice, first at the surface AB and then at the surface BC of the prism. Inside the prism, the velocity of different wavelengths differs. They travel with different velocities and start deviating away from the original direction of the incident beam. Energy of each wavelength decides the extent to which it gets deviated away from the incident beam. Since violet radiation is more energetic (because of shorter wavelength), it deviates the most. The red radiation being less energetic (because of longer wavelength), it deviates the minimum. Thus, for the same angle of incidence (i), the angle of deviation or more correctly the angle of dispersion (θ), for radiation of different wavelengths, is different. This is how colors get separated when a beam of light passes through a prism.

B) A Littrow prism

(i) A Littrow prism is a 30 degree prism since the prism angle (α) is 30 degree (**Fig. 2.32**).

(ii) It is made up of either a racemic mixture of quartz or crystalline quartz, i.e. dextrorotatory or levorotatory quartz.

(iii) Surface BC of this prism is made shiny.

A beam of radiation is incident on the surface AB at an angle of incidence (i). It gets refracted at surface AB and gets reflected back at the surface BC. This reflected beam is refracted once again at the surface AB. Thus, as shown in **Fig. 2.32**, unlike a Cornu prism, in case of a Littrow prism, incident beam undergoes refraction twice at

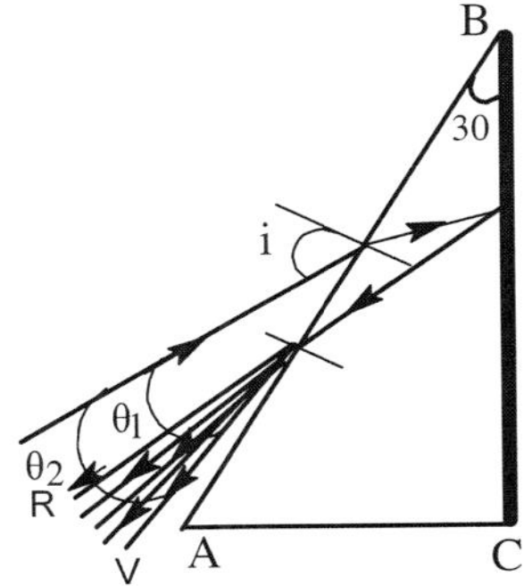

Fig. 2.32: A Littrow prism

the same surface (AB). In a Cornu prism, refraction occurs twice but at two different surfaces (AB and BC). Because of the reversal of the beam, polarization is also reversed in the Littrow prism and hence, either dextrorotatory or levorotatory quartz can be used.

In case of a Littrow prism also, different wavelengths travel with different velocities inside the prism. Thus, all the wavelengths get dispersed through different angles, which results in isolation of wavelengths from a polychromatic beam.

The performance of both the prisms is comparable but the Littrow prism provides a more compact system.

Spectral purity of radiation exiting from a prism monochromator decides the degree of isolation of different colors or wavelengths by the prism. The greater the isolation, the better is the efficiency of the prism as a monochromator. The spectral purity can be expressed quantitatively in terms of an angular dispersion by a prism. It is the rate of change of angle of dispersion (dθ) as a function of change of wavelength (dλ).

$$\therefore \text{Spectral purity} = \frac{d\theta}{d\lambda} \quad \ldots (2.15)$$

The quantity $\frac{d\theta}{d\lambda}$ can be resolved into two parts.

$$\frac{d\theta}{d\lambda} = \frac{d\theta}{dn} \times \frac{dn}{d\lambda}$$

where, $\frac{d\theta}{dn}$ is the change in the angle of dispersion (θ) as a function of refractive index (n) of the prism material, and $\frac{dn}{d\lambda}$ is the change in the refractive index (n) with the wavelength (λ).

The magnitude of $\frac{d\theta}{dn}$ is determined by the geometry of prism, i.e. the prism angle (α) and the angle of incidence (i). It increases rapidly with the prism angle (α) but the reflection losses are more for $\alpha > 60°$.

The magnitude of $\frac{d\theta}{d\lambda}$ depends on the material of construction of the prism.

The greatest dispersion for a given material is near its anomalous dispersion* region, which in turn is close to a region of absorption.

For getting higher spectral purity from the prism for the isolation of various spectral lines, the magnitude of dθ/dλ, i.e. the difference in the angle of dispersion for two different wavelengths, should be higher. For this to occur, the magnitudes of dθ/dn and dn/dλ should be higher.

Resolving power (R) of a prism monochromator is expressed as –

$$R = \lambda/d\lambda \quad \ldots (2.16)$$

where, λ is the average wavelength of two isolated wavelengths and dλ is the wavelength difference that can just be resolved.

2) Gratings as monochromators

A grating is a device which consists of a series of parallel and closely spaced grooves ruled either on some transparent material like glass or on some reflecting surface of a metal. Thus, there are two types of gratings.

A) Transmission gratings (**Fig. 2.33**), and
B) Reflection gratings (**Fig. 2.34**)

Each grating has relatively broad faces and narrow unused faces.

Gratings can be used in the IR, UV and visible regions. A grating suitable for the use in the UV-visible region has about 2000-6000 grooves per millimeter of its length. Gratings used in the IR requires very sophisticated equipment for its production. Hence, the production of gratings becomes an expensive process. This increases the cost of gratings and consequently of an UV

* In a *normal dispersion*, there is a gradual increase in the refractive index of the material with the increasing frequencies or decreasing wavelengths, whereas in an *anomalous dispersion*, there is a sharp decrease in the refractive index with the increase in the wavelengths.

spectrometer. These gratings, which are manufactured by making grooves directly on the material, are called *master gratings*.

In practice, *replica gratings* are used. For producing these replica gratings, master gratings are used as moulds. Hot, molten plastic material is poured into it. After cooling, a plastic replica grating, which is a transmission grating, is obtained. Instead of plastic, if hot, molten metal is poured into a mould of master grating, a metallic replica grating, which is a reflection grating, is obtained. These replica gratings are inferior to master gratings in performance but are quite adequate for day to day working.

Working

A number of beams are incident on a reflection grating or on a transmission grating at different points (A, B, C and D in **Figures 2.33** and **2.34**). The incident radiation in the reflection gratings is reflected back and in the transmission gratings, it is transmitted out from one of the faces of the grooves. Various points, A, B, C and D, act as new radiation sources. Different wavelengths get diffracted at different angles of diffraction (r) and get isolated from their mixture.

As shown in **Fig. 2.33**, when the beams are incident upon a transmission grating, each groove scatters the radiation and becomes opaque. The non-ruled portions thus behave as a series of closely spaced slits, each of which acts as a new radiation source. The radiation gets diffracted at each slit and undergoes either constructive interference or destructive interference. In order to select a particular wavelength from a mixture of wavelengths incident on a grating, the wave should undergo constructive interference.

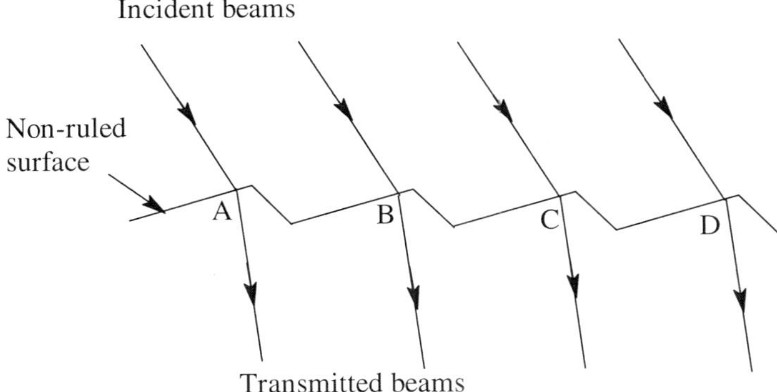

Fig. 2.33: A transmission grating

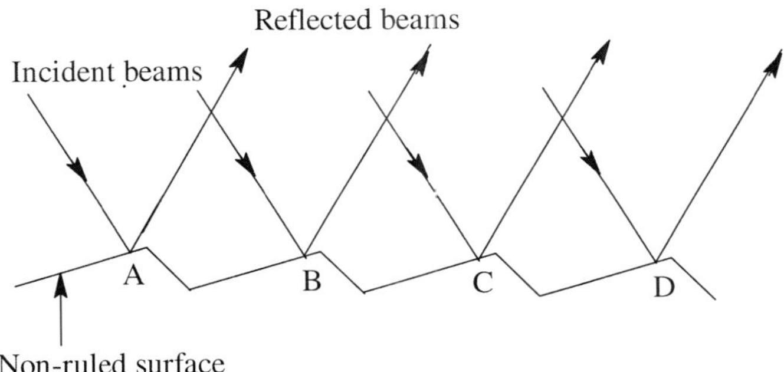

Fig. 2.34: A reflection grating

Diffraction is nothing but the bending of a wave-front when the waves pass by a sharp barrier or through a narrow opening, like a slit.

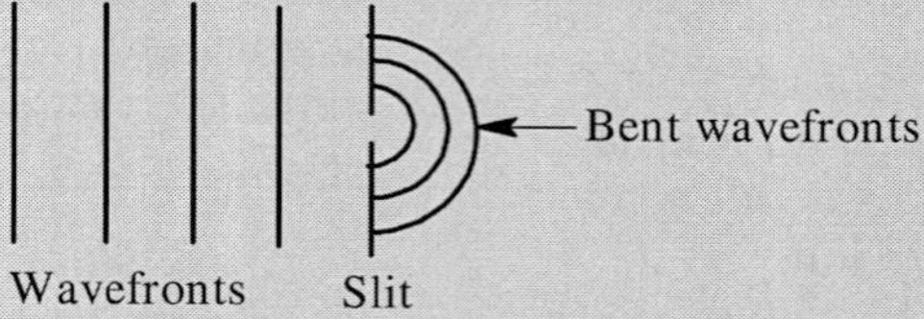

Interference is the overlapping or the superposition of waves from two or more origins or sources.

Constructive interference is the overlapping of crest of one wave on the crest of another wave and trough of one wave on the trough of another wave.

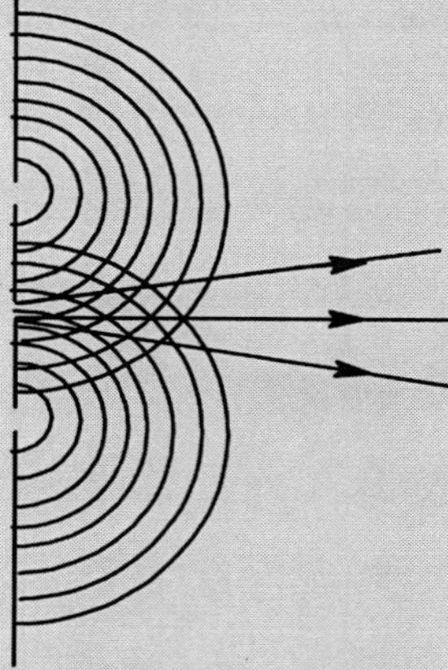

Destructive interference is the overlapping of crest of one wave on the trough of another wave and vice-versa.

Consider two parallel and monochromatic beams XA and YD, incident at two equivalent points on the successive grooves of a reflection grating, as shown in **Fig. 2.35**. Let angle of incidence of these beams with the grating normals, NN′ and NN″ be 'i'. The beams AF and DG represent the reflected beams for the corresponding incident beams, XA and YD, respectively. Let angle of reflection or angle of diffraction of these beams with the grating normal be 'r'. The distance AD = d, is the *grating spacing*, which is the distance between two equivalent points on the consecutive grooves of a grating.

In order to isolate a particular wavelength (λ) using a grating, it should undergo constructive interference. For constructive interference to occur between adjacent beams, it is necessary that their path lengths differ by an integral multiple (n) of the wavelength (λ) of the incident beam, i.e. the path difference between two beams should be equal to nλ.

In order to calculate the path difference, two perpendiculars, AC and DB, are drawn as shown in **Fig. 2.35**. The distance $\overline{CD}$ represents the additional distance traveled by the second incident beam YD and the distance $\overline{AB}$ represents the additional distance traveled by the first reflected beam AF. Thus, the path difference between the two consecutive beams, which are incident on and reflected back from a grating is

$(\overline{CD} - \overline{AB})$

The terms $\overline{CD}$ and $\overline{AB}$ are represented as vector quantities since the direction of their propagation is taken into consideration when the path difference is calculated. For the constructive interference to occur, this difference must be equal to nλ.

To find magnitudes of $\overline{CD}$ and $\overline{AB}$, the values of angles CAD and BDA are found out.

To find value of angle CAD

$\angle XAC = 90^o$

$\angle XAC = \angle i + \angle r + \angle x = 90^o$ ... (2.17)

$\angle N'AD = 90^o$

$\angle N'AD = \angle r + \angle x + \angle CAD = 90^o$ ... (2.18)

From **equations (2.17)** and **(2.18)**, it is clear that angle CAD should be equal to angle i.

$$\boxed{\angle CAD = \angle i}$$

To find value of angle BDA

In **Fig. 2.35**, angle GDB = 90 °, which is a sum of three angles, i, r and x.

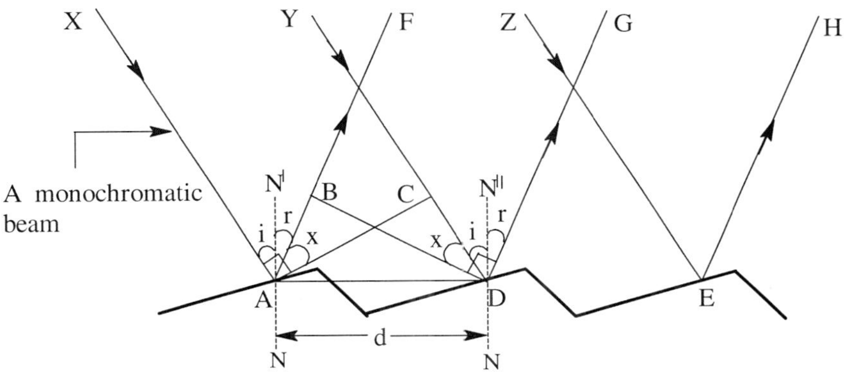

Fig. 2.35: Diffraction from reflection grating

$\angle GDB = \angle r + \angle i + \angle x = 90^o$ ... (2.19)

$\angle N''DA = \angle i + \angle x + \angle BDA = 90^o$... (2.20)

From **equations (2.19)** and **(2.20)**, it is clear that angle BDA should be equal to angle r.

$$\boxed{\angle BDA = \angle r}$$

The values of $\overline{CD}$ and $\overline{AB}$ can be written in terms of $\angle CAD$ and $\angle BDA$, respectively.

$\overline{CD} = AD \sin \angle CAD$

$= d \sin i$ ... (2.21)

Similarly,

$\overline{AB} = AD \sin \angle BDA$

$= - d \sin r$ ...(2.22)

The negative sign indicates the distance in the opposite direction for a reflected beam. Substituting for vector values of CD and AB from **equations (2.21)** and **(2.22)**, respectively, the path difference (PD) can be calculated as follows.

$$PD = (\overline{CD} - \overline{AB})$$

$$= d \sin i - (- d \sin r)$$

$$= d \sin i + d \sin r$$

This path difference should be equal to $n\lambda$ for the constructive interference to occur between the waves in two consecutive beams.

Hence, $d \sin i + d \sin r = n\lambda$

OR $d (\sin i + \sin r) = n\lambda$ ... (2.23)

In **equation (2.23)**, a grating spacing (d) is constant for a particular grating. If only the most intense, i.e. the first order line is selected, then n = 1, which is also a constant. If a beam containing, say two wavelengths, 600 nm and 800 nm, is incident at an angle 'i' on the grating, then the value of angle 'i', in **equation (2.23)**, is also same for both the wavelengths. Now, **equation (2.23)** has only two variables, 'r' and λ. Thus, in order to have two sides of **equation (2.23)** balanced, the angle of diffraction (r) should change if the λ is changed, i.e. the angle of diffraction (r) for each wavelength is different, even when the angle of incidence (i) is same. Hence, only one wavelength can be associated with a particular angle of diffraction, i.e. the radiation of a particular wavelength is collected along a particular angle of diffraction. Thus,

$$d (\sin i + \sin r_1) = n\lambda_1, \text{ and}$$
$$d (\sin i + \sin r_2) = n\lambda_2$$

Therefore, grating becomes a useful tool for isolating wavelengths from their mixture.

Drawback of gratings

Like interference filters, gratings also produce higher order spectra. This can be explained with the help of an **equation (2.23)**. For a definite angle of incidence (i) and angle of diffraction (r), left hand side of this equation would remain constant. Grating spacing (d) is also a constant. If the magnitude on the left side of **equation (2.23)** is 800, its right hand side can be written as follows.

$$d (\sin i + \sin r) = n\lambda = 1 \times 800$$
$$= 2 \times 400$$
$$= 4 \times 200$$

Thus, one can actually have a first order line of 800 nm or a second order line of 400 nm or a fourth order line of 200 nm. Similarly, when the gratings separate first order line of 600 nm, it also separates second order line of 300 nm, a third order line of 200 nm and fourth order line of 150 nm, as shown below.

$$n\lambda = 1 \times 600$$
$$= 2 \times 300$$
$$= 3 \times 200$$
$$= 4 \times 150$$

This suggests that several values of λ exist for a given angle of incidence and diffraction, but this is not a serious drawback of gratings since ordinarily, only the first order line is the most intense line and it is possible to design gratings that concentrate as much as 90 % of the incident intensity in this order. The higher order lines can generally be removed by using filters. For example, glass which absorbs radiation below 350 nm eliminates the higher order spectra associated with first order radiation in most of the visible region.

Dispersion by gratings

Like in prism monochromators, spectral purity in case of grating monochromators is also dependent on its capacity to isolate wavelengths from each other. The spectral purity in case of grating monochromators is expressed as the rate of change of angle of diffraction (dr) with respect to the change in wavelength ($d\lambda$.) and is expressed as dr /dλ. It can also be expressed as the difference in a linear distance (y_2 - y_1) between two isolated wavelengths (λ_1 and λ_2) per unit change in the wavelength. If a wavelength λ_2 is collected at a distance y_2 and a wavelength λ_1 is collected at a distance y_1, then -

$$\text{Linear dispersion} = \frac{(y_2 - y_1)}{(\lambda_2 - \lambda_1)} = \frac{dy}{d\lambda} \quad ...(2.24)$$

The greater the difference in the distance at which two wavelengths are collected, the greater is the spectral purity and the greater is the efficiency of the gratings as monochromator.

Figures 2.36 and **2.37** are the ray diagrams for the isolation of wavelengths by grating and prism, respectively.

Gratings vs. prisms as monochromators (Fig. 2.36 and Fig. 2.37)

1) For the grating monochromator, the angular dispersion of the wavelengths is because of the diffraction which takes place at the reflective surfaces. For the prism, the angular dispersion of the wavelengths is due to difference in velocities inside the prism.
2) In both the cases, the isolated radiation is focused on the focal plane AB, where it appears as two rectangular images of the entrance slit.

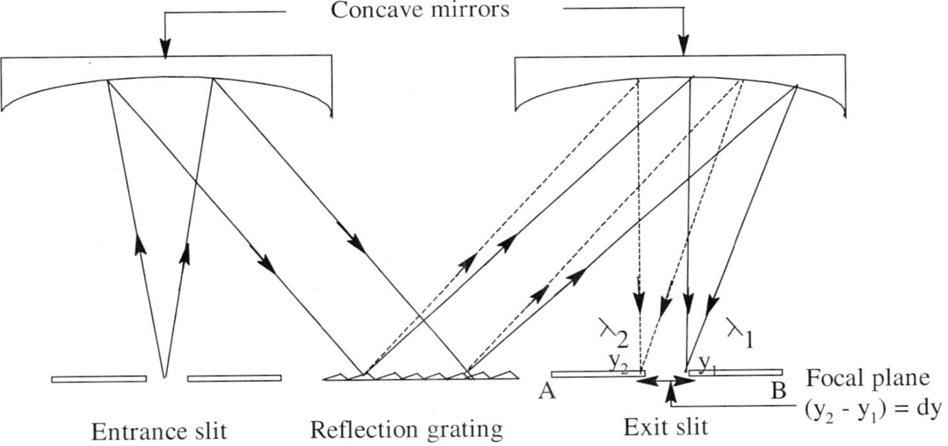

Fig. 2.36: Grating as a monochromator

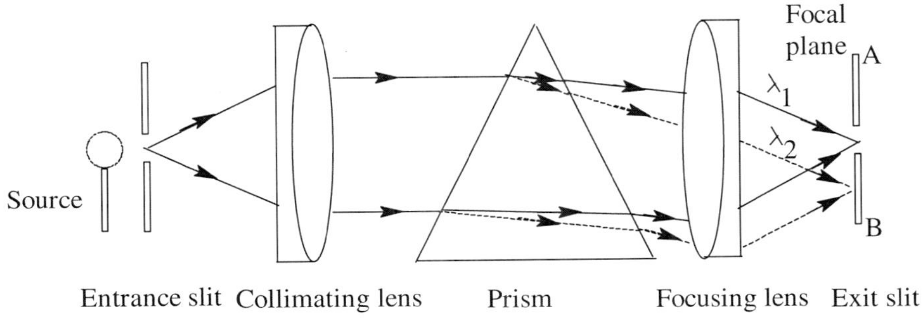

Fig. 2.37: Prism as a monochromator

By rotating the dispersing element, one band or the other, i.e. either λ_1 or λ_2, can be focused on the exit slit.

3) Dispersion of radiation by gratings is more than that by prisms. Hence, gratings are more efficient monochromators than prisms.
4) Manufacturing of gratings is tedious and involves a great skill. Hence, gratings are more costly as compared to prisms.
5) Dispersion by gratings is linearly related to the wavelength, which means that the position of a band along the focal plane for a grating varies linearly with its wavelength. For example, if a grating position is such that it produces a wavelength of 200 nm at exit slit, then to collect a wavelength of 250 nm at the same place (i.e. at the exit slit), if grating is to be moved by a distance of 10 units, then for collecting a wavelength of 300 nm at the same place, further displacement of a grating by 10 units would be required. This is not so in case of prisms, because in prisms, the shorter wavelengths are dispersed to a greater extent than the longer ones. This non-linear dispersion of radiation in prisms, makes designing of an instrument complicated. Thus, fabrication of instrument is less complex when gratings are used as monochromators as compared to prisms as monochromators.
6) Gratings provide wavelengths over a wider range and hence, can be used as monochromators in the entire UV, visible and IR regions. For using prisms in all these regions, one has to select prisms made up of different materials of construction, since glass absorbs in the range of 120 – 350 nm.

Though gratings are superior to prisms as monochromators, they suffer from disadvantages of producing somewhat greater amount of stray radiation and also of producing higher order spectra. Both these drawbacks are not the serious drawbacks since both can be taken care of by simple means. Stray radiation is mainly due to the reflection of the beams from various optical parts arising mainly because of mechanical imperfections. Scattering by dust particles on the

Table 2.2: Comparison between gratings and prisms

No.	Gratings	Prisms
1	The isolation of wavelengths is because of the diffraction of wavelengths.	The isolation of wavelengths is because of the difference in the velocities of wavelengths inside the prism.
2	Gratings are more efficient than prisms because of the higher degree of dispersion of radiation.	Prisms are less efficient than gratings because of the lower degree of dispersion of radiation.
3	Dispersion by gratings is linear. Hence, the fabrication of the instrument is easy.	Dispersion by prisms is non-linear. Hence, the fabrication of the instrument is difficult.
4	Manufacturing of gratings is tedious and involves a great skill. Hence, gratings are costlier compared to prisms.	Manufacturing of prisms is simple. Hence, prisms are cheaper compared to gratings.
5	Gratings are used in the UV, visible and IR regions.	Prisms are used mainly in the visible region.
6	Gratings produce higher order spectra.	Prisms do not produce higher order spectra.

surfaces of optical parts also causes stray radiation. The effect of stray radiation is minimized by proper designing of the instrument. Introduction of baffles in appropriate spots in the monochromator and coating of interior surfaces with a thin and uniform layer of black paint helps in reducing stray radiation. In addition, precautions are taken to restrict entry of dust particles in the instrument.

The higher order spectra can be easily eliminated by using a proper filter or a combination of filters to absorb unwanted wavelengths.

2.4.3. Sample Holders

The sample cells or *cuvettes* used for holding analytes or samples for analysis should fulfill following four conditions.

(1) They must be uniform in construction, i.e. the thickness of all the walls should be same and the surfaces facing the incident radiation must be absolutely flat so that the path length (b) remains constant over the entire cell.
(2) The material of construction should be inert to solvents as well as to analytes.
(3) The material of construction should transmit radiation after interacting with an analyte.
(4) The ideal cells or cuvettes have windows or walls, which are perfectly normal to the direction of the radiant beam in order to minimize losses due to reflection.

Glass does not satisfy all the above conditions since it is not transparent in the range of 120 - 350 nm, but quartz or fused silica satisfy the above conditions and hence, can be used for manufacturing sample cells.

In a double beam spectrometer (described under **Section 2.5.2**), two cuvettes or sample cells are used. One cell is for an analyte and another cell is for a blank solution, which is usually a solution devoid of an analyte. Thus, two cells, a *sample cell* and a *reference cell* (for a blank solution) are made use of. For higher accuracy, these two cells should be exactly identical to each other. Hence, always a "*matched pair*" of cells is to be purchased, even if only one cell is broken or cracked. The matched cells should be washed and dried properly before recording absorbance values since fingerprints, grease or any other deposits on the walls of the cells, alter the transmission characteristics of the cell considerably.

2.4.4. Detectors

A detector is a device which detects the energy of an incident beam and of a transmitted beam. The difference between the energy of these two beams indicates the energy absorbed by an analyte. This difference in the energy is converted into some parameters like current or voltage, which can be easily measured or read on a meter and can be used to calculate concentration of an analyte.

A detector should satisfy following conditions.

1) It should be *sensitive*. A sensitive detector can detect smaller concentrations of a substance. A highly efficient or sensitive detector can detect even traces of an analyte. Thus, sensitivity of a detector decides the lowest concentration of an analyte which can be detected accurately by it. The sensitivity of a detector increases as its capacity to detect lower concentration increases.
2) A detector should produce a *linear response* over a larger concentration range, i.e. if a detector produces a response of 10 μamp for a concentration of 10 μg/ml, it should produce a response of 20 μamp for 20 μg/ml or 30 μamp for 30 μg/ml and so on. When the detector produces such a linear response, plotting of a graph of current vs. concentration for a standard substance becomes easy. This standard graph can then be utilized in order to find the concentration of a substance in a sample.
3) A detector should be *non-destructive* in nature, i.e. it should not destroy the sample to be analyzed. This is important especially when a limited amount of sample is available for a number of tests. For example, when alkaloids are extracted from plant leaves, a large quantity of leaves results in a very small quantity of alkaloids. In order to confirm their structures after isolation, a number of tests are required to

be performed on such a limited quantity of the sample. In such a case, recovery of the sample after detection becomes very useful. Hence, as far as possible, a detector should be non-destructive in nature.

4) A detector should be *selective*, i.e. it should be able to detect one class of compounds or certain functional groups, selectively. This makes possible the detection of an analyte in the presence of other compounds, which are not detected by the detector. This avoids the separation of impurities from an analyte and provides accuracy in the measurements..

5) A detector should produce a *high signal-to-noise ratio*. A *signal* refers to a response produced by an analyte of interest, whereas a *noise*, which is an electrical noise, and not an auditory noise, refers to the signals produced by impurities or by some other factors. Noise results in the production of a number of unwanted peaks. A detector should produce a sharp and a strong peak for an analyte and very small peaks or no peaks for impurities. In such a case, the ratio of the height of a peak for a compound of interest to the height of an unwanted peak should be high or there should be sufficient difference between the signal given by the analyte and that given by an impurity or any other unknown source. In **Fig. 2.38**, h_1 is the height of the peak corresponding to the analyte of interest (signal) and h_2 is the height of the peak corresponding to some impurity (noise). The signal to noise ratio can then be expressed as the ratio of h_1 to h_2.

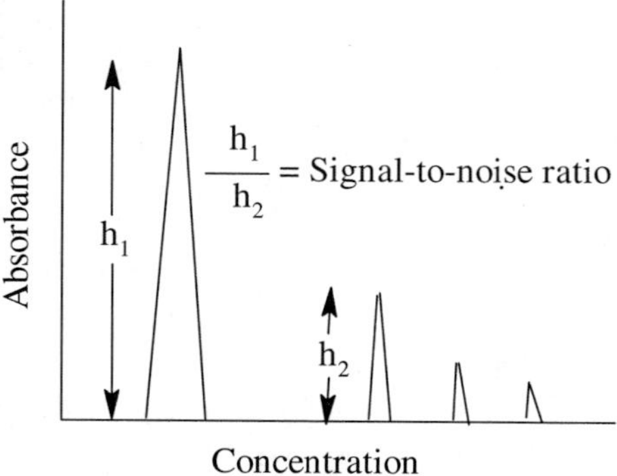

Fig. 2.38: Signal and noise in absorption spectrometry

Signal-to-noise ratio should be as high as possible for an efficient detector in order to get higher accuracy in analysis.

Following detectors are commonly used in UV spectrometry.

2.4.4.1.A Barrier Layer Cell or a Photovoltaic Cell

As shown in **Fig. 2.39**, in this detector, a barrier of a semi-conducting material such as selenium is present between two metallic blocks. This barrier layer restricts the conduction of electrons from one metallic block to the other. Hence, this detector is named as a barrier layer cell.

Construction

The barrier layer cell consists of a semiconductor such as selenium, which is deposited on a strong metallic block of iron or copper. Another surface of selenium is coated with a thin layer of silver or gold. The two metals form two electrodes of the detector. The entire assembly is enclosed in a transparent material. Both the electrodes are connected to an ammeter to record the current in the circuit.

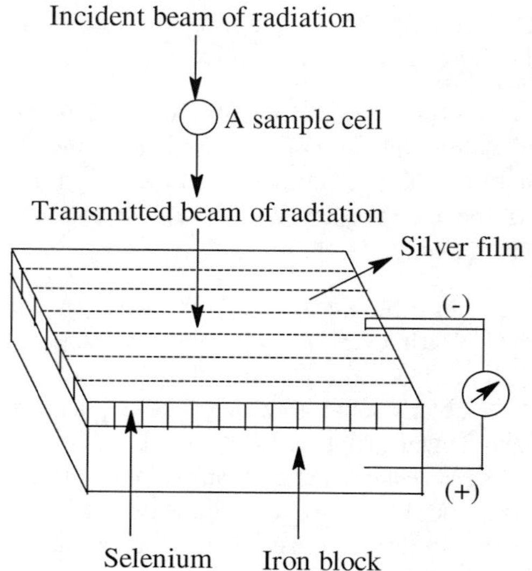

Fig. 2.39: A barrier layer cell or a photovoltaic cell

Working

After the interaction with the sample, when the transmitted radiation reaches the semiconductor, the covalent bonds in the latter are broken, as a result of which the electrons and the holes are liberated in the semiconductor. The electrons migrate towards the silver or the gold layer and the holes migrate towards the block of iron. The electrons do not pass through the semi-conducting selenium layer but are free to move through the external circuit into the iron block. When the two electrodes are connected to the ammeter, electrons accumulated on the silver layer start moving through the external circuit and produce electric current. The magnitude of the current produced depends on the number of electrons produced, which in turn depends on the energy of radiation reaching the detector. The energy of this radiation would be determined by the extent of interaction of the incident radiation with the sample, which in turn depends on the concentration of the sample. Thus, the current in the circuit is correlated to the concentration of an analyte. The higher the concentration of an analyte, the more is the interaction of the incident radiation with the sample and the less is the energy of the transmitted beam which falls on the detector. When the energy of the transmitted beam is low, a small number of electrons is generated and a smaller current is produced in the circuit. When a beam passing through a blank solution (a solution without an analyte) is incident on the detector, it produces larger current in the circuit because it is more energetic. Thus, the difference in the current produced by a blank and a sample solution increases as the concentration of the sample increases.

Advantages

(i) It is simple in design.
(ii) It does not require any external power supply.

Disadvantage

With time, the photovoltaic cell becomes useless because selenium layer loses its identity and starts conducting current or electrons through it. Under this situation, flow of electrons can occur from selenium layer to the iron block, which does not maintain any potential difference between the two metals (silver and iron). Hence, no current passes through an ammeter and thus, no signal is produced by the detector.

2.4.4.2. A Photocell

Construction

As shown in **Fig. 2.40**, this detector consists of two electrodes enclosed in an evacuated tube. Cathode is specially designed as a half cylinder and is coated from inside with a light sensitive material. Anode is in the form of a rod or a plate and is situated along the axis of the tube and opposite the cathode. Quartz or a fused silica window is provided for the passage of the transmitted beam through it.

Working

The radiation before and after the interaction with the sample are incident upon the photosensitive cathode. This results in the release of few electrons from its surface. These electrons are then attracted by an anode. This flow of electrons produces a definite magnitude of current in the circuit. The number of electrons released from the cathode depends on the energy of the beam incident on the detector, which in turn depends on the extent of interaction of the beam with the sample. The lower the concentration of a sample, the higher is the energy of the transmitted beam and the greater is the number of electrons ejected from the cathode and vice versa. The difference between the current produced by a blank and a sample solution increases with the increase in the concentration of the sample.

Advantages

Because of the semi-cylindrical shape of the cathode, the electrons ejected out when a transmitted beam strikes its photosensitive surface, undergo multiple reflections and further eject out a large number of electrons. Hence, a high degree of amplification is achieved by this detector. Therefore, a photocell is more sensitive than a photovoltaic cell. A detector with quartz or a fused silica window is useful over the entire UV-visible region.

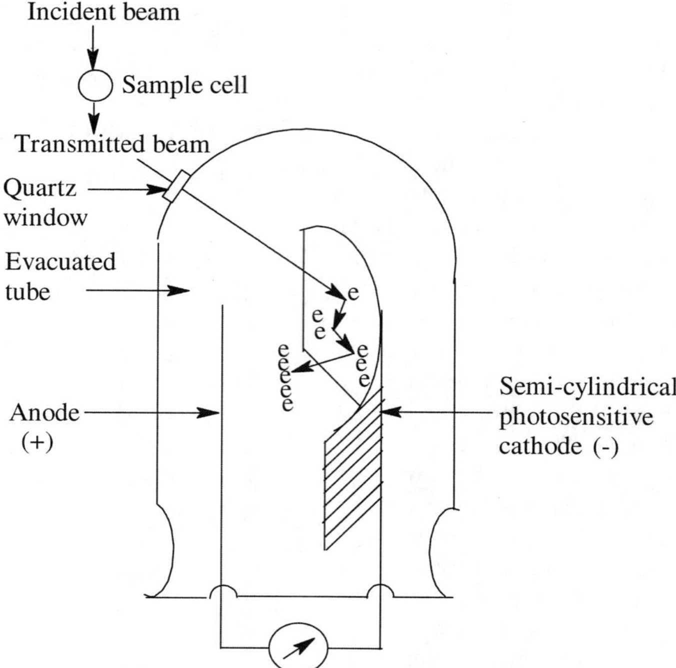

Fig. 2.40: A photocell

2.4.4.3. A Photomultiplier Tube

Construction

A photomultiplier tube, shown in **Fig. 2.41**, consists of one cathode (A) and 9-16 dynodes, enclosed in an evacuated tube. The cathode and all the dynodes are coated with a thin layer of a photosensitive material. Each dynode is made up of Be-Cu or of Cs-Sb. The successive dynodes are kept at higher and higher positive potentials with respect to the previous dynode. A collector is kept at the highest positive potential.

Working

A transmitted beam falling on the surface of a photosensitive cathode, results in the emission of electrons from its surface. These electrons are attracted towards the first dynode, which is kept at the positive potential. The electrons striking the first dynode again emit more electrons from its surface. These electrons are again attracted by the second dynode, where a similar effect is produced. For every quantum of light, approximately 10^6 electrons are produced. The process is repeated over all the dynodes in a tube and results in the production of a large number of electrons. All the

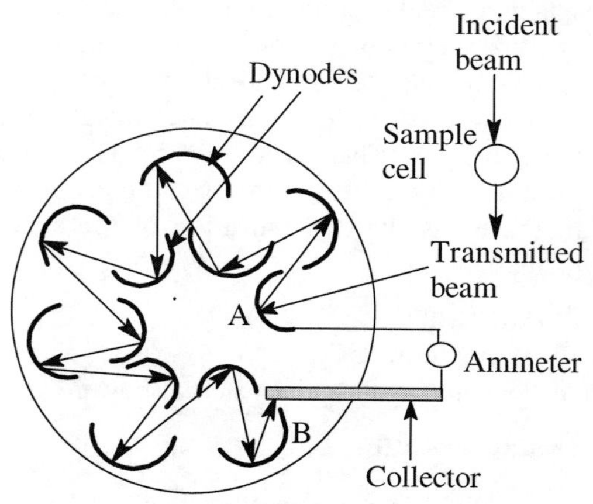

A = Photocathode and B = Anode

Fig. 2.41: A photomultiplier tube

electrons are ultimately collected by the collector and a current is produced in the circuit, which is responsible for producing a signal.

Advantages

(i) It is an extremely sensitive detector because of a very high degree of amplification, which results due to the release of a huge number of electrons at each dynode.

(ii) It is extremely fast in producing a response. The time gap between the impingement of a photon on a cathode and the arrival of a shower of electrons at the collector is hardly 1-10 seconds.

2.5. ULTRAVIOLET SPECTROMETERS

Ultraviolet spectrometers are of two types.

2.5.1. A single beam spectrometer

2.5.2. A double beam spectrometer

2.5.1. A Single Beam Spectrometer (Fig. 2.42)

A single beam spectrometer consists of the following components.

1) A source of radiation
2) An entrance slit
3) A wavelength selector – a filter or a monochromator
4) A cuvette or a sample holder
5) An exit slit
6) A photocell
7) A recorder

Working

In a single beam spectrometer, a beam of radiation travels in one direction only. Hence, only one reading at a time, i.e. either for a blank or a sample solution, can be recorded. Initially, a blank solution (all the reagents except for an analyte) is filled in the cuvette. The absorbance reading on a meter is adjusted to zero. If the percent transmittance is recorded, then it is adjusted to a full scale, i.e. to 100 %. Once the adjustment for the blank solution is done, the cuvette is emptied, washed with water, rinsed with the sample solution and ultimately filled with the sample solution. The reading on the meter is recorded for this solution. This absorbance or the transmittance reading is used for calculating the concentration of the sample.

Drawbacks

(i) Two separate readings, one for the blank and another for the sample, are required to be recorded in order to find concentration of an analyte.

(ii) The meter reading depends on the intensity of the beam transmitted by the blank solution and by an analyte solution. The intensity of transmitted beam depends on the intensity of the incident beam, which in turn depends on the voltage across the filament of the radiation source. Suppose that the reading for a blank solution is recorded when the voltage is 220 volts and because of the voltage fluctuation, if

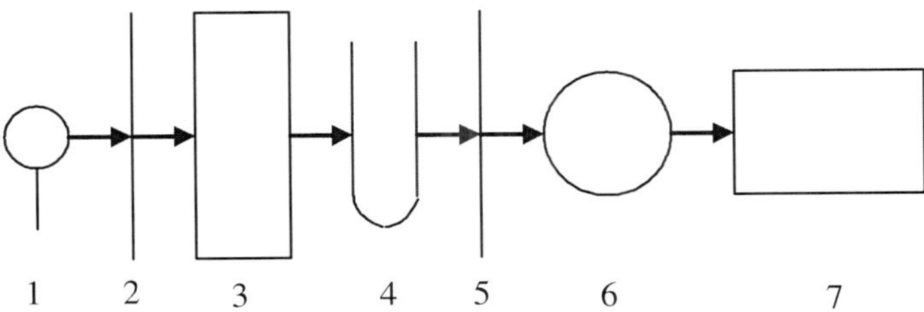

1. Source, 2. Entrance slit, 3. Monochromator, 4. Sample cell, 5. Exit slit 6. Photocell, 7. Recorder

Fig. 2.42: A single beam spectrometer

the reading for the test solution (an analyte) is recorded at 240 volts, the accuracy in the readings would not be obtained. This is because an incident beam is more powerful when the voltage is 240 volts than when the voltage is 220 volts. Automatically, the intensity or the power of the transmitted beam is also correspondingly higher when the voltage is 240 volts. Hence, even if the concentration of an analyte is more, the intensity of the transmitted beam remains higher than what it should have been if the voltage was 220 volts (If the concentration of an analyte is more, its interaction with the radiation is more and hence, the intensity of the transmitted beam is less. Correspondingly, the difference between the absorbance of a blank and an analyte solution is more). This gives smaller value of concentration of an analyte than the actual one, thereby leading to inaccurate results.

Fluctuation in the readings, with the variation in the source intensity, leading to an inaccuracy in the final result, is the major disadvantage of a single beam spectrometer. This defect can be minimized by using a storage battery as a current supply or by using a more expensive constant voltage transformer. The best remedy to avoid this inaccuracy is to use a double beam spectrometer.

2.5.2. A Double Beam Spectrometer (Fig. 2.43)

A double beam spectrometer consists of the following components.

1) A source of radiation
2) An entrance slit
3) A collimating lens
4) A wavelength selector- a filter or a monochromator
5) A beam splitter – a mirror
6) Two separate sample holders – one for the blank solution and another for the sample solution
7) Two photocells
8) A recorder

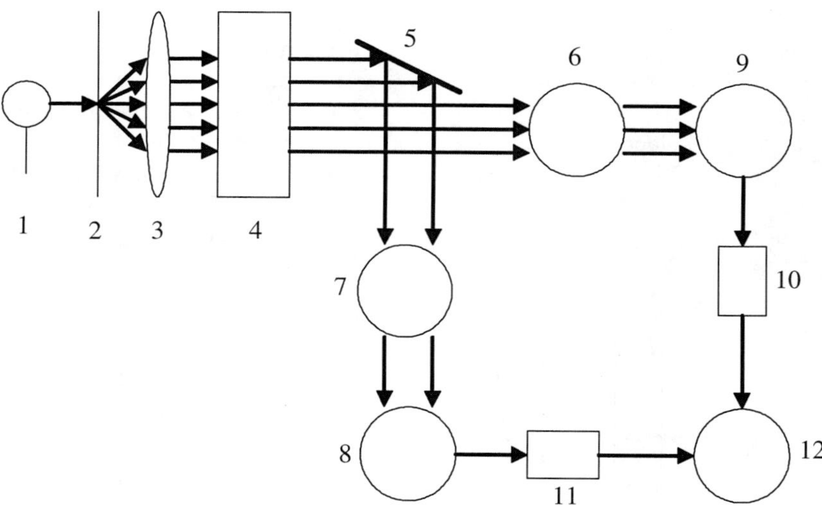

1. Source, 2. Entrance slit, 3. Collimating lens, 4. Monochromator,
5. Mirror-Beam splitter, 6. Sample cell, 7. Blank solution cell,
8, 9. Photocell, 10,11. Amplifiers, 12. Recorder

Fig. 2.43: A double beam spectrometer

Working

As the name suggests, in a double beam spectrometer, a beam of radiation is split into two directions. The beam coming out from the monochromator falls on a mirror, which is kept slanted at an angle. The mirror acts as a beam splitter and splits the beam into two directions by reflecting the incident beam. The beam in one direction falls on a cuvette containing a blank solution and the beam in another direction falls on a cuvette containing a sample solution. After interaction, the beams are focused on two separate detectors. The output of the detectors is connected to a phase sensitive amplifier, which responds to any change in the transmission through the sample and the blank. Ultimately, the phase sensitive amplifier transmits signals to the recorder.

Advantages

(i) Replacement of the blank solution with the sample solution is not required since two separate cuvettes are used in the instrument simultaneously. This helps in the rapid analysis.

(ii) Zero adjustment with the blank solution is not required since the recorder records the difference between the absorbance of the blank and the sample solutions.

(iii) Since the same beam is split into two, the beams of the same intensity are incident on the blank as well as sample solution at a particular moment. Therefore, even if the absorbance or the transmittance is recorded at different voltage values across the source, the net absorbance, i.e. the difference between the absorbance of the sample and that of the blank, always remains constant. This increases the reproducibility in the analysis.

2.6. APPLICATIONS OF UV-VISIBLE SPECTROMETRY

Ultraviolet spectrometry is mainly used for the quantitative analysis in order to find the amount of a substance in a sample. To some extent, it is used for qualitative analysis also, in order to characterize or identify a substance in a sample.

2.6.1. Qualitative Analysis

Every atom or a molecule has a definite energy level pattern associated with it. This energy level pattern of a species decides the amount of energy that can be absorbed by it when exposed to radiation. Every species shows the maximum absorption of energy at a specific wavelength (λ_{max}). This wavelength of maximum absorption is used as a qualitative parameter in case of UV-visible spectrometry.

In order to determine the value of λ_{max} of a species, the species is scanned in the UV-visible region, i.e. it is exposed to all the wavelengths from 200 to 800 nm and a graph of absorbance vs. wavelength is plotted. A little before the value of λ_{max} of the species, absorbance slowly goes on increasing, becomes maximum at λ_{max} value and goes on decreasing beyond λ_{max}. This results in the formation of a peak in the spectrum. The variation in the absorbance during scanning of a compound is shown in **Fig. 2.44**.

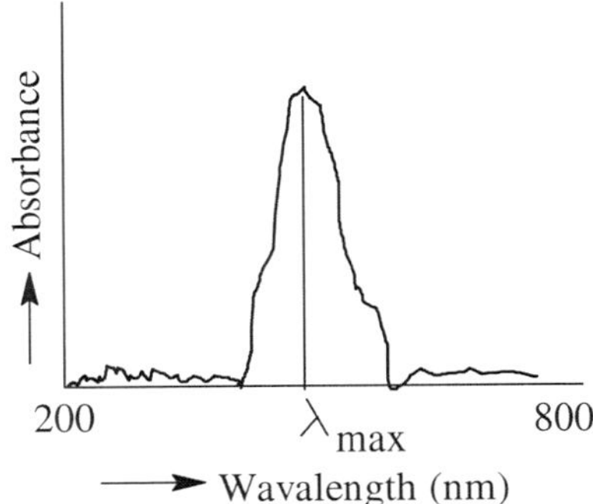

Fig. 2.44: Scanning in the UV-visible region to determine λ_{max} of a substance

A perpendicular dropped from the peak position on the wavelength axis provides the value of λ_{max} for that species. A species can be identified by comparing this value of λ_{max} with the value of λ_{max} reported in the literature.

2.6.2. Quantitative Analysis

Ultraviolet-visible spectrometry finds its maximum applications in the quantitative estimation. If a sample contains only one compound which absorbs in the UV-visible region, the system is called as a *single component system.* From the spectrometric point of view, a system is considered to be a single component one, if at the wavelength selected for the measurement, the determination of an analyte is not influenced by any other substance with the well defined spectrum or by any unidentified factor, usually referred to as the *background absorption*. In such a case, determination can be based on Beer-Lambert law, according to the following equation.

$$A = A^{1\%}_{1\,cm}\ b\ .\ c$$

where, 'A' is the absorbance of an analyte, 'b' is the path length, 'c' is the concentration of an analyte in g/100 mL and $A^{1\%}_{1\,cm}$ is the specific absorbance of an analyte.

In drug analysis, determination of the drug content from raw materials or drug formulations is required. In such cases, a stock solution of the sample is prepared by dissolution or extraction in a suitable solvent. It is diluted appropriately and the absorbance of the resulting solution is measured. The drug content is then determined by the following equation.

$$\text{Drug content (\%)} = \frac{\text{Dilution x stock volume (ml) x absorbance}}{A^{1\%}_{1cm} \text{ x sample weight (g) x cell thickness (cm)}}$$

2.6.2.1. Sample Preparation for Quantitative Estimation by UV-Visible Spectrometry

In order to carry out quantitative estimation of a single component system, sample solution is prepared by optimizing following parameters.

1) Solvent used for preparing solution of an analyte
2) Wavelength of maximum absorption (λ_{max}) of an analyte
3) Specific absorbance,
4) Concentration of an analyte
5) Linearity of the graph of absorbance vs. concentration for an analyte

Optimization of parameters

1) Solvent used for preparing solution of an analyte

The choice of solvents while preparing the sample solution is done based on the nature of an analyte. Few guidelines based on which a solvent is selected for UV-visible spectrometry are given below.

(i) A solvent must dissolve an analyte completely.
(ii) It should not interact chemically with an analyte.
(iii) It should not interact with the material of construction of a sample holder.
(iv) A solvent should not shift the peak of absorption beyond the UV-visible range.
(v) A solvent should be transparent over the range of absorption by an analyte.

Commonly used solvents for the UV-visible spectrometry include water, n-hexane, 95 % ethanol, diethyl ether, cyclohexane, 1,4-dioxane, benzene and acetone.

Table 2.3 gives the *cut off wavelengths* for the solvents below which they cannot be used because of the absorption by the solvents themselves. Any solvent, whose cut-off wavelength is shorter than the wavelength of

Table 2.3: Cut-off wavelengths for the solvents used in UV-visible spectrometry

Sr. No.	Solvent	Cut-off wavelength (nm)
1	Water	190
2	n-Hexane	195
3	Ethanol	210
4	Diethyl ether	210
5	Cyclohexane	210
6	1,4-Dioxane	220
7	Benzene	280
8	Acetone	330

maximum absorption (λ_{max}) of an analyte, should be used for the analysis. This ensures no interference from the solvent in the absorption of an analyte.

2) Wavelength of maximum absorption (λ_{max}) of an analyte

For the measurement of an absorbance in the UV-visible region, the wavelength of maximum absorption (λ_{max}) for that substance should be determined by scanning it in the wavelength region of 200 - 800 nm. The wavelength of maximum absorption (λ_{max}) is selected for the quantitative estimation of any compound for the following reasons.

(i) At λ_{max}, the method is most sensitive since the absorbance is highest.

(ii) The reproducibility of the wavelength setting is better at λ_{max} than on the edges of an absorption band.

(iii) For a given slit width, the variation of the absorbance within a spectral bandwidth, is the smallest at this point.

3) Specific absorbance

The specific absorbance value from the literature, may be used only if the cited experimental conditions (solvent, pH etc.) can be reproduced or otherwise its value can be determined from the slope of the curve for the absorbance vs. concentration, as explained under the calculation part (**Section 2.6.2.2**, **Fig. 2.45**).

4) Concentration of an analyte

A known weight of a sample, from which the concentration of an analyte is to be determined, is dissolved in a suitable solvent. The volume is made up to any arbitrary value (10, 100, 250 ml, etc.) and the absorbance of the resulting solution is recorded. The absorbance range of 0.3 to 0.8 is used to get the higher precision in the quantitative measurements. If the absorbance is more than 0.8, the solution is diluted. If the absorbance is lower than 0.3, the concentration of the solution is increased by dissolving more quantity of the sample in the solvent.

5) Linearity of the graph of absorbance vs. concentration for an analyte

It is absolutely essential for the sample solution to obey Beer-Lambert law in the range of concentration used for the analysis. In order to confirm that the sample obeys Beer's law, it is essential to confirm the linearity of absorbance with concentration. This is carried out by preparing a series of solutions for an authentic sample in the range of concentration of interest and recording their absorbance against the same reference solution at the selected wavelength. The absorbance can then be plotted on Y-axis with the concentration of the solutions on X-axis. This plot should be obtained as a straight line passing through origin (0, 0). Any intercept (either +ve or –ve) on the absorbance axis must be due to the experimental error (application of unsuitable reference solution).

More recently, the equation of regression line (A = a + bc), calculated from the measurement points, by means of the method of least squares, is obtained using computers. If the concentration is in terms of g/100 ml, the regression coefficients 'a' and 'b' of this equation are the intercept and the specific absorbance, respectively. The correlation coefficient (r) to get the best fit for the data, characterizes the deviation of the individual measurement points from the regression line. For good spectrometric methods, 'r' should be near about 0.999.

Once all these parameters are optimized for the solute, quantitative estimation of a sample can be undertaken.

2.6.2.2. Calculation Methods

In quantitative estimation, once the absorbance of a solution is recorded, its concentration can be found out using the following methods.

1) Using $A^{1\%}_{1\,cm}$ or molar absorptivity (ε) values

In the equation for Beer-Lambert law (A = a.b.c), the term 'a' is the absorptivity of a substance and it can be expressed either as $A_{1\,cm}^{1\%}$ or as molar absorptivity (ε). These values are reported in the literature for most of the organic compounds and can easily be used for the calculation of the concentration. Thus, absorptivity is a known parameter, most of the times. If it is not reported in the literature, it can be found out by recording absorbance for a series of dilutions of the same compound, either of 100 % purity or of known purity, i.e. if a compound 'B' is to be analyzed from a sample, then the same compound B should be available either in 100 % purity or its purity should be known. When a graph of absorbance vs. concentration is plotted for this substance, a straight line OD, as shown in **Fig. 2.45**, is obtained. The slope of this line is expressed as follows.

Slope of a line OD =

$$\frac{A_2 - A_1}{c_2 - c_1} = \frac{\Delta A}{\Delta c}$$

$$= \frac{\text{Difference in the absorbance}}{\text{Difference in the concentration}}$$

According to Beer-Lambert law,

$$A = a.\ b.\ c$$

$$\text{OR} \quad a = \frac{A}{b\,.\,c}$$

Since the path length, b = 1,

$$a = \frac{A}{c} = \text{Slope of a line OD}$$

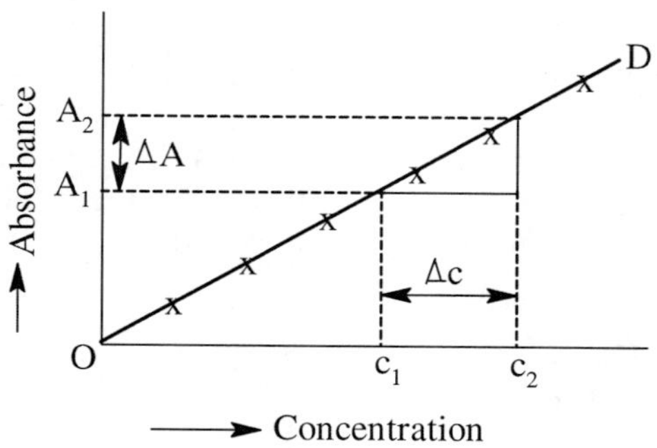

Fig. 2.45: Determination of an absorptivity of a substance

Thus, the slope of the line indicates the absorptivity of a sample.

$a = A_{1\,cm}^{1\%}$, if the concentration is in g/100 mL, and

$a = \varepsilon$ = molar absorptivity, if the concentration is in mol/L.

For calculating the concentration of a substance, therefore, it is necessary to find its absorbance (A).

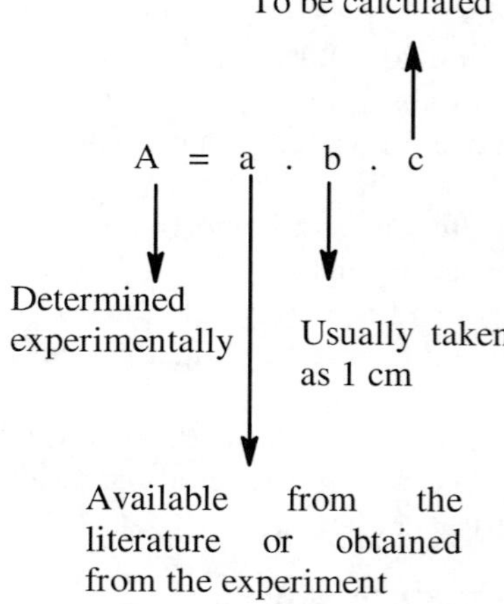

Thus, if the extinction coefficient (a) of a substance is known, its concentration in any sample can be calculated.

2) By using a calibration curve or a standard curve

Here, it is essential to have a calibration curve or a standard curve, as shown in **Fig. 2.46**, obtained by plotting absorbance values corresponding to various concentrations of a standard solution. A series of known concentrations is prepared by using a standard or a reference compound, which is of 100% purity or of known purity.

To analyze a sample with unknown concentration of a substance, the absorbance (A_u) of its solution is recorded. This absorbance is extrapolated to the line OD corresponding to a standard curve and a perpendicular is drawn from this point of intersection on the concentration axis so as to get the concentration (c_u) of the substance in the sample.

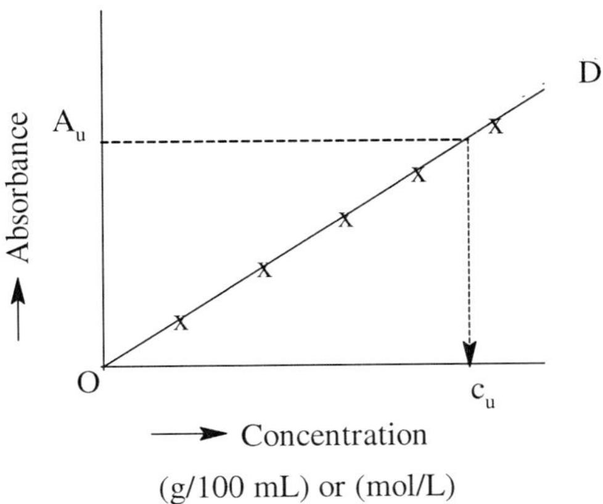

Fig. 2.46: Use of a standard curve for the quantitative analysis

Advantages

(i) This method does not involve any complexity in calculations.

(ii) The concentration of an analyte (c_u) in the sample is obtained directly from the graph.

Disadvantages

(i) This method involves preparation of a series of dilutions.

(ii) In addition, it is absolutely essential to have the reference compound, which is exactly identical chemically, as that of an analyte. Thus, the same compound should be available in the pure form or with the known purity. This may involve a lot of cost and effort in obtaining the compound in the pure form.

3) By recording absorbance values for a standard and a sample

In this method also, a reference or a standard compound of 100 % purity or of known purity, should be available for analyzing the substance from a sample.

A sample to be analyzed is dissolved in a suitable solvent. Its concentration is adjusted so as to get the absorbance in the range of 0.3 - 0.8. Similarly, a standard substance is also dissolved in a solvent to get the absorbance in the range of 0.3 - 0.8. The absorbance of both the solutions is recorded at the λ_{max} value of the compound. The Beer-Lambert law equations for these two solutions can be expressed by **equations (2.25)** and **(2.26)**.

$$A_{std} = a_{std}\, b\, c_{std} \quad \ldots (2.25)$$

$$A_{sample} = a_{sample}\, b\, c_{sample} \quad \ldots (2.26)$$

where, A_{std} = absorbance of a standard solution

A_{sample} = absorbance of a sample solution

b = 1 cm = path length for both the solutions, and

a = absorptivity, which is same for both the solutions since the standard and the sample solutions contain chemically identical substance.

$$\text{Hence, } a_{std} = a_{sample}$$

Dividing **equation (2.25)** by **equation (2.26)**, **equation (2.27)** is obtained.

$$\frac{A_{std}}{A_{sample}} = \frac{c_{std}}{c_{sample}} \quad \ldots (2.27)$$

In **equation (2.27)**, both the absorbance values, A_{std} and A_{sample}, are determined experimentally and the concentration of a standard (c_{std}) is known. Thus, the concentration of an analyte in the sample can be easily calculated.

Advantage

This method does not require plotting of a standard curve and requires only few readings to be recorded.

2.6.2.3. Areas of Applications

Principles of quantitative estimation by UV-visible spectrometry can be used for various applications.

1) To determine dissociation constant of acids and bases

Consider an acid HA, dissociating into H^+ ions and A^- ions as follows.

$$HA \rightleftharpoons H^+ + A^-$$

A dissociation constant (K_a) for this acid is expressed by the **equation (2.28)**.

$$K_a = \frac{[H^+][A^-]}{[HA]} \quad \ldots (2.28)$$

Taking the negative logarithm of all the terms in **equation (2.28)**, we get –

$$-\log_{10} K_a = -\log_{10} [H^+] - \log_{10} \frac{[A^-]}{[HA]}$$

but, $-\log_{10} K_a = pK_a$ and $-\log_{10} [H^+] = pH$

$$\therefore pK_a = pH + \log_{10} \frac{[HA]}{[A^-]} \quad \cdots (2.29)$$

Using a pH meter, pH of the solution can be determined. The concentration of either the undissociated acid (HA) in the solution at a particular pH or the concentration of A^- ions can be found out from the UV-visible spectrometry. Once the concentration of either HA or A^- ions is determined, the concentration of the remaining species can be calculated. For example, if an acid shows absorbance (A_{HA}) at some pH value of the solution, then the concentration (c_{HA}) of an undissociated acid, after its partial dissociation, can be found out by using **equation (2.30)**.

$$A_{HA} = a_{HA} \cdot b \cdot c_{HA}$$

$$c_{HA} = \frac{A_{HA}}{a_{HA} \cdot b} \quad \ldots. (2.30)$$

The initial concentration of an undissociated acid (HA) is known, since a definite quantity of the pure acid is used while preparing its solution. This initial concentration, minus the concentration of an undissociated acid (c_{HA}), remaining after partial dissociation, gives the amount of an acid dissociated and therefore, the concentration of A^- ions, i.e. $[A^-]$, in the solution can be found out. For example, if the initial concentration of the pure acid is 1 mol/L and after the partial dissociation, the concentration of an undissociated acid is 0.6 mol/L, then 0.4 mol/L of an acid is dissociated so as to produce 0.4 mol/L of A^- ions in the solution. Therefore, $[A^-]$ would be 0.4 mol/L. From the concentrations of undissociated and dissociated acids, the ratio of $\log_{10} [HA] / [A^-]$ can be found out.

Substituting its value in **equation (2.29)**, pKa of an acid can be calculated.

2) To determine the rate of a chemical reaction

Consider a following chemical reaction in which the reactants X and Y get converted to products R and S. Fixed quantities of X and Y are taken for the reaction and therefore, their concentrations are known.

$$X + Y \rightleftharpoons R + S$$

If the concentration of one of the products (R or S) is found out by recording the absorbance, then the concentration of the remaining product can be determined from the stoichiometry of the reaction. For example, in the above reaction, 1 mole of both the reactants X and Y, produce 1 mole each of R and S. If the concentration of R is found to be 0.01 moles after a particular reaction time, the reaction mixture should also contain 0.01 moles of S at the same time. Knowing the concentrations of all the four species, X, Y, R and S in the reaction mixture, the rate of reaction can be calculated by using **equation (2.31)**.

$$K = \frac{[R][S]}{[X][Y]} \quad \ldots (2.31)$$

3) As a detector

Most of the organic compounds are able to absorb UV radiation. Hence, UV spectrometry is very commonly combined with various chromatographic methods, such as column chromatography, HPLC, HPTLC, etc. The UV detector is very popularly used for detecting various organic compounds separated by the chromatographic techniques.

2.7. ANALYSIS OF A BINARY OR A MULTI-COMPONENT SYSTEM

2.7.1. Problems of Selectivity

The simplest way of checking whether the system under investigation is really a single component system from the spectrometric aspects is to record the spectra of the pure component, i.e. a standard [**Fig. 2.47(a)**] and the sample [**Fig. 2.47(b)**] to be analyzed (to confirm that the determination of an analyte does not include contribution by other substances).

1) As shown in **Fig. 2.47**, if the two spectra are

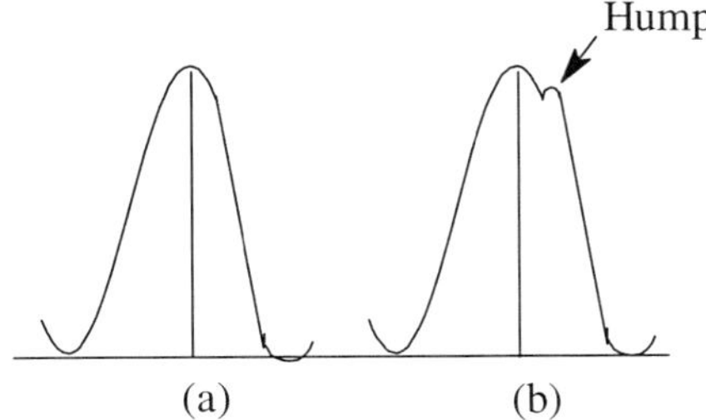

Fig. 2.47: (a) A normal peak for the standard and (b) a distorted peak for the sample in the UV spectrum

similar but the spectrum of the sample is distorted to a certain extent relative to the standard, a background problem (discussed in detail in **Section 2.7.2**) is probably responsible, which makes the direct analysis of a system as a single component system, impossible, but with the use of the mathematical methods - **background correction or other methods** - there is a chance for a solution of an appropriate precision.

2) If a well defined, extra band occurs in the system (**Fig. 2.48**), there is a possibility of another spectrometrically active component in the system. This problem can be solved by using a binary or a **multi-component system analysis** or by using a **derivative spectrometry**.

3) Sometimes, the sample solution contains

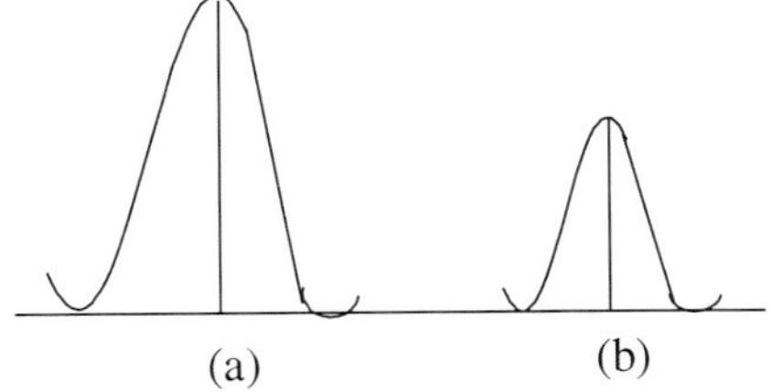

Fig. 2.48: A spectrum containing (a)a peak for an analyte and (b) an extra peak for the impurity

compounds with similar chromophores. For example, prednisolone is manufactured by dehydrogenation of hydrocortisone. There is a difference of only one double bond in their structures as shown in **Fig. 2.49**. Under this condition, the spectra of both the compounds closely resemble each other or they overlap because they have very similar absorption coefficients. Hence, even when the spectrum of the sample contains one normal peak, there is no guarantee that the system is a single component system.

Fig. 2.49: Dehydrogenation of hydrocortisone to prednisolone

Consequently, the selectivity of direct spectrometric methods should always be evaluated, and in the majority of cases, it is insufficient. To improve the situation, either selective absorption is produced by means of chemical reactions or the spectrometric measurement is made preceding chromatographic separation.

2.7.2. Background Correction Methods

In the spectrometric analysis of drugs, often there is an interference encountered due to absorption from other sources. This may be due to the presence of one or more substances, which can produce spectra, almost overlapping with the spectrum of an analyte. Hence, the measurement of the absorbance of the component of interest cannot be carried out directly.

Under this situation, the spectrum of an analyte is readily recognizable in the spectrum of the sample, but it is more or less distorted. The featureless and the unstructured spectrum, due to the presence of impurities, superimposed on a spectrum of an analyte, is called the *background*. The effect of absorption by the impurities on the absorption of an analyte is called the *background effect*.

The presence of the background may be due to the following reasons.

1) In case of plant extracts, along with the active component, many other impurities like starch, saponins, tannins, etc. also get extracted. The presence of such impurities can be the source of a background in case of substances like alkaloids, flavonoids, essential oils, etc. The products of animal origin, like insulin, also get contaminated due to the accompanying substances of the biological sample. Such impurities form a background for the spectrum of the active substances.
2) In case of drugs like penicillin or other antibiotics, which are manufactured by the process of fermentation, a similar situation may occur. The impurities from the fermentation broths, mother liquors or raw products, can form the background in this case.
3) In case of pharmaceutical formulations such as tablets, ointments or injections, the active ingredient is extracted along with the impurities such as excipients of tablets, base of an ointment and the oil component of the injection products. These extracted substances form the background in this case.
4) One more reason for the background is that an active principle of the pharmaceutical preparation produces a spectrum of relatively low intensity and one of the excipients in the formulation, present in a large excess, produces a well defined spectrum.

The interference due to background absorption can be eliminated by the advanced techniques like derivative spectrometry and difference spectrometry. In addition, there are also simpler techniques available, which have the common features that measurements are performed at other wavelengths as well as at the absorption maximum for an analyte, and the background corrections are done mathematically.

A number of methods are used to correct background effect.

1) Baseline method
2) Simple algebraic-geometric methods.
3) The method of orthogonal polynomials, and
4) The compensation method

2.7.3. Different Methods for the Analysis of a Multi-Component System

A number of drug formulations contain more than one active principle to be determined. Analysis of a mixture, containing two or more components, can be carried out in two ways.

1) Separate the components and then analyze them individually, or
2) Analyze the components in presence of each other without carrying out prior separation (spectrometric measurements).

The first method provides more sensitive and selective separation method, but it may involve longer time. Moreover, the separation method may not be very simple.

On the other hand, the analysis of components in presence of each other involves spectrometric determination, which is faster, but may involve complicated calculations. For mixtures containing more than two components, many simultaneous equations are generated, solving of which involves complicated calculations. These can be done routinely, only by means of computers. For mixtures containing two components also, lengthy calculations are involved.

The spectrometric measurement of multi-component systems is principally possible because the absorbance is an additive property in the concentration region usually applied in the UV-visible spectrometry. Thus, at a given wavelength, for a system containing several species, the measured absorbance is the sum of the absorbances of the individual species.

For the simultaneous determination of several components, all these components are required to be available in the pure form. Similarly, λ_{max} values of the pure components and their specific absorbance values, at λ_{max}, are required to be known.

2.7.3.1. Analysis of a Binary Mixture

In the analysis of binary mixtures, the spectra of both pure components are recorded first, and two λ_{max} values corresponding to the maximum absorption of both these compounds are determined. Then at the selected wavelengths, the specific absorbance values of both the components are determined. Analysis of different types of binary mixtures is discussed below.

1) Binary mixture analysis – Type 1

In a binary system, it can so happen that two components absorb radiation of totally different wavelengths in the spectra, where there is no interference at all from each other in the absorption measurements. This situation is shown in **Fig. 2.50**. In a mixture containing two compounds X and Y, let compound X absorb maximum energy at a wavelength λ_1 and compound Y absorb maximum energy at a wavelength λ_2. If $A_{x\lambda 1}$ is the absorbance of X at λ_1 and $a_{x\lambda 1}$ is its specific absorbance, then to find its concentration (c_x), **equation (2.32)** can be made use of. Similarly, the concentration of Y (c_y), can be found out from **equation (2.33)** by recording its absorbance, $A_{y\lambda 2}$, at λ_2 and by determining its specific absorbance, $a_{y\lambda 2}$. Thus, the concentration of the two components can be determined independently.

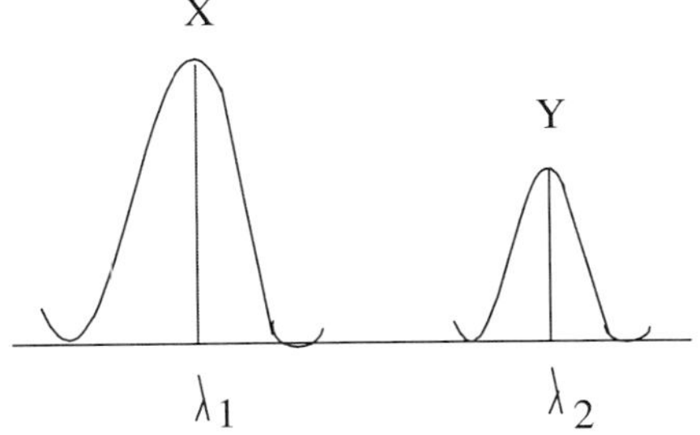

Fig. 2.50: Two components of a binary mixture absorbing at two different wavelengths

$$A_{x\lambda 1} = a_{x\lambda 1}.\ b.\ c_x \ \ldots (2.32)$$

$$A_{y\lambda 2} = a_{y\lambda 2}.\ b.\ c_y \ \ldots (2.33)$$

In practice however, such a case occurs very rarely.

2) Binary mixture analysis – Type 2

In most of the cases, it is observed that the spectra of the two components overlap in part. For

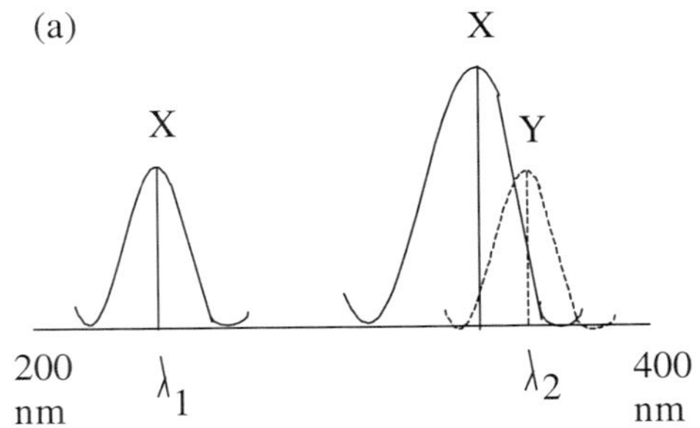

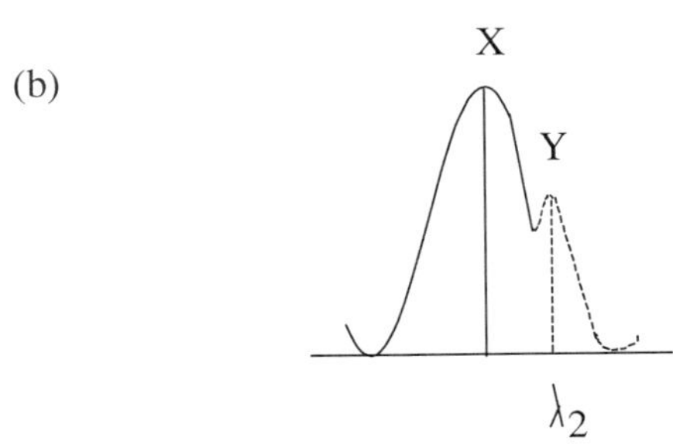

Fig. 2.51 (a): A spectrum of a binary mixture: Compound X absorbing at λ1 and compounds X and Y both absorbing at λ_2 (b): Actual appearance of the overlapping peaks for X and Y in their spectrum

example, out of the two components X and Y, only X has absorption at λ_1 but at λ_2, both X and Y absorb. This is shown in **Fig. 2.51(a)**. In the spectrum of a mixture, the overlapping peaks at wavelength λ_2 produce appearance as shown in **Fig. 2.51(b)**.

In such a case, the concentration of X can be found out by recording its absorbance ($A_{x\lambda 1}$) at λ_1. The absorptivity of X ($a_{x\lambda 1}$) at λ_1 can be found out, if it is not known, by the method mentioned earlier in this chapter (Method 1 under the **Section 2.6.2.2**). Using **equation (2.32)**, the concentration (c_x) of X can be found out.

To find concentration of Y (c_y), the absorbance ($A_{y\lambda 2}$) at the wavelength λ_2 is recorded. At this wavelength, both the compounds X and Y absorb, depending on their concentrations in the mixture. Since the absorbance is an additive property, the total absorbance ($A_{\lambda 2}$) of the mixture can be written as the sum of the absorbances shown by X ($A_{x\lambda 2}$) as well as by Y ($A_{y\lambda 2}$) at λ_2. Hence, the **equations (2.34)** and **(2.35)** can be written as -

$$A_{\lambda 2} = A_{x\lambda 2} + A_{y\ddot{e}2} \; \ldots \; (2.34)$$

$$A_{\lambda 2} = a_{x\lambda 2}.\ b.\ c_x + a_{y\lambda 2}.\ b.\ c_y \; \ldots \; (2.35)$$

In **equation (2.35)**, the value of $A_{\lambda 2}$ is known since net absorbance of the mixture at λ_2 is recorded. The absorptivities of X ($a_{x\lambda 2}$) and Y ($a_{y\lambda 2}$) at λ_2 can be found out. The concentration of X (c_x) is also calculated using **equation (2.33)**. The path length (b) is usually 1 cm. Thus, in **equation (2.35)**, all the terms, except for the concentration of Y (c_y), are known and hence, c_y can be calculated.

3) Binary mixture analysis – Type 3

Many a times, in a binary mixture, the spectra of two components completely overlap at λ_{max} values of both the components (**Fig. 2.52**). Under this situation, following two methods can be used to find the concentration of both X and Y.

(A) Simultaneous equation method

In this method, the absorbance of a mixture at λ_{max} value of the first component (λ_1) as well as at λ_{max} value of the second component (λ_2), is found out.

In order to find the concentration of both the

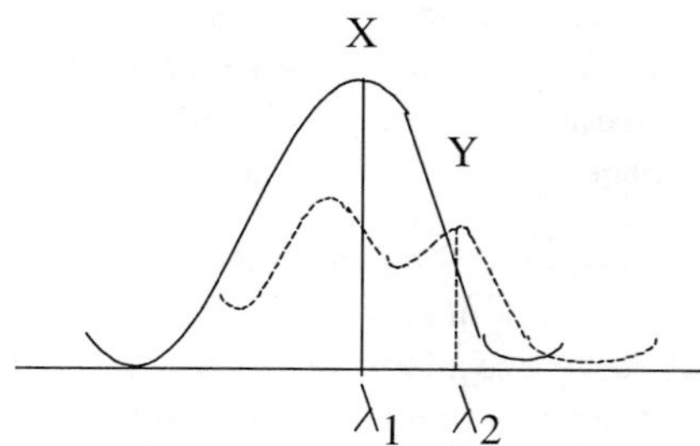

Fig. 2.52: A spectrum of a binary mixture showing overlapping of peaks for both the compounds at λ_{max} values of both the components

compounds X and Y in the mixture, the λ_{max} value of X (λ_1) and the λ_{max} value of Y (λ_2) should be found out by scanning pure compounds separately. Similarly, the absorptivities of X, ($a_{x\lambda 1}$) and ($a_{x\lambda 2}$), at the λ_{max} value of X (λ_1) and at the λ_{max} value of Y (λ_2), respectively, should be determined. Also, the absorptivities of Y, ($a_{y\lambda 1}$) and ($a_{y\lambda 2}$), at the λ_{max} value of X (λ_1) and at the λ_{max} value of Y (λ_2), respectively, should be determined. After getting this data, the absorbance values, ($A_{\lambda 1}$) and ($A_{\lambda 2}$), of the mixture of X and Y at λ_1 and λ_2 are found out. At both these wavelengths, the net absorbance is the sum of absorbances of X and Y. Hence, the two equations for the net absorbance of a mixture at λ_1 ($A_{\lambda 1}$) and the net absorbance of a mixture at λ_2 ($A_{\lambda 2}$), can be written. This leads to the **equations (2.36)** and **(2.37)**, respectively.

$$A_{\lambda 1} = A_{x\lambda 1} + A_{y\lambda 1}$$

$$A_{\lambda 2} = A_{x\lambda 2} + A_{y\lambda 2}$$

$$A_{\lambda 1} = a_{x\lambda 1} b\, c_x + a_{y\lambda 1}\, b\, c_y \; \ldots \; (2.36)$$

$$A_{\lambda 2} = a_{x\lambda 2} b\, c_x + a_{y\lambda 2} b\, c_y \; \ldots \; (2.37)$$

If b = 1, then -

$$A_{\lambda 1} = a_{x\lambda 1} c_x + a_{y\lambda 1} c_y \; \ldots \; (2.38)$$

$$A_{\lambda 2} = a_{x\lambda 2} c_x + a_{y\lambda 2} c_y \; \ldots \; (2.39)$$

To find values of c_x and c_y

Rearranging **equation (2.39)**, we get -

$$A_{\lambda 2} - a_{x\lambda 2}c_x = a_{y\lambda 2}c_y$$

$$\therefore c_y = \frac{A_{\lambda 2} - a_{x\lambda 2}c_x}{a_{y\lambda 2}} \quad \text{... (2.40)}$$

Substituting this value of c_y in **equation (2.38)**, we get -

$$A_{\lambda 1} = a_{x\lambda 1}c_x + a_{y\lambda 1}\left(\frac{A_{\lambda 2} - a_{x\lambda 2}c_x}{a_{y\lambda 2}}\right)$$

$$\therefore A_{\lambda 1}\, a_{y\lambda 2} = a_{x\lambda 1}c_x\, a_{y\lambda 2} + A_{\lambda 2}a_{y\lambda 1} - a_{x\lambda 2}\, c_x\, a_{y\lambda 1}$$

$$\therefore a_{x\lambda 2}\, c_x\, a_{y\lambda 1} - a_{x\lambda 1}c_x\, a_{y\lambda 2} = A_{\lambda 2}a_{y\lambda 1} - A_{\lambda 1}\, a_{y\lambda 2}$$

$$\therefore c_x\,(a_{x\lambda 2}\, a_{y\lambda 1} - a_{x\lambda 1}\, a_{y\lambda 2}) = A_{\lambda 2}a_{y\lambda 1} - A_{\lambda 1}\, a_{y\lambda 2}$$

$$\therefore c_x = \frac{A_{\lambda 2}a_{y\lambda 1} - A_{\lambda 1}\, a_{y\lambda 2}}{(a_{x\lambda 2}\, a_{y\lambda 1} - a_{x\lambda 1}\, a_{y\lambda 2})} \quad \text{... (2.41)}$$

Similarly, value of c_y can be expressed by **equation (2.42)**

$$c_y = \frac{A_{\lambda 1}\, a_{x\lambda 2} - A_{\lambda 2}a_{x\lambda 1}}{(a_{y\lambda 1}\, a_{x\lambda 2} - a_{y\lambda 2}\, a_{x\lambda 1})} \quad \text{... (2.42)}$$

In **equations (2.38)** and **(2.39)**, the values of the terms, $A_{\lambda 1}$, $A_{\lambda 2}$, $a_{x\lambda 1}$, $a_{y\lambda 1}$, $a_{x\lambda 2}$ and $a_{y\lambda 2}$, are known. Thus, there are two **equations (2.38 and 2.39)** and two unknowns (c_x and c_y). The values of these two unknowns can be found out by solving **equations (2.38)** and **(2.39)**, simultaneously. Thus, simultaneous equation method is commonly used for the overlapping spectra at different wavelengths. In this method, **equation (2.38)** is multiplied by the coefficient of c_x in **equation (2.39)** and **equation (2.39)** is multiplied by the coefficient of c_x in **equation (2.38)**. This makes the value of coefficients of c_x in both the equations exactly same. The subtraction of one equation from the other eliminates the term c_x and the value of c_y can be found out. The same procedure is followed to find the value of c_x. The simplified expressions for c_x and c_y are given in **equations (2.41)** and **(2.42)**, respectively. This method is restricted to a binary mixture or a mixture containing a limited number of components, since one has to solve 'n' number of equations to find the concentration of 'n' number of components in a mixture. The calculation becomes more complex as the number of components, and consequently, the number of equations, increases.

(B) Absorption ratio method

The absorption ratio method is a modification of simultaneous equation method. It is based on the principle that for any substance, which obeys Beer's law, the ratio of absorbance at two wavelengths is constant and is independent of its concentration or path length.

In case of analysis of a binary mixture by absorption ratio method, the absorbance of the mixture is measured at two wavelengths. One wavelength is the λ_{max} value of one of the components, either the λ_{max} of X (λ_2) or the λ_{max} of Y (λ_3), and another wavelength is an *iso-absorptive wavelength* (λ_1). An iso-absorptive wavelength is a wavelength at which both the substances exhibit the same absorbance. This is shown in **Fig. 2.53**. In order to determine the concentration of X and Y, two **equations**, **(2.43)** and **(2.44)** are constructed. Further derivation leads to **equation (2.50)**, which gives the concentration of X in a binary mixture.

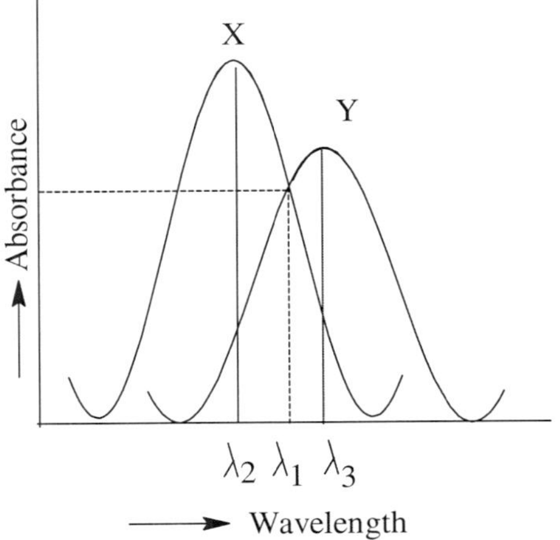

Fig. 2.53: An iso-absorptive wavelength (λ_1) for solutes X and Y

$$A_{\lambda 1} = A_{x\lambda 1} + A_{y\lambda 1}$$

$$A_{\lambda 2} = A_{x\lambda 2} + A_{y\lambda 2}$$

$$A_{\lambda 1} = a_{x\lambda 1} b c_x + a_{y\lambda 1} b c_y$$

$$A_{\lambda 2} = a_{x\lambda 2} b c_x + a_{y\lambda 2} b c_y$$

If b = 1, then -

$$A_{\lambda 1} = a_{x\lambda 1} c_x + a_{y\lambda 1} c_y \quad \ldots (2.43)$$

$$A_{\lambda 2} = a_{x\lambda 2} c_x + a_{y\lambda 2} c_y \quad \ldots (2.44)$$

λ_1 is an isoabsorptive wavelength and therefore, $a_{x\lambda 1} = a_{y\lambda 1}$.

$$\frac{A_{\lambda 2}}{A_{\lambda 1}} = \frac{a_{x\lambda 2} c_x + a_{y\lambda 2} c_y}{a_{x\lambda 1} c_x + a_{y\lambda 1} c_y}$$

Dividing each term by $(c_x + c_y)$, **equation (2.45)** is obtained.

$$\frac{A_{\lambda 2}}{A_{\lambda 1}} = \frac{\dfrac{a_{x\lambda 2} c_x}{c_x + c_y} + \dfrac{a_{y\lambda 2} c_y}{c_x + c_y}}{\dfrac{a_{x\lambda 1} c_x}{c_x + c_y} + \dfrac{a_{y\lambda 1} c_y}{c_x + c_y}} \quad \ldots (2.45)$$

Let $\dfrac{c_x}{c_x + c_y}$ be F_x and $\dfrac{c_y}{c_x + c_y}$ be F_y

$$\frac{A_{\lambda 2}}{A_{\lambda 1}} = \frac{a_{x\lambda 2} F_x + a_{y\lambda 2} F_y}{a_{x\lambda 1} F_x + a_{y_1} F_y} \quad \ldots (2.46)$$

Since $F_x + F_y = 1$, we get -

$$\frac{A_{\lambda 2}}{A_{\lambda 1}} = \frac{a_{x\lambda 2} F_x + a_{y\lambda 2}(1 - F_x)}{a_{x\lambda 1} F_x + a_{y\lambda 1}(1 - F_x)}$$

$$\frac{A_{\lambda 2}}{A_{\lambda 1}} = \frac{a_{x\lambda 2} F_x + a_{y\lambda 2} - a_{y\lambda 2} F_x}{a_{x\lambda 1} F_x + a_{y\lambda 1} - a_{y\lambda 1} F_x}$$

$$\frac{A_{\lambda 2}}{A_{\lambda 1}} = \frac{F_x (a_{x\lambda 2} - a_{y\lambda 2}) + a_{y\lambda 2}}{F_x (a_{x\lambda 1} - a_{y\lambda 1}) + a_{y\lambda 1}}$$

At λ_1, $a_{x\lambda 1} = a_{y\lambda 1}$ and $\therefore (a_{x\lambda 1} - a_{y\lambda 1}) = 0$

$$\therefore \frac{A_{\lambda 2}}{A_{\lambda 1}} = \frac{F_x (a_{x\lambda 2} - a_{y\lambda 2}) + a_{y\lambda 2}}{a_{y\lambda 1}}$$

$$\therefore \frac{A_{\lambda 2}}{A_{\lambda 1}} = \frac{F_x a_{x\lambda 2} - F_x a_{y\lambda 2} + a_{y\lambda 2}}{a_{y\lambda 1}}$$

$$\therefore \frac{A_{\lambda 2}}{A_{\lambda 1}} = \frac{F_x a_{x\lambda 2}}{a_{y\lambda 1}} - \frac{F_x a_{y\lambda 2}}{a_{y\lambda 1}} + \frac{a_{y\lambda 2}}{a_{y\lambda 1}} \quad \ldots (2.47)$$

Let $\dfrac{A_{\lambda 2}}{A_{\lambda 1}} = Q_M$, $\dfrac{a_{x\lambda 2}}{a_{x\lambda 1}} = Q_X$ and $\dfrac{a_{y\lambda 2}}{a_{y\lambda 1}} = Q_Y$

The **equation (2.47)** therefore takes the form –

$$Q_M = \frac{F_x a_{x\lambda 2}}{a_{y\lambda 1}} - F_x Q_Y + Q_Y$$

At an isoabsorptive wavelength, $a_{y\lambda 1} = a_{x\lambda 1}$

$$\therefore \frac{F_x a_{x\lambda 2}}{a_{y\lambda 1}} = \frac{F_x a_{x\lambda 2}}{a_{x\lambda 1}}$$

$$\therefore Q_M = F_x Q_X - F_x Q_Y + Q_Y$$

$$\therefore Q_M = F_x (Q_X - Q_Y) + Q_Y$$

$$\text{or } F_X = \frac{(Q_M - Q_Y)}{(Q_X - Q_Y)} \quad \ldots (2.48)$$

To find actual concentration, consider **equation (2.43)**, i.e..

$$A_{\lambda 1} = a_{x\lambda 1} c_x + a_{y\lambda 1} c_y$$

Since, $a_{x\lambda 1} = a_{y\lambda 1}$

$$A_{\lambda 1} = a_{x\lambda 1} c_x + a_{x\lambda 1} c_y$$

$$\therefore A_{\lambda 1} = a_{x\lambda 1}(c_x + c_y)$$

$$\therefore (c_x + c_y) = \frac{A_{\lambda 1}}{a_{x\lambda 1}} \quad \cdots (2.49)$$

From **equation (2.48)**,

$$F_x = \frac{Q_M - Q_Y}{(Q_X - Q_Y)} = \frac{c_x}{c_x + c_y}$$

$$\therefore \frac{c_x}{c_x + c_y} = \frac{Q_M - Q_Y}{(Q_X - Q_Y)}$$

$$\therefore c_x = \frac{Q_M - Q_Y}{(Q_X - Q_Y)}(c_x + c_y)$$

Substituting the value of $(c_x + c_y)$ from **equation (2.49)**, we get -

$$c_x = \frac{(Q_M - Q_Y)}{(Q_X - Q_Y)} \frac{A_{\lambda 1}}{a_{x\lambda 1}} \quad \ldots (2.50)$$

Once the concentration of X is known, concentration of Y can be calculated.

2.7.3.2. Analysis of a Multi-component System by Linear Combination

Modern mathematics and computer science offer simplicity in the analysis of a multi-component system. If the solution is based on the linear combination, the concentrations c_1, c_2, c_3, c_4,....... c_n, of 'n' components, should be determined by solving following equations.

At λ_1

$$A_{\lambda 1} = a_{1\lambda 1}\, b\, c_1 + a_{2\,\lambda 1}\, b\, c_2 + \ldots + a_{n\,\lambda 1}\, b\, c_n$$

At λ_2

$$A_{\lambda 2} = a_{1\lambda 2}\, b\, c_1 + a_{2\,\lambda 2}\, b\, c_2 + \ldots + a_{n\,\lambda 2}\, b\, c_n$$

$$\vdots$$

At λ_m

$$A_{\lambda m} = a_{1\,\lambda m}\, bc_1 + a_{2\,\lambda m}\, b\, c_2 + \ldots + a_{n\,\lambda m}\, b\, c_n$$

The terms, a_1, a_2, a_3,.....a_n, indicate absorptivities of the components and 'b' is the path length.

Thus, in this method, the number of equations in the system is 'm', equal to the number of wavelengths for which the absorbance values are recorded. The number of equations must be at least equal to the number of components. Equations (m) more than the number of components (n) of a mixture, increase accuracy of the measurement. The modern spectrometers are equipped with computers and hence, enable one to record a large number of data points, even at 'nm' intervals, in the spectral region of interest. This advancement of the introduction of computer in spectrometers has made possible the handling of a large number of equations.

In order to determine the concentration of a number of components in a mixture, the following conditions should be satisfied.

1) The spectra of all the pure components of a mixture must be available so as to have their λ_{max} values.
2) All the components should obey Bear-Lambert law in the wavelength region of interest.
3) The spectrum of the multi-component system must be representable as the sum of the spectra of the components.
4) Spectral data should be available in the digital form.
5) Appropriate computer and program for the calculations should be available.

When two or more components from any mixture are to be determined, the solutions of these pure compounds are prepared using the same concentration. In addition, two more concentrations, i.e. ± 10 % of the stated concentration, are also prepared. Then the individual spectra of these compounds are recorded. Also, a spectrum for a mixture, containing all these compounds, is recorded. By using these spectra, the concentration of each component in a mixture can be found out.

2.8. DERIVATIVE UV SPECTROMETRY

2.8.1. Theoretical Background

Derivative spectrometry is very commonly used for the background correction and for the selective analysis of compounds, producing overlapping bands in their UV spectra, when present in a mixture. In derivative spectrometry, a mathematical derivative of the absorbance with respect to the wavelength of radiation is calculated by the instrument itself, electronically or by using microcomputers. A spectrometer can calculate different orders of derivatives as follows.

(i) A *normal spectrum* is termed as a *zero order spectrum* and is represented as ^{o}D. It is a plot of absorbance (A) vs. wavelengths (λ).

(ii) The *first order spectrum* is obtained by calculating the first order derivative of an absorbance with respect to a wavelength so as to get the ratio, $dA/d\lambda$, and is represented as ^{1}D. It is a plot of $dA/d\lambda$ vs. wavelengths.

(iii) The *second order spectrum* is obtained by calculating the second order derivative of an absorbance with respect to a wavelength so as to get the ratio, $d^2A/d\lambda^2$, and is represented as ^2D. It is a plot of $d^2A/d\lambda^2$ vs. wavelengths.

(iv) The *third order spectrum* is obtained by calculating the third order derivative of an absorbance with respect to a wavelength so as to get the ratio, $d^3A/d\lambda^3$, and is represented as ^3D. It is a plot of $d^3A/d\lambda^3$ vs. wavelengths.

(v) The *fourth order spectrum* is obtained by calculating the fourth order derivative of an absorbance with respect to a wavelength so as to get the ratio, $d^4A/d\lambda^4$, and is represented as ^4D. It is a plot of $d^4A/d\lambda^4$ vs. wavelengths.

The nature of all these spectra is shown in **Fig. 2.54**. The derivatized spectra have following characteristics.

(i) In derivatized spectra, maxima and minima of the original function take zero values, and inflections are converted into maxima or minima, e.g. the first order derivative spectrum takes zero value at the maximum of the zero order spectrum.

(ii) The derivative spectra are more structured than the original spectra, since the number of peaks goes on increasing with the increase in the order of derivative. In the first order derivative spectrum, the original band splits into two. In the second order derivative spectrum, the original band splits into three. Thus, the number of peaks in a spectrum of order 'n' would be (n+1). Though the increase in the number of peaks helps in producing the spectral characteristic of a compound, it also increases the complexity of the spectrum.

The most widely used orders of derivative spectra are the second and the fourth, though sometimes, other derivatives are also used.

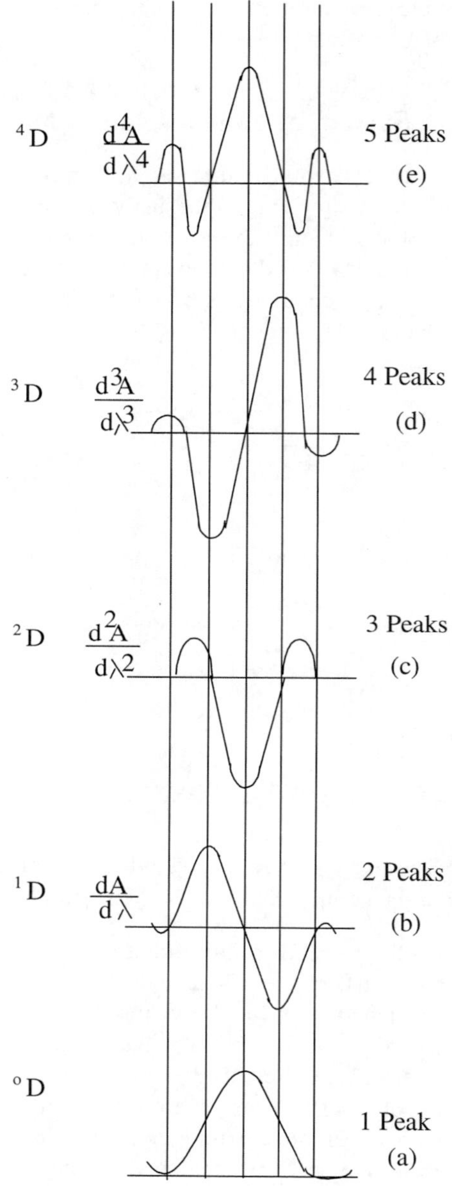

Fig. 2.54: (a) Zero (b) first (c) second (d) third and (e) fourth order derivative spectra

2.8.2. Applications of Derivative Spectrometry in Drug Analysis

Derivative spectrometry finds applications in the following fields.

1) Qualitative analysis

We have already seen that in derivative spectrometry, a single peak, corresponding to the zero order, splits into more peaks as the order increases and hence, the derivative spectra are more structured than the zero order spectra. This splitting pattern is slightly different for different compounds and is characteristic of that substance. From the splitting pattern, one can identify a compound, e.g. the zero order spectra of amphetamine and phenylethylamine are almost identical so that one cannot identify whether it is amphetamine or phenylethylamine. The second derivative spectra of two are also very similar, but the intensity ratios of certain side maxima have characteristic differences. This difference is made use of in the identification of individual compounds. The difference in the side bands is shown in **Fig. 2.55**.

effective than the other methods such as a *base-line method*, *algebraic-geometric methods*, *the method of orthogonal polynomials* and *compensation method.*

To solve relatively simple background problems, even the first derivative may prove sufficient, since with respect to short wavelength ranges, the background can be regarded as constant. A much more difficult background problem has been solved by means of the second or higher order derivative spectra.

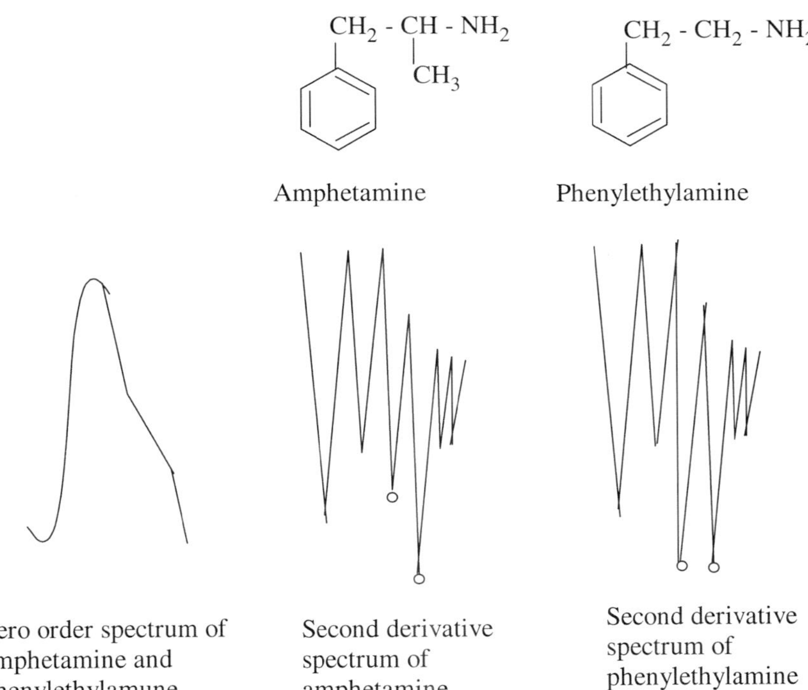

Fig. 2.55: Zero and second order spectra of amphetamine and phenylethylamine

2) Background correction in quantitative analysis

The sources for background effects are already discussed in this chapter earlier (**Section 2.7.2**). One of the most important applications of derivative spectrometry is the background correction, which in this case is simpler and more

As shown in **Fig. 2.56**, if the nature of the background is such that it shows a constant absorption (A = constant) over a wider range of wavelengths of interest, then the background effect is eliminated in the first derivative itself since, the first order derivative of a constant is zero, i.e. $dA/d\lambda = 0$.

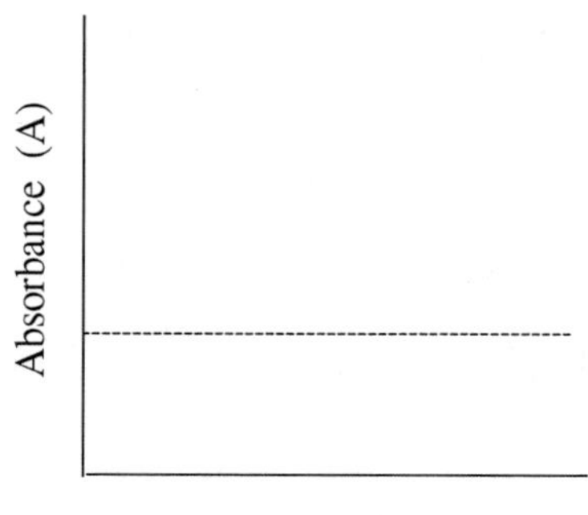

Fig. 2.56: A background showing constant absorption over a wider range of wavelengths

As shown in **Fig. 2.57** if the background is a linear function of wavelengths ($A = a + b\lambda$), then a second derivative will vanish, i.e., $d^2A/d\lambda^2 = 0$.

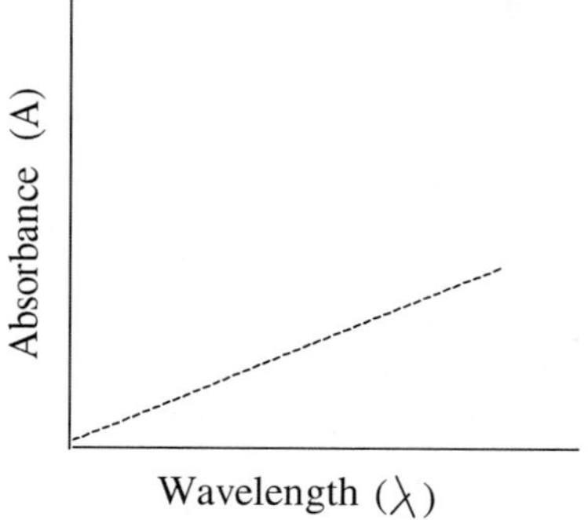

Fig. 2.57: A background showing linear relation of absorbance with wavelengths

Monotonous background curves, corresponding to the higher order functions, may also be eliminated, i.e. if $A = a + b\lambda + c\lambda^2 + g\lambda^3$, then $d^4A/d\lambda^4 = 0$.

Thus, by recording derivative spectra, the background effect can be eliminated. Elimination of the background effect in the analysis of a drug from its formulation is illustrated in **Fig. 2.58.**

Owing to the excipients, the apparent active principle content calculated from the normal or a zero order spectrum [**Fig. 2.58(a)**] of a methanol extract at 242 nm is more than 100 %. The generation of the first derivative spectrum [**Fig. 2.58(b)**] eliminates the background practically fully in the neighborhood of the maximum absorption and the active principle content calculated from the derivative spectrum is almost 100 %.

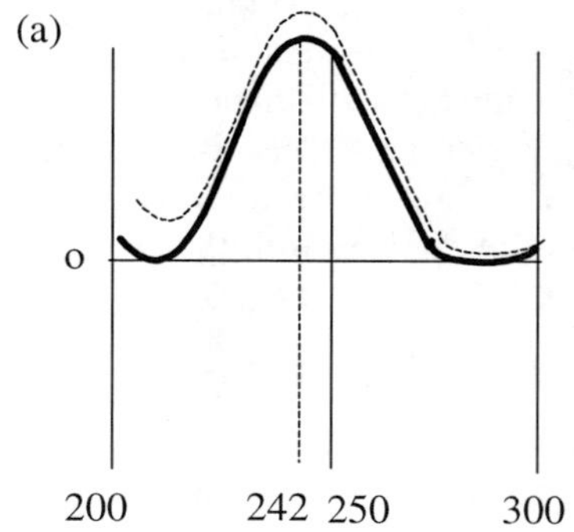

— Zero order spectrum of a pure drug

---- Zero order spectrum of a drug in formulation

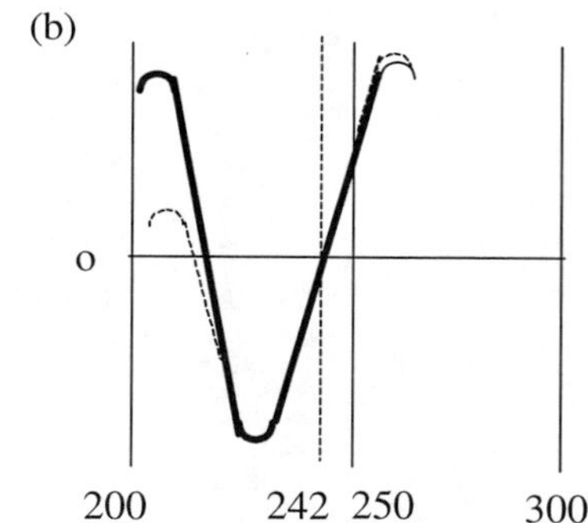

— First order spectrum of a pure drug

---- First order spectrum of a drug in formulation

Fig. 2.58: Elimination of the background effect in the analysis of a drug from its formulation

3) Elimination of an overlapping broad band in the quantitative estimation of substances with narrow bands

Derivative spectrometry provides an excellent selectivity for the analysis of a complex system in which a sharp band (for compound X) overlaps with a broad band (for compound Y) in a zero order spectrum. By generating an appropriately higher order derivative spectrum, the broad band can be eliminated because the intensity or amplitude or height of the originally broad band rapidly decreases with the increase in the order of the derivative as compared to the relative intensity of a sharp band.

Figure 2.59(a) shows a zero order spectrum (S) when X and Y are together. Individual peaks for X and Y are also shown. The compound X produces a narrow and a sharp peak in the spectrum, whereas the compound Y produces a broad band. In **Fig. 2.59(b)** and **(c)**, the second and the fourth order derivative spectra, respectively, of S, X and Y are shown.

stant, for the comparison purpose, it is assumed that –

$$A = \left(\frac{1}{W}\right)^n \quad ...(2.52)$$

Let us suppose that a sharp peak for X has the peak width corresponding to 2 units, whereas a broad peak for Y has the peak width corresponding to 8 units, in their zero order spectra. If the amplitude for these two peaks is calculated for the second and the fourth order spectra, the following values are obtained.

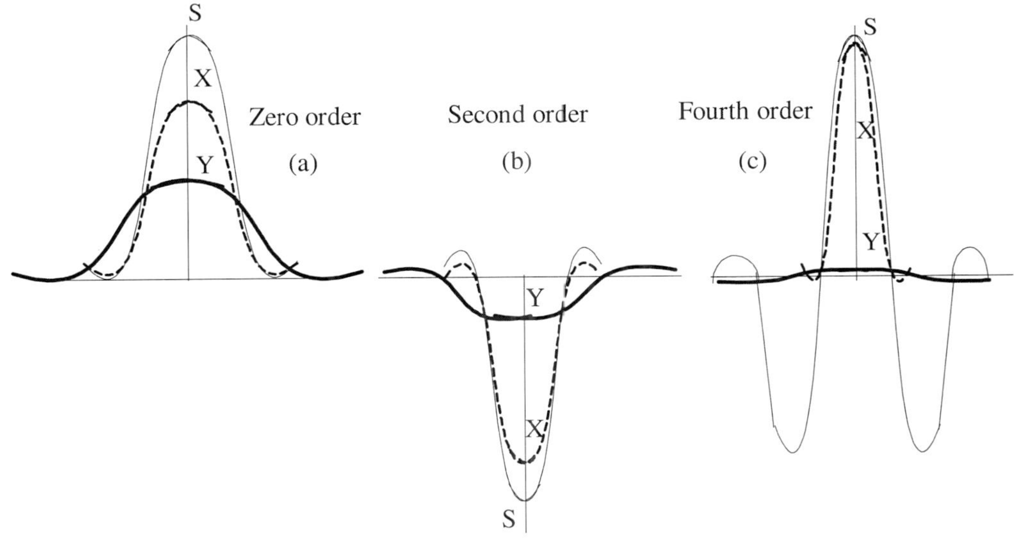

Fig. 2.59: Elimination of interference from a compound producing broad band in zero order spectrum

Amplitude (A) of a peak is found to be related to its width (W) by the **equation (2.51)**.

$$A = k\left(\frac{1}{W}\right)^n \quad ...(2.51)$$

where, n is the order of the derivative of the spectrum. Note that the value of 'k' being con-

For a sharp peak

(a) Second order spectrum:

$$A = \left(\frac{1}{2}\right)^2 = \left(\frac{1}{4}\right) = 0.25$$

(b) Fourth order spectrum:

$$A=\left(\frac{1}{2}\right)^4=\left(\frac{1}{16}\right)=0.0625$$

For a broad peak

(a) Second order spectrum:

$$A=\left(\frac{1}{8}\right)^2=\left(\frac{1}{64}\right)=0.0156$$

(b) Fourth order spectrum:

$$A=\left(\frac{1}{8}\right)^4=\left(\frac{1}{4096}\right)=0.00024$$

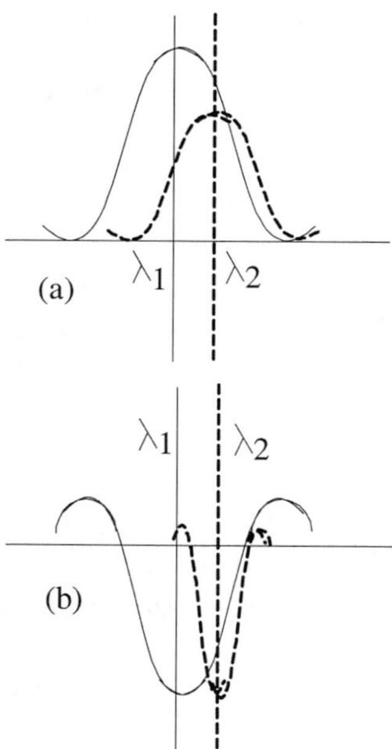

Fig. 2.60: (a) Overlapping of the zero order spectra of two compounds

(b) Separation of two peaks by the second order derivative spectrometry

Thus, it is clear that the amplitude for a broad peak is reduced drastically as compared to that for a sharp peak. Hence, the peak for Y merges almost completely into the baseline. Peaks for X and S coincide almost completely in the 2nd order and completely in the 4th order derivative spectra. Thus, the effect of a broad band on a sharp band is completely eliminated.

4) Analysis of a binary or a multi-component system by derivative spectrometry

In a binary mixture, if the zero order spectra of two components partially overlap, the two peaks can be separated in the second to the fourth derivative spectra, which can be utilized in the selective quantitative analysis of the two components from their mixture.

Figure 2.60(a) shows interference of two peaks at the wavelengths, λ_1 and λ_2. When the second order derivative spectrum [**Figure 2.60(b)**] is recorded, it is seen that at the wavelength λ_1, the absorbance from one component is maximum or

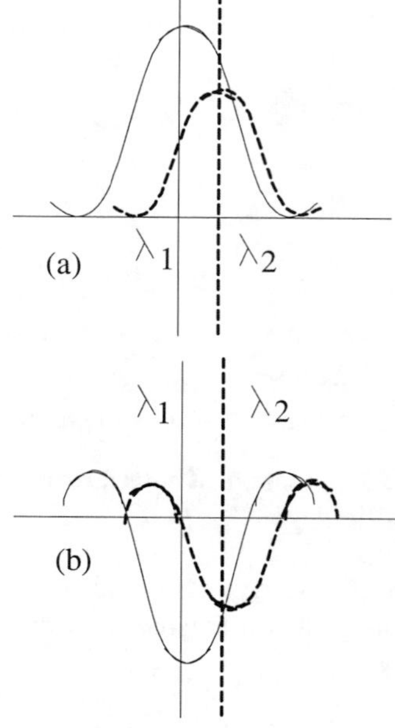

Fig. 2.61: Zero crossing method for analysis of a binary mixture

closely maximum and there is no interference from the second component. Such wavelengths can be used for the selective determination of the individual components.

Zero crossing method for the analysis of a binary mixture

Figure 2.61(a) shows zero order spectra of two compounds, both of which absorb at wavelengths λ_1 and λ_2. Hence, their selective analysis becomes difficult. When their higher order spectra are recorded, one can select a wavelength λ_1, where one compound shows maximum absorbance and another compound shows zero absorbance [**Figure 2.61(b)**]. Selection of such a wavelength makes possible analysis of a mixture without the interference of components with each other.

2.9. DIFFERENCE DERIVATIVE SPECTROMETRY

In the normal UV or colorimetric procedures, the *reference* and the *test* solutions are prepared in exactly the same manner, the only difference being that the reference solution does not contain an analyte. This increases the selectivity of the measurement of the absorbance of an analyte by decreasing or eliminating the effect of absorption by the solvent and the other reagents or by the impurities present therein.

In difference spectrometry, two solutions are used, both of which contain the same reagents in the same concentrations, including an analyte. Since an analyte is present in both the solutions, these solutions are not designated as the reference and the test solutions. The difference spectrometry makes use of chemical derivatization, whereas the difference derivative spectrometry makes use of chemical as well as mathematical derivatization. The simplest chemical derivatization includes change in the pH of a solution. The chemical derivatization of an analyte is carried out in one of the solutions, not necessarily the test solution. The difference in the absorbance of the two solutions is recorded and is plotted against the wavelengths.

Phenols or amines possess lone pairs of electrons on oxygen and nitrogen atoms, respectively. These substances interact with acids

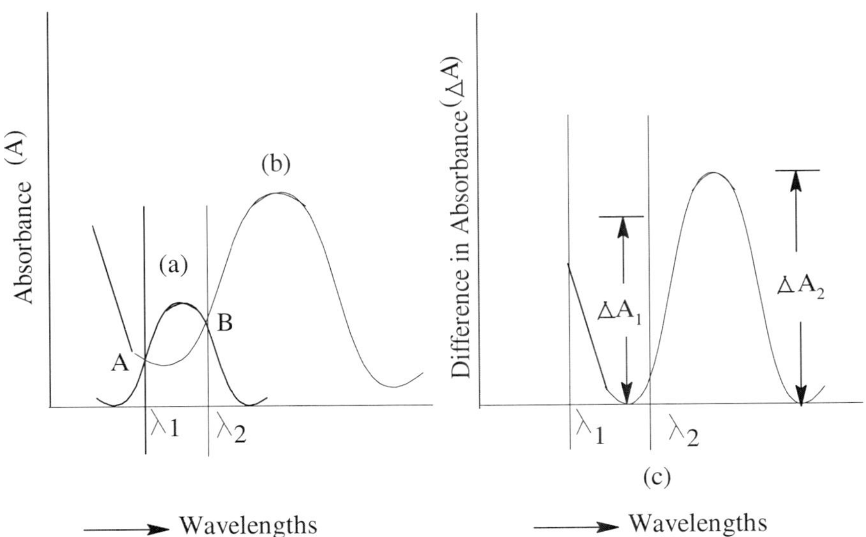

Fig. 2.62: Absorption of phenol in (a) acidic pH and in (b) alkaline pH (c) difference absorption spectrum of phenol

or bases, which brings about the change in the number of lone pairs of electrons in them, e.g. a molecule of phenol has two lone pairs of electrons on the oxygen atom. During analysis of phenol by difference spectrometry, when the pH of one of the solutions is increased by adding alkali to it, the number of lone pairs of electrons on the oxygen atom increases to three. These electrons are delocalized in the benzene ring and hence, a bathochromic shift, i.e. a shift in the absorption maximum towards a longer wavelength, is observed. The solution in another sample holder, however, shows the absorbance at a shorter wavelength only. The shift in the absorption wavelength of phenol with the change in the pH is shown in **Fig. 2.62**. In order to obtain the difference absorption spectrum, the difference between the absorbance of the solution in the alkaline and the acidic pH, is plotted against the wavelengths. In **Fig. 2.62**, the points A (λ_1) and B (λ_2) are the *isoabsorptive* or *isobestic points*, at which the absorbance in the acidic and the alkaline solutions, respectively, are same. Since the absorbance of phenol is higher in the alkaline pH as compared to that in the acidic pH, the difference in the absorbance at or beyond λ_2 is positive, but the difference is negative between λ_1 and λ_2.

The difference spectrometry can also be used for the selective analysis of compounds from a mixture of a neutral and an acidic or a basic compound, when they produce overlapping peaks. A bathochromic shift for an acidic compound makes possible the selective analysis of both the compounds. If the difference spectrometry does not provide the required selectivity, the difference derivative spectrometry is undertaken, which involves chemical as well as mathematical derivatization.

Thus, because of the ease of operation, economical methodology and wide applications, UV-visible spectrometry is very popularly used in the field of analysis.

CHAPTER 3

INFRARED SPECTROMETRY

The infrared (IR) radiation has longer wavelengths as compared to the ultraviolet (UV) and visible radiation and hence, it is less energetic. The UV region is in the range of 200-400 nm or millimicrons (mμ), the visible region is in the range of 400-800 nm or millimicrons (mμ), whereas the IR region is in the range of 800-10,000,00 mμ. In order to avoid the use of such large numbers, usually, the wavelengths in the IR region are expressed in micrometers (μm) instead of millimicrons (mμ).

1 μm = 1000 mμ = 1000 nm

Therefore, the range for the IR radiation is expressed as 0.8-1000 μm. The IR spectrum is divided into three regions.

1) Near IR region, which extends from 0.8 μm to 2.5 μm
2) Middle IR region, which extends from 2.5 μm to 50 μm and
3) Far IR region, which extends from 50 μm to 1000 μm.

Many a times, these three regions are described in terms of wavenumbers in cm^{-1}.

1) Near IR region ranging from 12,800 to 4000 cm^{-1}
2) Middle IR region ranging from 4,000 to 200 cm^{-1}, and
3) Far IR region ranging from 200 to 10 cm^{-1}

For practical purpose, most commonly, a region between 2.5 and 15 μm or 4000 cm^{-1} and 670 cm^{-1} is used. The IR spectrometry is used qualitatively as well as quantitatively, but its major application is in qualitative analysis to identify the functional groups such as amino, carboxylic, aldehyde, etc. from organic compounds. The UV radiation and the visible radiation being more energetic than the IR radiation, cause transition of electrons from one electronic state to the other. This is shown diagrammatically in **Chapter 1** (**Fig. 1.5**). When IR radiation is incident upon a molecule, it causes transition of electrons within the ground electronic state of a molecule, as shown in **Fig. 3.1**. Thus, IR radiation interacts with the substance and brings about transfer of electrons from lower rotational energy level (r) to the higher rotational energy level or from lower vibrational energy level (v) to the higher vibrational energy level, within the ground electronic state (E_o).

3.1. PRINCIPLE BEHIND ABSORPTION OF IR RADIATION

In a molecule, atoms do not remain stationary. Atoms either vibrate along the bond or rotate about a bond. If this vibrational or rotational motion of a pair of atoms in a molecule brings about net change in dipole moment, then it produces an alternating electric field. For example, in a hydrogen chloride molecule, a pair of electrons in a covalent bond between hydrogen and chlorine atoms is dragged more by an electronegative chlorine atom. Hence, the chlorine atom gains partial negative charge (δ-) and the hydrogen atom gains partial positive charge (δ+). This results in the formation of a dipole (two poles – one positive and another negative) and the molecule is said to be polar.

$$\overset{\delta+}{H} : \overset{\delta-}{Cl}$$

Thus, hydrogen chloride molecule possesses significant dipole moment. The magnitude of the dipole moment depends on the magnitude of charges on two atoms bound together and the distance between the centers of two charges. When atoms vibrate along a bond or rotate about a bond, regular fluctuations in the dipole moment occur. This fluctuating dipole moment produces an electric field which propagates in the form of waves. The frequency of these waves is equal to the natural frequency of vibration or rotation of atoms in a molecule. When IR radiation is incident upon a substance, only that radiation, whose frequency exactly matches with the natural vibrational or rotational frequency of a particular bond in a molecule, is able to interact with the molecule, i.e. a net transfer of energy from radiation to the molecule occurs resulting in a change in the amplitude of the molecular vibrations or rotations. Thus, molecule absorbs this radiation and produces a peak in its IR spectrum.

In homonuclear molecules like O_2, N_2 or Cl_2, molecules are not polar in nature, because both the atoms constituting these molecules drag electrons to the same extent towards them and hence, do not possess partial charges. Thus, they are not associated with any change in the dipole moment during the vibration or rotation. Such compounds do not produce their own electric field and hence, are not able to interact with IR radiation. Therefore, these compounds do not produce any peaks in IR spectrum and are called as IR inactive or IR transparent molecules.

O=O	N≡N	Cl—Cl
Oxygen	Nitrogen	Chlorine

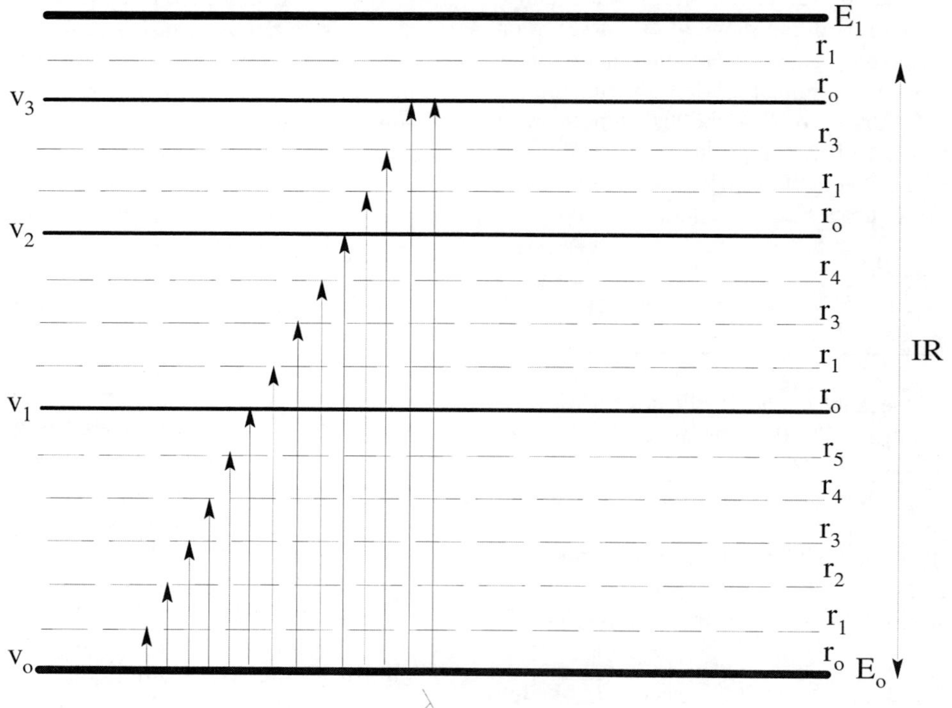

Fig. 3.1: Electronic, vibrational and rotational transitions in a molecule

3.1.1. Rotational Transitions

In a molecule, different atoms rotate about different bonds with different rotational frequencies, which depend on the masses of the two bonded atoms. When a molecule absorbs IR radiation, rotational frequency of a particular bond increases and electron is transferred from lower rotational energy level to the higher rotational energy level. The rotational transitions, which can be brought about by radiation of 100 μm or greater (far IR region), require low energy. This low energy can easily be lost to the adjacent molecules when they collide with each other. In liquids and solids, molecules are very close to each other and inter-molecular collisions occur frequently. Moreover, in liquids and solids, due to the availability of the limited space, rotation is highly restricted. Because of these factors, liquids and solids do not produce distinct peaks in this region of IR spectrum. Hence, this region is not used for their identification.

In gases, molecules remain far from each other and the inter-molecular collisions are rare. Because gaseous molecules are not closely spaced, atoms in gases can undergo rotation very easily. Hence, absorption by gases in this far IR region is characterized by discrete, well defined lines. This region of IR radiation is therefore, commonly used for the identification of gases.

3.1.2. Vibrational-Rotational Transitions

A molecule contains a number of bonds. All the atoms vibrate along a bond. Each bond in a molecule is therefore, associated with a definite vibrational frequency. With the absorption of IR radiation of appropriate energy, the vibrational frequency increases and electron gets transferred from one vibrational energy level to the other. Each vibrational energy level has several rotational energy states. Hence, vibrational transitions do involve rotational transitions as well. Therefore, these transitions are known as vibrational–rotational transitions. The amount of energy required for the vibrational–rotational transitions is more compared to that required only for the rotational transitions. This energy is supplied by the IR radiation, which falls in the range of 0.75-15 μm. In gases, molecules are apart from each other and atoms undergo rotation as well as vibrations freely. This results in the production of a series of closely spaced lines or a band spectrum, in this region. Therefore, this region is not suitable for the identification of gases. In liquids and solids on the other hand, rotation is highly restricted. Thus, peaks corresponding to the vibrational transitions only can be seen and vibrational-rotational transitions are not seen in their spectra. Hence, for the identification of solutions, liquids and solids, this range of IR spectrum is used.

3.2. MOLECULAR VIBRATIONS

In a molecule, atoms are not stationary but fluctuate continuously due to different types of vibrations. These vibrations are of two types.

3.2.1. Stretching vibrations
3.2.2. Bending vibrations

3.2.1. Stretching Vibrations

These vibrations involve a continuous change in the inter-atomic distance along the axis of a bond between two atoms. Stretching vibrations are of two types.

3.2 1.1. Symmetric stretching
3.2 1.2. Asymmetric stretching

3.2.1.1. Symmetric Stretching

Consider a tri-atomic molecule as shown in **Fig. 3.2**. In the symmetric stretching vibrations, as shown in **Fig. 3.2(a)**, two atoms bonded to a central atom, move away from the central atom simultaneously at one moment. The next moment, both the atoms move towards the central atom simultaneously. Thus, two bonds are stretched or compressed simultaneously, at one particular moment.

3.2.1.2. Asymmetric Stretching

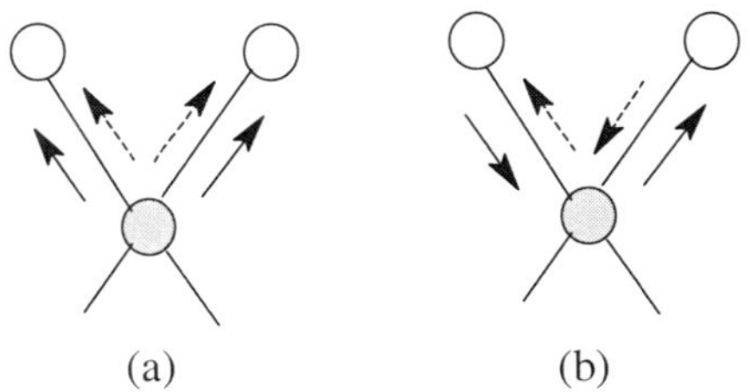

Fig. 3.2: Stretching vibrations

In the asymmetric stretching vibrations, as shown in **Fig. 3.2(b)**, out of two atoms bonded to a central atom, one atom moves away from the central atom, whereas another atom moves towards it and vice versa. Thus, at one particular moment, one bond is stretched and another bond is compressed.

3.2.2. Bending Vibrations

Bending vibrations are characterized by a continuous change in the angle between two bonds. These vibrations are of two types.

3.2.2.1. In-plane vibrations

3.2.2.2. Out-of-plane vibrations

These vibrations can also be explained with the help of a tri-atomic molecule.

3.2.2.1. In-plane vibrations

In these vibrations, all the three atoms of a triatomic molecule remain in the same plane even when bending of two bonds occurs. These vibrations are of two types.

1) Rocking
2) Scissoring

1) Rocking

As shown in **Fig. 3.3(a)**, in case of in-plane rocking vibrations, two bonds bend to the right simultaneously, at one moment and the next moment, they bend to the left simultaneously. This bending occurs in the same plane.

2) Scissoring

In case of in-plane scissoring, as shown in **Fig. 3.3(b)**, the movement of two bonds is similar to the movement of two blades of a scissor. Both the atoms come closer to each other at one moment and move away from each other, the next moment.

3.2.2.2. Out-of-plane vibrations

In these vibrations, the atoms which are in one plane initially, enter into different planes while bending. These vibrations are of two types.

1) Wagging
2) Twisting

1) Wagging

Wagging is similar to rocking but in rocking all the three atoms in a triatomic molecule remain in the same plane, while in wagging, the two bonded atoms leave the original plane. At one moment, both the bonded atoms go in front of the original plane and the next moment, both the atoms go behind the original plane. In **Fig. 3.4(a)**, the negative sign shows the original plane of the atoms and the positive sign indicates the plane in front or behind the original plane.

2) Twisting

In case of twisting vibrations, as shown in **Fig. 3.4(b)**, the central atom is in one plane, which is shown without any sign. The two bonded atoms bend the bonds in such a way that one atom enters the plane indicated by the positive sign and is in front of the original plane while another atom enters the plane indicated by the negative sign and is behind the original plane. This is similar to a twisting action and hence, the vibrations are referred to as the twisting vibrations.

Each vibration can produce a peak in the IR region. In a diatomic or a triatomic molecule, one

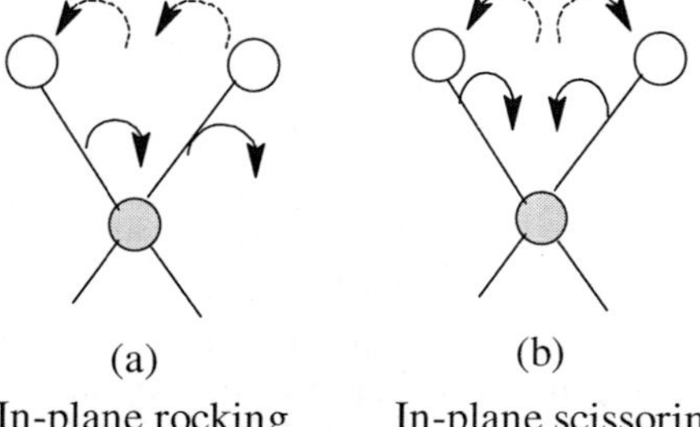

Fig. 3.3: In-plane vibrations

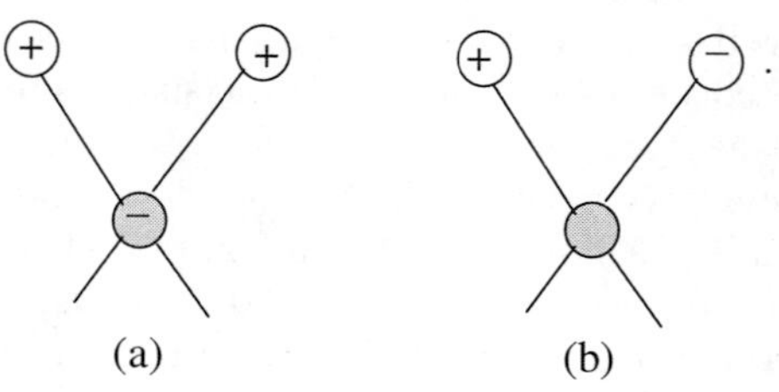

Fig. 3.4: Out-of-plane vibrations

can define the number and nature of such vibrations and can relate these to energies of absorption and correspondingly to the position of peaks in the spectrum. In case of polyatomic molecules, the number of vibrations is more. In addition, in polyatomic molecules, some more peaks are obtained because of the interaction among several atoms. Thus, apart from the peaks due to the individual vibrations, the interacting vibrations produce peaks in the spectrum and make it more complex.

3.3. INSTRUMENTATION

An IR spectrometer consists of the following components.

3.3.1. A source for IR radiation
3.3.2. A wavelength selector
3.3.3. A sample holder
3.3.4. A detector
3.3.5. A recorder

3.3.1. Sources for IR Radiation

For near IR region, the sources which are commonly used for UV-visible region are made use of. Hydrogen lamp, deuterium lamp, xenon arc or tungsten filament can produce radiation in the near IR region also.

For middle IR region, any inert solid heated to about 1500 to 2000 °K can be used. The following are the sources which are used commonly for the middle IR spectrometry.

3.3.1.1. The Nernst Glower

The Nernst glower consists of a cylinder of rare earth oxides, i.e. oxides of cerium, zirconium, thorium, yttrium, etc. As shown in **Fig. 3.5**, the cylinder is about 20 mm in length and 1-2 mm in diameter. The platinum leads are embedded at two ends of this cylinder for the passage of current.

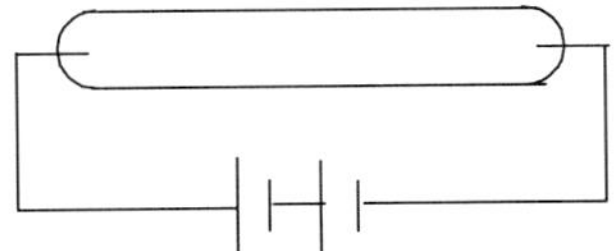

Fig. 3.5: The Nernst glower

When sufficient amount of current is allowed to flow through the cylinder, it gets heated up and produces radiation in the IR region.

The characteristic of the rare earth oxides is that they have a large negative temperature coefficient of electrical resistance. Hence, initially, when the temperature of the cylinder is low, it offers high resistance to the flow of current through it. This necessitates the initial external heating of the cylinder to dull red heat. When the temperature of the cylinder is increased sufficiently, its resistance to the flow of current is reduced. Thereafter, it allows conduction of current through it, which leads to further increase in the temperature. At temperature between 1500 and 2000 °K, the cylinder starts emission of IR radiation. With the increase in the temperature of the cylinder, its resistance is reduced considerably and a large amount of current flows through it. This excessive current can destroy the source. In order to avoid destruction of the source, the source circuit must be designed to limit the current.

3.3.1.2. The Globar Source

Like Nernst glower, the Globar source is also made up of a cylinder, but the material of construction is silicon carbide. The cylinder is 50 mm in length and 5 mm in diameter. The platinum wires embedded at two ends of the cylinder allow electrical heating of the cylinder.

Unlike the Nernst glower, this device has positive temperature coefficient of electrical resistance. Initially, when the temperature of the cylinder is low, its resistance is also low. Hence, in the beginning, it allows easy passage of current through it. With the passage of more and more current through the cylinder, its temperature increases considerably and the cylinder emits IR radiation. With the increase in the temperature of the cylinder, however, its resistance increases. This restricts the passage of excessive current that can flow through it and automatically protects the device. Sometimes, water cooling of electrical contacts is recommended to avoid arcing.

Spectral intensities of the Nernst glower and the Globar source are comparable but the

Globar source provides more intense radiation below 5 μm.

3.3.1.3. Incandescent Wire Source

As shown in **Fig. 3.6**, the incandescent wire source consists of a nichrome wire (an alloy of nickel and chromium) or a rhodium (Rh) wire, wound spirally on some inert material like a ceramic cylinder. When sufficient current is passed through the wire, it emits radiation in the IR region. It produces IR radiation of lower intensity as compared to those produced by the Globar source or by the Nernst glower, but this source lasts longer in their comparison.

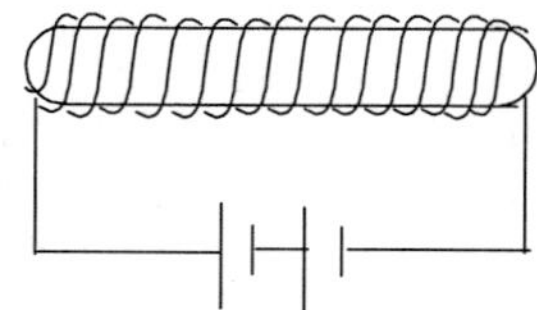

Fig. 3.6: Incandescent wire source

3.3.2. Wavelength Selectors

Like monochromators in the UV region, monochromators used in the IR region also consist of the following components.

1) An entrance slit
2) A dispersing element
3) An exit slit

A dispersing element is either a prism or a grating.

A) Prism as a dispersing element

As shown in **Table 3.1**, the material of construction of a prism used in the IR region varies as per the range of wavelengths required, since no material is transparent to IR radiation throughout its entire range.

(i) Quartz is used in the near IR region of 0.8-3 μm. Beyond 3 μm, quartz absorbs strongly. Lithium fluoride is also useful in the near IR region from 1 to 5 μm.

(ii) In the region between 5 and 15 μm, crystalline sodium chloride prism is used commonly, since it provides greater dispersion in this region. Beyond 20 μm, sodium chloride absorbs strongly and cannot be used.

(iii) Crystalline potassium bromide or cesium bromide prisms are suitable for the IR region between 15 and 40 μm. Except quartz, all other materials being alkali halides, are attacked easily by the moisture in the atmosphere. The condensation of moisture on them can however, be taken care of by using desiccants or heat. The polishing of the "*fogged*" surfaces also helps in getting rid of the problem of moisture condensation.

Table 3.1: Material of construction of prism in different IR regions

Near IR	Middle IR	
0.8-3 μm (Quartz) 1-5 μm (LiF)	5-15 μm (NaCl)	15-45 μm (KBr or CsBr)

B) Grating as a dispersing element

Like UV radiation, the dispersion of IR radiation can be brought about either by the transmission gratings or by the reflection gratings. For isolation of UV-visible radiation, gratings having grooves of the order of 2000-6000 per mm of its length are used, whereas for an IR region, gratings having only 10-100 grooves per mm of its length are used.

Gratings vs. prisms in the IR region

1) Reflection gratings provide better resolution, since there is less loss of the radiant energy than when a prism is used.
2) A grating provides linear dispersion.
3) A grating is resistant to the attack by water, since it is made up of either glass or plastic, coated with aluminium.
4) These three advantages of gratings are associated with one drawback. A grating

produces spectra of different orders because of the greater amount of the scattered radiation. This drawback is however, not a serious one, since the lines due to higher order spectra can be easily removed by using filters or occasionally, the prisms, in conjunction with a grating.

The comparison between the gratings and the prisms is given in the tabular form in **Chapter 2, Table 2.2**.

3.3.3. Sample Holders and Sample Preparation Techniques in IR Spectrometry

The choice of a sample holder used in the IR region depends on the type of sample used for recording the IR spectrum. The IR spectrum of a solution is very rarely recorded. It is very common to record the spectrum of a solid or a liquid in the IR region. This is because suitable solvents that are transparent throughout the entire IR region are not available. Hence, special techniques for preparing samples and special sample holders are required in the IR spectrometry.

3.3.3.1. Gaseous Samples

As shown in **Fig. 3.7**, the sample holder for the gaseous samples or the low boiling, i.e. volatile liquids, is an evacuated cell, which is few centimeters to several meters in length. In order to reduce the length of the cell, several baffles, i.e. the reflecting surfaces, can be introduced inside the cell so that the IR radiation entering the cell undergoes numerous reflections. This provides a longer path length in a compact cell.

3.3.3.2. Pure Liquids or Neat Liquids

It is a common practice to record an IR spectrum of a pure or a *neat* liquid without preparing its solution. The advantage of this method is that it requires hardly a drop of a liquid for recording a spectrum and it also saves the effort in preparing a sample. For recording the spectrum, a drop of a pure or a "*neat*" liquid is squeezed between two rock salt plates so as to get a thickness of 0.01 mm or less. The two plates are held together by a frame. The whole assembly is mounted in the path of IR radiation.

This technique suffers from the drawback that it does not provide reproducible transmittance data and therefore, makes the accurate determination of molar absorptivity difficult though not impossible. None the less, the resulting spectra are usually satisfactory for qualitative purpose.

In case of a poor transmittance by a liquid, it can be dissolved in a suitable solvent so as to prepare its solution. The details of the solvents and the cell used are described under the solid samples (**Section 3.3.3.3**).

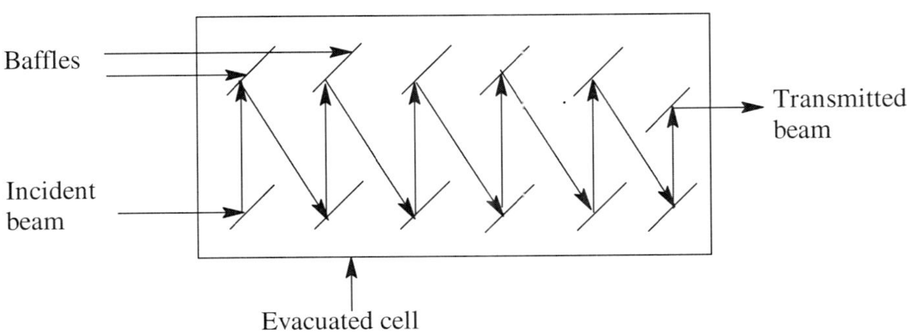

Fig. 3.7: A sample holder for the gaseous sample

3.3.3.3. Solids

The IR spectrum of a solid is recorded by using the following methods.

1) By preparing solution of a solid
2) By using a mull method (Nujol and KBr pellet methods)

1) Infrared analysis by preparing solution of a solid

(i) Solvents

A solution of a solid can be prepared if a suitable solvent which is transparent throughout the IR region is available. This solution can then be filled in cells in order to record its spectrum.

In UV spectrometry, water, methanol or ethanol are commonly used to prepare solutions. In IR spectrometry, these solvents are used very rarely, mainly because of two reasons. The first reason is that these solvents absorb strongly in the middle IR region and the second reason is that they attack alkali metal halides, the most commonly used material of construction of the cell windows.

The choice of solvents in the IR region is limited because no single solvent is transparent throughout the entire middle IR region. The commonly used solvents and their range over which they are transparent to IR radiation are listed in **Table 3.2**.

Solvents like carbon tetrachloride, chloroform, carbon disulfide, dimethylformamide, dioxane, cyclohexane, benzene, etc. can be used in the IR region. A care must be taken to dry all these solvents, since traces of moisture in them can attack alkali halide windows of the cell.

Table 3.2: Infrared solvents and their useful range

Wavelength (μm)	Solvent
2-6	CCl_4
4-8	$CHCl_3$
8-12	CCl_4
8-16	CS_2

(ii) Cells

In the IR spectrometry, the cells used for filling the solution, whose spectrum is to be recorded, possess following characteristics.

(a) Material of construction of the cells is either quartz or glass with sodium chloride window for the passage of IR radiation.
(b) The cells are demountable and the path length can be varied, as per the requirements, with the help of Teflon spacers.
(c) Since most of the solvents absorb IR radiation, a path length of the order of 0.01 to 1 mm is commonly used in IR spectrometry as against 1 cm path length in the UV-visible spectrometry. Thus, IR cells are usually much narrower as compared to those used in the UV-visible spectrometry.
(d) Since the cells are narrow, the solution of an analyte is introduced in the cell by a hypodermic syringe.
(e) The concentration of a sample is in the range of 0.1 to 10 %.
(f) The cells require special maintenance, since the sodium chloride windows absorb moisture from atmosphere and their surface becomes "*fogged*". The original surface can be recovered back by polishing the fogged surface with *buffing powder*.

2) Infrared analysis by a mull method

A *mull* is a two phase mixture, e.g. a mixture of a solid and a liquid or a mixture of two solids. If the solid to be analyzed is not soluble in an IR transparent solvent, then the solid is dispersed in a liquid to prepare a semi-solid mass called mull.

(i) Preparation of a mull using Nujol

Around 2-5 mg of the solid to be analyzed is finely ground. The particle size of the suspended solid should be smaller than 2 μm or smaller than the wavelength of the IR radiation (2.5 – 50 μm) incident on it. If this condition is not satisfied, then the considerable amount of radiation is lost due to scattering. The sample is further ground in the presence of one to two drops of heavy hydrocarbon oil, *nujol*. Hydrocarbons produce peaks around 3000 cm^{-1} in their IR spectrum. If a substance to be analyzed by IR spectrometry, i.e. an analyte, also produces peaks in the same area, then the hydrocarbon, nujol, is replaced by another liquid, *fluorolube*, which is a halogenated polymer. A semi-solid mass thus obtained is referred to as *mull*. Mull is then squeezed between two rock salt plates so as to get a thin film. The whole assembly is mounted on a holder and a spectrum is recorded.

The care should be taken to prepare a mull, which can provide transmittance of more than 50 %. This produces sharp peaks in the IR spectra.

(ii) Preparation of a potassium bromide (KBr) pellet

In the nujol method, a mull is prepared by mixing a solid and a liquid. In the KBr pellet method, a mull is prepared by dispersing one solid into another solid, i.e. by dispersing an analyte in dried potassium bromide powder.

One milligram or less, of the analyte, is finely ground using a small agate mortar and pestle. It is intimately mixed with about 100 mg of dried potassium bromide powder. This mixture is then filled in a special stainless steel die. When the pressure of about 10,000 to 15,000 pounds per square inch is applied to this die, a transparent disk or a mull or a pellet is formed due to the presence of a directly compressible material, potassium bromide. In order to remove any entrapped air or entrapped moisture from the pellet, vacuum can be applied. This helps in providing better results. The disk is removed from a die and mounted on a holder which can be held in the path of IR radiation in the instrument. If care is not taken to remove moisture from the pellet, the absorbed moisture produces peaks at around 3500 and 1640 cm^{-1}, corresponding to O-H stretching and bending, respectively.

3.3.4. Detectors

All the detectors used in the IR spectrometry make use of the capacity of IR radiation to produce heat. More energetic radiation is able to produce more heat and vice versa. This heat can be converted to some electric parameters for the measurement purpose. The element which absorbs heat produced by the IR radiation should neither absorb heat from any other external sources or environment nor dissipate its heat to the surrounding. Hence, this element is encapsulated or shielded from the surrounding environment. In order to increase the capacity of this element to absorb heat supplied by the IR radiation as completely as possible, it is fabricated in the form of a number of small sized and thin fragments or wires. The following detectors are commonly used in the IR spectrometry.

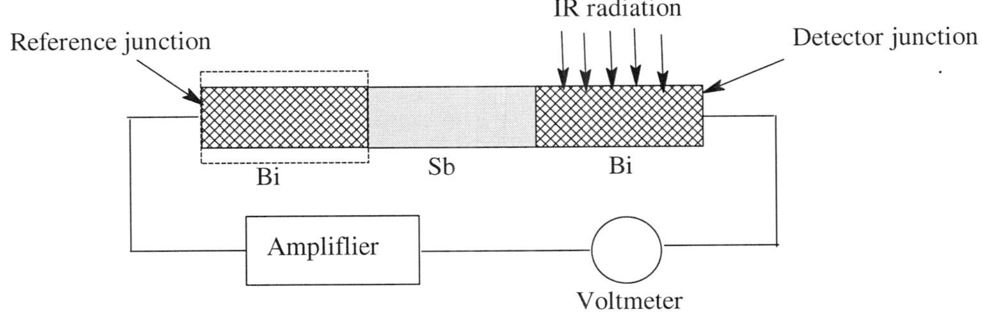

Fig. 3.8: A thermocouple

3.3.4.1. Thermocouples

A thermocouple consists of a pair of junctions. As shown in **Fig. 3.8,** two junctions are formed by connecting two pieces of a similar metal like bismuth (Bi) to either ends of a dissimilar metal such as antimony (Sb) or a semi-conducting alloy. One junction is used as a *reference junction* and another junction is used as a *detector junction.* A potential difference is developed across the two junctions depending on the difference between their temperatures.

1) A reference junction

Temperature of a reference junction need not be kept constant since the difference between the temperatures of the junctions is required to determine the intensity of a signal. Still, most of the times, to get the accurately measurable difference between the temperatures of the two junctions, the temperature of the reference junction is kept more or less constant by cooling it in ice. The greater the difference in the temperatures of the two junctions, the higher is the sensitivity of the method and the higher is the accuracy of the measurement. The reference junction has relatively large heat capacity, i.e. a large amount of heat is associated with the minute change in the temperature of the reference junction. In order to protect or shield the reference junction against the radiation incident on the detector junction, it is housed in an insulating chamber.

2) A detector junction

A detector junction or the junction for detecting intensity of IR radiation transmitted after the interaction with an analyte should be designed so as to have complete absorption of heat from the IR radiation incident on it. Hence, special care is taken to design this junction from very fine wires of metals such as platinum, silver, antimony or bismuth. Fine wires increase the surface area of the junction and help in complete absorption of heat from the IR radiation. It can also be formed by depositing a thin layer of metal on a non conducting material. Since black bodies absorb the heat maximum, the junction is blackened. All these factors improve heat absorption capacity of the junction. The detector junction is designed so as to have a small heat capacity which enables the recording of minute changes in the temperature with small changes in the heat supplied to it by the incident IR radiation. The detector junction is sealed in an evacuated chamber having IR transparent window.

An efficient thermocouple detector can produce sufficiently large signal for a temperature as low as 10^{-6} °K. Several thermocouples can be connected in series in order to enhance the sensitivity of the measurement. The detector in such a case is referred to as a *thermopile.*

3.3.4.2. A Bolometer

A bolometer, shown in **Fig. 3.9**, makes use of a material whose resistance changes with the change in its temperature. The change in the resistance of the material allows different magnitudes of current to pass through it. Hence, a bolometer is also called as a *resistance thermometer.*

A responsive element of this thermometer is made up of strips of metals like platinum or nickel or of a semiconductor. When a semiconductor is used in the detector, the device is called as a *thermister.* The responsive element is purposely made smaller

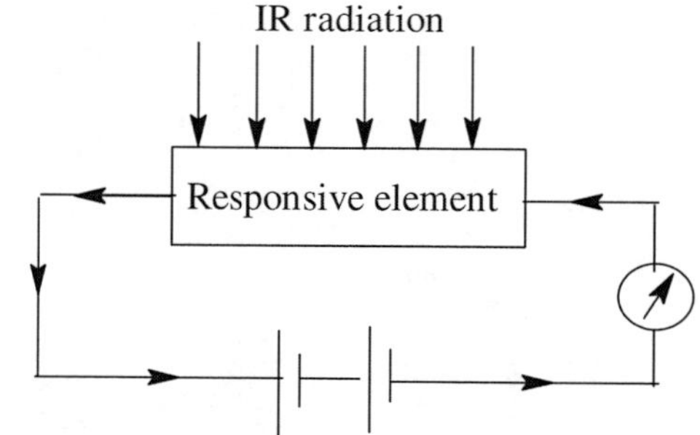

Fig. 3.9: A bolometer

in size and is blackened. This helps in the complete absorption of heat provided by the IR radiation. When heat is absorbed by the responsive element, its temperature changes, which in turn results in the change in its resistance and consequently, in the change in the magnitude of current flowing through it. The greater the current passing through it, the greater is the response produced by the detector.

A bolometer is not very extensively used as an IR detector because of limited sensitivity towards the measurement of intensity of IR radiation.

3.3.4.3. A Golay Cell

A Golay cell, shown in **Fig. 3.10**, is also called as a *gas thermometer*. It consists of a cylindrical chamber, filled with xenon gas. Walls of this chamber are blackened for the complete absorption of heat supplied by the IR radiation incident on it. One end of this cylinder is fitted with an IR transparent window. Another end contains a flexible diaphragm which is silvered from outside. The chamber also contains a phototube.

When the IR radiation enters this chamber, the blackened walls absorb heat provided by the radiation. This in turn heats the xenon gas inside the chamber. The xenon gas expands and exerts pressure on the flexible diaphragm. The curvature of the diaphragm depends on the increase in the temperature of the xenon gas, which in turn depends on the heat absorbed by it, which further

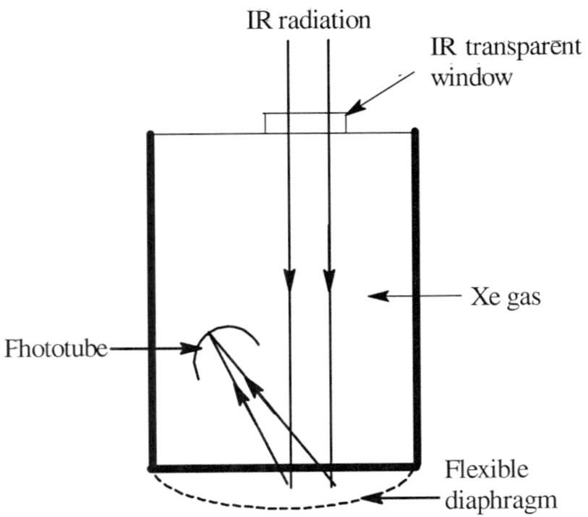

Fig. 3.10: A Golay cell

depends on the intensity of the incident IR radiation. When the IR radiation falls on the silvered diaphragm, they reflect back in the chamber and fall on the photosensitive surface of a phototube. Depending on the curvature of the flexible diaphragm, a definite fraction of the reflected beam strikes the active surface of a phototube. This leads to a change in the photocurrent, which can be related to the power of IR radiation. A Golay cell finds its special use

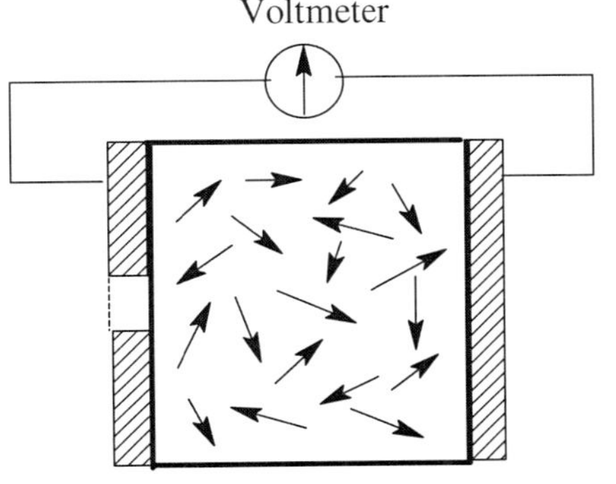

(a) Randomly oriented dipoles
(At room temperature)

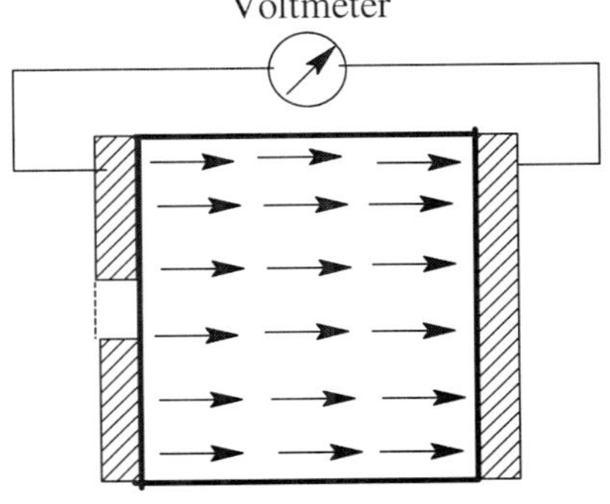

(b) Aligned dipoles
(Above room temperature & below Curie temperature)

Fig. 3.11: A pyroelectric detector

above 50 μm, i.e. in the far IR region, where radiation is less energetic. In the near and the mid IR regions, its sensitivity is comparable with the other less expensive heat detectors.

3.3.4.4. Pyroelectric Detectors

Pyroelectric substances are the dielectric materials having special thermal and electrical properties. Certain crystals such as lithium tantalate, barium titanate and triglycine sulfate possess pyroelectric property, i.e. they produce temperature sensitive dipole moments. To construct a pyroelectric detector, a pyroelectric substance is placed between two electrodes, one of which has an IR transparent window. Two electrodes are connected to each other via a voltmeter.

Molecular dipoles in a pyroelectric substance are randomly oriented at room temperature, as shown in **Fig. 3.11(a)**. When the IR radiation falls upon a pyroelectric substance, it absorbs energy from the radiation. This energy is utilized in aligning the molecular dipoles of the pyroelectric substance. The extent of alignment

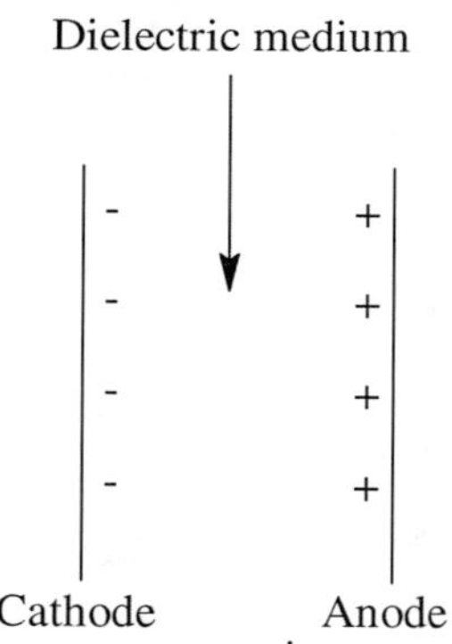

Fig. 3.12: A capacitor or a condenser

depends on the energy of the incident IR radiation. As shown in **Fig. 3.11(b)**, when dipoles are aligned, the two poles in all the molecules are oriented in one direction only. Since this crystal is sandwiched between two electrodes, the alignment of the dipoles results in the deposition of the positive charge on one electrode and the negative charge on another electrode. This charge distribution across the crystal, results in the formation of a capacitor, as shown in **Fig. 3.12**.

When two electrodes are connected, a current starts flowing through the circuit. The magnitude of this current depends on the extent of orientation of dipoles, which in turn depends on the amount of heat supplied by the IR radiation.

Thus, a pyroelectric substance is a temperature-dependent capacitor. It responds fast enough to the changes in its temperature. It loses its polarization or the alignment of dipoles in it when it is heated to a temperature called a *Curie point*. Above Curie point, a pyroelectric substance does not behave as a capacitor and cannot be used for the detection. For triglycine sulphate, the Curie point is 47 °C.

3.3.4.5. Photo-conductivity Detectors or Semi-conductor Detectors

The photo-conducting detectors consist of a semi-conducting material such as lead sulfide, cadmium telluride, indium antimonide or germanium doped with traces of copper or mercury, deposited on a non-conducting material like glass. The whole assembly is enclosed in an evacuated chamber. With the absorption of the IR radiation, the non-conducting valence electrons are promoted to higher energy levels, where they become conducting. Thus, an electrical resistance of a semiconductor is reduced. This change in the resistance depends on the energy of IR radiation incident on the detector. The change in the resistance produces voltage difference or current in the circuit, which can be measured to find the power of IR radiation incident on the detector.

For the near IR region in the range of 1 to 3 μm, lead sulfide is the semiconductor of choice, whereas for the mid and the far IR regions, mercury or cadmium telluride can be used as a semi-conducting material. Thus, though this detector is the fast responding and the most sensitive detector among all others, it can be used only over a limited range of wavelengths.

3.4. FOURIER TRANSFORM INFRARED (FT-IR) SPECTROMETRY

The conventional or the ordinarily used instruments for the IR spectrometry are either the *non-dispersive* instruments, which make use of a series of narrow band filters of the appropriate wavelengths or the *dispersive* instruments, which make use of monochromators like prisms or gratings.

The non-dispersive instruments are usually used for the quantitative analysis of alkali metals by exposing the sample to an appropriate wavelength by choosing appropriate filters sequentially. These instruments are simple to operate, cheaply available, give good signal to noise ratio, but do not provide important spectral details over a wide range of wavelengths, which are particularly important for the qualitative analysis and the structure elucidation.

The conventional spectrometry is termed as *frequency domain spectrometry* because the changes in the radiant power are recorded with the changes in the frequencies, whereas the Fourier Transform (FT) spectrometry is termed as *time domain spectrometry* because the changes in the radiant power are recorded with the changes in time. Time domain spectrum of a source consists of several wavelengths reaching the detector simultaneously.

In the dispersive instruments, rotation of a dispersive element makes available sequentially, all the wavelengths in the region of interest. The speed of the motion of the dispersive element decides the time required for completing the scan. In this method, since the sample is exposed to all the wavelengths sequentially, much time is wasted in scanning spectral regions that contain little or no information. Hence, analysis becomes time consuming.

The FT instruments are the special instruments, which make use of multiple detectors or channels to obtain information about different parts or elements of the spectrum simultaneously.

3.4.1. Advantages of Fourier Transform Instruments

1) The FT instruments provide very high signal-to-noise ratio (S/N) because of two reasons. The first reason is that they provide extremely accurate and precise wavelengths for analysis. Secondly, these instruments have few optical components and no slits to attenuate radiation. Both these factors allow the greater power of the radiation to reach the sample. The higher signal-to-noise ratio provided by these instruments helps in isolating weak peaks from noise.
2) The most important advantage of FT instruments is that all the elements of the source reach the detector simultaneously. This makes possible the recording of a spectrum in a small time period (0.5 – 1 sec).

The time domain spectra cannot be generated by using radiation of the frequency range that is associated with the optical spectrometry (10^{12} to 10^{15} Hz). This is because the transducers that can respond to the power variations at these enormous frequencies are not available. A typical transducer does not produce periodic variation in frequencies but yields a signal that corresponds to the average power of a high

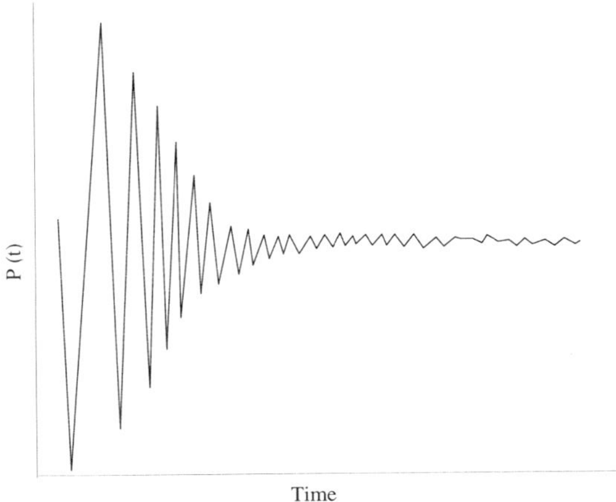

Fig. 3.13: A time domain spectrum of a source made up of several wavelengths

frequency. A time domain spectrum of a source made up of several wavelengths is shown in **Fig. 3.13**.

To obtain time domain spectrum, as shown in **Fig. 3.13**, one has to convert a high frequency signal to a signal which is measurable, in such a way that these modified frequencies are directly proportional to those in the original signal. This conversion of a high frequency to a measurable frequency is termed as *modulation*. A number of methods can be used for signal modulation. The Michelson interferometer is very commonly used for this purpose in the optical region.

3.4.2. A Michelson Interferometer

Michelson interferometer consists of the following components.

1) A source of IR radiation
2) A beam splitter
3) A fixed mirror
4) A movable mirror

As shown in **Fig. 3.14**, a collimated beam of radiation coming out from the source, when falls on a beam splitter, splits into two beams. One beam falls on the fixed mirror, which is kept at a distance F from the center of the beam splitter. Another beam falls on a movable mirror, which is kept perpendicular to the fixed mirror. The movable mirror moves horizontally through a definite distance every time. Two beams reaching a fixed mirror and a movable mirror get reflected back on the beam splitter. Half of each reflected beam is now directed towards the sample and the detector

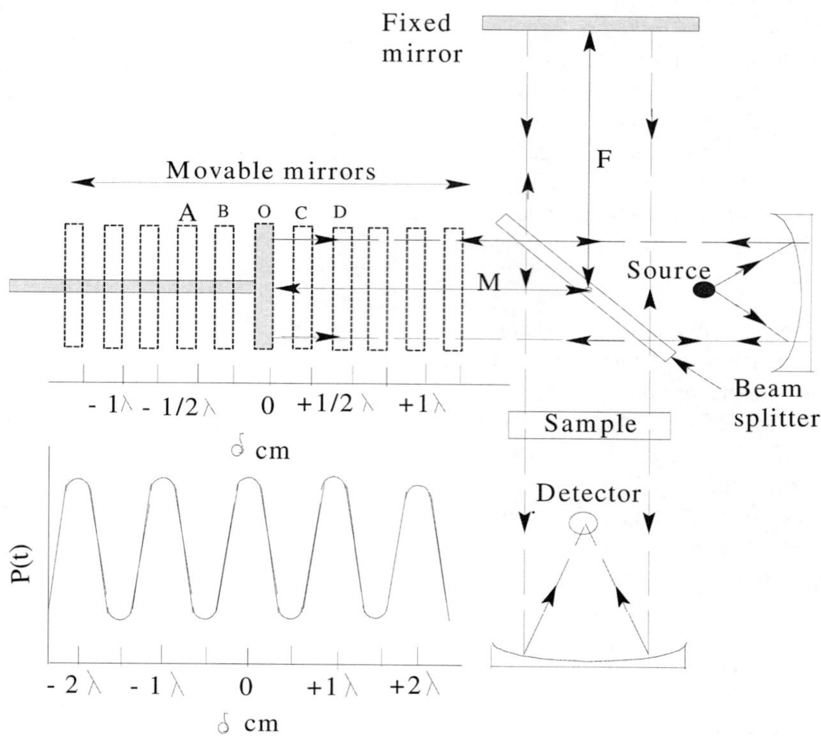

Fig. 3.15: An interferogram

Fig. 3.14: A Michelson interferometer

and another half of both the beams is directed towards the source. The two halves reaching the detector are used for the analysis of a sample.

In **Fig. 3.14**, F is the distance of the fixed mirror from the centre of the beam splitter and M is the distance of the movable mirror from the centre of the beam splitter. The difference in the path lengths for the two beams is (2M - 2F) and is referred to as the *retardation* (δ, delta, Gr.).

When the two mirrors are equidistant from the beam splitter, M = F (position O in **Fig. 3.14**) and the path difference (2M - 2F) between the two beams is zero. Under this situation, both the reflected beams would be in phase. Hence, these two beams would undergo constructive interference and would provide the beam of maximum power.

If the movable mirror is moved through a distance + λ/4 or - λ/4, i.e. towards or away from the beam splitter (positions C and B, respectively, in **Fig. 3.14**), for a reflected beam, this distance would become + λ/2 or - λ/2. Thus, for a distance M = F + λ/4, the distance 2M = 2F + λ/2. Hence, the path difference (2M – 2F) would be equal to λ/2 and hence, the two beams would be out-of-phase. Thus, these two beams would undergo destructive interference and would provide the beam of zero power.

If the mirror is further moved by a distance + λ/2 or -λ/2 (positions D and A, respectively, in **Fig. 3.14**), then the path difference between the beams would become equal to λ and once again the beams would undergo constructive interference and would produce a beam of maximum power.

When the output power P(t) from the detector is plotted against the path difference (2M – 2F) or retardation (δ), the cosine curve, as shown in **Fig. 3.15**, is obtained. This plot, in general, is called an *interferogram*.

Once the radiation comes out of the Michelson interferometer, its frequency is reduced. The relation between the two frequencies, before striking the interferometer and after coming out of the interferometer, can be deduced as follows. As shown in **Fig. 3.15**, one cycle of the signal occurs when the mirror is moved through a distance λ/2. If the mirror is moving with a velocity V_M and if it takes time T to move through this distance, then **equation (3.1)** can be derived as follows.

$$\text{Velocity} = \text{Distance/Time}$$

$$V_M = \lambda/2 \ / \ T$$

$$T\ V_M = \lambda/2$$

$$\text{Frequency, } f = 1/T$$

$$\text{Hence, } f = 1/T = V_M \ / \ \lambda/2$$

$$f = 2\ V_M \ / \ \lambda$$

$$\text{Since } \lambda = c \ / \ í$$

$$f = (2\ V_M\ í) \ / \ c \ .... (3.1)$$

where, ν is the frequency of radiation entering an interferometer, which is also called as an *optical frequency*, 'f' is the frequency of radiation coming out of an interferometer, which is also called as an *interferometer frequency* or *modulated frequency*, V_M is the velocity of the mirror and 'c' is the velocity of light (3×10^{10} cm/sec).

If velocity of the mirror is 0.2 cm/sec, then for IR radiation of (1.9×10^{13} Hz) the modulated frequency can be calculated by using **equation (3.1)** as follows.

$$2\ V_M \ / \ c = f \ / \ \nu$$

$$\text{Therefore, } f = (2\ V_M \ / \ c) \times \nu$$
$$f = (2 \times 0.2 \ / \ 3\times 10^{10}) \times 1.9 \times 10^{13}$$

$$f = 0.1333 \times 10^{-10} \times 1.9 \times 10^{13}$$

$$\therefore f = 253 \text{ Hz}$$

3.4.3. The FT-IR Instruments

In the olden days, the FT-IR spectrometers were very bulky and expensive. Nowadays, these instruments are made very compact and are available at the reasonable cost. Hence, these instruments are slowly replacing the dispersive instruments.

3.4.3.1. Components of the FT-IR Spectrometers

The FT-IR spectrometers are usually single beam spectrometers. Most of the FT-IR spectrometers work based on the principle of Michelson interferometer. Various components of the FT-IR spectrometer are as given below.

1) A drive mechanism

For recording a good FT-IR spectrum, it is absolutely essential to have very precise movement of the movable mirror. The fine, accurate and a constant movement of this mirror is achieved by means of a motor-driven micrometer screw, especially in the far IR region (50 -1000 ìm or 200 - 10 cm^{-1}). For achieving more precise movement of the mirror, the mirror mount is floated on the air cushions, held within the close-fitting stainless steel sleeves. The mount is connected to an electromagnetic coil. Increasing current in this coil, brings about a constant, accurate and precise movement of the mirror. This ultimately helps in producing a good interferogram and subsequently, a good spectrum.

The movement of mirror should occur at regular retardation intervals. Also, mirror should be occupying the point of zero retardation in order to permit signal averaging. If this point is not known precisely, the signals in the consecutive sweeps would not be fully in phase. In order to achieve precise signal sampling and signal averaging, three interferometers are arranged on the same mirror mount.

2) A beam splitter

A beam splitter splits the beam into two. Both these beams should be of equal intensity. This can happen only if the proper material of construction with appropriate refractive index is selected, which allows 50 % radiation to get reflected and 50 % radiation to get transmitted. The materials which satisfy this requirement are mentioned in **Table 3.3**.

3) Sources

The sources used in the FT-IR spectrometers are the same as the sources used for the conventional IR spectrometry.

4) Detectors

The FT-IR spectrometers require more sensitive and fast responding detectors compared to the conventional IR spectrometry. Hence, the FT-IR spectrometers make use of pyroelectric detectors having triglycine sulphate. The slow responding and less sensitive thermal detectors do not find place in the FT-IR spectrometry.

Table 3.3: Material of construction of a beam splitter in various IR regions

Sr. No.	IR Region	Material of construction of a beam splitter
1	Far IR	Thin film of Mylar, sandwiched between two plates of a low refractive index solid
2	Middle IR	Thin films of germanium or silicon deposited on cesium iodide or bromide, sodium chloride or potassium bromide
3	Near IR	A film of ferric oxide deposited on calcium fluoride

3.5. APPLICATIONS OF IR SPECTROMETRY

The IR spectrometry is mainly used qualitatively in order to find the presence or the absence of certain functional groups. Unlike the UV-visible spectrometry, its quantitative application is very limited.

3.5.1. Qualitative Applications of IR Spectrometry

For identification of organic compounds, spectra are recorded in the mid IR region, the commonly used region being 2 to 15 μm (5000-600 cm^{-1}). Unlike an UV spectrum, an IR spectrum contains a large number of peaks. In order to identify an organic compound, only certain peaks or certain group frequencies in the IR spectrum are observed. An approximate frequency at which the organic functional groups such as –OH, -NH_2, C=O, NO_2, etc. absorb IR radiation can be calculated from the masses of the atoms and the force constant of a bond between them. **Equation (3.2)**, used to calculate a wavenumber (or group frequencies) associated with a particular bond, is as given below.

$$\sigma = 2\ \pi\ c\ [\ (k/\ \mu)\ ]\ ^{1/2}$$

$$= 1/\ 2\ \pi\ c\ [(k\ (m_1 + m_2)\ /\ m_1\ m_2]\ ^{1/2} \quad ...(3.2)$$

where, σ = wavenumber of an absorption peak,

c = velocity of light,

k = force constant, and

m_1 and m_2 = masses of two atoms bonded together.

These calculated wavenumbers are not absolutely constant for a particular functional group because to some extent they also depend on the rest of the structure of a molecule. Since the remaining structure of a molecule affects these group frequencies to a lesser extent, a range of frequencies is assigned to a particular functional group. If a peak is obtained in that region, then it is more probable to have that functional group in a molecule.

The group frequencies for various functional groups, which are calculated by using **equation (3.2)**, are summarized in charts known as *correlation charts*. In the literature, many correlation charts are available. These may show minor variation in different group frequencies but still all these correlation charts enable us to guess the presence or the absence of the functional groups in a molecule. It is very common to describe position of a peak in the IR spectrum of a molecule in terms of wavenumbers instead of wavelengths. Wavenumber is the reciprocal of the wavelength. Hence, a region of 2 to 15 μm is described as a region of 5000 cm^{-1} to 670 cm^{-1}. The value of a wavenumber (in cm^{-1}) corresponding to a wavelength of 2 μm is calculated as follows.

1 cm =10 mm

1mm=10^3 μm

Therefore, $\lambda = 2\ \mu m = (2 \times 10^{-3})$ mm

$= (2 \times 10^{-4})$ cm

Wavenumber $= 1/\lambda = [1/\ (2 \times 10^{-4})]\ cm^{-1}$

$= [10^4\ /\ 2]\ cm^{-1}$

$= 10{,}000\ /\ 2\ cm^{-1}$

$= 5{,}000\ cm^{-1}$

Similarly, λ =15 μm is equal to 666 cm^{-1}

or approximately equal to 670 cm^{-1}.

The shorter the wavelength, the more energetic it is. Hence, the IR radiation of 2 μm (5000 cm^{-1}) is more energetic than the IR radiation of 15 μm (670 cm^{-1}). In an IR spectrum of a molecule, the more energetic radiation corresponds to the stretching vibrations of bonds and the less energetic radiation corresponds to the bending vibrations of bonds.

For simplicity, the mid IR region is divided into four parts.

1) A hydrogen stretching region [3700 cm^{-1}-2700 cm^{-1}]

In this region, the peaks are obtained due to stretching of a bond between the hydrogen atom and another atom bonded to it. The stretching of a bond is mainly by the hydrogen atom since it is the lighter of the two atoms and hence, the absorption is not appreciably affected by the rest of the molecule. Secondly, the hydrogen stretching frequency is much higher than that for the other chemical bonds and hence, no interaction of this vibration is observed with other vibrations.

The major stretching vibrations and consequently, the functional groups, which can be identified in this region, are as follows.

A) O-H stretching

(i) Alcohols and phenols

Monomeric alcohols and phenols produce peaks corresponding to the stretching of the bond between the oxygen atom and the hydrogen atom (O-H stretching) in the range of 3650 to 3590 cm^{-1}. Hydrogen bonded alcohols and phenols show peaks at lower wavenumbers, i.e. in the range of 3550 to 3450 cm^{-1}. The intermolecular hydrogen bonding in alcohols (R-OH) is shown in **Fig. 3.16(a)**.

The extent of hydrogen bonding increases with the increase in the concentration and also in the presence of a polar solvent. The intermolecular and the intramolecular hydrogen bonding [**Fig. 3.16(b)**] can be differentiated based on the IR spectrometry. The peak for O-H stretching shifts towards the higher wavenumber in case of intermolecular hydrogen bonding, when the solution is diluted with a solvent, whereas there is no change in the peak position for O-H stretching, after dilution, in case of intramolecular hydrogen bonding. This is because dilution is able to break intermolecular hydrogen bonding, but not the intramolecular hydrogen bonding.

(a) (b)

Fig. 3.16: (a) Intermolecular and (b) intramolecular hydrogen bonding

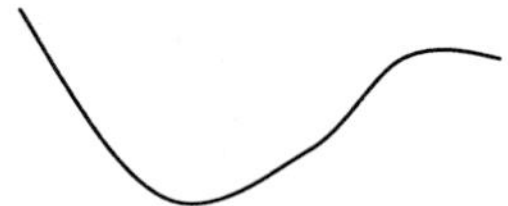

Fig. 3.17: A broad peak for O-H stretching in carboxylic acids in the IR region

(ii) Carboxylic acids

Carboxylic acids show peak corresponding to O-H stretching in the range of 3650 cm^{-1} - 3500 cm^{-1}. The peak is broad and typical in shape, which itself can sometimes suggest the presence of a carboxylic group in a compound. This is shown in **Fig. 3.17**. The O-H bands are often broader than N-H bands and appear only in dilute non-polar solvents.

Fig. 3.18: Dimer of an acid

Acids usually exist in the form of a dimer as shown in **Fig. 3.18**. The hydrogen bonding tends to broaden the peaks and move them towards lower wavenumbers because of the reduction in the vibrational frequency in the presence of hydrogen bonding. The hydrogen bonded carboxylic acids produce peak in the range of 2700-2500 cm^{-1}.

If a sample is not dried properly before recording a spectrum, then also a peak is seen in this region due to O-H stretching in water. This may mislead in elucidating the structure of a molecule. Hence, a sample should be dried properly before recording its IR spectrum.

B) N-H stretching

(i) Primary and secondary amines and amides

As shown in **Fig. 3.19**, the primary amines (R-NH_2) and amides (R-CO-NH_2) produce two peaks corresponding to the symmetric and the asymmetric N-H stretching vibrations, one around 3450 cm^{-1} and another around 3350 cm^{-1}. The secondary amines (R-NH-R') and amides (R-CO-NH-R') produce only one peak at around 3400 cm^{-1}, corresponding to N-H stretching.

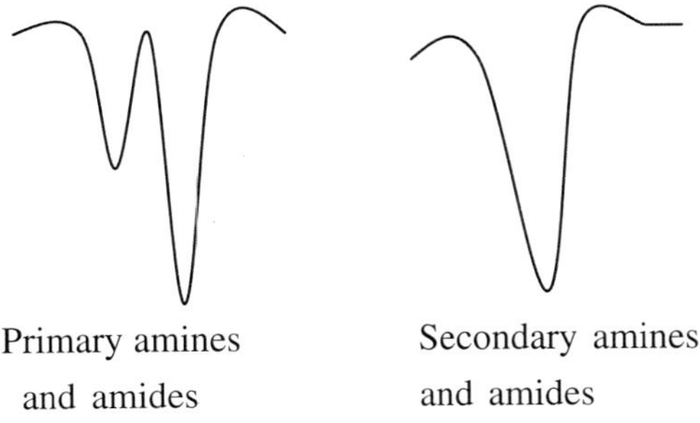

Fig. 3.19: Peaks for N-H stretching in amines and amides in the IR region

C) C-H stretching

(i) **The aliphatic compounds** have a sufficient number of C-H bonds. They show a prominent peak between 3000 and 2850 cm^{-1} due to C-H stretching.

(ii) **An acetylenic C-H bond** ($\equiv$ C—H) is recorded at about 3300 cm^{-1}.

(iii) **An aldehydic C-H stretching** $\left[-\overset{\overset{\large O}{||}}{C}-H \right]$ produces a distinct peak in the range of 2745-2710 cm^{-1}.

If the hydrogen atom in any of the above functional groups is replaced by deuterium, then the peaks shift to the lower wavenumbers because of the reduction in the frequency of vibrations when the heavier deuterium is present in place of a lighter hydrogen atom.

2) A triple bond region [2700-1850 cm^{-1}]

Any peak in this region can confirm the presence of a particular functional group, especially a nitrile group ($C\equiv N$), since a limited number of groups absorb in this region of a spectrum. Nitriles show a very strong peak in the range of 2280-2210 cm^{-1} due to stretching. Alkynes also produce a peak in the range of 2260-2100 due to ($C\equiv C$) stretching, but its intensity may vary. Sometimes, the peak is strong and sometimes, it is medium in the intensity.

Apart from a triple bond stretching, peaks for the S-H stretching ($\approx$ 2600 cm^{-1}), the P-H stretching ($\approx$ 2400 cm^{-1}) and the Si-H stretching ($\approx$ 2200 cm^{-1}), are also seen in this region. These occur less commonly in organic compounds.

3) A double bond region [1850-1550 cm^{-1}]

This is an important region in the IR spectrum, since a number of organic compounds such as ketones, aldehydes, amides, carboxylic acids, esters, anhydrides and so on, get recorded here.

(i) Ketones, amides and aldehydes show C=O stretching at around 1660 cm^{-1}.

(ii) Carboxylic acids show C=O stretching at around 1700 cm^{-1}.

(iii) For esters, acid chlorides and acid anhydrides, C=O stretching is recorded at higher wavenumbers. Esters get recorded at around 1720 cm^{-1}, whereas acid chlorides and acid anhydrides get recorded at still higher wavenumbers corresponding approximately to 1760 cm^{-1}.

Since C=O stretching from various functional groups gets recorded in this region, one cannot determine the type of a carbonyl group that is present in a molecule, solely on the basis of the peak position in this region. However, C=O stretching along with some other characteristic peaks in other regions, may help in confirming the presence of a particular group in a molecule. For example, aldehydes show C=O stretching along with C-H stretching at about 2700 cm^{-1}. Esters show C=O stretching along with C-O-R stretching at about 1200 cm^{-1}. Similarly, for carboxylic acids, apart from C=O stretching, an additional peak at 1300 cm^{-1} due to carboxylate anion stretching, is also seen.

(iv) A peak due to C=N stretching is obtained between 1660-1600 cm^{-1}.

(v) Olefins show peaks for C=C stretching, usually in the range of 1640-1580 cm^{-1}.

(vi) Aromatic compounds with a low degree of substitution exhibit four peaks, approximately near 1600, 1580, 1500 and 1460 cm^{-1}.

4) A finger print region [1480-910 cm^{-1}]

This region contains a large crowding of peaks. Even then, the region between 1480 cm^{-1} to 910 cm^{-1}, commonly known as a *fingerprint region*, is very important in order to confirm the identical structural features as in case of an authentic substance. The peaks in this region for two substances would match exactly with each other if and only if these two substances are exactly identical. The small structural differences in two substances would not allow exact overlapping of the peaks in this region, e.g. o-nitrophenol and p-nitrophenol would show the peaks for a nitro group as well as for a phenolic hydroxy group in the appropriate regions. Hence, these two substances can be identified based on the peaks they produce in the fingerprint region only. The small differences in the structures of molecules result in significant changes in the distribution of absorption peaks in this region of the spectrum. This is because in this region, the peaks obtained are due to single bonds, almost all of which are of the same energy. The absorption bands in this region, therefore, depend upon the overall skeletal structure of the molecule. Thus, though the spectrum in this region is highly complex, it is this complexity and uniqueness of the spectrum, which proves usefulness of this region to the final identification of a substance.

A nitro group also shows two distinct peaks in this region, at around 1550 cm^{-1} and 1350 cm^{-1} due to symmetric and asymmetric stretching vibrations of the double bonds in N(=O)=O group.

Similarly, two bands at around 1300 cm^{-1} and 1100 cm^{-1} are recorded for a sulfone (SO_2) group.

3.5.2. Quantitative Applications of IR Spectrometry

The quantitative use of IR spectrometry is very limited because it is very difficult to get the reproducible data from IR spectra. In order to make the IR spectrometry quantitative, an IR spectrum of a definite concentration of a standard is recorded. The concentration along with the percent transmittance for this standard substance decides the heights of the peaks produced in its IR spectrum. If a spectrum is recorded for some concentration of a sample, it is very difficult to adjust percent transmittance of this sample to exactly the same value as that of the standard. Since, the peak heights do not solely depend on the concentration factor, the quantitative estimation by IR spectrometry becomes difficult. In order to make IR spectrometry quantitative, one can adjust the percent transmittance of a standard and a sample to the same value, but this task is difficult though not impossible. Hence, quantitative use of IR spectrometry is limited.

Moreover, the instrumental deviations from Beer's law are more common than with visible and UV wavelengths because the IR bands are relatively narrower. Similarly, the low intensity of sources and the low sensitivity of detectors in the IR region, require wide monochromator slit widths. Thus, the band widths employed are frequently of the same order of magnitude as the widths of absorption peaks. All these facts lead to a non-linear relationship between absorbance and concentration. Hence, IR spectrometry is not commonly used for quantitative estimation.

A list of common functional groups that can be identified by IR spectrometry and the vibrations associated with them are mentioned in **Table 3.4**. These common frequencies can be used to identify the functional groups in organic compounds, which help to elucidate the structures of different molecules.

Table 3.4: The modes of vibrations and the approximate associated frequencies for the functional groups

No.	Functional group	Mode of vibration	Approximate frequency (cm^{-1})
1	Alcohols and Phenols	O-H stretching	3550
2	Carboxylic acids	O – H stretching, C = O stretching $-C(=O)O^-$ stretching	3550 1700 1300-1200
3	Primary amines and amides Secondary amines and amides Amines and amides	N – H stretching N – H stretching N – H bending	2 peaks at 3450 and 3350 1 peak at 3400 1650-1620
4	Nitriles	C≡N	2280
5	Alkynes	C≡C	2260
6	Hydrocarbons	C – H stretching	3000
7	Aldehydes	C – H stretching C = O stretching	2700 1660
8	Ketones	C = O stretching	1660
9	Nitro	$N(=O)=O$ symmetric and asymmetric stretching	1550 and 1350
10	Sulfones	$S(=O)=O$ symmetric and asymmetric stretching	1300 and 1100
11	Aromatic ring	C = C stretching	1600, 1550, 1500 and 1450

CHAPTER 4

NUCLEAR MAGNETIC RESONANCE SPECTROMETRY

The main difference between the ultraviolet (UV)-visible spectrometry, the infrared (IR) spectrometry and the nuclear magnetic resonance (NMR) spectrometry is that the former two methods deal with the excitation of *electrons*, whereas the latter method deals with the excitation of a *nucleus* from the lower energy level to the higher one.

A static charge produces only the electric field, but a moving charge produces its own electric as well as magnetic field. A nucleus is positively charged and it spins about an axis. Therefore, it produces its own electric and magnetic fields. In short, a nucleus acts as a tiny bar magnet.

When a nucleus or a molecule is not kept in an external magnetic field, it possesses a definite amount or a quantum of energy. If a molecule is kept in a strong external magnetic field, the energy level of certain nuclei splits into two or more quantized energy levels. Thus, energy levels in a nucleus are magnetically induced. The transition of a nucleus from the lower energy level to the higher one can be brought about by the absorption of an electromagnetic radiation (EMR) of a suitable frequency range of 4 to 600 MHz (or a suitable wavelength range of 0.6-10 meters), which is in the radiofrequency portion of the electromagnetic spectrum. The study of absorption of radiofrequency by nuclei is called the *nuclear magnetic resonance* (NMR) *spectrometry*.

4.1. PROPERTIES OF A NUCLEUS

1) It is assumed that the nuclei rotate about an axis and thus, have a property of spin.
2) Each spinning nucleus possesses angular momentum (p), the value of which depends on the orientation of a nucleus in the external magnetic field. The maximum value of the angular momentum of a nucleus is given by the **equation (4.1)**.

$$p=\left(\frac{h}{2\pi}\right)\sqrt{I\,(I+1)} \quad \ldots (4.1)$$

where, I is the spin quantum number of the nucleus, and h is the Plank's constant.

3) Each spinning nucleus acts as a bar magnet. Hence, it produces a magnetic dipole moment (μ, mu, Gr.= Greek), whose direction is along the spin axis and its magnitude is given by the **equation (4.2)**.

$$\mu = \gamma\, p \ldots (4.2)$$

where, γ (Gamma, Gr.) = magnetogyric ratio, which is a characteristic of a particular nucleus, and p = angular momentum of a nucleus. The magnitude of γ is expressed as-

$$\gamma = \frac{\mu}{I\,\hbar}$$

where, $\hbar$ is the modified Plank's constant, which is equal to (h/2π).

Since, a nucleus possesses different magnitudes of angular momentum (p), it is associated with different magnitudes of magnetic dipole moments. Thus, a nucleus is present in various magnetic quantum states, described by the magnetic quantum number (m), the magnitude of which is given as m = I, (I-1), (I-2),….,-I.

4) In the absence of an external magnetic field, all the orientations of the nucleus have identical energies. When a molecule is kept in an external magnetic field of strength (B_o), a single energy level splits into (2I+1) energy levels. Each energy level can be assigned a particular magnetic quantum number. For any nucleus

with spin quantum number, I = 1/2, a single energy level splits into (2I+1) = (2x½+ 1) = 2 energy levels. The magnetic quantum numbers associated with these two energy levels are, m = +1/2 and m = -1/2. For a nucleus having I = 1, a single energy level splits into (2I+1) = (2x1 + 1) = 3 energy levels. The magnetic quantum numbers associated with these three energy levels are, m = +1, m = 0 and m = -1. The energy of a nucleus in these orientations or quantum states is given by **equation (4.3)**.

$$E = -\left(\frac{m\,\gamma\,h}{2\pi}\right)B_o$$

Or

$$E = -\,m\,\gamma\,\hbar\,B_o \ldots (4.3)$$

For I = ½, m= + ½ and m= - ½. Hence, the energy of two energy levels of a nucleus is + ½ $\gamma\,\hbar\,B_o$ and - ½ $\gamma\,\hbar\,B_o$. Thus, the energy difference (δE) between the two energy levels is -

$$\delta E = (+\tfrac{1}{2}\gamma\,\hbar\,B_o) - (-\tfrac{1}{2}\gamma\,\hbar\,B_o)$$

Therefore, $\delta E = \gamma\,\hbar\,B_o$

4.1.1. Magnitude of Spin Quantum Number (I)

The value of a spin quantum number (I) depends upon a particular nucleus. It can be zero, a half integral or an integral multiple, i.e. I = 0, 1/2, 1, 3/2, 2 and so on. For assigning the value of I to a particular nucleus, the following rules are used.

1) The value of I is zero, when both the atomic mass and atomic number are *even*, e.g. nuclei of ${}_6C^{12}$, ${}_8O^{16}$, ${}_{16}S^{32}$, etc.
2) The value of I is a half integral multiple, i.e.1/2, 3/2, 5/2, etc. when the atomic mass is *odd* and atomic number is *odd* or *even*, e.g. nuclei of ${}_1H^1$, ${}_6C^{13}$, etc.
3) The value of I is an integral multiple, i.e. 1, 2, 3, etc. when the atomic mass is *even* and atomic number is *odd*, e.g. nuclei of ${}_1H^2$, ${}_7N^{14}$, etc.

This information is tabulated in **Table 4.1**.

Table 4.1: Values of spin quantum number for various nuclei

Value of I	Atomic Mass	Atomic Number	Examples of nuclei
0	Even	Even	${}_6C^{12}$, ${}_8O^{16}$, ${}_{16}S^{32}$
1/2, 3/2	Odd	Odd/Even	${}_1H^1$, ${}_6C^{13}$
1, 2	Even	Odd	${}_1H^2$, ${}_7N^{14}$

4.2. PROTON (¹H) MAGNETIC RESONANCE (PMR) SPECTROMETRY

4.2.1. Principle

Very commonly, the NMR spectrometry is applied to the nuclei having I= ½ (e.g. ${}_1H^1$, ${}_6C^{13}$, ${}_7F^{19}$and ${}_{15}P^{31}$). When this technique is applied to protons (${}_1H^1$), the technique is referred to as *proton magnetic resonance* (PMR) *spectrometry*.

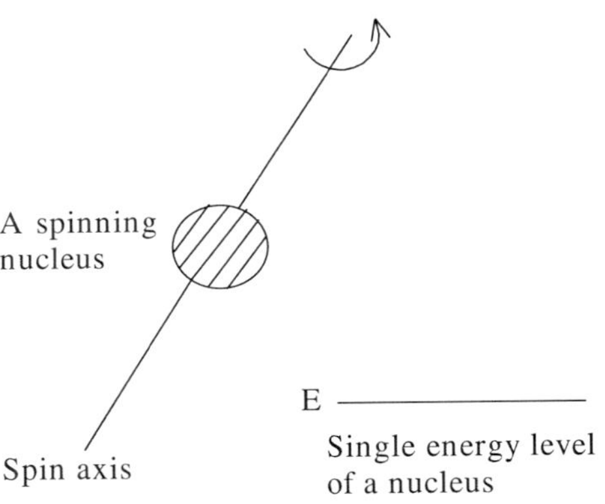

Fig.4.1: Spinning of a nucleus in the absence of an external magnetic field

This chapter deals with the studies involving nuclei with I = 1/2. Consider a spinning nucleus in the absence of an external magnetic field. It is associated with energy E, as shown in **Fig. 4.1**. This nucleus, when placed in an external magnetic field, the initial single energy level splits into (2I+1) energy levels, i.e. into (2 x 1/2 +1) = 2 energy levels. These two energy levels are assigned the magnetic quantum numbers, m = +1/2 and m = -1/2. This is shown in **Fig. 4.2**. Thus, the external magnetic field provides different energy levels, which are required for the transition of a nucleus. It should be noted that the external magnetic field does not cause transition of a nucleus from one energy level to the other, but just splits the original energy level into two energy levels for a nucleus with I = 1/2.

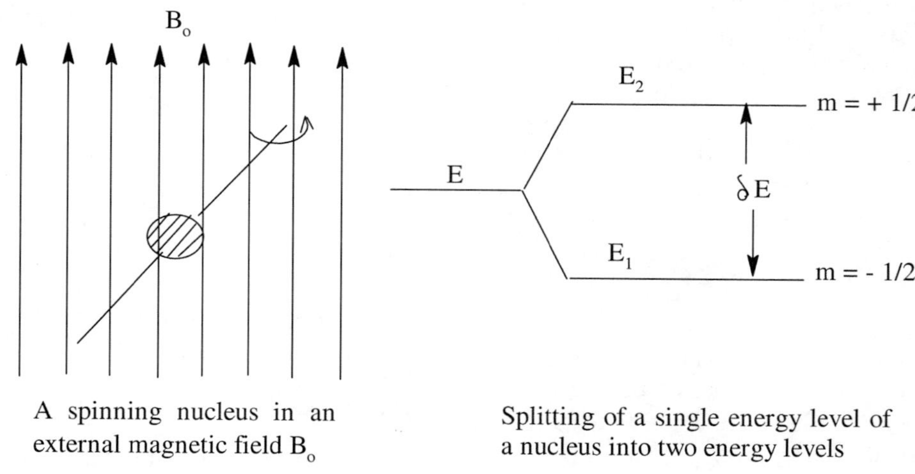

A spinning nucleus in an external magnetic field B_o

Splitting of a single energy level of a nucleus into two energy levels

Fig.4.2: Spinning of a nucleus in the presence of an external magnetic field

Another effect that is produced by applying the external magnetic field is that of a *torque*. The spinning nucleus, when kept in an external magnetic field of strength B_o gauss, experiences B_o as a torque about an axis perpendicular to the spinning axis. (A torque is nothing but the two forces of exactly the same magnitude, acting in directions opposite to each other. This is shown in **Fig. 4.3**). This causes the spin axis to precess about the direction of the field, i.e. the field B_o constantly pushes the spinning axis of the nucleus, because of which along with the spin motion, a nucleus starts performing a *gyroscopic motion* or a *precessional motion*, as shown in **Fig. 4.3**.

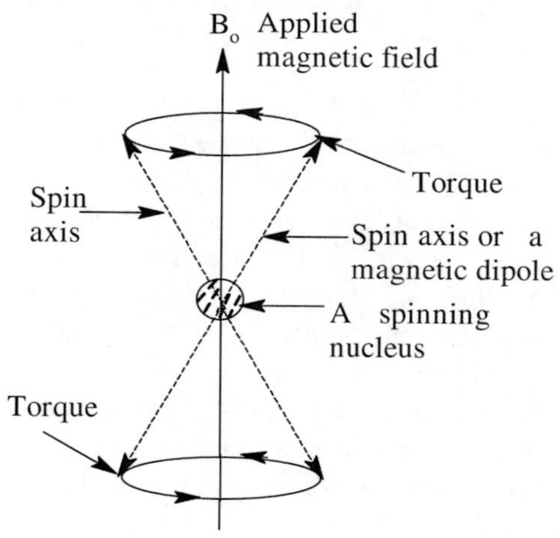

Fig.4.3: Precessional motion of a nucleus in the presence of an external magnetic field

The frequency with which a nucleus precesses when kept in an external magnetic field is called its *precessional frequency* or the *Larmour frequency*. If a nucleus completes 10 cycles in 1sec, its precessional frequency is said to be 10 cps or 10 Hz. The actual precessional frequency depends on the strength of the external magnetic field (B_o). If the strength of the external magnetic field is increased, the precessional frequency of a nucleus also increases, and vice versa. Thus, a nucleus precessing 10 times/sec, when the magnetic field applied is B_o, may precess 15 times/sec (15 Hz) at the magnetic field higher than B_o and may precess 5 times/sec (5 Hz) at the field lower than B_o. The precessional frequency (ν_o), is thus, directly proportional to the strength of the external magnetic field. The expression for ν_o is given by **equation (4.4)**.

$$\nu_o \propto B_o$$

$$\text{or} \quad \nu_o = \left(\frac{\gamma}{2\pi}\right) B_o \quad \ldots (4.4)$$

where, ($\gamma/2\pi$) is a constant of proportionality and γ is a magnetogyric ratio and is unique for each isotope.

If **equation (4.4)** is multiplied by Plank's constant (h), the following equation is obtained.

$$h\nu_o = \left(\frac{h}{2\pi}\right) \gamma B_o$$

Replacing the term ($h/2\pi$) by $\hbar$, i.e. by the modified Plank's constant, **equation (4.5)** is obtained.

$$h\nu_o = \hbar \gamma B_o \quad \ldots (4.5)$$

The term, $h\nu_o$ is the energy difference (δE) between the two energy levels obtained after splitting. Thus, **equation (4.5)** can be written as -

$$\delta E = \hbar \gamma B_o \ldots (4.6)$$

Since $\delta E \propto B_o$, the energy gap between the two energy levels would increase with the increase in the strength of the external magnetic field. This is shown in **Fig. 4.4**. If a nucleus in the magnetic field is exposed to *radio-waves* (λ= 0.6 - 10 meters), then the radio-wave of the correct frequency, whose energy corresponds to the energy gap between the energy levels of a nucleus, is absorbed. This absorption of energy ultimately results in the transition of a nucleus from the lower energy level to the higher one.

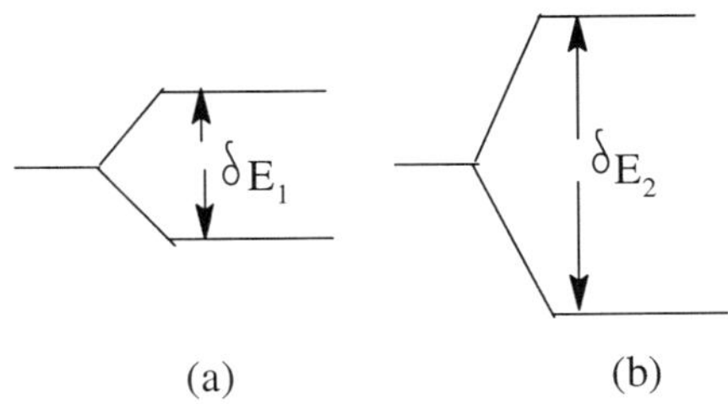

Fig.4.4: Energy gap between the energy levels (a) at lower and (b) higher magnetic fields

Role of External Magnetic Field in NMR Spectrometry

1) The External magnetic field splits the energy of the nucleus into two or more energy levels, depending on the spin quantum number (I) of a nucleus.
2) For I = 1/2, the magnetic quantum number m = + 1/2 or − 1/2. Hence, there are two energy levels present in such nuclei.
   For I = 1, m = + 1, 0, and -1. Hence, there are three energy levels present in such nuclei.
3) Magnetic field induces the precessional motion in a nucleus.
4) The magnitude of the external magnetic field decides the *precessional* or the *Larmour frequency* (ν_o) of a nucleus.
5) The Magnetic field also decides the magnitude of the energy gap (δE) between the consecutive energy levels of a nucleus
6) The higher the magnitude of the external magnetic field, the larger is the energy gap between the consecutive energy levels.
7) Note that, the magnetic field does not bring about the transition of a nucleus from the lower energy level to the higher energy level.
8) The transition of a nucleus from the lower energy level to the higher energy level is brought about by the radio-waves.

4.2.2. Signal in NMR Spectrum

The transition of a nucleus from the lower energy level to the higher energy level occurs due to the absorption of energy supplied by the radio-waves of the correct frequency and that in the reverse direction is due to an emission of energy. When the transition of a nucleus occurs in any direction, it is associated with a reversal of the spin orientation, i.e. if a nucleus is spinning clockwise in the lower energy level, after the absorption of energy, it occupies the higher energy level and starts spinning anticlockwise. The change in the direction of spinning also occurs when the nucleus comes down from the higher energy level to the lower energy level, by giving out the absorbed energy. Both the transitions are equally probable. Most of the times, the number of nuclei in the lower energy level (N_α) is more as compared to that in the higher energy level (N_β). Hence, the absorption of energy from the irradiating field is dominant. This absorption is observed as a signal, whose intensity is proportional to the population difference (N_α - N_β). Since the difference (N_α - N_β) depends on the total number of spins in the sample, the intensity of a peak depends on the concentration of the sample. If the population of the nuclei in the lower and the higher energy levels is equal, i.e. if $N_\alpha = N_\beta$, the absorption and emission processes cancel each other and no signal is observed. This condition is known as *saturation*.

The energy required for the transition of a nucleus from the lower energy level to the upper energy level is provided by the radiofrequency (ν). The absorption of energy occurs only when this radiofrequency matches exactly with the Larmour frequency of the precessing nucleus. This phenomenon is known as *resonance*. Thus, resonance is essential for the signal to be seen in the NMR spectrum. When resonance occurs or when the radiofrequency matches exactly with the Larmour or precessional frequency of a nucleus, the radio-waves provide energy which is exactly equal to the energy gap between the higher and the lower energy levels of a nucleus. Thus, at resonance, the exact amount of energy, which is required for the transition of a nucleus, is absorbed by the nucleus.

4.2.3. Different Methods of NMR Measurements

Two methods to achieve resonance between the precessional frequency of a nucleus and the radiofrequency (RF) are as mentioned below.

4.2.3.1. A continuous wave method

4.2.3.2. A pulsed method

4.2.3.1. A Continuous Wave Method

A continuous wave method uses a continuous or an uninterrupted radiofrequency power. It was used up to about the end of 1960s. It is adequate for recording the spectra of nuclei with high natural abundance and with large magnetic moments, e.g. ^1H, ^{19}F and ^{31}P. Sufficient concentration of the nuclei is also essential for recording peaks with adequate intensities. The resonance condition is satisfied by using either a *radiofrequency sweep method* or by using a *magnetic field sweep method.*

1) Radiofrequency (RF) sweep method

In a RF sweep method, the nucleus is kept in the constant magnetic field B_o. This makes the nucleus to precess with the precessional frequency ν_o. The magnetic field (B_o) also splits the energy level of a proton into two, corresponding to the energy gap (δE_o). This nucleus is exposed to the radio-waves of increasing frequencies, which are generated by using an oscillating field B_1, applied perpendicular to B_o, as shown in **Fig. 4.5(a)**.

At one particular moment, the RF (ν) of radio-waves becomes exactly equal to the precessional frequency (ν_o) of the nucleus. When these two frequencies match, the resonance occurs and the radio-waves supply exact amount of energy (δE_o), which is required for the transition of a nucleus from the lower energy level to the higher energy level. When the transition occurs, the nucleus '*flips*' and the reversal of the spin orientation is observed. This is shown in **Fig. 4.5(b)**. In the process of flipping, the nuclear magnet produces a current in the

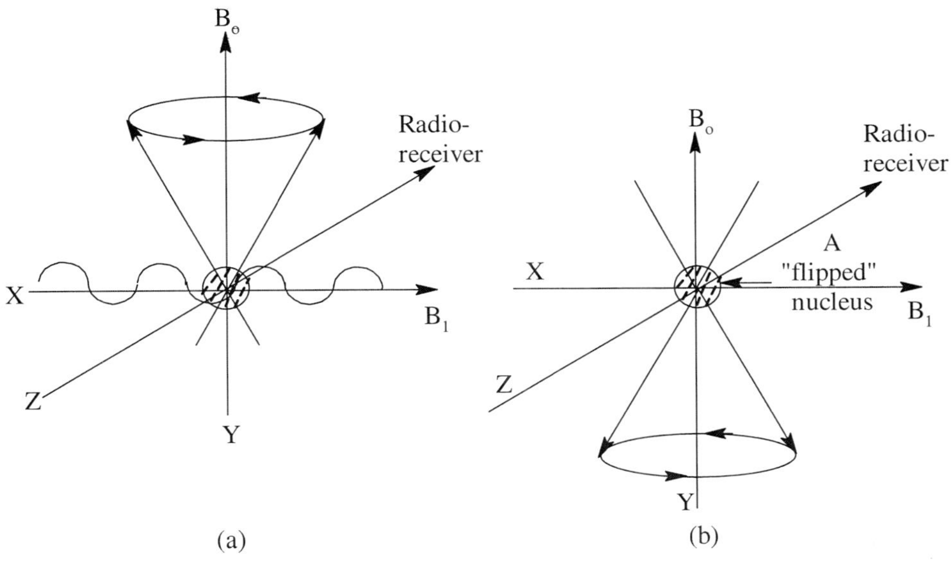

Fig. 4.5: (a) Perpendicular arrangement of an external magnetic field (B_o), an oscillating magnetic field (B_1) and a radio-receiver (b) a flipped nucleus

radio-receiver which is oriented perpendicular to the two fields B_o and B_1 [**Fig. 4.5(b)**].

For a nucleus having the spin quantum number of 1/2, the absorption of energy from the RF involves flipping of the magnetic moment or a magnetic dipole that is oriented in the field direction to a state in which the moment is in the opposite direction.

2) Magnetic field sweep method

In case of a magnetic field sweep method, the RF (ν) is kept constant. The sample is kept between two poles of a strong magnet. An additional varying magnetic field is produced by passing the slowly increasing magnitudes of current through the coil surrounding the sample (**Fig. 4.6**). As the current passing through the coil is increased, the higher and higher magnetic field is produced. The increasing magnetic field slowly increases the precessional frequency and also the energy gap between the consecutive energy levels of a nucleus. At a particular value of current in the coil, and therefore of the magnetic field, the precessional frequency (ν_0) of a nucleus matches with the RF (ν). The resonance between the two frequencies causes a nucleus to flip and sends a signal to the radio-receiver. A peak thus, appears in the spectrum for that nucleus.

4.2.3.2. A Pulsed Method

A continuous wave method is neither useful for the insensitive nuclei nor for the nuclei

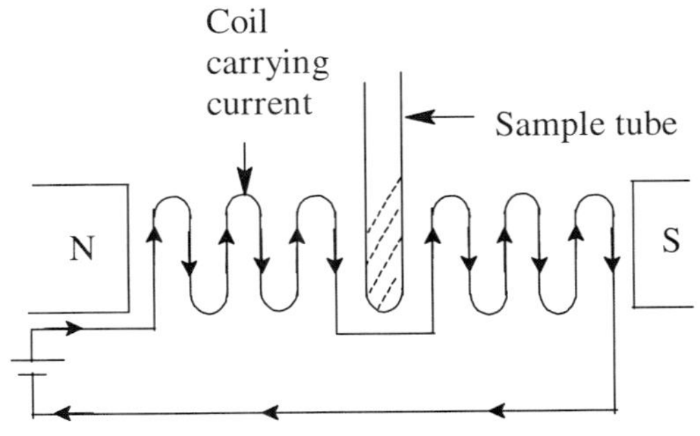

Fig. 4.6: Coils for generating variable magnetic field

with the low natural abundance. Also, it cannot be used for the routine measurements of very dilute solutions. Such nuclei require new measurement techniques. A '*pulsed NMR spectrometry*' provided a solution for such nuclei. It forms the basis of modern NMR spectrometry.

In the pulsed method, all the nuclei of one species in the sample, i.e. all the protons (^1H) or all the ^{13}C nuclei, are excited simultaneously by a RF *pulse* or a *band*, i.e. the sample is exposed to a number of radiofrequencies simultaneously, as against the exposure of the sample either to a fixed RF or to a slowly increasing radiofrequencies, in a continuous method. The following terms are of importance in the pulsed NMR spectrometry.

(i) A pulse

A RF generator usually operates at a fixed frequency (ν). However, if it is switched on only for a short time (T_p), a pulse is obtained which contains not only the frequency 'ν' but a continuous band of frequencies, symmetrical about the frequency ν. Only a part of the frequency band is effective in exciting transitions. This frequency band is approximately proportional to $1/T_p$.

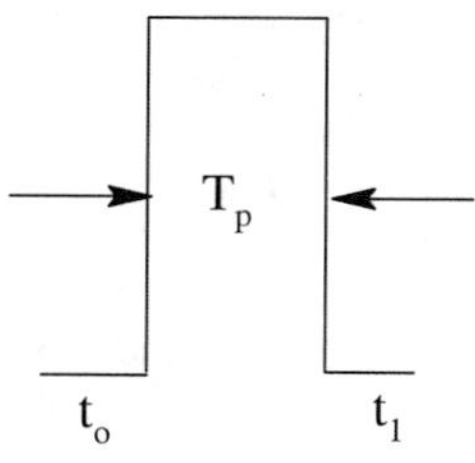

Fig. 4.7: A schematic diagram of a pulse

As shown in **Fig. 4.7**, the RF generator is switched on at time t_o and switched off at time t_1 to obtain the pulse duration, (T_p) of the order of several microseconds (μs). The choice of the generator frequency (ν) is determined by the strength of the external magnetic field (B_o) and the nuclei to be observed. For example, for the protons, at B_o = 4.7 Tesla, the value of ν is 200 MHz. For ^{13}C resonances, at B_o = 4.7 Tesla, the frequency ν is 50.3 MHz (**Table 4.2**).

Table 4.2: ^1H and ^{13}C frequencies at different magnetic flux densities (B_o)

B_o (Tesla, T)	Resonance frequency (MHz)	
	^1H	^{13}C
1.41	60	15.1
1.88	80	20.1
2.11	90	22.63
2.35	100	25.15
4.70	200	50.3
5.87	250	62.9
7.05	300	75.4
9.40	400	100.6
11.74	500	125.7
14.09	600	150.9
17.62	750	188.2
18.79	800	201.2

(ii) Pulse duration

The pulse duration required for the experiment depends on the width of the spectrum, e.g. if $T_p = 10^{-5}$ seconds, the frequency band is about 10^5 Hz wide. If ν is the generator frequency, then it is observed at the centre of the band. Two ends of the band correspond to the frequencies-

$$\nu + \frac{1}{T_P} \text{ and } \nu - \frac{1}{T_P}$$

If ν is correctly chosen, then all the frequencies in the spectrum to be recorded are contained in this band. The amplitude (i.e. the height of the pulse or how strong pulse is to be applied) of the frequency components of a pulse decreases with the increasing separation from ν. Usually, the hard pulses, i.e. the short pulses of high power, are used so as to irradiate all the nuclei in the sample equally. The pulse duration is so chosen that the frequency band exceeds the width of the spectrum by one to two powers of ten.

(iii) Pulse angle

A nucleus with I = $^1/_2$ precesses about the field axis (i.e. about B_o or Z - axis) on the surface of a double cone, as shown in **Fig. 4.3**. If Z-components of all the nuclear magnetic moments in a sample are added, a macroscopic magnetization (M_o) is obtained along the field direction, since $N_\alpha > N_\beta$. The vector M_o plays an important role in the pulsed NMR spectrometry.

To induce the transition of nuclei from the lower energy level to the upper, the RF pulse (i.e. a band of radiofrequencies) is applied to the sample along the direction of X-axis by using a linear oscillating or an alternating magnetic field (B_1). The magnetic vector of this electromagnetic radiation is able to interact with the nuclear dipoles, and therefore, with M_o. The linear alternating magnetic field oscillates clockwise and anticlockwise. The linear alternating magnetic field along X-direction would be represented by two vectors with the same magnitude (B_1), rotating in the XY-plane with the same frequency (ν), the one which rotates clockwise is B_1(r), while the other, which rotates anticlockwise is B_1(l). These are shown in **Fig.4.8**.

The sum of these two vectors gives the alternating magnetic field along the X-direction, its maximum value being $2B_1$. Of the two rotating magnetic field components, only the one, which has the same direction of rotation as the precessing nuclear dipoles, can interact with them

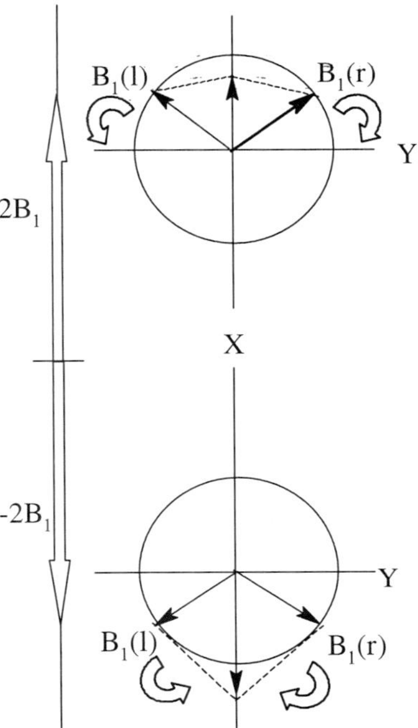

Fig. 4.8: Representation of a linear alternating field (max $2B_1$) as the sum of the two rotating fields B_1 (r) (clockwise) and B_1 (l) (anticlockwise)

and thus with M_o. The effect of this interaction is that the macroscopic magnetization (M_o), which is along the field direction B_o (i.e. along Z-axis), is tipped away from the Z-axis (**Fig. 4.9**). This tilting occurs in a plane which is perpendicular to the direction of B_1. Since the magnetic field B_1 is rotating and since the X-axis of the rotating coordinating system is normally defined as being along the direction of B_1, the effect of B_1 is to turn the vector M_o about the X' axis, i.e. in the $Y'Z$ plane, where X' and Y' refer to the *rotating coordinate system* (X', Y' and Z), which rotates with the same frequency as B_1. The angle (è) through which the vector (M_o) is tipped, is called the *pulse angle*. It is expressed as follows.

$$\theta = \nu B_1 T_p \quad \ldots (4.6)$$

where, B_1 is the rotating magnetic field of an oscillator, ν is the RF and T_p is the length of time for which the pulse is applied.

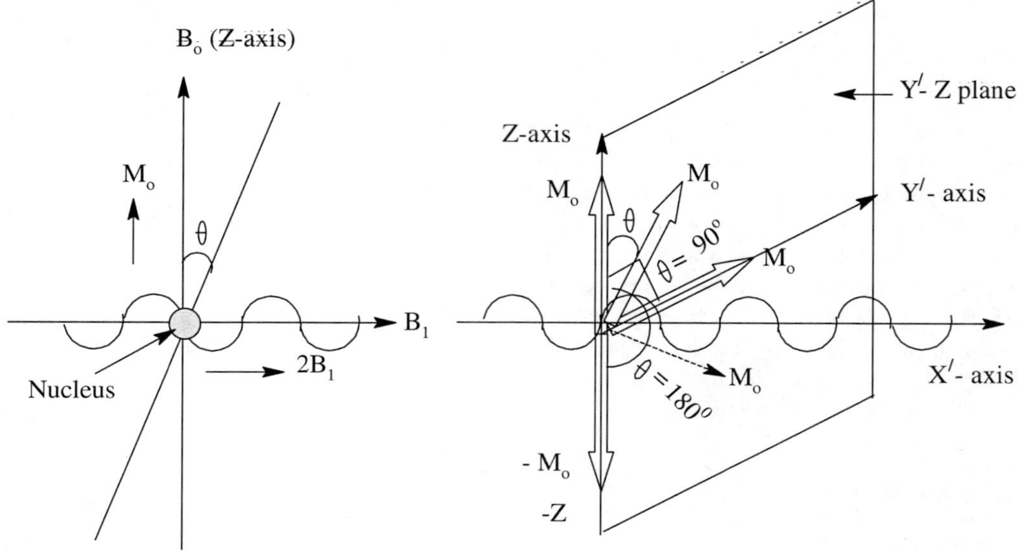

Fig. 4.9: Tilting of macroscopic magnetization M_o to $Y'Z$ plane and rotation of M_o in $Y'Z$ plane about X'-axis from +Z to ˘Z when RF is applied along X-axis

From **equation (4.6)**, it is clear that the pulse angle (θ) increases with the following two factors -

(a) The increase in the amplitude of the component of the RF pulse (**Fig. 4.10**) at the frequency ν_i (i.e. one particular RF from the band of radiofrequencies, symmetrical about the centre frequency ν_i) of the nuclear resonance transition.

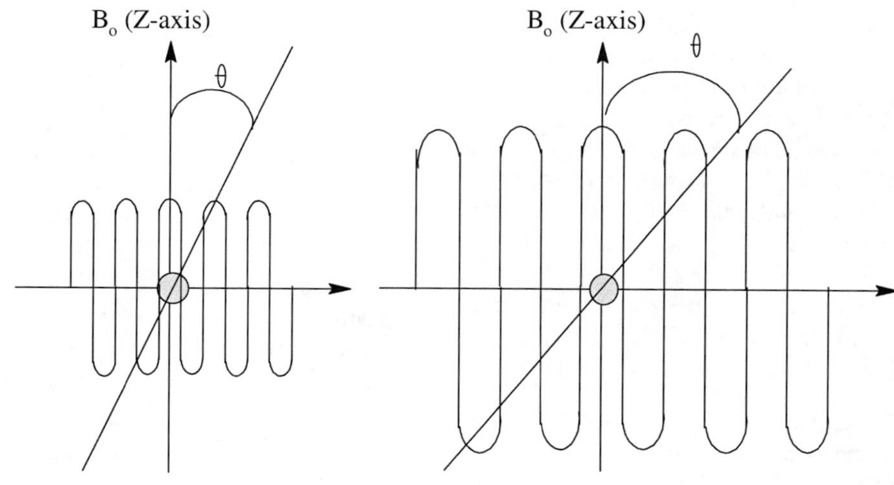

Fig. 4.10: Increase in the pulse angle (θ) with the increase in the amplitude of the RF

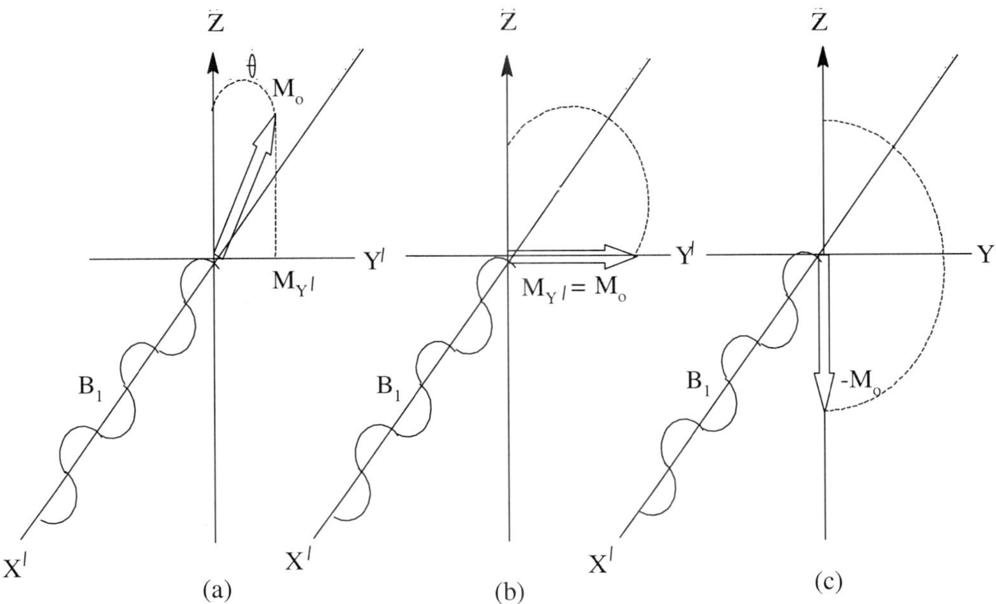

Fig. 4.11: Direction of the macroscopic magnetization vector (M_o) in the rotating coordinate system (a) after a pulse of arbitrary angle θ X′ (b) after a pulse of 90° X′ (c) after a pulse of 180° X′

(b) With the increase in the length of time (T_p) for which the pulse is applied.

In the pulsed NMR technique, the experiments with pulse angles of 90° and 180° are commonly used.

A wavy line about X′-axis in **Fig. 4.11** indicates the direction of the effective field B_1. When the RF or B_1 is applied along X′-axis and the magnetization vector M_o is shifted from the direction along +Z-axis to Y′-axis, the pulse angle is referred to as q = 90° X′, and when the vector M_o is shifted from the direction along + Z-axis to –Z-axis, the pulse angle is referred to as θ =180° X′.

If B_1 is along the direction of the Y′-axis (as used for certain experiments, **Fig. 4.12**), the motion of the vector M_o is in the X′ - Z plane about Y′ axis. In this case, when the vector is along X′ - axis, the pulse angle is described as q= 90° Y′, and when the vector is along –Z-axis, q = 180° Y′.

The perpendicular distance of the vector M_o from the Z-axis [**Fig. 4.11(a-c)**] indicates its magnitude, i.e. the number of nuclei contributing to the transition from the lower to the higher energy level at a particular value of an angle of pulse. From the vector diagrams [**Fig. 4.11 (a-c)**], it is clear that the transverse distance (M_{Y}'), when M_o is tilted from +Z to Y′ axis, increases and it decreases when the vector is shifted from Y′ to –Z-axis. This means that M_{Y}' has the maximum value at the pulse angle 90° X′ and is zero for $\theta_{X'}$ = 0° or 180°. The transverse component M_{Y}' is crucial for the observation of an NMR signal, since the receiver coil, which records the current generated due to flipping of the nuclei or due to resonance phenomenon, is oriented with its axis along the Y-direction. A signal proportional to M_{Y}' is induced in the receiver coil. Thus, the signal is maximum for a 90° X′ pulse, whereas for the 180° X′ pulse, no signal can be observed.

As seen before, the pulse angle can be increased either by increasing the amplitude of the pulse component or by increasing the pulse duration T_p [since as per the **equation (4.6)**, $\theta = n B_1 T_p$]. If the amplitude of the RF is kept constant and the pulse duration T_p is increased in stages of 1 μs,

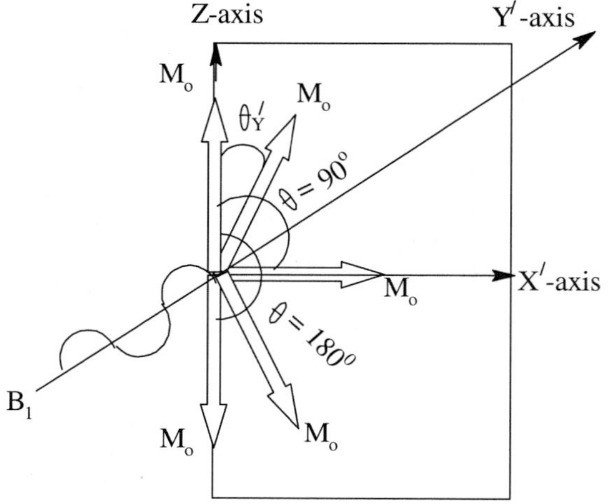

Fig.4.12: Rotation of the vector M_o in X′ - Z plane about Y′-axis from - Z to X′ and from X′ to ˘ Z, when RF is applied along Y′-axis.

a sigmoid signal, as shown in **Fig. 4.13**, is obtained. The amplitude of the signal passes through a maximum and then becomes zero. The maximum corresponds to a pulse angle of 90° and the zero amplitude corresponds to a pulse angle of 180°. Similarly, the time (T_p) required for the 180° pulse is double the time required for the 90° pulse. For all the values of T_p greater than 20 μs (**Fig. 4.13**), a signal is again observed, but with the negative amplitude. For a pulse angle greater than 180°,

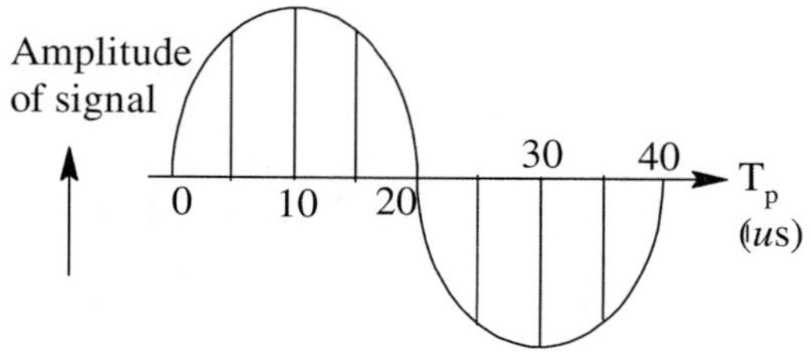

Fig.4.13: A sigmoid signal

which corresponds to the negative transverse component (= $M_{Y'}$), a negative current is induced in the receiver coil.

Thus, it is clear that if the pulse duration is changed, the nuclei are exposed to different values of the pulse angle. The reason for the change in the amplitude or the intensity of the NMR signal with the change in the pulse duration or pulse angle can be explained on the basis of the individual spins ($N = N_\alpha + N_\beta$), which together make up M_o. When the pulse of 180° is applied, the NMR signal is not obtained because the populations N_α and N_β have been exactly reversed, so that there are more nuclei in the upper than in the lower energy level. For a 90° pulse, there are more nuclei in the lower energy level as compared to that in the upper level. This is because the magnetization is in the Y′ direction, whereas for the zero signal or for the saturation ($N_\alpha = N_\beta$), the magnetization is in the Z-direction (either +ve or –ve).

4.2.4. Relaxation Processes

Relaxation processes are the deactivation processes by which excited nuclei from the higher energy level come back to the ground state by giving out energy. In order to get a peak in the NMR spectrum, it is essential to have a slight excess of nuclei in the lower energy level (N_α).

The Boltzmann statistics (**equation 4.7**) provides the distribution of nuclei between different energy states in the thermal equilibrium for a macroscopic sample, such as that in an NMR sample tube. For nuclei with I = 1/2, if the number of nuclei in the lower energy level is represented by N_a and that in the upper energy level as N_b, then –

$$\frac{N_\beta}{N_\alpha} = e^{-\delta E / kT}$$

$$\approx 1 - \frac{\delta E}{kT}$$

$$= 1 - \frac{h \nu B_o}{kT} \quad \ldots (4.7)$$

where, k is the Boltzmann constant (k = 1.3805 x 10^{-23} JK^{-1}) and T is the absolute temperature in °K. For protons and other nuclei, the energy difference (δE) is very small compared to the average energy (kT) of the thermal motions, i.e. kT >> δE. Hence, (1 - δE / kT) is very near to 1 or marginally smaller than 1. Consequently, the ratio (N_β / N_α) ≈ 1 and therefore, the populations of the two energy levels are nearly equal. The excess in the lower energy level is only in the region of parts per million (ppm). Hence, the peak in the NMR spectrum is weak. Usually, the rate of relaxation processes is slightly higher than the Boltzmann distribution and therefore, at any temperature, there is a slight excess of nuclei in the ground state. Thus, the relaxation processes avoid saturation of the energy levels ($N_\beta = N_\alpha$) and play an important role in determining the intensity of the peaks in the NMR spectrum. One way of transition of a nucleus from the higher energy level to the ground state is to give out the absorbed energy in the form of radiation. Since the probability of a spontaneous re-emission of photons varies as the cube of frequency for radiowaves (being too small since radiowaves are too long) absorbed by a sample in the NMR region, this process does not occur to a significant extent. Hence, in the NMR studies, the *radiative* relaxation is of no importance.

The major mechanism of relaxation in the NMR region is therefore, *non-radiative* in nature. The two non-radiative nuclear relaxation processes are as described below.

4.2.4.1. Spin Lattice Relaxation

A sample for NMR spectrometry is in the form of a number of molecules. The collection of the entire mass of the sample along with its environment is termed as *lattice*. Thus, a lattice contains a number of nuclei. In a solid sample, these nuclei do not rotate or vibrate freely. In case of a liquid or a gaseous sample, various nuclei in the lattice constantly undergo vibrational or rotational motion. Any charged species in motion, produces electric and magnetic fields. The phase and the frequency of the magnetic field or an electric field produced by different nuclei depend on the frequency of vibration or rotation of the nuclei. If the frequency of rotation or vibration of any nucleus in the lattice, matches with the precessional frequency of some other nucleus in the lattice, the transfer of energy takes place and the nucleus from a higher spin state comes back to a lower spin state. The absorbed energy increases the amplitude of thermal vibrations or rotations in sample molecules, which results in a minuscule increase in the temperature of the sample. This relaxation process brings down a nucleus from the higher energy level to the ground state and thus, helps in increasing the number of nuclei in the ground state (N_α). The life time (T_1) of an excited state determines an efficiency of the nucleus to return back from the excited state to the ground state. Liquids and gases have short relaxation time ((T_1 = 1 sec or less) and hence, the transfer is very efficient. They produce broader resonance bands. Solids have larger relaxation time (T_1 > 1 hr) and therefore, result in narrow absorption bands.

4.2.4.2. Spin-Spin Relaxation

In the sample, certain nuclei have the identical precessional frequencies, but they are present in different magnetic quantum states. In case of spin-spin relaxation, a mutual exchange of spins between an excited nucleus and a neighboring nucleus occurs. Since the nucleus in the lower spin state gets excited at the cost of the nucleus in the higher energy state, this relaxation process does not help in increasing the number of nuclei in the lower energy state, i.e. there is no net change in the relative spin state population. Hence, this relaxation process does not help in increasing the intensity of an NMR peak. The life time (T_2) of an excited state determines an efficiency of spin-spin relaxation. The large values of T_2 result in narrow resonance lines. This relaxation process mainly occurs in solids.

4.2.5. Chemical Shift

The difference between the absorption position of a proton in the test compound and the absorption position of the protons of a reference compound is known as *chemical shift*.

Why do different protons in the same molecule produce peaks at different positions in the NMR spectrum though the same external magnetic field is applied to all?

The NMR technique would not be of any use if all the protons in a molecule get recorded at the same place. In the NMR spectrometry, the protons in the same chemical environment (*chemically equivalent protons*) get recorded at the same place or at the same chemical shift values. The protons in different chemical environments produce peaks at different values of chemical shift.

The peak in the NMR spectrum is produced when there is a resonance between the Larmour or the precessional frequency (ν_o) of a nucleus and the applied RF (ν). While recording an NMR spectrum, an isolated nucleus is not made use of. Instead, a molecular sample is exposed to the external magnetic field. The precessional frequencies of all the protons in the molecule are decided not only by the magnetic field *applied* externally but also by the magnetic field which is *experienced* by them. The magnetic field experienced by the proton depends on the chemical environment of the protons and also on the strength of the applied magnetic field. The nuclei are always surrounded by electrons and other atoms. In diamagnetic molecules, the electrons around each nucleus, when influenced by the external magnetic field (B_o), circulate in such a way as to create a small local magnetic field of their own, which opposes B_o. Thus, the resultant field (B_{eff}) experienced by the nucleus can be expressed as follows.

$B_{eff} = B_o$ – (The field induced or generated by the circulating electrons)

This can be expressed by **equation (4.8)**.

$$B_{eff} = B_o - \sigma B_o \quad \ldots (4.8)$$

where, σB_o is the *induced magnetic field* or a *diamagnetic shielding* and σ is the *shielding constant* or a *screening constant*, which is dimensionless and is of the order of 10^{-5} for protons, but reaches a larger value for the heavy atoms, since the shielding increases with the number of electrons. The value of σ does not depend on the applied magnetic field but is determined solely by the electronic and the magnetic environment of the nuclei.

The resonance frequency (σ_o) is given by the **equation (4.9)**.

$$\nu_o = \frac{\gamma}{2\pi} B_{eff}$$

$$\text{or } \nu_o = \frac{\gamma}{2\pi}(B_o - \sigma B_o)$$

$$\text{or } \nu_o = \frac{\gamma}{2\pi}(1 - \sigma) B_o \quad \ldots (4.9)$$

where, γ is the magnetogyric ratio of the nucleus.

Thus, the resonance frequency or the precessional frequency (ν_o) is proportional to the magnetic field B_o and to the *shielding factor* ($1 - \sigma$). Since the shielding constant σ is different for different protons, depending on their chemical environments, their precessional frequencies differ. It should be noted that the degree of electronic shielding (σ) is clearly dependent on the electron density around a proton. Hence, the higher the electron density around a proton, the higher is the magnitude of σ and correspondingly of σB_o. This means that the higher field is induced by the surrounding electrons in the direction opposite to that of the external magnetic field (B_o). This results in the greater cancellation (σB_o) of the magnetic field and provides the lower value of B_{eff}. The higher the cancellation of the field, the higher is the additional magnetic field to be applied so as to make it feel the magnitude of the applied magnetic field or to achieve the production of a signal in the NMR spectrum.

Thus, though the same magnetic field B_o is applied to all the protons, all of them do not precess with the same precessional frequency, since their precessional frequency is decided by the magnitude of the magnetic field (B_{eff}) which is actually experienced by the protons in a molecule, which in turn depends on their chemical environment. It is this precessional frequency which should match with the RF obtained from the oscillating magnetic field B_1. Hence, the chemically non-equivalent protons produce separate resonance signals in the NMR spectrum.

This can be well explained with the example of ethanol, which contains three kinds of protons (protons in three different chemical environments). The chemical environment for the methyl protons ($-CH_3$), the methylene protons ($-CH_2$) and the field (B_0) and a constant radio-frequency (ν) in a non-protonated solvent containing a reference standard tetramethylsilane (TMS). All the three peaks for ethanol are *downfield*, i.e. on the left side of TMS. In TMS, silicon is electropositive relative to carbon and carbon is electronegative compared to hydrogen. Thus, dragging of electrons away from the protons is almost negligible. Hence, the electron density around the protons of TMS is high. The higher the electron density around the proton, the higher is the shielding and the higher is

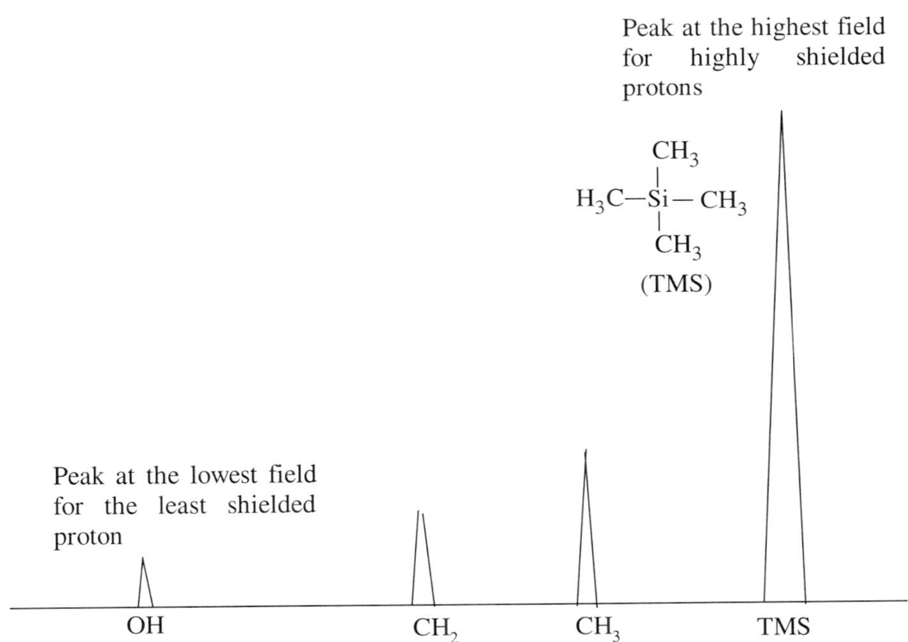

Fig. 4.14: Position of protons in ethanol with respect to TMS

hydroxy proton (-OH) in a molecule of ethanol (CH_3CH_2OH) is different. Hence, their σ values are different. Therefore, the magnetic fields (B_{eff}) which are actually experienced by the methyl protons ($-CH_3$), methylene protons ($-CH_2$) and the hydroxy proton (-OH) in a molecule of CH_3CH_2OH are different. Hence, the NMR spectrum of ethanol produces three major peaks. In order to explain the appearance of these three peaks let us assume that the spectrum is recorded using a variable magnetic the field (higher τ or lower δ) at which the protons absorb. Therefore, TMS protons are highly shielded and appear at the highest field (**Fig. 4.14**).

In CH_3-CH_2-OH, the three protons in the methyl (CH_3) group are chemically equivalent and produce a single peak at the same place in the spectrum. Both the protons in the methylene ($-CH_2$) group are chemically equivalent and produce a single peak at the same position in the spectrum, but since, the chemical environment for the methylene protons is different than that for the methylene protons , the peaks for the methyl and the methylene protons appear at two different positions in the spectrum. The oxygen bound proton appears at the lowest magnetic field, i.e. it requires the lowest magnetic field to induce the transition (because B_{eff} is the maximum for it). Hence, its peak appears to the extreme left of TMS, followed in order by the methylene protons and the methyl protons.

Though the applied magnetic field is B_o, it is not experienced by all the protons in ethanol because of the difference in the shielding factor. As seen before, the electrons around the proton, under the influence of a magnetic field, circulate and generate their own magnetic field so as to oppose the applied external magnetic field B_o. This results in the cancellation of the external magnetic field to some extent.

In case of a hydroxyl proton, the oxygen being electronegative in nature attracts electrons towards itself. This is responsible for reducing an electron density around a proton attached to it, considerably. Hence, a hydroxyl proton is the least shielded proton in ethanol. The reduction of the external magnetic field by this proton is the least and therefore, the effective field experienced by it is the maximum.

The methylene protons are in the vicinity of the oxygen atom, but they are not directly linked with the oxygen atom. Hence, the reduction in the electron density around methylene protons is not to the extent to which it is observed in a hydroxyl proton. Because of little higher electron density around methylene protons, as compared to that of a hydroxyl proton, the reduction in the magnetic field experienced by the methylene protons is more than that for a hydroxyl proton. Hence, these protons are more shielded compared to a hydroxyl proton and experience lower magnetic field as compared to the hydroxyl proton.

The methyl protons, being farthest from the hydroxyl proton, experience the least withdrawal of electrons away from them. The electron density around the methyl protons being the highest of all, they experience maximum shielding. Since the shielding is maximum, the reduction in the magnetic field is also maximum and they experience the least magnetic field.

The magnitude of shielding in protons in TMS and protons in ethanol is in the following order.

All the 12 protons in TMS > 3 methyl protons > 2 methylene protons > 1 hydroxyl proton

Because of the maximum shielding in TMS, its peak appears at the extreme right in the NMR spectrum (upfield to all the peaks or the lowest δ value). The minimum shielding is observed in the hydroxyl proton and hence, its peak appears at the extreme left in the NMR spectrum (downfield to all the peaks or the highest δ value). The methyl protons are downfield to TMS but upfield to the hydroxyl and the methylene protons. The methylene protons are downfield to TMS and methyl protons but upfield to a hydroxyl proton.

Let the sample of ethanol and TMS be kept in the external magnetic filed B_o. Let B_{eff} (TMS), B_{eff} (CH_3), B_{eff} (CH_2) and B_{eff} (OH) be the fields experienced by the protons in TMS, and by the methyl protons, the methylene protons and the hydroxyl proton in ethanol, respectively. Let σ(TMS), $\sigma(CH_3)$, $\sigma(CH_2)$ and σ(OH) be the shielding constants for the protons in TMS and for the methyl, methylene and the hydroxyl protons in ethanol. The magnitude of the effective field felt or experienced by these protons is given by the following equations.

$$B_{eff}(\text{TMS}) = B_o - \sigma(\text{TMS})B_o$$

$$B_{eff}(CH_3) = B_o - \sigma(CH_3)B_o$$

$$B_{eff}(CH_2) = B_o - \sigma(CH_2)B_o$$

$$B_{eff}(\text{OH}) = B_o - \sigma(\text{OH})B_o$$

Since,

$$\sigma(\text{TMS}) > \sigma(CH_3) > \sigma(CH_2) > \sigma(\text{OH})$$

$$B_{eff}(\text{OH}) > B_{eff}(CH_2) > B_{eff}(CH_3) > B_{eff}(\text{TMS})$$

Since, the field experienced by the TMS protons is the least, they precess with the lowest frequency, ν(TMS), whereas the field experienced by the hydroxyl proton being maximum, it precesses with the highest precessional frequency, ν(OH). The precessional frequency for the CH_2, ν(CH_2), and that for the CH_3 protons, ν(CH_3), is in between ν(TMS) and ν(OH). The order of the precessional frequencies of different protons is as follows.

$$\nu\,(OH) > \nu(CH_2) > \nu(CH_3) > \nu(TMS)$$

The effective field felt by the protons not only decides their precessional frequencies but also the energy difference between the lower and the higher energy levels of these nuclei. The higher the magnitude of the effective field felt by a proton, the higher is its precessional frequency and the higher is the energy gap between the lower and the higher energy levels. This is shown diagrammatically in **Fig. 4.15.**

In **Fig. 4.15**, ν(1) is the RF which corresponds to the energy, δE(1). In order to have a peak for different protons in an NMR spectrum, the precessional frequency of different protons should match with this RF, ν(1), i.e. their energy gaps should be widened so as to match them with the energy of the RF, δE(1). Because of the maximum shielding in TMS protons, their precessional frequency and the energy difference δE (TMS) is the least among all. In order to have the resonance between the precessional frequency of TMS protons and the applied RF ν(1), an additional magnetic field is required to be applied to TMS. This additional field to be applied to the TMS protons, to attain the field that induces

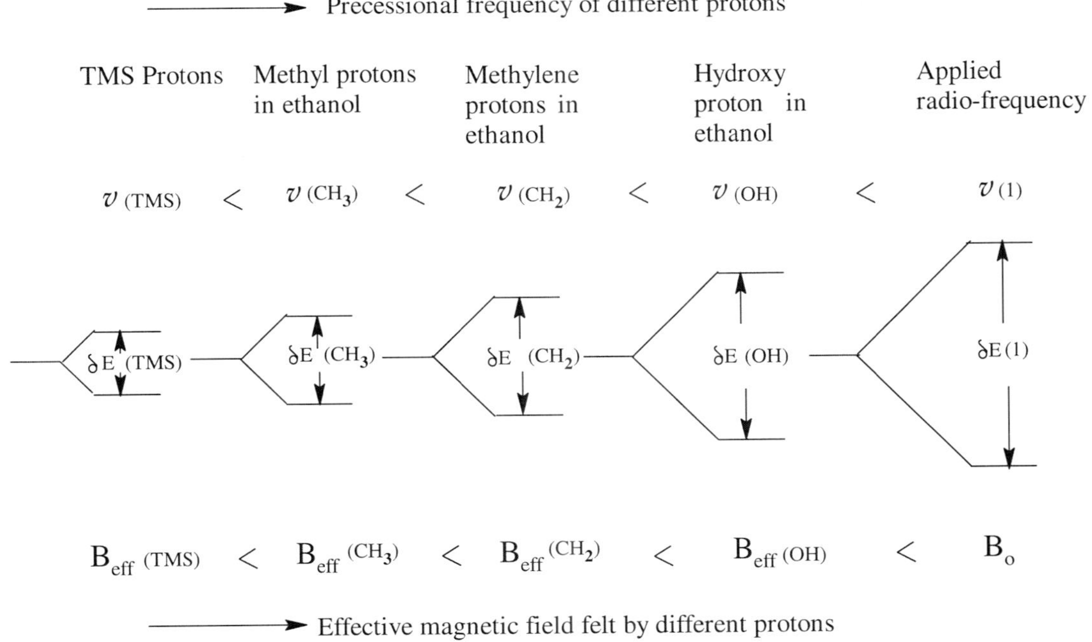

Fig. 4.15: The energy gap, the effective magnetic field experienced and the precessional frequency of protons in ethanol and TMS along with the applied RF, ν(1) in the external magnetic field B_o

a transition, is the maximum among all the protons and hence, its peak is produced *upfield* to all the protons. The hydroxyl proton experiences the least shielding and therefore, the resonance between the precessional frequency of a hydroxyl proton ν(OH) and the applied RF ν(1) occurs after applying only the little additional magnetic field. Hence, the peak for OH proton appears at the lowest field or it is to the extreme left of the spectrum. The reference compound, TMS, absorbs at the higher field than almost all the organic protons. Hence, usually, there is no peak upfield to TMS in the NMR spectrum.

Thus, the chemically non-equivalent protons get recorded at different positions in the NMR spectrum but chemically equivalent protons get recorded at the same place.

4.2.5.1. Measurement of Chemical Shifts

The position of the signals in the NMR spectrum is measured with respect to the position of a reference compound. Before each measurement, the reference compound is added to the sample to be analyzed. In such cases, the standard is called as an *internal standard*. In proton (^1H) and ^{13}C NMR spectrometry, tetramethylsilane (TMS) is usually employed for this purpose.

Advantages of TMS as an internal standard

1) Tetramethylsilane contains 12 equivalent protons and hence, it produces a single and a sharp peak. Therefore, only a small amount of the reference standard is required to be added.
2) All the 12 protons in TMS are highly shielded and hence, its peak is at the higher field than the most other protons.
3) Tetramethylsilane is chemically inert, magnetically isotropic and non-associating.
4) Its low boiling point (26.5 °C) makes possible easy recovery of the sample.

Tetramethylsilane is insoluble in water. In such cases it cannot be used as the internal standard. A different reference compound is then added to the sample and the results are converted to the TMS scale. Occasionally, an external standard is used. This is a reference compound which is sealed into a capillary and its resonance is recorded along with the sample. Special co-axial sample tubes, which are available commercially, are used for this purpose. However, in case of an external standard method, the nuclei at the position of the reference standard, experience a different shielding from those in the sample.

4.2.5.2. Scales of Measurement of Chemical Shift

Why absolute scale cannot be used for the measurement of chemical shift?

If the spectrum is recorded by keeping the magnetic field (B_o) constant, then the precessional frequencies of the protons in the sample, though different, remain fixed. For the lower values of B_o, protons precess with the lower precessional frequencies and for the higher values of B_o, protons precess with the higher precessional frequencies. Thus, for the higher magnetic field, the match between the precessional frequency of a proton and the radiofrequency would occur at the higher value of RF.

When the sample is exposed to a range of radiofrequencies and when the precessional frequencies of the protons in the sample match with the RF, a peak is obtained in the spectrum.

If the spectrum is recorded for a mixture of bromoform ($CHBr_3$), methylene bromide (CH_2Br_2), methyl bromide (CH_3Br) and TMS, by using a constant value of $B_o = 2.11$ T (Tesla), then the peak for TMS is obtained exactly at 90,000,000 Hz, i.e. at 90 MHz.

The signal for CH_3Br is obtained at 90,000,237 Hz.

The signal for CH_2Br_2 is obtained at 90,000,441 Hz.

The signal for $CHBr_3$ is obtained at 90, 000,614 Hz.

Thus, the proton in bromoform has the highest measured resonance and the proton in the TMS, the lowest. This indicates that the protons are least shielded in bromoform and most shielded in TMS, i.e.

$$\sigma(CHBr_3) < \sigma(CH_2Br_2) < \sigma(CH_3Br) < \sigma(TMS)$$

Thus, at B_o = 2.11 T (21,100 gauss), the protons require RF of the order of 90 x 10^6 Hz, i.e. 90 MHz. If B_o = 1.41 T (14,100 gauss), then the RF required for matching the precessional frequencies of protons is of the order of 60 x 10^6 Hz, i.e. 60 MHz.

If the frequency differences ($\Delta\nu$) for protons in CH_3Br, CH_2Br_2 and $CHBr_3$ are measured from TMS, then the values obtained are, 237, 441 and 614 Hz, respectively (**Fig. 4.16**).

The $\Delta\nu$ values for most of the protons in the usual types of organic compounds are spread over about 900 cycles per sec (cps), i.e. over 900 Hz, when the external magnetic field is about 21,100 Gauss or 2.11 Tesla. The actual precessional frequencies of the protons are in terms of 90 x 10^6 Hz. If the position of absorption of a given proton is to be determined with an accuracy of about ±1 cps, i.e. if the precessional frequencies 90,000,000 and 90,000,001 are to be measured accurately, then the instrument used should be able to discriminate frequencies of the order of 1 part in 10^8. In order to achieve this, an equally accurate system for the measurement of the applied magnetic field is necessary. Since, the strength of the applied magnetic field cannot be determined so accurately, the absolute position of absorption of a proton cannot be obtained directly from the instrument. However, the relative proton frequencies can readily be determined with an accuracy of about ±1 cps. Since only the relative absorption values can be obtained accurately, the use of TMS is absolutely essential for determining the chemical shift values.

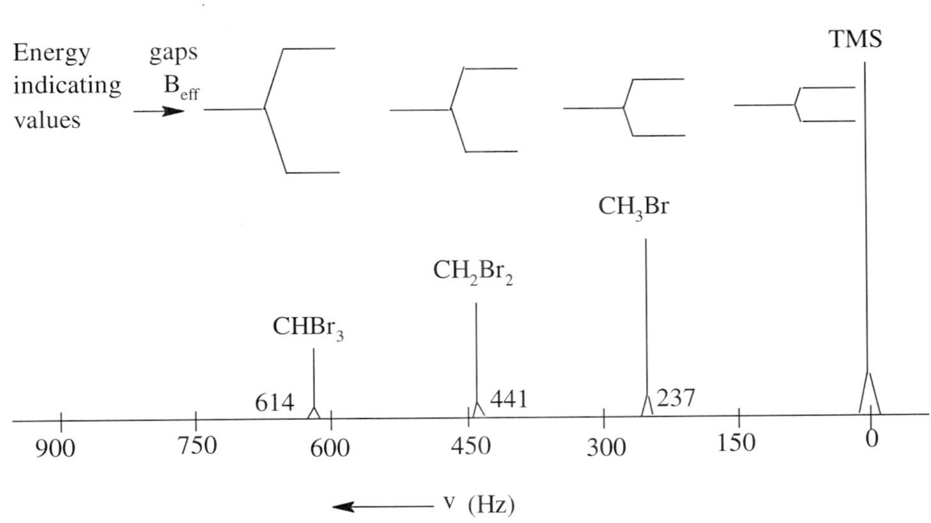

Fig. 4.16: ^{1}H-NMR spectrum of a mixture of $CHBr_3$, CH_2Br_2, CH_3Br and TMS at 90 MHz

Three scales are used for expressing the chemical shift values. They are as follows.

1) Frequency (ν) scale (Hertz or cps)

In this case, the chemical shift is quoted in Hertz (Hz) or cycles per second (cps). The frequency difference (Δν) is obtained for a particular proton from TMS, after recording to NMR spectrum.

The values of Δν depend on the following two factors.

(i) The magnitude of the external magnetic field (B_o) used, and

(ii) The RF used

By using an equation, $\nu = (\gamma / 2\pi) B_o$, the chemical shift of a proton in terms of frequency (ν) can be calculated from the magnetic field required to be applied to make the precessional frequency (ν) of a proton equal to the applied RF .

Consider a proton in the sample which gets recorded at the chemical shift of 120 Hz downfield to TMS when the RF of 60 MHz is used. If the spectrum is recorded at 90 MHz, then the chemical shift for the same proton changes and becomes equal to 180 Hz. This is calculated as follows.

$$\nu = \frac{90}{60} \times 120 = 180 \text{ Hz}$$

Thus, as the operating RF is increased, the peak for a proton is shifted more away from TMS. Hence, whenever chemical shift is to be quoted in terms of hertz, the operating frequency of the instrument should also be mentioned.

2) δ (Delta, Gr.) scale

Since the chemical shift values in terms of hertz are dependent on the magnetic field used, there was no uniformity in their values when the same sample was analyzed on different instruments. In order to have the field independent scale, a dimensionless parameter, δ, was introduced. The magnitude of ä is calculated as follows.

$$\delta = \frac{B_{reference} - B_{sample}}{B_{reference}} \times 10^6 \text{ ppm}$$

where, B_{sample} = field strength for the resonance of protons of the sample, and

$B_{reference}$ = field strength for the resonance of protons of the reference compound.

The factor 10^6 is introduced to simplify the numerical values. Hence, δ values are always expressed in parts per million (ppm).

The chemical shift in δ can also be expressed as -

$$\delta = \frac{\upsilon_{sample} - \upsilon_{reference}}{\upsilon_{reference}} \times 10^6$$

where, $\nu_{sample} - \nu_{reference}$ is Δν,

$\nu_{reference}$ is the operating frequency and is given by the instrument manufacturer.

$$\therefore \delta = \frac{\Delta \nu}{\text{operating frequency of the instrument in cps or Hz}} \times 10^6$$

As seen before, for a particular proton, the chemical shift value, (Δν) of 120 Hz, at the operating frequency of 60 MHz, becomes 180 Hz if the spectrum is recorded at 90 MHz. If d values for this proton are recorded on two different instruments, with the operating frequencies of 60 MHz and 90 MHz, then the following values are obtained.

For the operating frequency of 60 MHz, Δν = 120 Hz.

$$\therefore \quad \delta = \frac{120}{60 \times 10^6} \times 10^6 = 2$$

For the operating frequency of 90 MHz, $\Delta \nu = 180$ MHz

$$\therefore \quad \delta = \frac{180}{90 \times 10^6} \times 10^6 = 2$$

Thus, δ values do not change from instrument to instrument. They remain same even when the operating frequencies are different. Hence, the chemical shift values expressed in terms of δ are independent of the strength of the magnetic field used or the RF used for the measurement.

Delta (δ) value for TMS is taken as zero since in this case, $\Delta\nu = 0$. Delta (δ) scale extends from 0-10. At the higher values of δ, protons experience the higher magnetic field (B_{eff}) and vice versa.

3) τ (Tau, Gr.) scale

The term, τ, is defined in terms of δ, as follows -

$$\tau = 10 - \delta$$

For TMS, $\delta = 0$. Hence, $\tau = (10 - 0) = 10$. Thus, on the τ scale, TMS peak appears at 10. As the value of τ increases, the protons require higher magnetic field to produce a peak in the spectrum. For protons with higher τ values, the value of B_{eff} is lower and vice versa.

4.2.6. Spin-Spin Coupling

When the NMR spectrum of a molecule is recorded using a low resolution NMR spectrometer, the peaks for the chemically non-equivalent protons are recorded at different chemical shift values. All these peaks are recorded as *singlets*.

When the NMR spectrum of the same molecule is recorded by using a high resolution NMR spectrometer, the splitting of the singlet into a doublet, triplet, quartet, quintet, sextet, septet, octet or a multiplet, is observed, i.e. a *fine structure* of the spectrum is seen. The multiplicity in the peaks arises because of the fact that the neighboring magnetic dipoles in the molecule interact with each other. The phenomenon of the splitting of a peak or a resonance band into a multiplet, in order to produce the fine structure of the spectrum, is called *spin-spin coupling* or *spin-spin splitting*.

4.2.6.1. Coupling to One Neighboring Nucleus (A-X spin system)

In order to understand how splitting of a resonance band occurs, consider a simple molecule, represented in **Fig. 4.17**, containing two protons, H_A and H_X, adjacent to each other.

```
      HA     Hx
      |      |
R1 —  C  ——  C — R4
      |      |
      R2     R3
```

$$R_1 \neq R_2 \neq R_3 \neq R_4 \neq H$$

Fig.4.17: A molecule representing A-X spin system

In this molecule, since four different groups are attached to two carbon atoms, the protons on these carbon atoms are chemically non-equivalent. Hence, the two protons produce signals at two different values of chemical shift. Under the low resolution, these protons produce two singlets, as shown in **Fig. 4.18(a)**. Under the high resolution, both the protons produce doublets. The fine spectrum is shown in **Fig. 4.18(b)**.

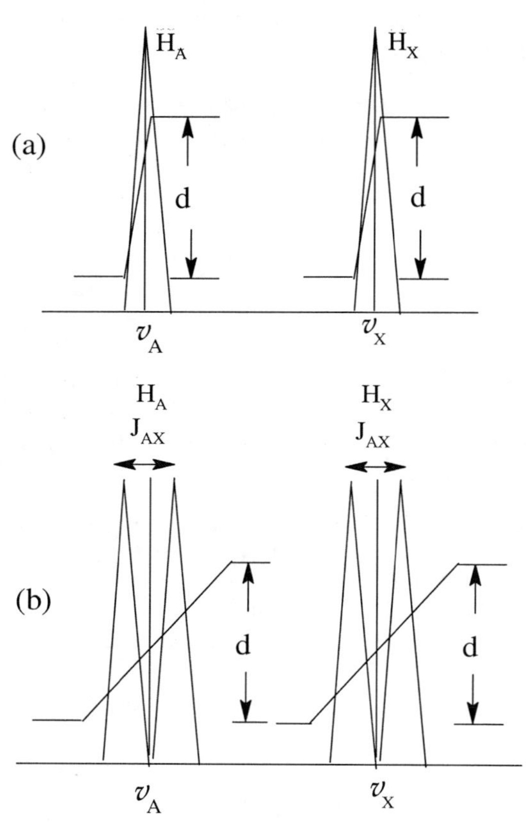

Fig. 4.18: (a) Low resolution and (b) high resolution NMR spectra for a molecule with A-X system

Each singlet which appears in the low resolution spectrum, splits into two peaks or a doublet in the high resolution spectrum. The distance between the two peaks of each doublet is called a *coupling constant* (J_{AX}).

(i) The coupling constant (J) is usually measured in Hertz (Hz)

(ii) Since the splitting is due solely to the nuclear magnetic moments [Refer to **equations (4.1)** and **(4.2)**] - unlike the chemical shift - it does not depend on the field strength used and therefore, does not differ from instrument to instrument. An increase in the field strength causes ν_A and ν_X to shift further apart but the value of J_{AX} remains the same for particular protons in a particular molecule.

(iii) For two interacting protons like H_A and H_X (**Fig. 4.17**), the value of J_{AX} is exactly same.

(iv) It should be noted that the chemical shift always corresponds to the middle of a doublet or a multiplet, which would be the position of the signal if there were no coupling.

Thus, the measurement of the chemical shift (δ) of protons gives idea of the chemical environment of protons, while J value gives idea about which two protons are interacting with each other. **Table 4.3** gives J values for different protons.

In **Fig. 4.18(a) and (b)**, the distance 'd' is obtained by integrating the peaks. It shows the number of protons responsible for producing that peak. Since, for both the peaks, the distance 'd' is same, both the peaks are produced due to equal number of protons (one proton in this case).

An explanation to the splitting of the resonance band into a doublet or an explanation to the spin-spin coupling phenomenon is given on the basis of the spin states of each proton with respect to that of its neighbor.

Consider the same molecule as shown in **Fig. 4.17**, containing two adjacent protons H_A and H_X in different chemical environments. Each proton H_A and H_X can spin either clockwise or anticlockwise. Hence, the two *spin orientations* or *states* are associated with both the protons. The spin states of two protons H_A and H_X can be represented diagrammatically, as shown in **Fig. 4.19**. The magnetic field experienced by a proton on one carbon atom is influenced by the spin states of the proton on the adjacent carbon atom. Proton H_A has two spin states and hence, it is associated with two magnetic fields, which are experienced by the adjacent proton H_X. Similarly, proton H_X has two spin states and hence, it is associated with two magnetic fields, which are experienced by the adjacent proton H_A. The magnitude of the two magnetic fields associated with each proton depends on their chemical environment. Hence, the two magnetic fields experienced by both the protons, H_A and H_X, are different. Therefore, each proton is associated with two precessional frequencies, ν_1 and ν_2 (for proton H_A) and ν_3 and ν_4 (for proton H_X).

Table 4.3: Spin-spin coupling constant (J) values for different protons

Sr. No.	Type of protons	J (Hz)
1.	H H R— C — C — R' R'' R'''	5 - 8
2.	Geminal protons on saturated carbon atom C (H)(H)	12 - 15
3.	Geminal protons on unsaturated carbon atom C= C (H)(H)	0.5 - 3
4.	Cis protons H C= C H	7 - 12
5.	Trans protons H C= C H	13 - 18
6.	Aromatic protons H H H H H H (benzene ring)	Ortho - 6 – 9 Meta - 1 – 3 Para - 0 - 1

Thus, if the spectrum is recorded at a constant magnetic field (B_o) and the sample is exposed to a mixture of radiofrequencies, one peak appears for a proton H_A, when ν_1 matches with the RF and another peak appears when ν_2 matches with the RF. Since there is little difference in these two frequencies (ν_1 and ν_2), the two peaks get recorded closer to each other. This results in a doublet for the proton H_A. Similarly, for the proton H_X, one peak appears when ν_3 matches with the RF and another peak appears when ν_4 matches with the RF. Thus, a doublet is seen for the proton H_X also.

From **Fig. 4.19**, it is clear that the statistical probabilities of the occurrence of the two spin states in both the protons is same (1:1) and therefore, the intensity of both the peaks in a doublet or all the four peaks in two doublets is equal.

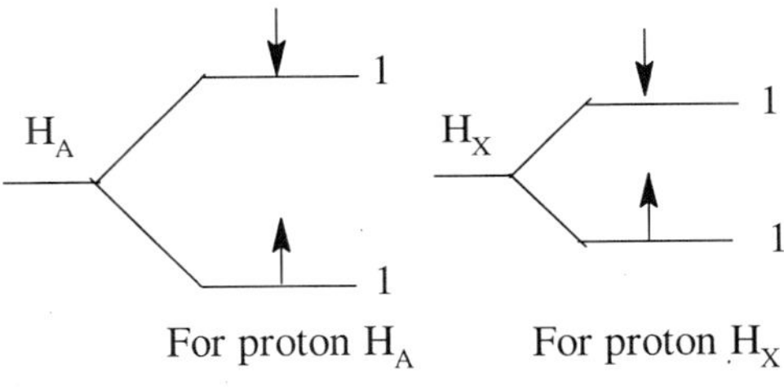

Fig. 4.19: Spin orientation of protons H_A and H_X for an AX system

4.2.6.2. Coupling to Two Equivalent Neighboring Nuclei (AX_2 spin system)

Under the low resolution, the NMR spectrum of the compound shown in **Fig. 4.20**, produces two peaks of different integrations (d and 2d, as shown in **Fig. 4.21**), whose ratio is 1: 2.

Under the high resolution, the same molecule shows a fine spectrum as shown in **Fig. 4.21(b)**. The proton H_A appears as a triplet. The two protons, H_{X1} and H_{X2}, are chemically equivalent and appear as a doublet. When these peaks are integrated, an integration corresponding to a distance, 'd', is obtained for the peak for C-H proton (H_A) and the integration corresponding to a distance, '2d', is obtained for the peak for CH_2 protons (H_{X1} and H_{X2}). The appearance of a doublet and a triplet can be explained based on the spin states of the nuclei H_A, H_{X1} and H_{X2}.

For a single proton H_A, as seen before, the parallel (clockwise) and antiparallel (anticlockwise) spins are possible, as shown in **Fig. 4.19**. Since the

H_A H_{X1}

R_1—C—C—R_3

R_2 H_{X2}

$R_1 \neq R_2 \neq R_3 \neq H$

Fig. 4.20: A molecule representing AX_2 spin system

proton H_A produces two different fields, these two fields are experienced by the two protons H_{X1} and H_{X2}, adjacent to it. Hence, these two protons precess with the precessional frequencies ν_1 and ν_2 and therefore, protons H_{X1} and H_{X2} appear as a doublet. Since, two protons are responsible for producing this doublet, the integration of this peak is '2d'.

For two protons H_{X1} and H_{X2}, there are three different spin combinations as follows.

(i) As shown in **Fig. 4.22**, two protons, H_{X1} and H_{X2}, can be parallel to each other and can spin along the direction of the field (α, α orientation).

(ii) The two protons, H_{X1} and H_{X2}, can be parallel to each other and can spin in the direction opposite to the direction of the field (β, β orientation).

(iii) The two protons, H_{X1} and H_{X2}, can be antiparallel to each other with (α, β orientation) or (β, α orientation).

(iv) Since the two protons, H_{X1} and H_{X2}, assume three different orientations, they produce three different magnetic fields, which are experienced by the adjacent proton H_A. Since, this proton H_A experiences three fields, it precesses with three different precessional frequencies, ν_3, ν_4 and ν_5. Hence, it resonates with three different radiofrequencies and produces three peaks.

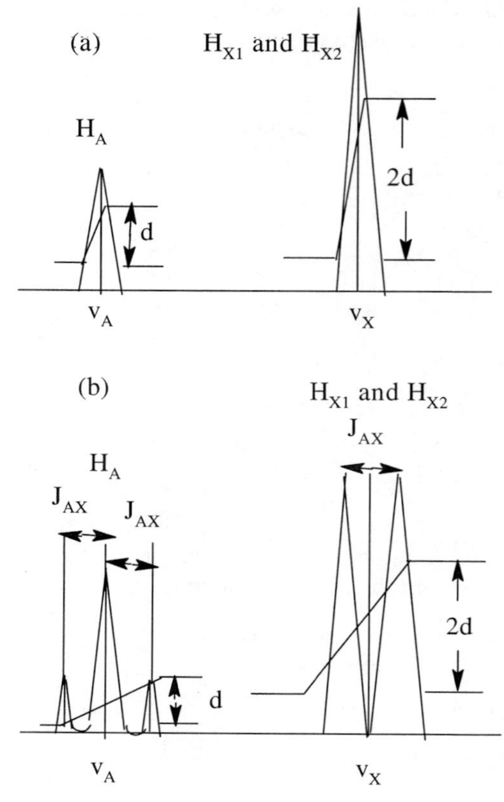

Fig. 4.21: (a) Low resolution and (b) high resolution NMR spectra for a molecule with AX_2 system.

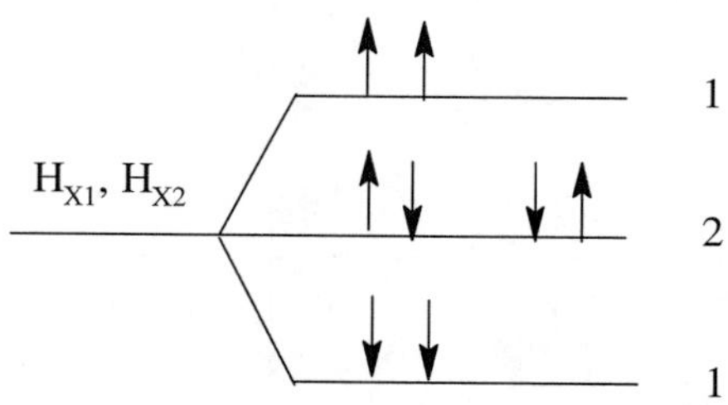

Fig. 4.22: Spin combination of protons H_{X1} and H_{X2} for an AX_2 system

If the spins of H_{X1} and H_{X2} are antiparellel, [(α, β) or (β, α)], then their magnetic fields get cancelled with each other and they do not contribute to any additional field. Hence, the resonance signal corresponding to that orientation is in the position which would occupy if there were no coupling. Two parallel spin arrangements [(α, α)) or (β, β)] provide two different magnetic fields and contribute to two more resonance signals. A triplet is thus observed for the proton H_A. Since the probability of getting antiparellel spins, ((α, β) or (β, α), is double the probability of getting parallel spins, (α, α)) or (β, β), the ratio of the intensities of the three peaks in a triplet is 1: 2:1. Since H_A, H_{X1} and H_{X2} are interacting, the distance between the two peaks (J_{AX}) in a doublet for H_{X1} and H_{X2} and for two consecutive peaks in a triplet for H_A is same. Since a triplet is obtained for one proton (H_A), the integration for the triplet peak corresponds to a distance, 'd'.

4.2.6.3. Coupling to Three or More Equivalent Neighboring Nuclei (AX_n spin system)

Consider a molecule shown in **Fig. 4. 23.**

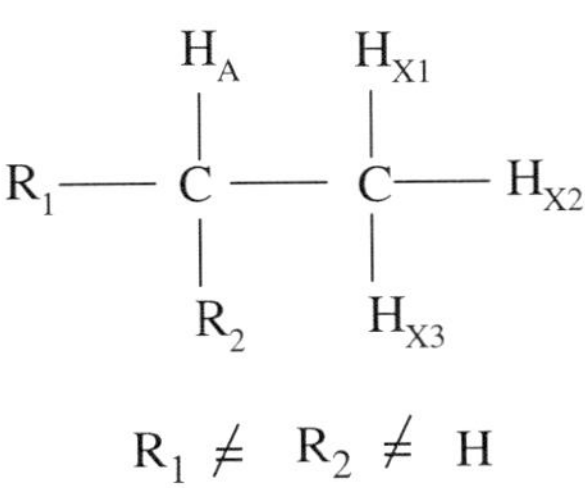

Fig. 4.23: A molecule representing AX_n spin system

Under the low resolution, the NMR spectrum of this compound shows two peaks of different heights as shown in **Fig. 4.24(a),** whose ratio is 1: 3.

Under the high resolution, this molecule shows a fine structure as shown in **Fig. 4.24(b)**. The proton H_A can spin clockwise and anticlockwise. Thus, it can produce two fields, one in the direction of the external magnetic field and another in the direction opposite to that of the external magnetic field. These two fields produced by H_A are felt by all the three protons H_{X1}, H_{X2} and H_{X3}, which are present on the adjacent carbon atom. Hence, a doublet is obtained for these three methyl protons, the integration for which is '3d'.

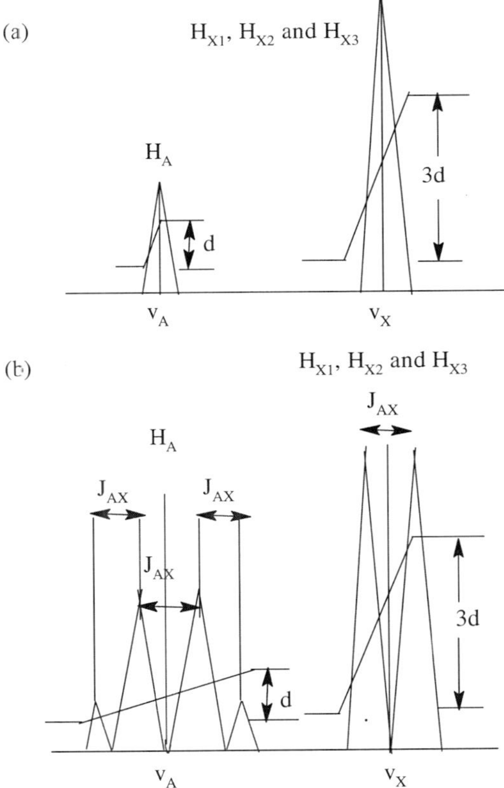

Fig. 4.24: (a) Low resolution and (b) high resolution NMR spectra for a molecule with AX_n system

The three methyl protons, H_{X1}, H_{X2} and H_{X3}, can assume four spin orientations as shown in **Fig. 4.25**. Because of these four orientations, the three methyl protons produce four magnetic fields, which are experienced by the neighboring proton, H_A. Hence, this proton H_A can assume four different precessional frequencies, ν_3, ν_4, ν_5 and ν_6, each of which when corresponds to the applied RF, produces a peak. Thus, the proton H_A appears as a quartet. As shown in **Fig. 4.25**, since the probability of assuming four orientations is in the ratio of 1: 3: 3: 1, the intensity of four peaks in the quartet is also in the ratio of 1: 3: 3: 1. Since the quartet is produced for one single proton, the integration for the quartet corresponds to the distance 'd'.

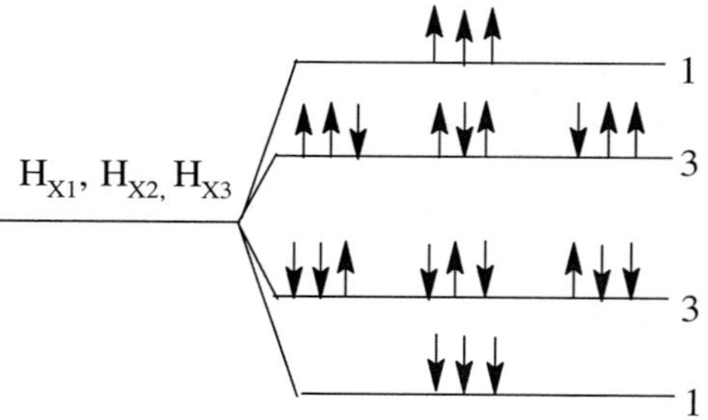

Fig. 4.25: Spin orientation of protons H_{X1}, H_{X2} and H_{X3} in AXn system

4.2.7. Chemical Exchange

Consider a molecule of ethanol as shown in **Fig. 4.26**.

```
     H     H
     |     |
  H—C — C—OH
     |     |
     H     H
```

Fig. 4.26: A molecule of ethanol

Under the low resolution, the spectrum of ethanol appears as three singlets. One singlet is for the methyl protons (CH_3), whose integration corresponds to 3 protons, another singlet is for the methylene protons (CH_2), corresponding to the integration of 2 protons and the third one is for the hydroxyl proton (OH), corresponding to the integration of 1 proton. This is shown in **Fig. 4.27(a)**.

Under the high resolution, because of the spin-spin coupling, the fine structure of the spectrum is seen as shown in **Fig. 4.27(b)**. The fine spectrum shows a triplet for the methyl protons (CH_3), a quartet for the methylene protons (CH_2) and a singlet for the hydroxyl proton (OH). Three methyl protons orient in four different states as shown in **Fig. 4.25** and they produce four magnetic fields, which are felt by the neighboring methylene protons. Hence, a quartet is obtained for the two methylene protons. The two methylene protons orient in three different manners as shown in **Fig. 4.22**. Therefore, they produce three magnetic fields, which are felt by the neighboring methyl protons and hence, methyl protons appear as a triplet.

Three different magnetic fields produced by the methylene protons are experienced by the hydroxyl proton (OH) as well, but the expected multiplicity of the hydroxyl proton is not observed in the high resolution NMR spectrum of ethanol, which usually contains acidic or basic impurities. The expected multiplicity for the hydroxyl proton is observed only if the sample of ethanol is extremely pure. This is shown in **Fig. 4.27(c)**.

The reason for not getting the expected multiplicity for OH proton in a molecule of ethanol is explained based on the phenomenon called *chemical exchange*. The protons attached to the oxygen (O-H), nitrogen (N-H) or sulphur (S-H) atoms can form hydrogen bonds, they can undergo exchange and they possess varying degrees of acidic character. Such protons are called *easily exchangeable protons*. The term *chemical exchange* is used to indicate the presence of a particular proton in different molecules of the same sample. For example, at a given period of time, the

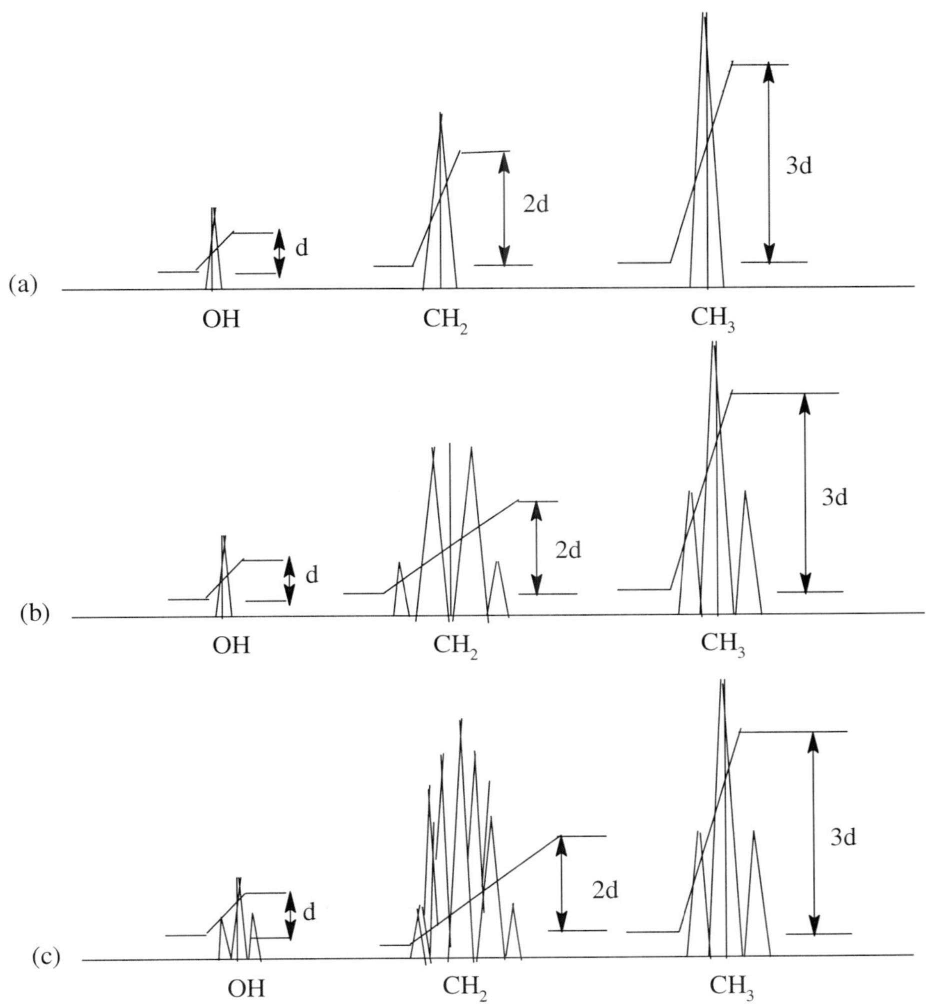

Fig. 4.27: (a) Low resolution and (b) high resolution NMR spectra for ethanol (c) high resolution NMR spectrum of extremely pure ethanol

hydroxyl proton from one molecule of ethanol can get associated with the other molecules of ethanol from the same sample. This is shown in **Fig. 4.28**.

$$2CH_3\,CH_2\,OH \longrightarrow CH_3CH_2O^- + CH_3\,CH_2\,\overset{+}{O}H_2$$

Non-protonated ethanol — Protonated ethanol

Fig. 4.28: Chemical exchange in ethyl alcohol

The rate of transfer of this proton from one molecule to the other, i.e. the rate of chemical exchange, in highly purified sample of ethyl alcohol is relatively slow, but this rate is markedly increased by the acidic or basic impurities. These impurities, which are usually present in ethanol, catalyze the exchange of hydroxyl protons between ethanol molecules. If the rate of chemical exchange is very slow, the hydroxyl proton remains on the oxygen atom for the sufficient period and can experience the three magnetic fields produced by the two methylene protons. Under this situation, the hydroxyl proton shows an expected triplet. The peak for CH_2 protons is also split by the hydroxyl proton and the methylene protons appear as a multiplet. On the contrary, if the chemical exchange is rapid, the O-H proton can remain in association with many ethyl alcohol molecules. The same proton is present in two chemical environments, either in a non-protonated ethyl alcohol molecule (CH_3-CH_2-OH) or in the protonated ethyl alcohol molecule (CH_3-CH_2-$^{+}OH_2$.). Thus, this proton appears as a sharp singlet and the chemical shift for this proton is determined by the average chemical environment it experiences in the protonated and the non-protonated molecules. Similarly, the peak for the methylene protons will not be split by the hydroxyl proton if the rapid chemical exchange of O-H proton occurs and it would appear only as a quartet and not as a multiplet.

If the rate of chemical exchange is much slower than the frequency separation of the components of the multiplet, in the absence of exchange, the anticipated multiplicity of both, the hydroxyl and the methylene protons, will be observed. When the rate of chemical exchange is of the same order of the magnitude as the frequency separation of the components of the multiplet, in the absence of exchange, the instantaneous spin orientations are only partially averaged and a broad peak results. The maximum width of this broad peak is the width of the multiplet observed in the absence of rapid chemical exchange.

4.2.8. Multiplicity Rules

The splitting of a peak into a number of peaks in the NMR spectrum of a molecule takes place according to the certain rules, discussed below.

1) The chemically and magnetically equivalent nuclei do not interact or couple. Hence, they produce a singlet. Protons are said to be magnetically equivalent when they have identical screening constant (σ.) Most of the times, such protons are also chemically equivalent. For example, three protons in a methyl group (CH_3) in propyne CH_3–C≡H are equivalent, but the three protons in a methyl group and one proton in –C≡H group are chemically non-equivalent. Though they are chemically non-equivalent, they are magnetically equivalent because of the presence of a triple bond in a molecule. Hence, a separate peak for C≡H proton, downfield to the methyl protons, is not observed, but a singlet at δ =1.8, corresponding to all the four protons is observed. Thus, magnetically equivalent protons produce peak at the same δ value.
2) The multiplicity M, i.e. the number of lines in a multiplet can be calculated by using **equatation (4.8)**.

$$M = 2nI + 1 \quad \ldots (4.8)$$

where, n is the number of equivalent neighboring nuclei and I is the spin quantum number. For nuclei with I = 1/2 (e.g. proton), the above equation reduces to M = n + 1.
For couplings to nuclei with I = 1/2, the signal intensities within each multiplet correspond to the coefficient of the binomial series, which can be obtained from *Pascal's triangle*, shown in **Table 4.4**.
3) If the protons have interacting protons on both the adjacent atoms, as shown in the molecule in **Fig. 4.29**, then the multiplicity of protons (*CH_2), is expressed as follows.

$$M = (2\, n_A I_A+1)\,(2n_B\, I_B +1)$$

where, n_A and n_B are the number of interacting protons on either side of protons and I_A and I_B are the spin quantum numbers. Since $I_A = I_B$ =1/2 for protons, the above formula reduces to-

$$M \equiv (n_A + 1)(n_B + 1)$$

Since $n_A \equiv n_B \equiv 2$ for $*CH_2$ protons in the molecule shown in **Fig. 4.29**, M = (2 + 1) (2 + 1) = 3 x 3 = 9.

Thus, $*CH_2$ protons appear as nine lines or as three triplets.

(A) (B)

$$R - CH_2 - {*CH_2} - CH_2 - R'$$

Fig. 4.29: A molecule having interacting protons on both the sides

If $R = R'$ i.e. if R and R′ are identical, then the protons A and B are chemically and magnetically equivalent. In this case, the $*CH_2$ protons appear as a pentet (quintet).

$$M = (n + 1) = 4 + 1 = 5$$

4.2.9. Signals for Easily Exchangeable Protons

The protons bonded to electronegative elements like O, N or S can be easily characterized from the NMR spectra of the corresponding deuterated samples. For example, when deuterium oxide (D_2O) is added to ethanol, the hydroxyl proton of ethanol is replaced by deuterium, as shown in **Fig. 4.30**. This is termed as *deuterium exchange*. Deuterium exchange is not very common with protons attached to carbon atoms since these protons are not easily replaceable by deuterium. Protons on carbon atoms can be deuterated, only if they are present on the carbon atom, alpha to a keto (CO) group or a nitrile group (CN).

$$C_2H_5OH + D_2O \rightleftharpoons C_2H_5OD + DHO$$

Fig. 4.30: Deuterium exchange in ethanol

The rate of exchange of a proton depends on the electronegativity of the element attached to it. The more the electronegativity of an element, the higher is the rate of exchange. Hence, the rate of exchange of N-H and S-H protons in the non-aqueous media is much slower than that of O-H protons. The peak for DHO, obtained during deuterium exchange with ethanol protons, occurs at about $\delta = 4.88$.

There is no definite range for the chemical shift values (δ) of the easily exchangeable protons like O–H, N–H and S–H, since their chemical shifts are subjected to considerable variations. These chemical shifts are influenced by the solvent used

Table 4.4: Pascal s triangle indicating signal intensities within each multiplet

n = 0 (singlet)							1						
n = 1 (doublet)						1		1					
n = 2 (triplet)					1		2		1				
n = 3 (quartet)				1		3		3		1			
n = 4 (quintet)			1		4		6		4		1		
n = 5 (sextet)		1		5		10		10		5		1	
n = 6 (septet)	1		6		15		20		15		6		1

to dissolve an analyte, the concentration of an analyte, the temperature of the solution, and the impurities such as water, present in the analyte solution. The measured δ values are reproducible only under the well defined experimental conditions. The signals for the O–H protons may be found anywhere in the spectrum, whereas the signals for the S–H and N–H protons usually fall within narrower regions. The exchange of N–H protons in amides usually does not occur so readily and hence, these protons can couple with the neighboring protons, thereby bringing about the splitting of the peaks in their NMR spectrum. The chemical shift ranges for the O–H, N–H and S–H protons in different functional groups are given in **Table 4.5**.

Table 4.5: Chemical shift ranges for O–H, N–H and S–H protons in different functional groups

Types of proton	Functional group	δ (H) ppm
O–H	Alcohols	1-5
	Phenols	4-10
	Acids	9-13
	Enols	10-17
N–H	Amines	1-5
	Amides	5-6.5
	Amido Group in Peptides	7-10
S–H	Thiols-Aliphatic	1-2.5
	Thiols-Aromatic	3.4

4.2.10. Spin–Spin Decoupling

The spin–spin coupling occurs because of the interaction of the magnetic fields of the adjacent protons. It is observed only under high resolution. It produces the fine structure of the spectrum, i.e. the multiplicity of the peaks for protons is observed. Because of the multiplicity, the spectrum under high resolution becomes complex. This complexity in the spectrum can be removed by *spin-spin decoupling*. This can be achieved in two ways.

1) Isotope exchange

The protons attached to the electronegative atoms, such as oxygen, nitrogen or sulphur, can be easily replaced by deuterium. The isotope exchange, i.e. the replacement of active or easily exchangeable protons in an analyte by deuterium, reduces the number of protons in the compound. This automatically reduces the number of peaks in the NMR spectrum and makes a complex spectrum a simple one.

2) Nuclear magnetic double resonance technique (NMDR)

In the nuclear magnetic double resonance technique, a nucleus is subjected to two radiofrequencies, one is called an *applied frequency* (ν_1) and the other one is called an *irradiation frequency* (RF). For an AX system (**Fig. 4.17**), if a constant magnetic field B_o, is applied, then the proton H_A precesses with the frequency ν_A and the proton H_X precesses with the frequency ν_X. In the normal spectrum, (**Fig. 4.18**) two doublets are seen for both these protons when the sample is exposed to a mixture of radiofrequencies and the resonance is obtained for the match of ν_A and ν_X, separately.

In the double resonance technique, apart from the RF, the molecule is irradiated with a second RF signal (ν_X), which corresponds to the precessional frequency of H_X. When this RF is applied, the proton Hx flips and undergoes rapid changes in its spin state. Under this condition, the neighboring proton H_A, is aware of only one equivalent spin state of H_X and therefore, H_A shows only a singlet. Thus, the double irradiation of H_X effectively decouples the signal from H_A [**Fig. 4.31(b)**]. Similarly, if the proton H_A is irradiated with a second frequency (ν_A), which matches with its precessional frequency, the signal for H_X appears as a singlet [**Fig. 4.31(c)**]. Thus, the simplicity in the spectrum is observed after irradiating the nucleus with double frequencies.

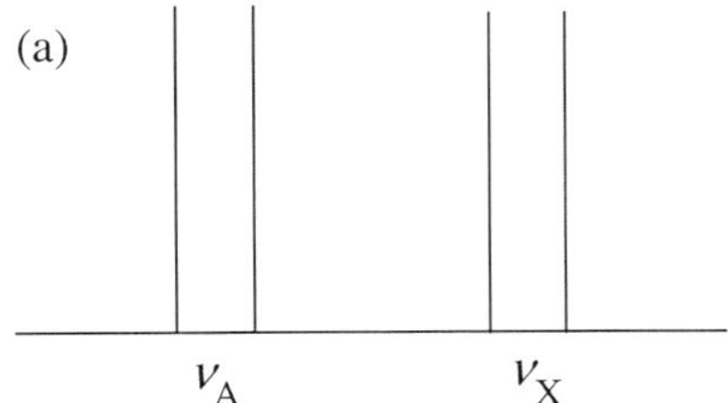

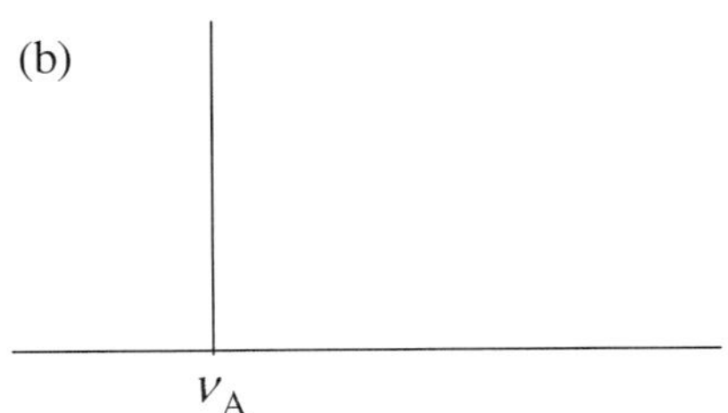

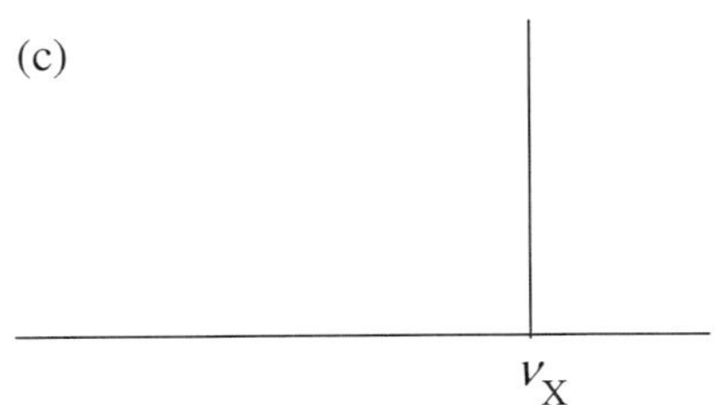

Fig. 4.31: (a) A normal spectrum for A-X system (b) double irradiation of H_X (c) double irradiation of H_A

4.2.11. Applications of NMR Spectrometry

The NMR spectrometry has continued to develop so rapidly because of the number of applications. Some of the applications are mentioned below.

4.2.11.1. General Applications

1) The chemical shift values in the NMR spectrum of a compound provide an excellent means to predict the chemical environment of various protons in the molecule.
2) The total number of protons in a molecule can be found out from the electronic integration of all the peaks in the NMR spectrum of a compound.
3) The easily exchangeable or active protons in a molecule can be identified by performing deuterium exchange.
4) The NMR spectrometry can be used to monitor the chemical reactions by distinguishing between the peaks for the reactants and products of the reaction. For example, nitrobenzene would produce peaks in its NMR spectrum only in the range of $\delta = 6 - 8$, a range characteristic of the aromatic protons. When it is reduced to get aniline, the additional broad peak for two protons in an amino group, is observed in the range of $\delta = 4 - 5.5$.
5) From the rate at which the products are formed or the reactants disappear, the rates of chemical reactions can be found out.

4.2.11.2. More Specific Applications

1) To study rotation about C-C single bond when both the carbon atoms have sp^3 hybridization

The rotation between the two sp^3 hybridized carbon atoms in ethane is so fast that it cannot be slowed down even at low temperatures and hence, it cannot be studied. The rotation between the two sp^3 hybridized carbon atoms in the halogenated ethanes (**Fig. 4.32**) and t-butyl-substituted ethanes is not very fast and can be slowed down by reducing the temperature and hence, can be studied.

Fig. 4.32: Fixed configuration of chloroethane (I)

The NMR spectrum of chloroethane [**Fig. 4.33(a)**] at room temperature, would show two peaks, one for 3 equivalent methyl protons and another for 2 equivalent methylene protons. This is because at room temperature, the rotation about C-C single bond is so fast that the three methyl protons and the two methylene protons experience the average chemical environment. The average chemical environment experienced by the three methyl protons is different than that experienced by the two methylene protons since a chloro group is attached directly to the methylene group, whereas the methyl group is attached directly to the methylene group. Hence, the two distinct peaks are obtained for the methyl and the methylene protons at different values of ä. If the rotation around C-C single bond is frozen by lowering down the temperature, a fixed configuration [**Fig. 4.32 (I)**] would be observed. This would create the non-equivalence within the three methyl protons and also within the two methylene protons. This leads to a more complex NMR spectrum [**Fig. 4.33(b)**], in which the methyl protons appear as a triplet and the methylene protons appear as a quartet. From the temperature at which the fine structure of the spectrum is seen, the values of free enthalpy of activation (Δ G) can be calculated. With this data, the rate of rotation and the energy barrier to rotation can be calculated.

2) To study rotation about a partial double bond

Dimethylamides are most suitable to study rotation about a partial double bond from the NMR

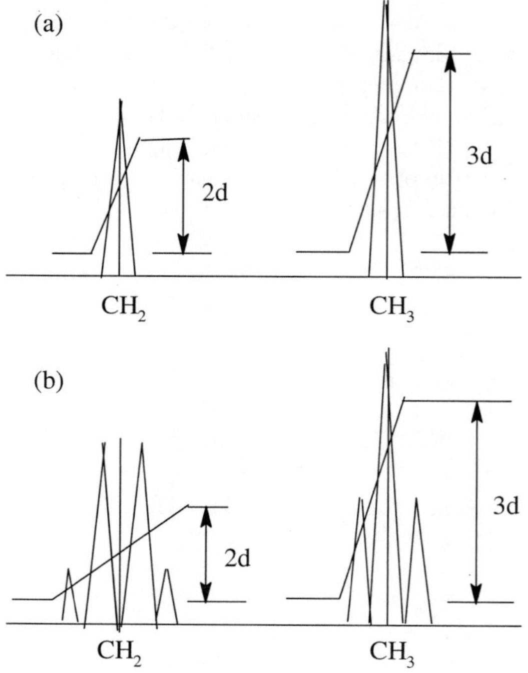

Fig. 4.33: Spectrum of chloroethane (a) at room temperature and (b) at temperature lower than room temperature

spectrometry. The highest free enthalpy of activation for dimethyl formamide [**(II), Fig. 4.34**] can be found from its NMR spectrometric data. Delocalization of an electron pair on the N atom of dimethylformamide leads to the formation of a resonating form, in which a double bond exists between carbon and nitrogen atoms.

Fig. 4.34: Dimethylformamide (II)

The free rotation of the $N(CH_3)_2$ group about N – C single bond is very fast at high temperatures. Because of this, both the methyl groups on the nitrogen atom become equivalent. This produces a sharp singlet corresponding to six protons in the NMR spectrum of N, N-dimethylformamide. As the temperature is lowered down, the rotation of the $N(CH_3)_2$ group about N – C single bond is slowed down. Therefore, each methyl group spends enough time in a particular chemical environment. One methyl group is on the side of oxygen atom attached to the adjacent carbon atom, whereas another methyl group is on the side of hydrogen atom attached to the adjacent carbon atom. Thus, the chemical environments of the two methyl groups are different and hence, these two methyl groups become magnetically and chemically non-equivalent. Thus, with the lowering of the temperature, a sharp peak slowly goes on broadening first. As the temperature is lowered down further, two broad peaks start appearing. Finally, below 60 °C, two sharp resonance signals for two methyl groups appear in the spectrum. The peaks for two CH_3 groups in the NMR spectrum of N, N-dimethylformamide at various temperatures are shown in **Fig. 4.35**. The free enthalpy of activation (ΔG) is found to be 20.9 ± 0.2 Kcal mol^{-1}

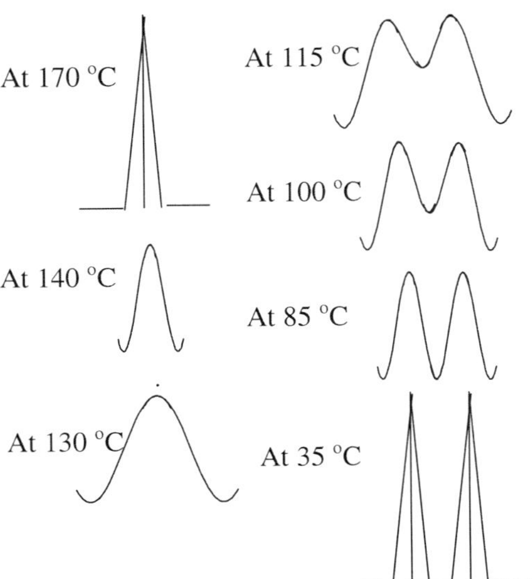

Fig. 4.35: The peaks for two CH_3 groups in the NMR spectrum of N, N- dimethylformamide at various temperatures

at T = 393 K. With this data, the rate of rotation and the energy barrier to rotation can be calculated.

In thioamides **(III)**, shown in **Fig. 4.36**, the ΔG values are 2 - 4 Kcal mol^{-1} higher than in the amides with the same substituents.

Fig. 4.36: Thioamide (III)

3) To study the rate of inversion of nitrogen atom

Consider a trivalent nitrogen atom with three different substituents on it. Such a compound has pyramidal structure. When all the three substituents attached to such a nitrogen atom are different, this compound exists as two enantiomers as shown in **Fig. 4.37**.

The system **(IV)**, as shown in **Fig. 4.37**,

Fig. 4.37: Enantiomers of a compound with trivalent nitrogen in system (IV)

undergoes rapid inversion. The spectra of these two enantiomers are identical in achiral solvents and hence, the inversion cannot be studied. In order to study the inversion, a prochiral group, such as a benzyl (Ph-CH_2) or an isopropyl group [-CH $(CH_3)_2$], should be introduced into a molecule. In system **(IV)**, if R_1 is the benzyl group, R_2 is the methyl group and R_3 is the methoxy group, then a molecule as shown in system **(V)** in **Fig. 4.38** is obtained. In these two enantiomers, the rate of inversion is temperature dependent. As the temperature is lowered, the two benzylic protons, H_A and H_B, experience different chemical environments and can produce different peaks. The ΔG value at this stage is recorded as 12.7 Kcal.mol^{-1} at the temperature of 257 K. The rate of inversion can then be calculated from this data.

Fig. 4.38: Enantiomers of a compound with trivalent nitrogen in system (V)

4) To study keto-enol tautomerism

Keto-enol tautomerism is best studied with the help of a molecule of acetylacetone **(VI)**. It is an example of a β-diketone, which forms stable enols.

Fig. 4.39: Keto-enol tautomerism in acetylacetone (VI)

At room temperature, acetylacetone remains in the ketone as well as in the enol form in 1:4 ratio. The proportion of the enol form is more since it is stabilized by the intramolecular hydrogen bonding as shown in **Fig. 4.39**. The rate of conversion of a keto form to an enol form is very fast at higher temperatures, but as the temperature is lowered below 43 °C, the conversion is slowed down. Hence, below this temperature, the signal of the olefinic proton H_A in the enol, is seen at $\delta = 5.62$, and the methylene protons, H_A and H_B, in the ketone, are seen at $\delta = 3.66$ (**Fig. 4.40**). The comparison of the intensities for the olefinic proton (CH) and for the methylene protons (CH_2) shows that the equilibrium mixture contains more molecules in the enol form than in the keto form. The ratio of the tautomers is best determined from the ratio of the integration of the signal for methyl groups in enol to the integration of the signal for methyl groups in the keto form. This ratio is found to be about 80: 20. As shown in **Fig. 4.40**, the methyl protons in the enol form appear at $\delta = 2.0$ and that in the keto form appear at $\delta = 2.2$. The signal of the strongly acidic hydrogen bonded OH proton is obtained at $\delta = 15.5$. If the temperature of the mixture is increased, then the methyl protons appear at the average δ value for both the forms.

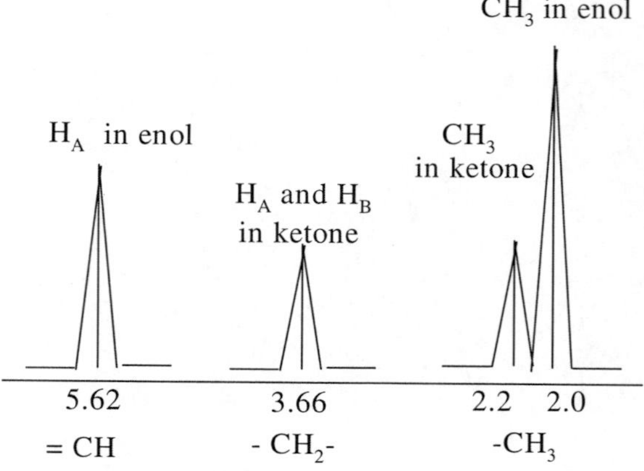

Fig. 4.40: Peaks for different protons in keto and enol forms of acetylacetone in the ^{1}H NMR spectrum at low temperature (20 °C)

Similarly, the peaks for the olefinic (CH) proton and for the methylene (CH_2) protons are also averaged. If triethylamine is added to the mixture, the keto form entirely gets converted to the enol form, since the enol form is stabilized by a strong hydrogen bonding between the amine nitrogen and the hydroxyl proton.

5) To study conformational isomerism

At room temperature, the cyclohexane molecule undergoes rapid inter-conversion from one chair form **(VII a)** to another **(VII b)**. This inter-conversion is shown in **Fig. 4.41**.

When this conversion takes place, the proton which is axial (H_a*) in one chair form, **(VII a)**, becomes equatorial (H_e*) in another chair form, **(VII b)**, because of flipping of the ring. Similarly, the proton which is equatorial in **(VII a)** becomes axial in **(VII b)**.

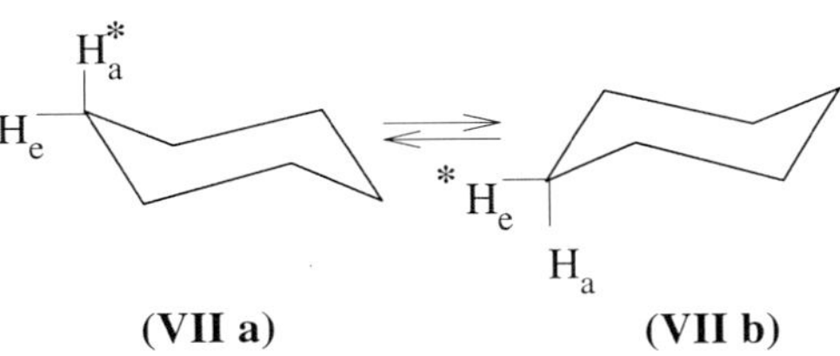

Fig. 4.41: Chair forms of cyclohexane

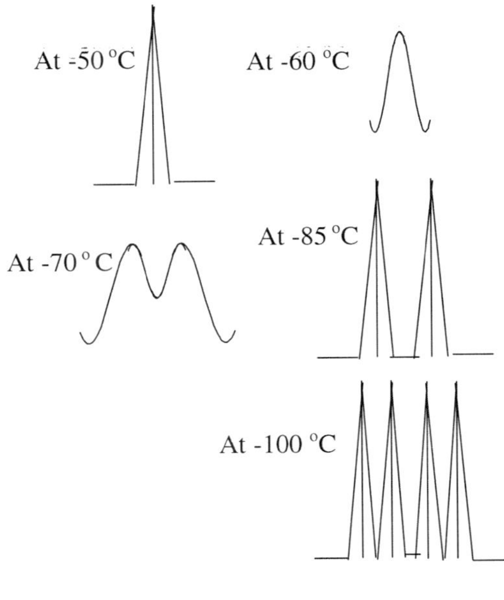

Fig. 4.42: The NMR spectrum of cyclohexane at different temperatures

At temperatures above -50 °C, this inter-conversion is so fast that one cannot differentiate between the axial proton and the equatorial proton. Hence, only a sharp singlet is seen at a chemical shift which corresponds to the average environment experienced by each proton. As the temperature is lowered down, the sharp singlet goes on broadening. With the further lowering of the temperature to -70 °C, two broad peaks start appearing, one peak corresponding to an axial proton and another corresponding to an equatorial proton. At -85 °C, two sharp singlets are observed. Ultimately, as shown in **Fig. 4.42**, at -100 °C, these two singlets appear as two doublets. The spin-spin coupling occurs between the axial and the equatorial protons, which appear as two doublets. A doublet appearing more downfield (away form TMS), corresponds to the equatorial protons and that appearing upfield (more towards TMS), corresponds to the more shielded axial protons.

6) To differentiate between cis and trans isomers

This can be well explained with the example of 2,6-dimethyl-1-benzylpiperidine, as shown in **Fig. 4.43**.

In the trans isomer, there is no plane of symmetry since one methyl group is in front of the plane and another methyl group is behind the plane. Hence, the two protons H_A and H_B in the benzylic methylene group are magnetically non-equivalent. Since only one methyl group is responsible in splitting the peaks for benzylic methylene group, a resonance peak in the form of a quartet (3+1), corresponding to the integration of 2 protons, at ä = 3.41 and J = 13.2 Hz, is observed [**Fig. 4.44(b)**].

H_3C N CH_3 H_B C H_A (a) Cis

H_3C N CH_3 H_B C H_A (b) Trans

Fig. 4.43: 2,6-Dimethyl-1-benzylpiperidine

In the cis isomer, because of the plane of symmetry, the protons on both the methyl groups are magnetically equivalent. Hence, benzylic methylene protons appear as a sharp singlet at δ=3.47, corresponding to the integration of 2 protons [**Fig. 4.44(a)**].

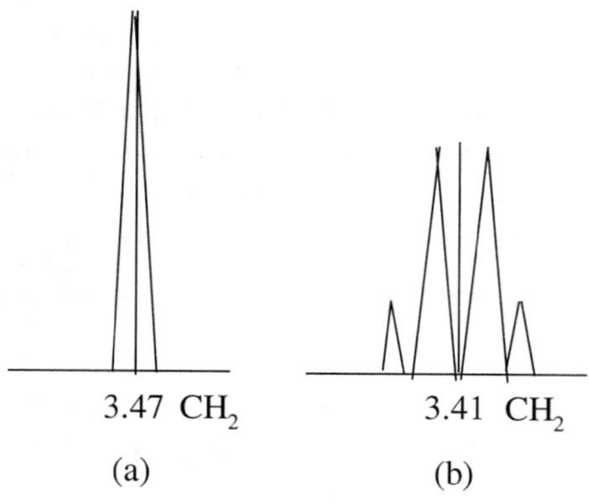

Fig. 4.44: Differentiating peaks for (a) cis form and (b) trans form of 2,6 dimethyl-1-benzylpiperidine in the NMR spectrum

4.2.12. Sample Preparation in NMR Spectrometry

Liquids and solids are commonly analyzed by NMR spectrometry. *Neat* or pure liquids can be analyzed directly if they are less viscous, but viscous liquids need dilution with a proper solvent. The sample size for NMR spectrometry is 35-50 mg of solid or 0.35 to 0.5 ml of liquid. The solvent used to dissolve sample should satisfy the following conditions.

1) It should be chemically inert.
2) It should be magnetically isotropic.
3) It should be volatile in nature so that the sample can be easily recovered after the analysis.
4) It should not produce any peak in the NMR spectrum, i.e. the solvent should be devoid of any protons. The solvents containing protons should be deuterated so that the protons are replaced by deuterium.
5) The solvents such as carbon tetrachloride (CCl_4), deuterated chloroform ($CDCl_3$), water (D_2O), methanol (CD_3OD), dimethyl sulphoxide (CD_3SOCD_3), acetic acid (CD_3COOD), etc. can be used for recording NMR spectra.

The sample solution is filled in the NMR sample tubes. In order to keep all the protons in the sample, in the homogeneous magnetic field, the sample is kept spinning at a speed of around 30 rps. If the spinning speed is lower than this, the field averaging is incomplete and broad resonance lines occur. If the speed is higher than 30 rps, it results in the *ringing effect*, producing peaks even on the negative side of the base line, as shown in **Fig. 4.45**.

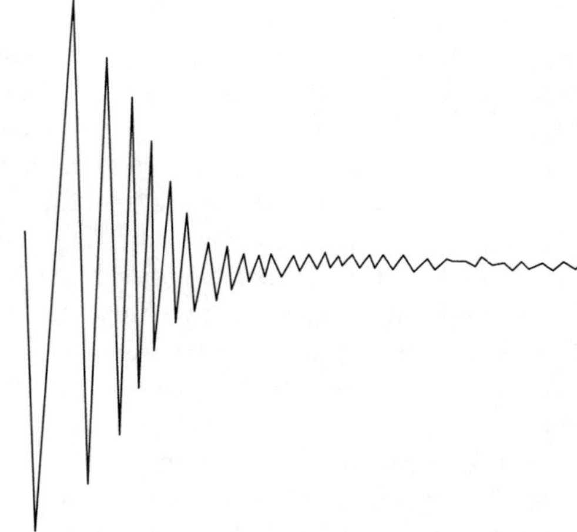

Fig. 4.45: Ringing effect in NMR spectrum

4.2.13. The Time Domain and the Frequency Domain–Fourier Transformation

Whenever the quantity of a sample or the solubility of a sample in a suitable solvent is limited, Fourier Transform (FT) NMR spectrometry is of special importance. We have seen that when the sample is kept in the external magnetic field (B_o), the nuclei distribute themselves in the upper and the lower energy levels, based on the Boltzmann statistics. The nuclei in the upper level produce magnetization in the opposite direction of the field and the nuclei in the lower level, produce magnetization in the direction of the external magnetic field. Since the number of nuclei in the lower level (N_α) is more than the number of nuclei in the upper level (N_β), the net macroscopic magnetization (M_o) is along the direction of the field.

When the pulse is applied and then switched off, the magnetization vector M_o, is deflected from its equilibrium position through an angle θ. The angle, through which it is deflected, depends upon the time period (T_p) for which the pulse is applied. The vector, M_o, like the individual spins, precesses about the Z-axis with the Larmour frequency, ν_L. Its orientation at any instant is specified in the stationary co-ordinate system by the three components, M_X, M_Y and M_Z, which vary with time. This is as shown in **Fig. 4.46**.

During relaxation, the spin system reverts to its equilibrium state with M_Z increasing slowly to its original value M_o, while M_X and M_Y approach zero.

When a rotating co-ordinate system X', Y' and Z' is considered, after the pulse, M_o lies along Y' axis at the instant t = 0, as shown in **Fig. 4.48(a)** and hence, $M_o = M_{Y'}$. As the Y' axis rotates at the Larmour frequency of the nuclei, the transverse magnetization in the Y' direction remains constant. The magnitude of $M_{Y'}$ depends on the number of nuclei contributing to the precession in the direction of the magnetic field. As the nuclei start relaxing, they flip and change the orientation of spin, thereby reducing the value of $M_{Y'}$ with time. Thus, when the pulse is applied, the nuclei, i.e. dipoles, bunch together or get concentrated in one particular region, as shown in **Fig. 4.47**. When the relaxation process starts, they gradually fan out or disperse in different directions as shown in **Fig. 4.48(b)** and **(c).** Since, fewer nuclei now contribute towards

Fig. 4.46: Three components of M_o after applying pulse in the stationary co-ordinate system

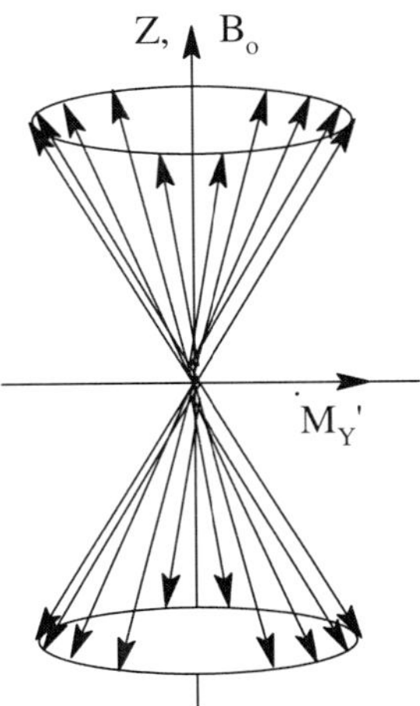

Fig. 4.47: Bunching of nuclear spins precessing about Z-axis after 90 ° pulse

M_Y', the magnitude of M_Y' becomes smaller and smaller and ultimately becomes zero.

The signal detected by the NMR spectrometer, following a pulse, is determined by M_Y' but it does not normally look like the typical decay curve as shown in **Fig. 4.48(d)**. A typical decay curve would be obtained only if the generating frequency (ν_1) and the precessional frequency of the nuclei in the sample coincide exactly, i.e. when the sample has all equivalent protons whose precessional frequency (ν_L) is exactly same as the applied RF (ν_1). This is true for a sample of CH_3I. In this molecule, there is only one resonance frequency for the three equivalent protons of the methyl group. In **Fig. 4.49**, the envelope of the curve corresponds to the steeply reducing part AB in the exponential decay curve of **Fig. 4.48(d)**. In **Fig. 4.49(a)**, the time interval between the successive maxima is $1/\Delta\nu$, where, $\Delta\nu$

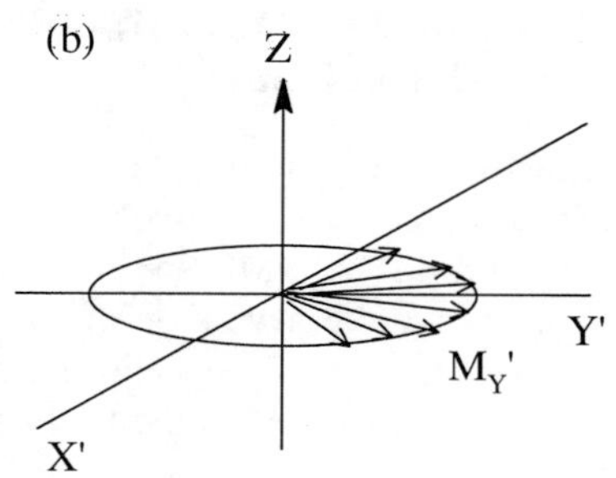

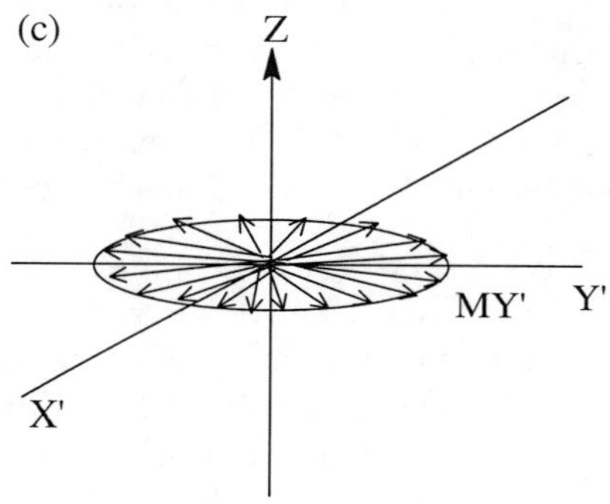

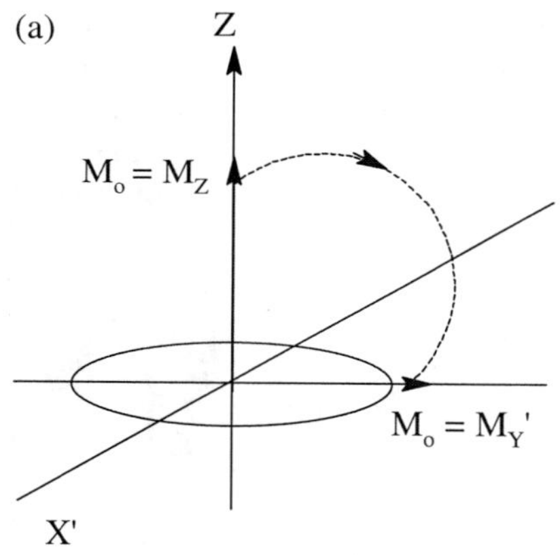

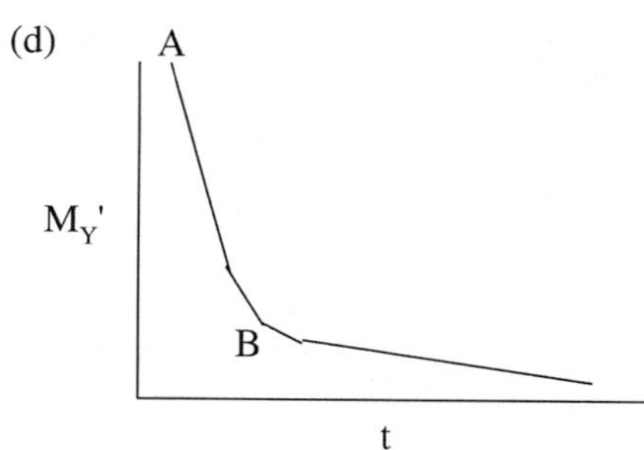

Fig. 4.48: Transverse or spin-spin relaxation

is the difference between the generating frequency ν_1 and the resonance frequency ν_L of the nuclei. This decay of the transverse magnetization is detected in the receiver and is called as the *free induction decay* (FID).

In the pulsed method, a band of frequencies is applied to the sample. If the sample contains nuclei with different resonance frequencies or if the spectrum consists of a multiplet as a result of spin-spin coupling, the decay curves of different transverse magnetization components are superimposed and interference between the FIDs occurs, which is recorded as an *interferogram*. **Figure 4.50** shows such an interferogram for the ^{13}C resonance of

$^{13}CH_3OH$. This interferogram contains the resonance frequencies and intensities, which are of interest to us. However, this interferogram cannot be analyzed directly, since the spectra are usually interpreted in the frequency domain rather than in the time domain. Nevertheless, the two spectra can be derived from each other, by a mathematical operation called the *Fourier Transformation* (FT). The ^1H NMR spectrum of CH_3I consists of a singlet [**Fig. 4.49(b)**], whereas the ^{13}C spectrum of $^{13}CH_3OH$ is a quartet [**Fig. 4.50(b)**], due to coupling of ^{13}C nucleus with three protons of the methyl group.

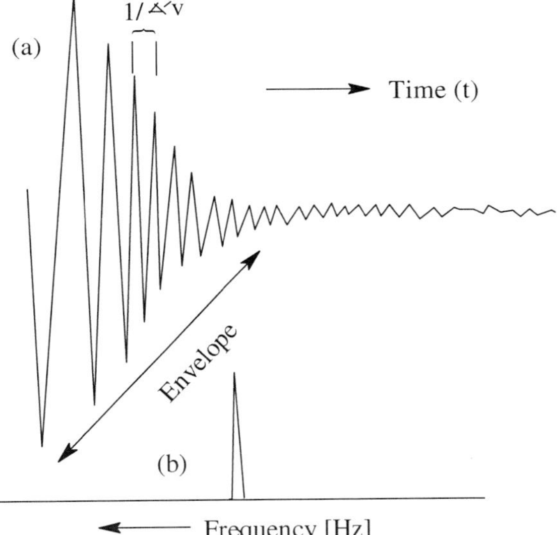

Fig. 4.49: ^1H NMR spectrum of methyl iodide (a) Time domain spectrum [FID] (b) Frequency domain spectrum obtained by Fourier Transformation of (a)

Usually, the intensity of an individual FID is so weak that after FT, the signals are very small compared to the noise. This is especially true for the nuclei like ^{13}C or ^{15}N, having low natural abundance and therefore, low sensitivity, or for samples which are very dilute. Therefore, FIDs of many pulses are added together in the computer and then transformed to get a spectrum. This phenomenon is called as *spectrum accumulation*. This process increases the signal–to-noise ratio (S: N) in proportion to the square root of the number of scans [NS], i.e.

$$S : N \propto \sqrt{NS}$$

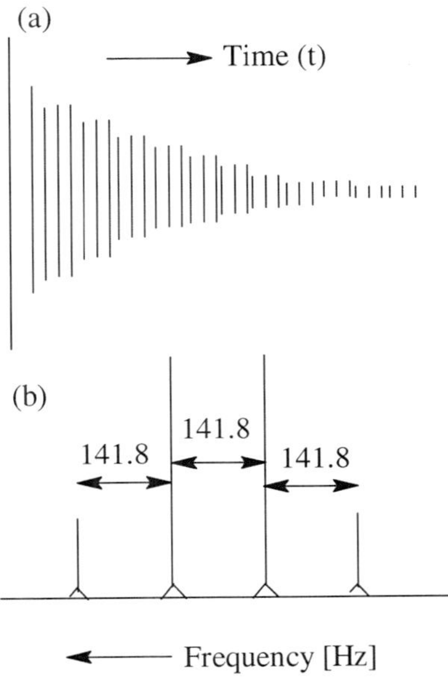

Fig. 4.50: ^{13}C NMR spectrum of methanol (a) Time domain spectrum (b) Frequency domain spectrum

4.2.14. Instrumentation

The pulsed NMR spectrometer

Different components of the pulsed NMR spectrometer, as shown in **Fig. 4.51**, are as follows.

1) A magnet
2) A probe head
3) A sample container
4) A transmitter
5) A receiver

1) A magnet

The magnitude of an external magnetic field decides the strength of resonance signals. Hence, the magnetic field should be very strong and homogeneous. Three types of magnets can be used in the NMR spectrometers.

(i) Permanent magnets

These magnets provide a homogeneous and a stable magnetic field but the field variation is not possible with these magnets.

(ii) Electromagnets

These magnets can be used when the variation in the field strength is required. These magnets do not produce a stable magnetic field. Hence, the use of a field stabilizer is absolutely essential whenever electromagnets are used. This adds up to the cost of instrumentation.

Permanent magnets and electromagnets were used until the early 1960s. They produce the lower magnetic fields, the maximum field strength being 1.41 T (Tesla), at which most of the protons possess precessional frequency around 60 MHz. With this frequency, spectra at low resolution can be recorded.

(iii) Cryomagnets

All the modern instruments are equipped with cryomagnets. These magnets provide the magnetic field, which is along the axis of the sample tubes, and is as high as 19 T, giving a frequency of 800 MHz for protons. With this frequency, spectra can be recorded at high resolution and hence, detail information about the structure of a molecule can be obtained.

2) The probe head

The sample tube is inserted in the probe head, which contains the transmitter, the receiver coils, the coils for generating field gradients, the coils for decoupling and also a preamplifier. It also contains the turbine for spinning the sample and the shim coils for optimizing the field homogeneity. In the latest instruments, the field homogeneity is so good that the sample spinning is not always necessary. This has helped in performing experiments with pulsed field gradients.

3) A sample container

A sample tube is usually made up of glass. The length of this tube is 20 cm and the external diameter is 5 mm. This tube is introduced into the probe head with the help of a sample changer. The sample tube is rotated about its longitudinal axis, which improves the field homogeneity.

4)) A transmitter

The transmitter consists of a RF generator. The radiofrequencies are generated by using a quartz crystal oscillator. It provides various frequencies needed for recording NMR spectra. It also produces pulses of the required duration and power.

5) A receiver

Depending on the magnitude of the transverse magnetization (M_X), a RF voltage is induced in the receiver coil. In the pulsed method, the transmitter pulse can excite nuclear spins which are in a band, symmetrical about the centre frequency (ν_1). The induced voltage does not have a pure single frequency, but a spread of frequencies determined by the chemical shifts, which are within a narrow range of a few kilo hertz (KHz) above or below the transmitter reference frequency (ν_1).

If the absolute values of the differences between the signal and the reference frequencies are fed to the receiver coil, the system cannot distinguish between a signal at a frequency higher than ν_1 and one at a frequency lower than ν_1, by the same amount. Thus, if two signals had frequencies equidistant from ν_1, one higher and another lower, only one signal would be obtained. To avoid this, the reference frequency (ν_1) can be positioned at one end of the spectrum rather than in the middle of it. This has two disadvantages.

(i) One half of the frequency band, determined by the pulse duration (T_p), remains unused.

(ii) The second disadvantage is that the unused band frequencies cause electronic noise.

Because of these two drawbacks, the sensitivity

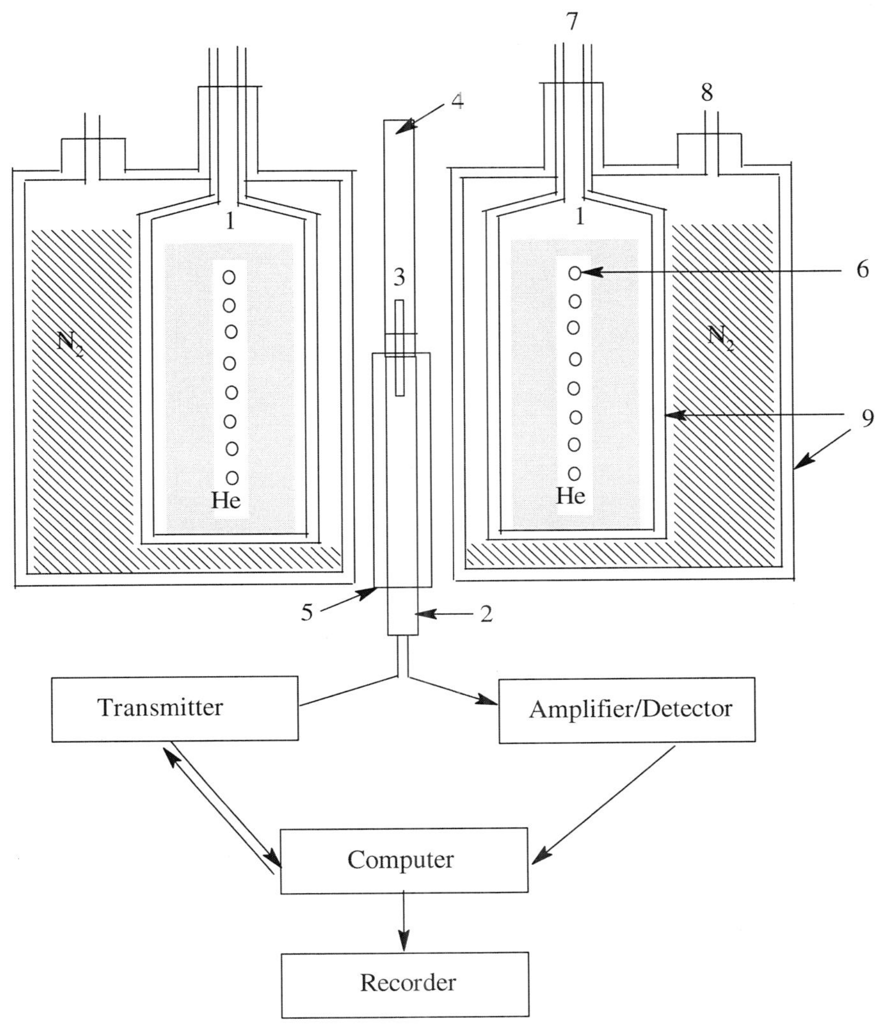

1. Magnet, 2. Probe head, 3. Sample tube, 4. Sample changer. 5. Shim coils, 6. Magnet coils, 7. Filling column for liquid helium, 8. Filling column for liquid nitrogen, 9. Vacuum jackets of inner and outer vessels

Fig. 4.51: Components of NMR spectrometer

of the measurement is reduced considerably.

To avoid this loss in the sensitivity by this measurement system, the modern NMR pulse spectrometers use *quadrature detection*. In this method, two phase sensitivity detectors are used. One detector measures the Y' component of the (M_{Y}') magnetization vector and another detector simultaneously measures the X' component (M_{X}'), which is at 90° to the Y' component. The measurement of these two components in two different phases with the Fourier transformation, makes it possible to differentiate between the signals whose frequencies lie above and below the reference frequency. Thus, this measurement system allows ν_1 to be positioned in the middle of the spectrum to be observed, thereby increasing the sensitivity by a factor of $\sqrt{2}$.

CHAPTER 5

MASS SPECTROMETRY

5.1. PRINCIPLE

In mass spectrometry, a sample in the form of vapor state is bombarded with a high energy electron beam. As a result, usually one electron is knocked off from the molecule. This results in the formation of a molecular ion, which has a positive charge on it and one free electron. For example, when a beam of electrons is bombarded on the vapor of a ketone, one of the electrons from the lone pairs of electrons on the oxygen atom is lost by the ketone, thereby producing a molecular ion $(M)^+$ with a positive charge on the oxygen atom and one free electron. The extra energy dissipates throughout the molecular ion. Hence, the molecular ion in turn, produces further fragments (F_1^+ and F_2^+). This is illustrated by the following example.

:O: Bombardment of electrons -e → :O:+ (C–R, C–R') → :O+ ≡C–R + R'•

(M)$^+$ (F$_1$)$^+$

OR

:O: Bombardment of electrons -e → :O:+ (C–R, C–R') → :O+ ≡C–R' + R•

(M)$^+$ (F$_2$)$^+$

The arrow (⌒) in the above reactions is termed as a *fish hook arrow* and is used to indicate the *homolytic fission* of a bond. A bond between two atoms contains two electrons. In homolytic fission of a bond, two electrons are equally shared by the two bonded atoms so that each atom bears one single electron. In a *heterolytic fission* (indicated by an arrow⌒, not shown in above reactions) both the electrons of a bond reside on one of the two bonded atoms and another atom gains the positive charge.

A mass spectrometer separates and detects either the positive or the negative ions, depending upon the polarity selected in the instrument, based on their mass to charge (m/z) ratio. The molecular ion $(M)^+$ and the two fragment ions $(F_1)^+$ and $((F_2)^+$ have definite mass depending on the groups R and R′. The charge (z) is 1 on all the ions here. These ions are subjected to the electric and the magnetic fields and are collected at the collector depending upon their m/z values. All the three species, the molecular ion $(M)^+$ and the two fragment ions $(F_1)^+$ and $((F_2)^+$, have different m/z values, on the basis of which they are separated and detected in mass spectrometry. The neutral molecules are pumped away and are not detected.

5.2. BASIC COMPONENTS OF MASS SPECTROMETERS

A mass spectrometer has the following four components-

5.2.1. A sample inlet
5.2.2. An ion source
5.2.3. An analyzer
5.2.4. A detector

5.2.1. A Sample Inlet

1) The sample must be introduced in the vapor state into the ion chamber of a mass

spectrometer. The operating pressure of an ion source is 10^{-7} mm of Hg. The minimum vapor pressure should be about 10^{-6} mm of Hg.

2) The gases and the volatile liquids are introduced into a mass spectrometer through a leak from a gas reservoir. Since the sample is to be introduced in the reservoir, the sample size increases almost to 1mg.
3) The samples having low volatility, e.g. peptides or amino acids, are introduced on the bakelite tip of a direct–insert-probe. In this case, the sample size is reduced considerably and is as low as 0.1 mg. The probe is directly inserted into an ion-source. When heated by a platinum wire, the sample vapor is produced in the form of a '*plug*', which is bombarded by the electrons.

5.2.2. Ion Source

The sample in the vapor form, when introduced in the ion source, is converted into ions using various techniques. These are described below.

5.2.2.1. Electron Impact (EI) Method
5.2.2.2. Chemical Ionization (CI) Method
5.2.2.3. Field Ionization (FI) Method
5.2.2.4. Fast Atom Bombardment (FAB) Method
5.2.2.5. Matrix Assisted Laser Desorption Ionization (MALDI) Method
5.2.2.6. Inductively Coupled Plasma (ICP) Ionization Method

5.2.2.1. Electron Impact (EI) Method

The mass spectrometry, which makes use of an EI method, is termed as Electron Impact Mass Spectrometry (EIMS). In an EI method, a beam of electrons is produced by using a hot metal filament. The electrons produced are highly energetic and hence, they can bring about excessive fragmentation so as to leave no molecular ion in the sample. This problem can be overcome sometimes, by using less energetic beam of electrons. Thus, in an EI method, the intensity of the molecular ion $(M)^+$ is nil or very low. Hence, this method cannot be used to find the molecular weight of an analyte. The EI method is used for volatile and thermally stable compounds with small molecular weight (800 Da). It provides information about the fragmentation pattern of a molecule and therefore, of the structure of a compound. The EI spectra are generally reproducible and hence, are used very commonly for the finger printing purpose.

5.2.2.2. Chemical Ionization (CI) Method

The mass spectrometry, which makes use of a CI method, is termed as Chemical Ionization Mass Spectrometry (CIMS). In a CI method, a gaseous sample is mixed with a large excess of an ionizing gas such as methane, isobutane or ammonia. This mixture is fed to an ion chamber. The pressure inside the ion chamber is as low as1mm of Hg (1 Torr). The mixture is bombarded with electrons of about 100 eV. Since the ionizing gas is in large excess, the electron bombardment results in its ionization, producing a number of positive ions or *primary ions*. This is shown below with the help of methane as an ionizing gas.

$$CH_4 + e \longrightarrow CH_4^{\bullet +}$$

$$CH_4^{\bullet +} \longrightarrow CH_3^{+} + H^{\bullet}$$

$$CH_4^{\bullet +} + CH_4 \longrightarrow CH_5^{+} + CH_3^{\bullet}$$

$$CH_3^{+} + CH_4 \longrightarrow C_2H_5^{+} + H_2$$

These positively charged primary ions (CH_5^+ and $C_2H_5^+$) react with an analyte (AH). When an analyte AH contains electronegative atoms like oxygen, nitrogen or sulphur, it reacts with the primary ions by accepting a proton (H^+) from them. Thus, an analyte acquires a positive charge (AH_2^+) along with the formation of an uncharged hydrocarbon (CH_4 or C_2H_4). Sometimes, a prominent peak is obtained because of a hydride ion ($H:^-$) abstraction from an analyte, thereby producing a cation of an analyte $(A)^+$ and a neutral molecule (C_2H_6), by the primary ion. The reactions of an analyte with the primary ions are shown below.

$$CH_5^{+} + AH \longrightarrow \underset{(M+1)^+}{AH_2^{+}} + CH_4$$

$$C_2H_5^{+} + AH \longrightarrow \underset{(M+1)^+}{AH_2^{+}} + C_2H_4$$

$$C_2H_5^{+} + AH \longrightarrow \underset{(M-1)^+}{A^{+}} + C_2H_6$$

Because of the conversion of an analyte, either to AH_2^+ ion or A^+ ion, the molecular ion (AH^+), is often weak in the CI spectra. However, the base peak, i.e. the most intense peak, is because of either $(M + 1)^+$ ion, i.e. AH_2^+ ion, or because of $(M-1)^+$ ion, i.e. A^+ ion. These ions are usually known as *quasi-molecular ions*.

If the ionizing gas like isobutane having high proton affinity is used, it causes little or no fragmentation of the sample and thus, results in an uncomplicated spectrum of the sample with an intense quasi-molecular ion, A^+. Hence, CI spectra are relatively easy to interpret. Like an EI method, the CI method is also used for the volatile and the thermally stable compounds with small molecular weight (800 Da) but it provides information about molecular weight of a compound.

5.2.2.3. Field Ionization (FI) Method

The mass spectrometry, which makes use of a FI method, is termed as Field Ionization Mass Spectrometry (FIMS). By this technique, the positive ions are generated using low energy. A very high positive potential is applied to a pointed or a sharp metallic wire which is either platinum or tungsten. A very high potential gradient, of the order of 10^7 to 10^8 volts/cm, is applied between the analyte and the metallic wire. Because of the high potential, a molecule loses its electron to the anode. The positive ions formed are repelled by the anode and are accelerated into the mass spectrometer.

In this method, since only 12-13 eV is available for the ionization of the sample, there is very little or no fragmentation of the molecular ion and hence, the molecular ion is very intense. This makes the mass spectrum very simple. Therefore, this mode is preferred when the molecular weight of an analyte or the structures of the large molecules are to be found out. The sensitivity of the source in the FI mode is almost 1/10th to 1/100th of an EI mode.

When the compound is non-volatile or thermolabile, its solution is prepared in a volatile solvent and is applied to the field ion emitter. The solvent is allowed to evaporate. The sample is then subjected to the high electric field. This modification of the FI is called field desorption (FD). This technique is useful for the nucleotides and the quaternary ammonium salts.

5.2.2.4. Fast Atom Bombardment (FAB) Method

The mass spectrometry, which makes use of a FAB method, is termed as Fast Atom Bombardment Mass Spectrometry (FABMS). In this technique, a beam of electrons is produced by heating a metallic element. These electrons are bombarded on an argon gas. This results in the ionization of an argon gas. The Ar^+ ions thus generated are accelerated by applying electric field. The beam of accelerated Ar^+ ions is then passed through a chamber containing argon gas at 10^{-3} to 10^{-4} mm of Hg. The accelerated Ar^+ ions exchange their charge to Ar atoms and thus produce a beam of fast moving argon atoms. These accelerated Ar atoms then bombard the sample dissolved in a solvent. This results in the production of sample ions which are fed to the mass spectrometer.

$$Ar \xrightarrow{-e} Ar^{+}$$

$$\underset{\text{Fast moving Ar+ ions}}{Ar^+} + Ar \longrightarrow \underset{\text{Fast moving Ar atoms}}{\overrightarrow{Ar}} + Ar^{+}$$

In contrast to an EI or a CI method, the FAB is useful for the non-volatile, polar, and thermally unstable compounds with high molecular weight up to 5,000 Da, e.g. insulin, aminoglycosides, nucleotides, phospholipids, vitamin B, etc. Hence, this technique is suitable for proteins, peptides and biopolymers. However, this technique is now superseded by the Matrix Assisted Laser Desorption Ionization (MALDI) method, which is described below.

5.2.2.5. Matrix Assisted Laser Desorption Ionization (MALDI) Method

Weak organic acids strongly absorb UV laser radiation. In the MALDI technique, an organic acid is used as a matrix material. When an analyte is co-crystallized with a large excess of such a matrix, a homogeneous mixture of an analyte and a matrix is obtained. When a pulse of UV laser radiation is applied to this analyte-matrix mixture, the matrix absorbs energy supplied by the radiation very strongly. This brings about the vaporization of an analyte. The absorption of laser energy by matrix also results in the donation of a proton from the matrix to an analyte or acceptance of a proton by the matrix from an analyte. This brings about an ionization of an analyte to produce either positive or negative ions, respectively.

Because of a homogeneous mixture of an analyte with the matrix, the transfer of energy from the matrix to an analyte, is very efficient. Hence, the MALDI technique provides high yields of ions of the analyte and high sensitivity, which enables the accurate measurements to the subpicomole level. In addition, MALDI technique does not destroy analytes during vaporization and ionization.

Like FAB, MALDI technique is also used for non-volatile, polar and thermally unstable compounds with high molecular weight upto 5,000 Da, but it provides 100-1000 times higher sensitivity compared to FAB. The concentrations, as low as picogram or fentogram levels, can be analyzed with great accuracy using this technique.

5.2.2.6. Inductively Coupled Plasma (ICP) Ionization Method

In this case, energy required for the ionization of an argon gas is obtained by using an inductive coupling of high-frequency. This energy produces argon ions or plasma. When the analyte solution is injected in the form of an aerosol into these argon ions, the aerosol droplets are vaporized and ionized. The analyte ions generated from the high energy, inductively coupled plasma (ICP) source are directed into the mass analyzer. This technique is an efficient tool in many areas such as electronics, medicine and biology.

5.2.3. Analyzer

The third component of a mass spectrometer is an analyzer. In the mass analyzer, ions are separated based on their mass-to-charge (m/z) ratios by applying electric field or magnetic field or both. The ions are analyzed by measuring the electric field or the magnetic field or both, required for getting a peak in the spectrum, or by measuring the time they take to travel a fixed distance. Accordingly, mass spectrometers are of two different kinds.

5.2.3.1. Field instruments
5.2.3.2. Time of Flight instruments

5.2.3.1. Field Instruments

In the field instruments, by scanning the field strength (electric or magnetic or both), all the ions produced in the ion source are sequentially focused at the detector.

5.2.3.2. Time of Flight (TOF) Instruments

When ions are accelerated using an electric potential, all the ions have the same amount of kinetic energy. Even then, different ions reach the detector at different times. This is because the lighter ions have the smaller mass and the higher velocity, whereas the heavier ions have the larger mass and the smaller velocity. Hence, the smaller ions reach the detector first and the larger ions take a longer time. The time taken by an ion to reach the detector (Time of Flight) is thus directly related to their mass-to-charge ratios. The time of flight for an ion is measured accurately in order to determine its mass. This is commonly used with the MALDI technique. **Figure 5.1** shows the components of the Time of Flight instrument.

potential difference of about 3000-6000 volts. The accelerated ions enter the magnetic field (H) which is applied perpendicular to the direction of motion of ions. This produces a force which is

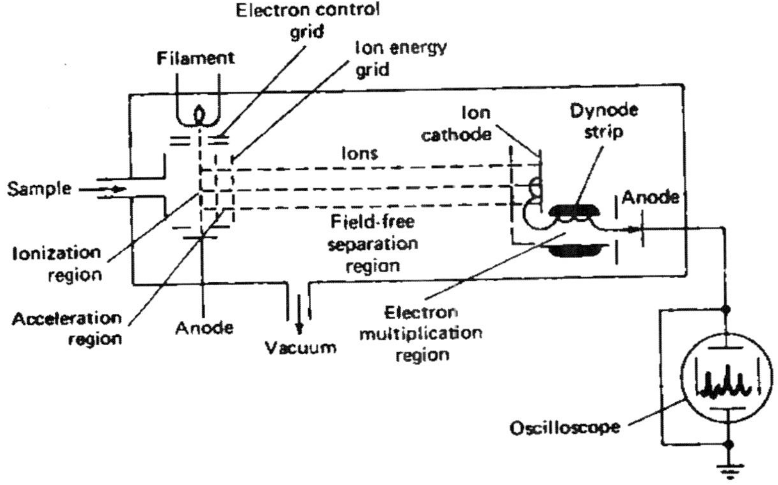

Fig. 5.1: Time of Flight instrument

perpendicular, both to the direction of motion of electrons and also to the direction of the applied magnetic field. This force causes the deflection of ions based on their mass to charge ratio (m/z). Then the ions pass through an exit slit or a collector slit and impinge upon a collector. The signal received is then amplified and recorded in the form of peaks in the mass spectrum.

The ions of different m/z values follow paths of different curvatures or radii in the analyzer. In the electric field, all the ions acquire the same kinetic energy. The kinetic energy of ions is expressed as $^{1}/_{2}mv^2$ (m is the mass of an ion and v is its velocity). The velocity of the heavier ions is lesser as compared to the lighter ions. Because of the higher mass, the heavier ions resist the change in the direction of motion. Also, they are accelerated to a lesser extent as compared to the lighter ions. Therefore, they follow the path of the greater curvature. Because of the smaller mass, the lighter ions get deflected easily. Also, they are

5.2.4. A Detector

A detector in mass spectrometry is nothing but a photomultiplier or a scintillation counter. When the energetic ions coming out of an analyzer impinge upon the detector, they generate a number of electrons. These electrons are further amplified and produce a current in the circuit, which is then recorded in the form of a signal in the mass spectrometer.

5.3. THEORY BEHIND MASS SPECTROMETRY

The theory behind mass spectrometry can be explained with the help of a single focusing mass spectrometer, shown in **Fig. 5.2**.

The sample is introduced into the ion source of a mass spectrometer in the vapor form and is bombarded by electrons of about 70 eV. The positive ions formed in the ion source are accelerated by using plates which are kept at a

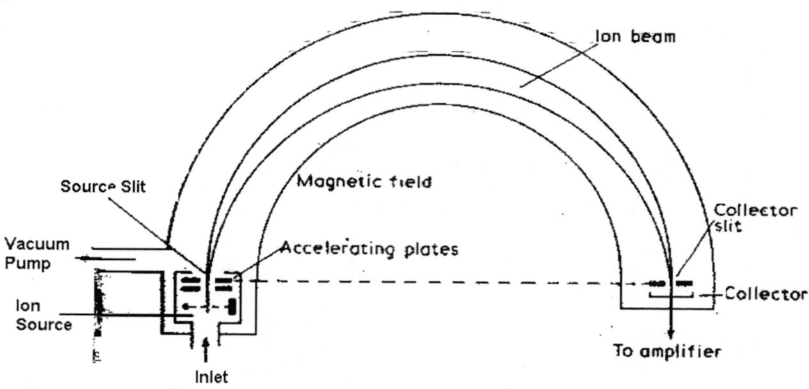

Fig. 5.2: A single focusing mass spectrometer

accelerated more compared to the heavier ions. Therefore, they follow the path of a smaller curvature and reach the detector faster than the heavier ions. By changing either the accelerating voltage (V) or the magnetic field (H), the radius of the ion path can be changed, which allows ions of different mass to charge ratios (m/z) to impinge upon the collector at the same point.

The variation in the magnetic field provides a wide range of ions to be covered in a single sweep, but the voltage sweep makes the scanning very rapid.

The relation between the magnetic field (H), the accelerating voltage (V), the radius (r) of the ion path and the m/z value of an ion can be obtained as follows:

In an electric field, the potential energy (P. E.) of an ion is converted to its kinetic energy (K. E.), i.e.

P. E. = K. E.

$$zV = \frac{1}{2} mv^2 \quad .... (5.1)$$

where, z = charge on an ion

V = accelerating voltage

m = mass of an ion, and

v = velocity of an ion

In the magnetic field, ions follow semicircular path and hence, the centripetal force (CPF) is balanced by the centrifugal force (CFF), i.e.

$$CPF = CFF$$

$$\text{Or } Hzv = mv^2 / r \; .... (5.2)$$

$$\text{Or } v = Hzr / m \; .... (5.3)$$

By putting the value of v from **equation (5.3)** in **equation (5.1)**, an **equation (5.4)** for the m/z value of an ion can be obtained.

$$zV = \tfrac{1}{2} m (Hzr / m)^2$$

$$= \tfrac{1}{2} H^2z^2r^2 / m$$

$$V = \tfrac{1}{2} H^2zr^2 / m$$

$$\text{Hence, } m/z = H^2r^2 / 2V .... (5.4)$$

Equation (5.4) shows that the radius (r) of the ion path varies for ions having different m/z values, if the values of H and V are kept constant. If all the ions of different m/z values are to be collected at the same point on the detector, the value of 'r' should be kept constant. This makes the fabrication of a mass spectrometer much simpler and allows the collection of different ions at one point, without the need for the change in the position of a collector slit. This can be achieved by changing either the magnitude of the electric field (V) or the magnetic field (H) or both.

In some mass spectrometers, the magnetic field (H) is kept constant and the accelerating potential (V) is gradually increased. In **equation (5.4)**, the left hand side (m/z) is constant for a particular ion. If H and r are kept constant on the right hand side of this equation, then the value of m/z is inversely proportional to V, i.e. the heavier ions can be collected by applying smaller accelerating potentials and vice versa. If V and r are kept constant, then the value of m/z is directly proportional to H. In this case, at lower values of H, ions with smaller m/z values would be collected, and as we increase the value of H, ions of higher m/z values would get recorded.

5.4. A DOUBLE FOCUSING MASS SPECTROMETER

In a single focusing mass spectrometer, the curvature in the ion path is obtained by applying the magnetic field in the direction perpendicular to the direction of the motion of ions. The ions with the higher m/z values follow the path of a larger radius and the ions with the lower m/z values follow the path of a smaller radius. Hence, the time taken by the particles of the smaller m/z value to reach the collector is shorter as compared to that required by the particles of the higher m/z values. Thus, in the magnetic field, the ions are separated based on their m/z values.

In a double focusing mass spectrometer, shown in **Fig. 5.3**, an additional electrostatic field is applied at right angles to the direction of the motion of ions between the ion accelerating chamber and the magnetic analyzer. The additional electrostatic analyzer selects the ions based on their energy. Thus, it brings about the separation of ions based upon their energies and sends them in sequence in the magnetic analyzer, where further separation of ions having very narrow range of energy occurs based on their m/z values. This increases the resolution of a double focusing mass spectrometer to 30,000 from 3,000, as attainable in the single focusing spectrometer.

5.5. A QUADRUPOLE MASS SPECTROMETER OR A QUADRUPOLE MASS FILTER

The quadruple instruments are the *field instruments*, which incorporate the combination of a radiofrequency (RF) and a direct current field.

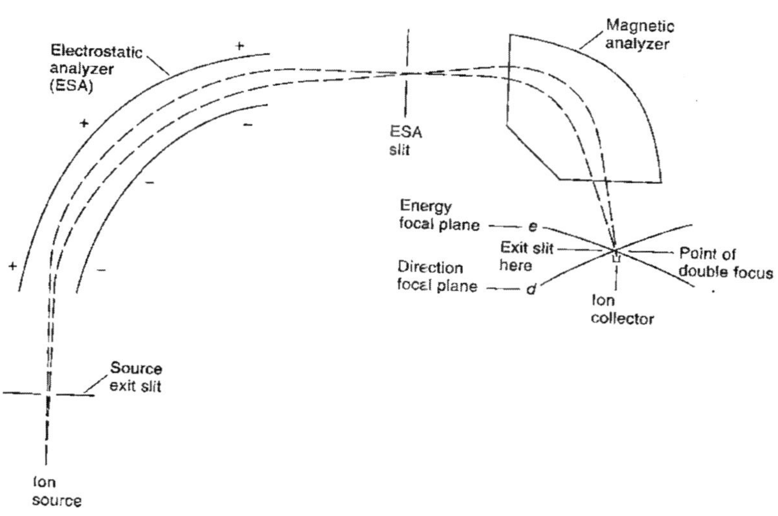

Fig. 5.3: A double focusing mass spectrometer

In a quadrupole mass spectrometer, shown in **Fig. 5.4**, the focusing of ions after their acceleration from the ion source is brought about by the process of filtration. A quadrupole filter consists of four parallel tungsten rods or poles. Across one pair of tungsten rods, a direct current voltage (V_{dc}) is applied and across another pair of tungsten rods, a RF voltage (V_{rf}) is applied. When the ions produced in the ion source enter the area between two pairs of rods, they travel with a constant velocity in the direction parallel to the poles. Because of the application of the RF voltage (V_{rf}), the polarity of the two tungsten rods constantly changes. Hence, the positively charged ions moving through the space available between the rods are attracted by the negatively charged rod at one moment, but the next moment, when the same rod acquires the positive charge, the ions are repelled away from it. This continues and results in the complex oscillations in X and Y directions. The force of attraction exerted by the negatively charged tungsten rod on the positively charged ions is so great for certain ions that the ions collide with the rod and loose their charge. Thus, the ions of certain m/z values do not get recorded at a particular value of V_{rf}. Only a *stable oscillation*, for an ion having a definite m/z value, is allowed to pass from one end of the quadrupole to the other, without striking the poles. Thus, an ion of only one m/z value can pass through the filter at a particular value of V_{dc} and V_{rf}. All the other ions possess unstable oscillations and strike the poles and are lost. By varying V_{dc} and V_{rf}, the ions of different m/z values are allowed to pass through the filter sequentially. The lower voltages allow ions of smaller m/z values to pass through the filter.

A quadrupole mass spectrometer uses a very low accelerating voltage of the order of 5-30 V as against 3000-6000 V in a single focusing spectrometer. Hence, the pressure, as high as 10^{-4} to 10^{-5} mm of Hg, can be maintained in an ion source as against a low pressure of the order of 10-7 mm of Hg in the ion source of a single focusing spectrometer, to prevent arcing. This is particularly found to be advantageous in GC/MS combination.

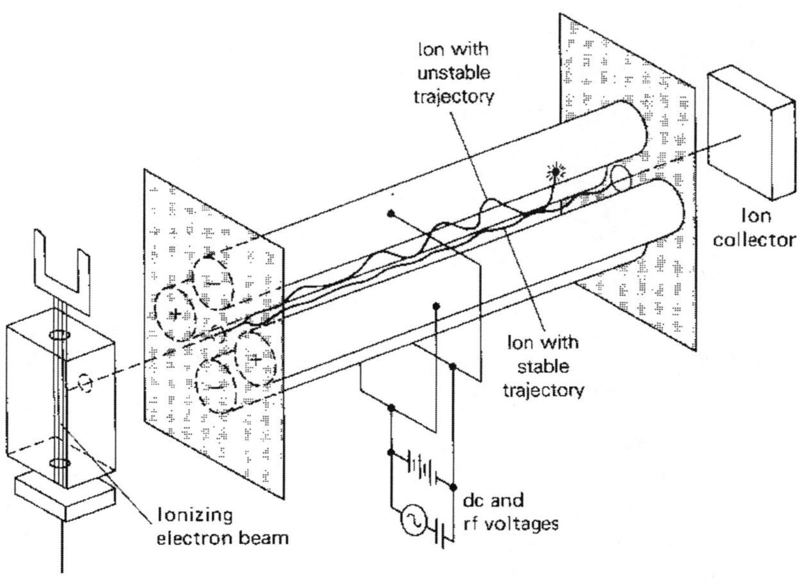

Fig. 5.4: A quadrupole mass spectrometer

A quadrupole mass spectrometer provides a very high resolving power and can record peaks for species with 1000 atomic mass units (amu).

5.6. RESOLVING POWER OF A MASS SPECTROMETER

The resolving power of a mass spectrometer is determined by the **equation (5.5)**.

$$\text{Resolving power} = \frac{m_1}{m_2 - m_1} \quad \ldots (5.5)$$

$$= \frac{m_1}{\Delta m}$$

where, m_1 and m_2 are the masses of two ions getting separated in the mass spectrometer and Δm is the mass difference between them. Hence, the resolution of a mass spectrometer is defined as its ability to distinguish between the ions having different mass to charge ratio values. This means that a high resolving power spectrometer is able to produce distinct peaks even when the difference between the masses (m_1 and m_2) is small, i.e. a low resolving power mass spectrometer can separate a mass of 300 from 300.1 and a high resolving mass spectrometer can resolve a mass of 300 from 300.01. High resolution can provide determination of mass up to four decimal points.

5.7. TANDEM MASS SPECTROMETRY OR MULTI-STAGES MASS SPECTROMETRY (MS/MS)

The *tandem mass spectrometry* is described as MS/MS and is abbreviated as MS^n, where n is the number of mass spectrometers used in a series. The tandem mass spectrometry is used when an analyte is a mixture of a number of components. In this method, an analyte is introduced in the first mass spectrometer, wherein the milder method of ionization such as MALDI, brings about the gentle ionization and converts various components of a mixture into the corresponding molecular ions. These molecular ions are sent sequentially to the second mass spectrometer, where they are fragmented and analyzed. In the second mass spectrometer, the fragmentation is achieved by inducing the collisions of the selected ions or molecules with a collision gas, usually argon or helium. This process is known as collision induced dissociation (CID) or collision activated dissociation (CAD). Thus, the technique of MS/MS is similar to LC/MS or GC/MS. The only difference is that MS/MS isolates the components in the form of molecular ions, whereas the chromatographic techniques isolate the components in the molecular form. The tandem mass spectrometry is generally used to obtain the structural information.

5.8. GAS CHROMATOGRAPHY AND MASS SPECTROMETRY (GC/MS)

The gas chromatography is an efficient tool for the separation of components of a mixture. The mass spectrometry helps in the identification of the fractions eluted in the gas chromatography. If the fraction which is eluted out from the column is fed directly to a mass spectrometer, the separation as well as the identification of the components of a mixture is achieved simultaneously. Thus, a GC/MS technique is commonly used for structure elucidation.

In gas chromatography, the concentration of the compound in the eluate is very low because of the larger amount of the carrier gas. This reduces the sensitivity of the method and records the additional peaks in the mass spectrum. In order to increase the sensitivity and reduce the complexity of a mass spectrum, it is essential to remove the carrier gas from the eluate and enrich the eluate with the compound.

The concentration of a compound in the eluate can be achieved in two ways.

1) When the eluate of a gas chromatograph, which is always in the vapor form, is allowed to condense in a capillary or on a small metal surface, the vapor of the sample gets condensed, but the carrier gas escapes. Once the eluate is enriched with the compound, it is introduced in normal manner into the mass

spectrometer. This procedure is repeated for every compound that is eluted out from the column.

2) Another way to remove the carrier gas from the eluate is to use an *interface* or a *separator*. This helps in the enrichment of a compound. Three different kinds of interfaces are used for the removal of the carrier gas from the eluate of a compound.

5.8.1. Watson–Biemann Effusion Separator

This separator consists of a simple sintered glass tube kept in an evacuated chamber. The eluate from the column is allowed to pass over the separator. As shown in **Fig. 5.5**, the carrier gas preferentially passes through it and the eluate gets concentrated almost 100 times with respect to a compound on the other side of the separator. One more separator in a series, further enriches the eluate with respect to a compound.

5.8.2. Ryhage Jet Separator

As shown in **Fig. 5.6**, this jet separator consists of two tubes with small apertures at their tips, kept apart at a distance. The two tubes are aligned so as to have the apertures of both the tubes at the same level. The eluate containing a compound along with the carrier gas is passed at a high speed through an orifice. Because of the venturi action, the gases coming out through a small orifice, when expand suddenly, get cooled. The carrier gas diffuses on the sides of the tubes without any condensation but the heavier compound concentrates at the center of the gas jet. Because of the high speed of an eluate, the concentrate passes through the second orifice and then into the ion source of a mass spectrometer. Two jet separators in a series, concentrate the compound, number of folds in the eluate.

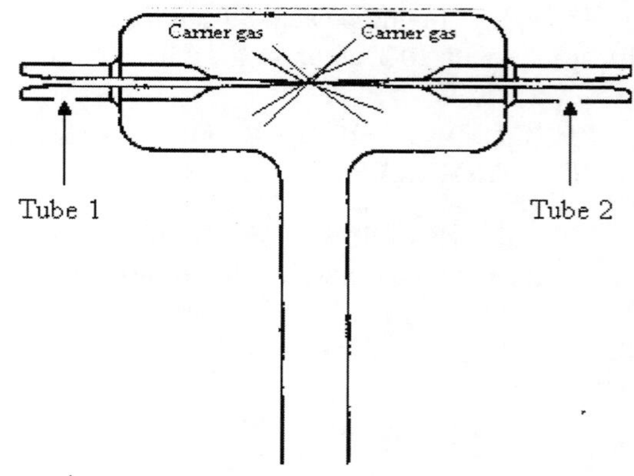

Fig. 5.6: A Ryhage jet separator

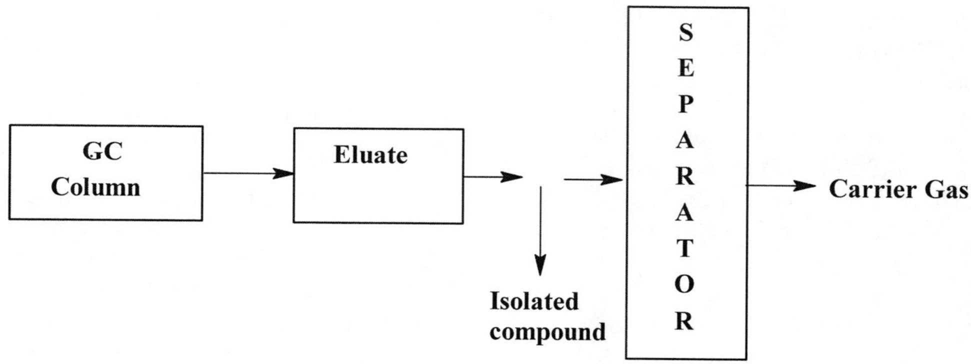

Fig. 5.5: Enrichment of an isolated compound using Watson–Biemann effusion separator

5.8.3. Llwellyn–Littlejohn separator

This separator, shown in **Fig. 5.7.** makes use of an elastomer membrane. The membrane is chosen in such a way that a separated compound has higher solubility in it compared to that of the carrier gas. Because of the higher solubility of the compound in the elastomer membrane, it diffuses through the membrane at higher rate but the carrier gas does not permeate through it. The compound interacts with the membrane and permeates through it on the other side, thereby enriching the eluate with the compound. The vapor of an organic compound being lighter compared to the carrier gas passes through the membrane much faster than the carrier gas. The concentrated eluate is passed through another semi-permeable elastomer membrane, thereby further enriching the eluate with the compound.

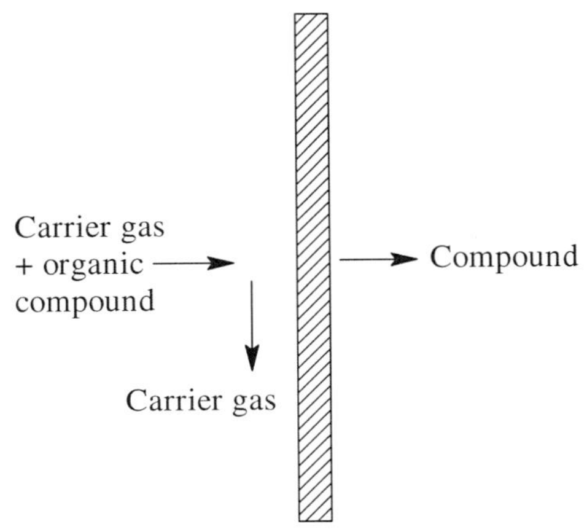

Fig. 5.7: Llwellyn–Littlejohn separator

5.9. HIGH PRESSURE LIQUID CHROMATOGRAPHY AND MASS SPECTROMETRY (HPLC/MS)

In case of GC/MS, the eluate contains a carrier gas and the vapor of an organic compound. In HPLC/MS, the eluate from a chromatograph contains a compound dissolved in the liquid mobile phase. To enrich the compound in the eluate, the liquid mobile phase is to be removed. This can be done in three ways.

1) In the first method, an eluate is passed over a conveyer belt and is exposed to the IR radiation. Because of the heat provided by the IR radiation, the liquid mobile phase evaporates, whereas the compound in the liquid or solid form gets deposited on the bed, which enters the ion source of a mass spectrometer.
2) Another way to remove the mobile phase is to pass the mixture of an organic compound and the liquid mobile phase through a *jet separator* (**Fig. 5.6**). Because of the ventury action, there is sudden cooling of the mobile phase. This reduces the solubility of the compound in the mobile phase and the compound separates out. This separated compound is then fed into the ion source of a mass spectrometer. Instead of a jet separator, the eluate can be passed through a vacuum nebulizer, wherein the eluate with a high speed, passes through a capillary, producing the small droplets at its tip. Due to the applied vacuum, the mobile phase evaporates and the compound is left behind in the capillary. This separated compound is then fed to the ion source of a mass spectrometer.

The HPLC/MS technique is commonly used for the peptide analysis and for the separation of drugs from their mixture or formulations.

5.10. TERMS USED IN MASS SPECTROMETRY

1) Molecular ion peak

An electron impact on the vapor of any molecule results in the removal of an electron from it and leads to the formation of a positive ion, i.e. the intact molecule (M) less one electron. This positive ion produced is referred to as the molecular ion $(M)^+$. The peak corresponding to the molecular ion in the mass spectrum is called the *molecular ion peak*.

2) Base peak

The most intense peak in the mass spectrum is called the *base peak*. The molecular ion peak may sometimes be the base peak.

3) Isotope peaks

The isotope peaks are obtained when a molecule contains heavier isotopes of certain atoms than the common isotopes. Commonly seen isotope peaks are $(M+1)^+$ peaks or $(M+2)^+$ peaks. **Table 5.3** lists the elements existing as isotopes and their relative abundance in nature.

4) Intensity of isotope peaks and relative abundance

Intensity of an isotope peak is much lesser than that of the $(M)^+$ peak except when Cl or Br is present in the molecule. The intensity of an isotope peak depends on the relative abundance of that isotope in nature. The relative abundance of an isotope is calculated on the basis of 100 molecules. From the relative abundance, the intensity of $(M+1)^+$ or $(M+2)^+$ peaks can be determined. For a compound containing one carbon atom, out of every 100 molecules, 98.892 molecules contain C^{12} isotope and 1.108 molecules contain C^{13} isotope. Hence, the intensity of $(M+1)^+$ peak is about 1.1 % of the intensity of the $(M)^+$ peak and the ratio of the intensities of M^+ and $(M+1)^+$ peaks is 98.892: 1.108.

For compounds containing silicon, the intensities of $(M)^+$ peak corresponding to Si^{28} isotope, $(M+1)^+$ peak corresponding to Si^{29} isotope and $(M+2)^+$ peak corresponding to Si^{30} isotope are in proportion of their relative abundance in the nature, i.e. 92.18: 4.71:3.12. For compounds containing sulphur, the ratio of intensities of $(M)^+$: $(M+2)^+$ peaks, corresponding to S^{32} and S^{34} isotopes is 95.018: 4.215. The height of the peak is the measure of intensity of that peak. Fluorine and iodine have only one naturally occurring isotope corresponding to atomic mass of 19 and 127, respectively. Hence, they produce only one peak corresponding to $(M)^+$ ion.

5) Metastable ion peak

The formation of a molecular ion $(M)^+$ and the further fragmentation to produce fragment ions $(F)^+$ occur in the ion source of the mass spectrometer. They produce distinct peaks in the mass spectrum when both are formed in the ion source itself. On the contrary, if a molecular ion does not cleave in the ion source to produce the fragment ion but cleaves during its acceleration in the electric field or during its flight in the magnetic field, then the fragment ion $(F)^+$ is recorded at the lower mass than the actual mass of $(F)^+$. The ion $(F)^+$, when gets recorded at the lower mass, is designated as m^* and called as a *metastable ion*.

When the fragment ion is formed after the acceleration, it has lesser kinetic energy than the ion which is formed in the ion source and accelerated in the electric field, because some of the kinetic energy received by the molecular ion during the acceleration is carried off by the neutral fragment. Hence, its peak (m^*) occurs at the lower mass than $(F)^+$. This peak is usually broad in nature and low in intensity. The actual position (m/z value) of this metastable ion is expressed in terms of m/z values of $(M)^+$ and $(F)^+$ by the **equation (5.6)**.

$$m^* = \frac{[(F)^+]^2}{(M)^+} \quad ...(5.6)$$

The recent advanced mass spectrometers produce computer displays which normally omit metastable ion peaks.

6) Nitrogen Rule

This rule states that the molecular ion having even molecular weight must possess either no nitrogen or an even number of nitrogen atoms and a molecule with odd molecular weight should contain an odd number of nitrogen atoms.

7) Atomic weight / Molecular weight

The atomic weight is the average of the weights of all the natural isotopes of an element.

The molecular weight of a compound is determined by adding the atomic weights of atoms constituting a molecule.

8) Atomic mass / Molecular mass

The atomic mass is the exact mass of the most abundant isotope of an element. The molecular mass of a compound is obtained by adding exact masses of the most abundant isotopes of elements constituting a molecule.

5.11. APPLICATIONS OF MASS SPECTROMETRY

1) Determination of molecular weight of compounds

The mass spectrum of a compound is a line spectrum obtained by plotting m/z values on X-axis and the intensity of peaks or lines with respect to a base line, on Y-axis. A peak of 100 % intensity is considered as a base peak.

A molecule losing a single electron after a milder ionization method produces a molecular ion. This ion corresponds to the m/z value, which is exactly equal to the molecular weight of that compound. While recording a mass spectrum, components of air, such as H_2O (m/z = 18), N_2 (m/z = 28), O_2 (m/z = 32), Ar (m/z = 40) and CO_2 (m/z = 44) can be recorded as the reference peaks, if the traces of air are introduced in the instrument. These compounds or the final ion C^+ (m/z = 12) can also be used for the calibration of a mass spectrometer.

When the molecular weight of a compound is found by counting the number of lines from a reference line, the *nearest whole number* value of molecular weight is obtained. An accurate molecular weight determination up to 4 or 6 decimal points is carried out by a *peak matching process* or by an *isotope abundance ratio method*. These methods also help in finding the exact molecular formula or a fragment formula.

2) Determination of a molecular formula or a fragment formula

The correct molecular formula or the elemental composition of a compound can be determined if the exact mass of atoms up to 4 or 6 decimals is known. This is possible with a high resolution spectrometer or a double focusing spectrometer. For example, four different molecules, viz., CO, N_2, CH_2N and C_2H_4 have a nearest whole number molecular weight equal to 28. Hence, it is difficult to find the exact molecular formula of compounds from the nearest whole number molecular weight. If their exact molecular weight up to 4 or 6 decimal points is calculated, the values differ from each other for all the four molecules. This helps in deriving the correct molecular formula of the molecules. **Table 5.1** gives the exact mass and weight of atoms up to 4 decimal points.

Table 5.1: Atomic mass and atomic weight of atoms up to four decimals

Element	Atomic mass up to 4 decimals	Atomic weight up to 4 decimals
Hydrogen	1.0078	1.0079
Carbon	12.0000	12.0111
Nitrogen	14.0031	14.0067
Oxygen	15.9949	15.9994

The calculation of the molecular mass up to 4 decimal points for all the four molecules is shown in **Table 5.2**.

Thus, in a high resolving mass spectrometer, the peaks are observed at different m/z values for the molecular ions of these compounds and hence, these m/z values can be used to confirm their molecular formulae.

A peak matching process can help the comparison of the peak position of a sample with that of a reference. A fluorocarbon in that mass region can be used as a reference. Use of an oscilloscope for this purpose permits determination of the molecular mass up to six decimal places on a double focusing mass spectrometer. This establishes the identity and the elemental composition of individual ions or compounds.

Table 5.2: Calculation of the molecular mass

CO	N_2	CH_2N	C_2H_4
12.0000	14.0031	12.0000	12.0000
+ 15.9949	+ 14.0031	+ 2 x 1.0078=2.0156	12.0000
= 27.9949	= 28.0062	+ 14.0031	+ 4 x 1.0078 = 4.0312
		= 28.0187	= 28.0312

3) Determination of molecular formula or elemental composition of ions by isotope abundance ratio method

The compounds containing elements, which exist in the form of isotopes, produce additional peaks in the mass spectrum. The compounds containing elements like ^{13}C, ^{2}H, ^{15}N and ^{33}S contribute to a mass peak $(M)^+$ and a mass plus 1 peak $(M+1)^+$. The compounds containing elements like ^{18}O, ^{30}Si, ^{34}S, ^{37}Cl and ^{81}Br contribute to a mass peak $(M)^+$ and a mass plus 2 peak $(M+2)^+$. **Table 5.3** lists the elements existing as isotopes and their relative abundance in nature. The ratio of the intensities of the $(M)^+$ and $(M+1)^+$ peaks or the ratio of the intensities of the $(M)^+$ and $(M+2)^+$ peaks for these elements is approximately equal to the ratio of their natural isotopic abundance.

In methyl chloride (CH_3Cl), for different isotopes of C, the possible compositions are- $^{12}CH_3{}^{35}Cl$ and $^{13}CH_3{}^{35}Cl$. Hence, the former molecule would produce the $(M)^+$ peak at m/z = 50, i.e. (12+3+35) and the latter molecule would produce the $(M)^+$ peak at m/z = 51, i.e. (13+3+35). Hence, the two peaks, $(M)^+$ and $(M+1)^+$, are obtained because of the presence of isotopes of C.

Table 5.3: Relative abundance of isotopes

Sr. No.	Isotopes	Relative Abundance	Peak
1	$^{1}H:^{2}H$	99.985 : 0.015	(M+1)
2	$^{12}C:^{13}C$	98.892 : 1.108	(M+1)
3	$^{14}N:^{15}N$	99.635 : 0.365	(M+1)
4	$^{16}O:^{17}O:^{18}O$	99.759 : 0.037 : 0.204	(M+1) & (M+2)
5	$^{28}Si:^{29}Si:^{30}Si$	92.18 : 4.71 : 3.12	(M+1) & (M+2)
6	$^{32}S:^{33}S:^{34}S$	95.018 : 0.75 : 4.215	(M+1) & (M+2)
7	$^{35}Cl:^{37}Cl$	75.529 : 24.471	(M+2)
8	$^{79}Br:^{81}Br$	50.52 : 49.48	(M+2)

For any compound containing one carbon atom, e.g. CH_3Cl, out of 100 molecules, 98.892 molecules would possess ^{12}C isotope and 1.108 molecules would possess ^{13}C isotope. Hence, the ratio of the heights or the intensities of the $(M)^+$ to $(M+1)^+$ peaks is 98.892 : 1.108 or approximately equal to 99:1.

Similarly, for different isotopes of Cl in CH_3Cl, the possible compositions are - $^{12}CH_3{}^{35}Cl$ and $^{12}CH_3{}^{37}Cl$. Hence, the former molecule would produce the $(M)^+$ peak at m/z = 50, i.e. (12+3+35) and the latter molecule would produce the $(M)^+$ peak at m/z = 52, i.e. (12+3+37). Hence, the two peaks, $(M)^+$ and $(M+2)^+$, are obtained because of the presence of isotopes of Cl.

For any compound like CH_3Cl, containing one chlorine atom, out of 100 molecules, 75.529 molecules would possess ^{35}Cl isotope and 24.471 molecules would possess ^{37}Cl isotope. Hence, the ratio of the heights or the intensities of the $(M)^+$ to $(M+2)^+$ peaks is 75.529 : 24.471 or approximately equal to 75:25 or 3:1.

For methyl bromide (CH_3Br), for different isotopes of C, the possible compositions are - $^{12}CH_3{}^{79}Br$ and $^{13}CH_3{}^{79}Br$. Hence, the former molecule would produce the $(M)^+$ peak at m/z = 94, i.e. (12+3+79) and the latter molecule would produce the $(M)^+$ peak at m/z = 95, i.e. (13+3+79). Hence, the two peaks, $(M)^+$ and $(M+1)^+$, are obtained because of the presence of isotopes of C.

Similarly, for different isotopes of Br, the possible compositions are - $^{12}CH_3{}^{79}Br$ and $^{12}CH_3{}^{81}Br$. Hence, the former molecule would produce the $(M)^+$ peak at m/z = 94, i.e. (12+3+79) and the latter molecule would produce the $(M)^+$ peak at m/z = 96, i.e. (12+3+81). Hence, the two peaks, $(M)^+$ and $(M+2)^+$, are obtained because of the presence of isotopes of Br. Since the isotopic abundance for bromine is approximately equal to 50:50, the ratio of the heights or the intensities of the $(M)^+$ to $(M+2)^+$ peaks is approximately equal to 50:50 or 1:1.

Hence, in the mass spectrum of the molecules having these isotopes, the patterns as shown in **Fig. 5.8** are observed.

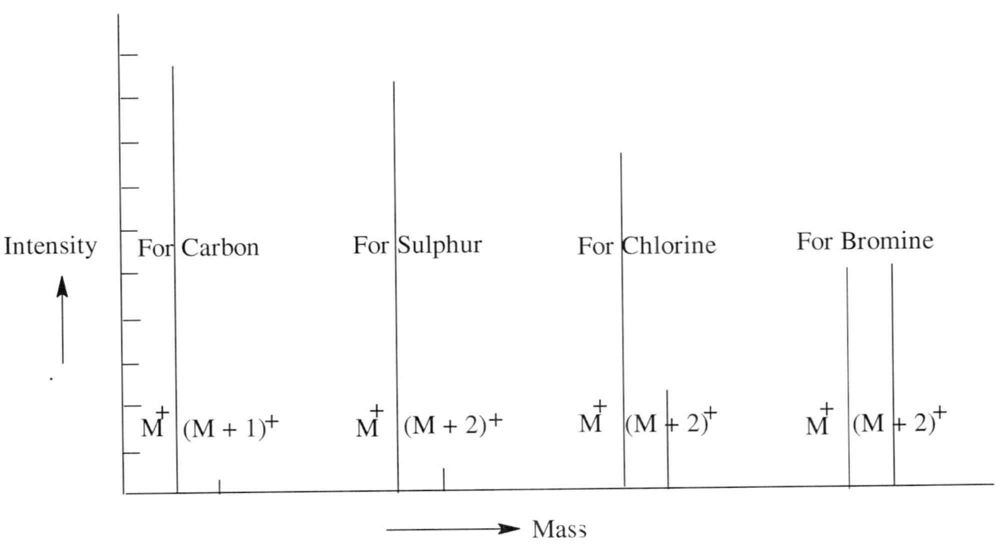

Fig. 5.8: The ratio of intensities of parent peak to the isotopic peak for different elements

The ratio of the intensities of the $(M)^{+}$: $(M+1)^{+}$ peaks and the $(M)^{+}$: $(M+2)^{+}$ peaks gives the idea about the elemental composition of the molecular ion. Hence, to determine the elemental composition of a molecule or a fragment, the intensity ratios of the molecular ion peak to the $(M+1)^{+}$or $(M+2)^{+}$ peak are determined. From **Table 5.3** of isotope abundance ratios, the presence of a particular element is confirmed.

5.12. FRAGMENTATION IN MASS SPECTROMETRY

In the ion source, if the excess of energy is provided during the ionization of a molecule, the molecular ion $(M)^{+}$ undergoes further fragmentation to form the fragments characteristic of a molecule. The sequence of the fragmentation and the fragmentation pattern provide the valuable information about the structure of the parent compound. The general paths observed in molecules during the fragmentation in mass spectrometry are summarized below.

To indicate various fragmentation processes, two types of arrows are commonly used. As mentioned earlier, the one indicating the transfer of only one of the electrons of a bond is shown by a *fish hook arrow* (⌒). Another normal arrow (⌒) indicates the transfer of both the electrons of a bond.

5.12.1. Hydrocarbons

5.12.1.1. Straight Chain Saturated Hydrocarbons

In the straight chain saturated hydrocarbons, there is a possibility of the breakage of a number of C-C bonds. This results in the production of a number of peaks in its mass spectrum.

(i) In case of a n-hexane (**Fig. 5.9**), the parent peak $(M)^{+}$ is the most intense peak.

(ii) The molecular ion can lose one CH_3 radical, giving rise to $(M-15)^{+}$ peak, when C_1-C_2 band is cleaved.

(iii) A cleavage of C_2-C_3 single bond results in the loss of a mass corresponding to one C_2H_5 group. Hence, this cleavage produces a peak at the mass $(M-29)^{+}$.

(iv) The loss of one CH_2 unit contributes to a mass loss of 14 units. Hence, the cleavage after 'n' number of carbon atoms in a straight chain saturated hydrocarbon gives mass loss of (14 x n + 1) units.

$$\overset{1}{CH_3}—\overset{2}{CH_2}—\overset{3}{CH_2}—\overset{4}{CH_2}—\overset{5}{CH_2}—\overset{6}{CH_3}$$

n-Hexane C_6H_{14} (C_nH_{2n+2})

↓

$$[CH_3—CH_2—CH_2—CH_2—CH_2—CH_3]^{\bullet +}$$

Molecular ion, $(\overset{+}{M})$, m/z = 86

→ $^{\bullet}CH_3 + {}^{+}CH_2—CH_2—CH_2—CH_2—CH_3$
(I) C_5H_{11} m/z = $(M - 15)^{+}$

→ $CH_3—\dot{C}H_2 + {}^{+}CH_2—CH_2—CH_2—CH_3$
(II) C_4H_9 m/z = $(M - 29)^{+}$

→ $CH_3—CH_2—\dot{C}H_2 + {}^{+}CH_2—CH_2—CH_3$
(III) C_3H_7 m/z = $(M- 43)^{+}$

Fig. 5.9: Fragmentation in n-hexane

(v) Thus, the fragmentation of the straight chain saturated hydrocarbons results in the formation of peaks corresponding to the mass of C_nH_{2n+1} units, where 'n' is the total number of carbon atoms in that fragment. These peaks are indicated by the compounds (**I**), (**II**) and (**III**) in **Fig. 5.9**.

(vi) The mass spectrum of these hydrocarbons also shows the peaks corresponding to C_nH_{2n} units (loss of CH_2 units – not shown in **Fig. 5.9**).

(vii) For all the hydrocarbons containing more that 8 carbon atoms, the mass spectrum appears almost the same. The identification of the individual hydrocarbon is then based on the molecular ion peak.

5.12.1.2. Branched Chain Hydrocarbons

In case of the branched hydrocarbons, the cleavage occurs at the bond adjacent to the branching. The positive charge is retained by a species so that a more stable carbocation is formed after cleaving. Thus, a tertiary carbocation is formed in preference to a secondary one and a secondary carbocation is formed in preference to a primary one. As shown in **Fig. 5.10**, in case of 2,2,3-trimethylpentane, the cleavage occurs at C_2-C_3 bond and the positive charge resides on a fragment, which leads to the formation of a tertiary carbocation. The electron releasing methyl or alkyl substituents tend to reduce the positive charge at

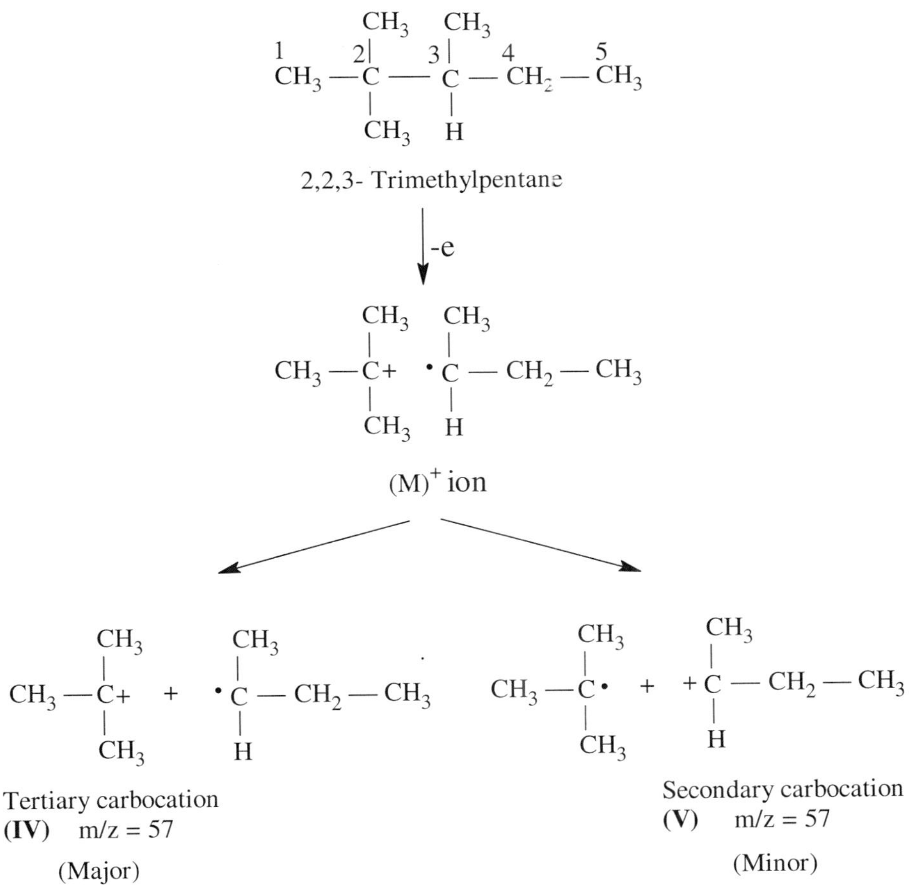

```
        CH3   CH3
1      2|    3|     4       5
CH3 —C —— C — CH2 — CH3
        |     |
        CH3   H
```

2,2,3- Trimethylpentane

↓ -e

```
        CH3   CH3
        |     |
CH3 —C+    • C — CH2 — CH3
        |     |
        CH3   H
```

$(M)^+$ ion

```
   CH3          CH3                            CH3         CH3
   |            |                              |           |
CH3 —C+   +   • C — CH2 — CH3        CH3 —C•   +   + C — CH2 — CH3
   |            |                              |           |
   CH3          H                              CH3         H
```

Tertiary carbocation
(**IV**) m/z = 57
(Major)

Secondary carbocation
(**V**) m/z = 57
(Minor)

Fig. 5.10: Fragmentation in 2,2,3-trimethylpentane

the electron deficient carbon. In doing so, the alkyl substituent itself becomes somewhat positive. This dispersal of charge stabilizes the tertiary carbocation (**IV**). Hence, in case of 2,2,3-trimethylpentane, a secondary carbocation (**V**) is not formed as a predominant ion.

Another example is of 2-methypentane. As shown in **Fig. 5.11**, in this case, a more stable secondary carbocation (**VI**) is formed in preference to a primary carbocation (**VII**).

5.12.1.3. Cycloalkanes

In cycloalkanes (C_nH_{2n}), the cleavage is accompanied by the loss of hydrogen radical. As shown in **Fig. 5.12**, cyclohexane (C_6H_{12}) shows a peak at m/z for $(C_6H_{11})^+$, i.e. $(C_nH_{2n-1})^+$ ion and at $(C_6H_{10})^+$, i. e. $(C_nH_{2n-2})^+$ ion. The fragmentation of these species is further continued in (C_nH_{2n-1}) and in (C_nH_{2n-2}) series.

Apart from these two series, cyclohexane, as shown in **Fig. 5.13**, shows an intense peak by the cleavage of two C-C bonds and by losing an ethylene (C_2H_4) molecule.

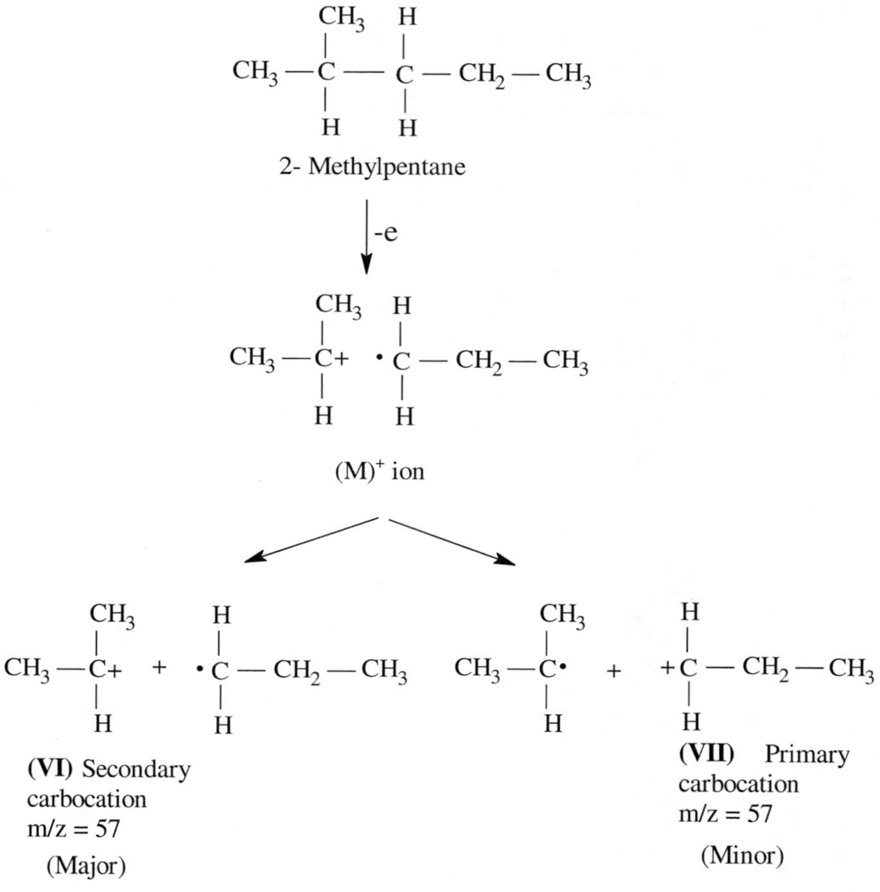

```
         CH3   H
          |    |
   CH3 — C  —  C — CH2 — CH3
          |    |
          H    H
      2- Methylpentane

            | -e
            v

         CH3   H
          |    |
   CH3 — C+   • C — CH2 — CH3
          |    |
          H    H
         (M)+ ion

           /        \
          v          v

     CH3        H                       CH3          H
      |         |                        |           |
CH3 — C+  +  • C — CH2 — CH3      CH3 — C•   +   +C — CH2 — CH3
      |         |                        |           |
      H         H                        H           H
(VI) Secondary                                  (VII) Primary
carbocation                                     carbocation
m/z = 57                                        m/z = 57
(Major)                                         (Minor)
```

Fig. 5.11: Fragmentation in 2- methypentane

Cyclohexane

-e

M^+ ion corresponding to C_nH_{2n} $(C_6H_{12})^+$

$+ \cdot H$

Ion corresponding to C_nH_{2n-1} $(C_6H_{11})^+$

$+ H^\bullet + {}^\bullet H \rightarrow H_2$

Ion corresponding to C_nH_{2n-2} $(C_6H_{10})^+$

Fig. 5.12: Fragmentation in cyclohexane by C-H bond cleavage

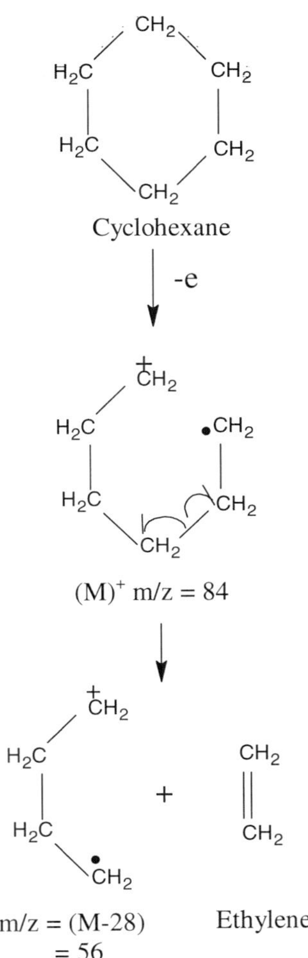

Fig. 5.13: Fragmentation in cyclohexane by C-C bond cleavage

15.12.1.4. Alkenes

1) Olefins

(i) A compound containing only one double bond and having three carbon atoms undergoes the cleavage of the bond adjacent to a double bond, e.g. propene undergoes fission as shown in **Fig. 5.14**.

(ii) Compounds with a carbon – carbon double bond having more than three carbon atoms show fragmentation pattern so as to form a more stable allylic carbocation. As shown in **Fig.**

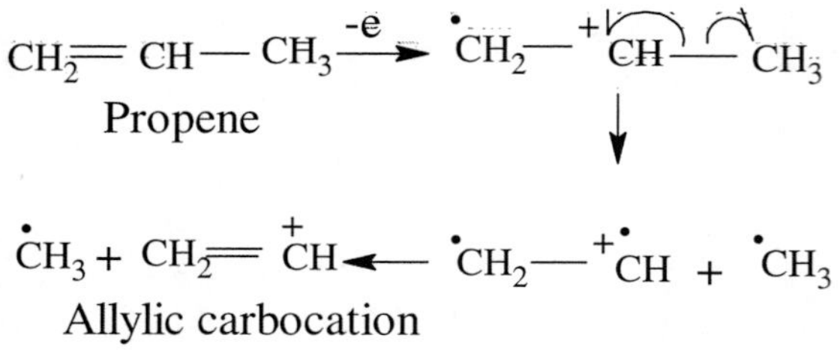

$CH_2{=}CH{-}CH_3 \xrightarrow{-e} \dot{C}H_2{-}\overset{+}{C}H{-}CH_3$ (Propene)

$\downarrow$

$\dot{C}H_3 + CH_2{=}\overset{+}{C}H \leftarrow \dot{C}H_2{-}\overset{+\bullet}{C}H + \dot{C}H_3$

Allylic carbocation

Fig. 5.14: Fragmentation in 1-propene

5.15, the bond between the unsaturated group and the α-carbon atom is termed as a *vinylic* bond. The bond between the α- and β- carbon atoms, is termed *allylic* in aliphatic systems and *benzylic* in the aromatic systems. The cleavage of the vinylic bond occurs relatively infrequently, whereas the cleavage of an allylic bond is commonly encountered.

If an olefin has no γ- carbon atom (e.g. 1-butene, **Fig. 5.16**), then the homolytic cleavage of a single bond between the α- and β carbon atoms

>C=C–C–C–C–

α β γ

Vinylic Allylic

C₆H₅–C–C–C–

α β γ

Vinylic Benzylic

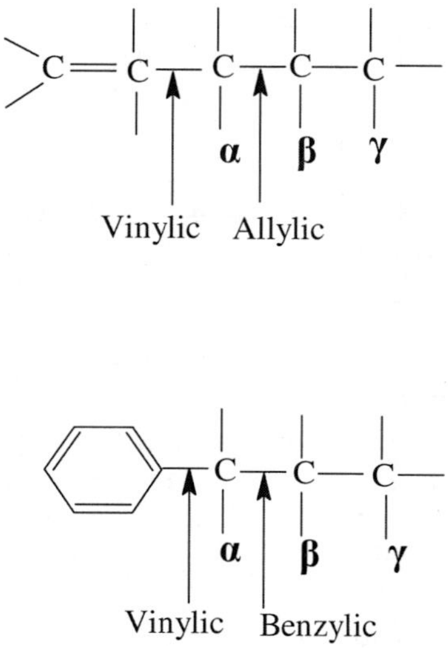

Fig. 5.15: Types of bonds in unsaturated systems

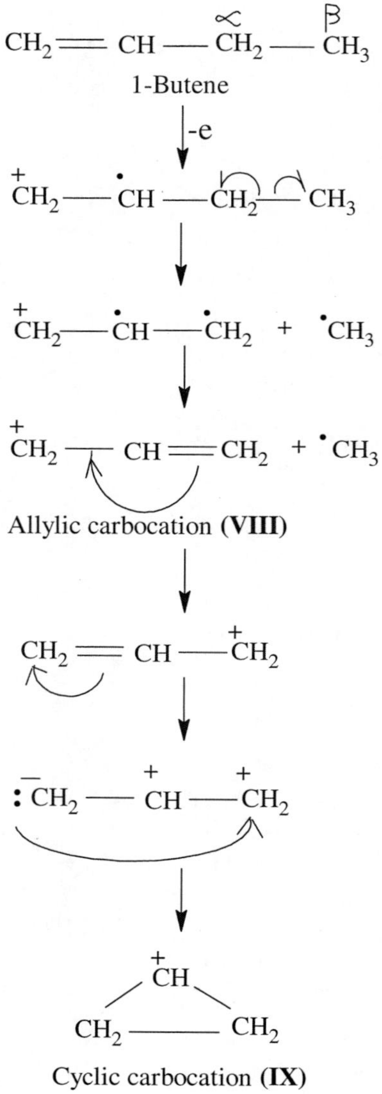

results in the formation of a stable carbocation (**VIII**). Further, the heterolytic cleavage of a double bond induces cyclization, thereby producing a more stable cyclic carbocation (**IX**).

(iii) In long chain olefins containing 5 or more than 5 carbon atoms in a chain, the fragmentation is associated with the cleavage of an allylic bond

$CH_2{=}CH{-}\overset{\alpha}{C}H_2{-}\overset{\beta}{C}H_3$

1-Butene

$\downarrow$ -e

$\overset{+}{C}H_2{-}\dot{C}H{-}CH_2{-}CH_3$

$\downarrow$

$\overset{+}{C}H_2{-}\dot{C}H{-}\dot{C}H_2 + \dot{C}H_3$

$\downarrow$

$\overset{+}{C}H_2{-}CH{=}CH_2 + \dot{C}H_3$

Allylic carbocation (**VIII**)

$\downarrow$

$CH_2{=}CH{-}\overset{+}{C}H_2$

$\downarrow$

$:\overset{-}{C}H_2{-}\overset{+}{C}H{-}\overset{+}{C}H_2$

$\downarrow$

$\overset{+}{C}H$ / $CH_2{-}CH_2$

Cyclic carbocation (**IX**)

Fig. 5.16: Fragmentation in 1-butene

and transfer of the γ-H to the ionized double bond. This fragmentation process is termed as *McLafferty rearrangement*. For example, in **Fig. 5.17**, the fragments for 1-pentene are formed according to McLafferty rearrangement. This involves homolytic fission of the bonds. The rearrangement involving transfer of a hydrogen atom from one part of an ion to another, via a six membered transition state, is termed as McLafferty rearrangement.

The heterolytic fission of the bonds in 1-pentene leads to the formation of the fragments as shown in **Fig. 5.18**.

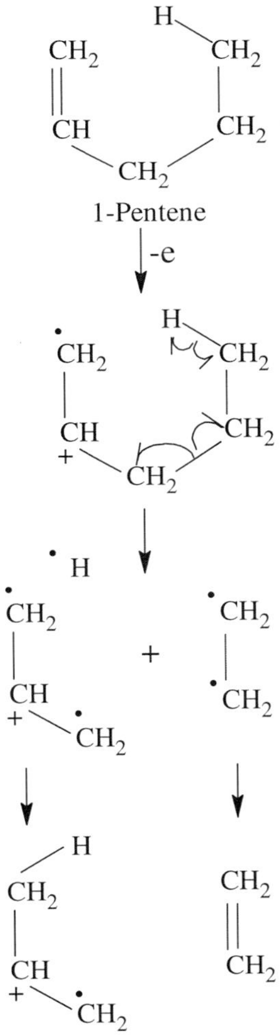

Fig. 5.17: Homolytic fission in 1-pentene

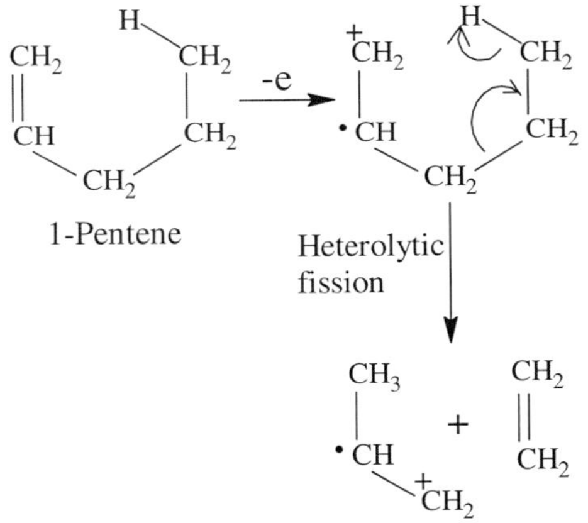

Fig. 5.18: Heterolytic fission in 1-pentene

In 2-hexene (**X**) or 3-heptene (**XI**) and 1-hexene (**XII**) or 1-heptene (**XIII**) (**Fig. 5.19**), the fragmentation would occur to produce a stable allylic carbocation by the cleavage at the bond between the α- and β -carbon atoms.

2) Cycloalkenes

The cycloalkenes undergo a characteristic retro-Diels-Alder fission. The fragmentation pattern for cyclochexene is shown in **Fig. 5.20**. This fragmentation pattern is seen in case of terpenes and steroids.

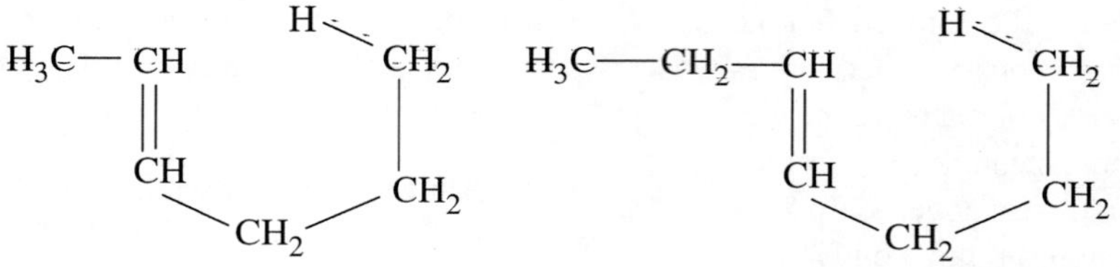

2-Hexene (**X**)

3-Heptene (**XI**)

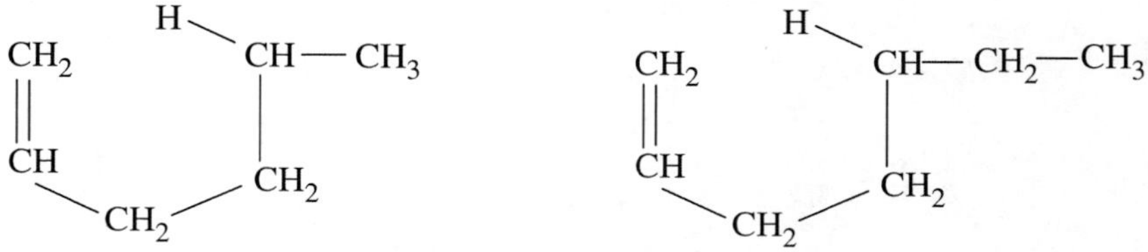

1-Hexene (**XII**)

1-Heptene (**XIII**)

Fig. 5.19: Structures of long chain alkenes

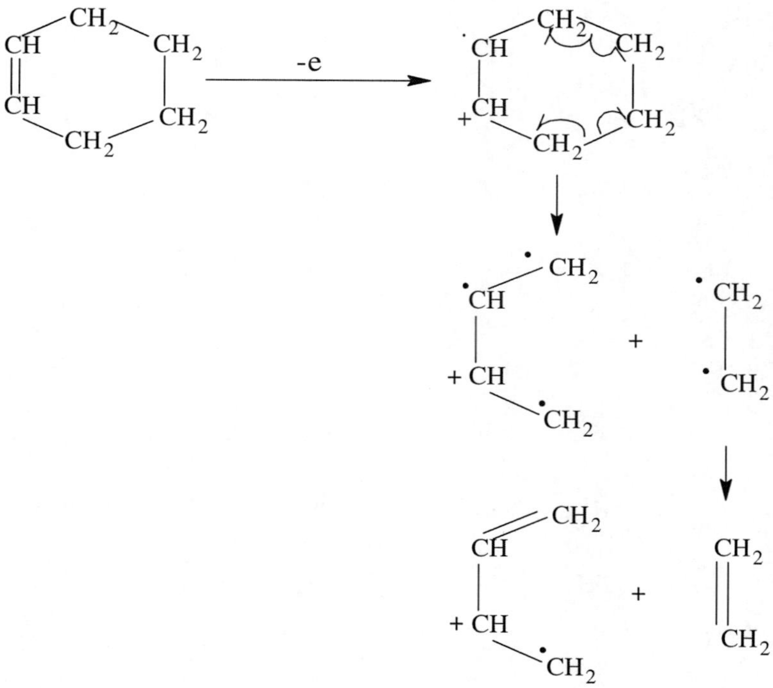

Fig. 5.20: Fragmentation in cyclohexene

3) Alkylbenzenes

The alkylbenzenes like toluene or ethylbenzene, cleave at the C-C bond β- to the aromatic ring, i.e. a bond between the α- and β - carbon atoms is cleaved in this case also. This cleavage can lead to the formation of a benzylic cation (**XIV**) or a tropylium ion (**XV**), the latter being more stable. Fragmentation in toluene is illustrated in **Fig. 5.21**.

5.12.2. Alcohols, Amines and Ethers

A common fragmentation process, which occurs in the cation radicals of alcohols, amines and ethers, is the cleavage of the bond between the α - and β -carbon atoms. This α, β - cleavage results in the formation of an oxonium or immonium ion. The molecular ions for alcohols, amines and ethers are shown in **Fig. 5.22**.

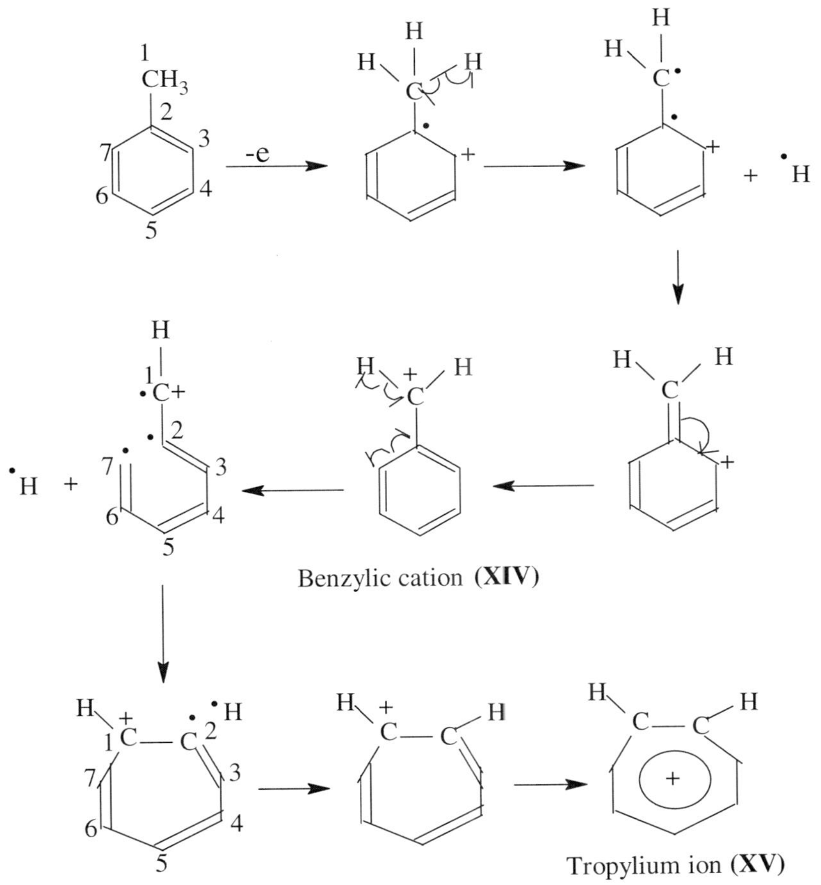

Benzylic cation (**XIV**)

Tropylium ion (**XV**)

Fig. 5.21: Fragmentation in toluene

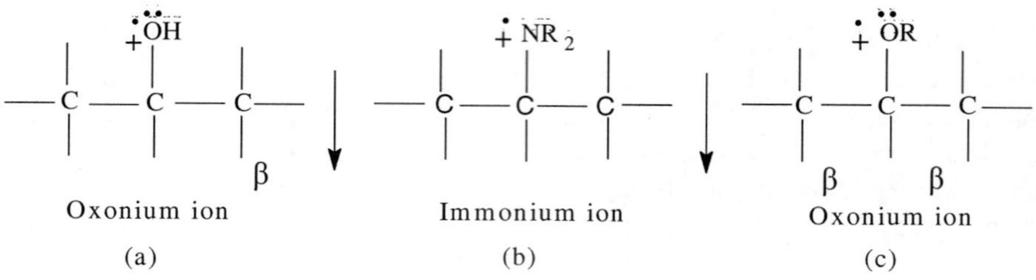

Oxonium ion (a) Immonium ion (b) Oxonium ion (c)

Fig. 5.22: Molecular ions for (a) alcohols, (b) amines and (c) ethers

5.12.2.1. Alcohols

In alcohols, the fragmentation occurs either by the α, β- cleavage or by the elimination of a water molecule.

1) Fragmentation by the α, β- cleavage

Fragmentation in ethanol is shown in **Fig. 5.23**. For 2-methyl-2-butanol, the fragmentation occurs by the two α, β-cleavages as shown in **Fig. 5.24**.

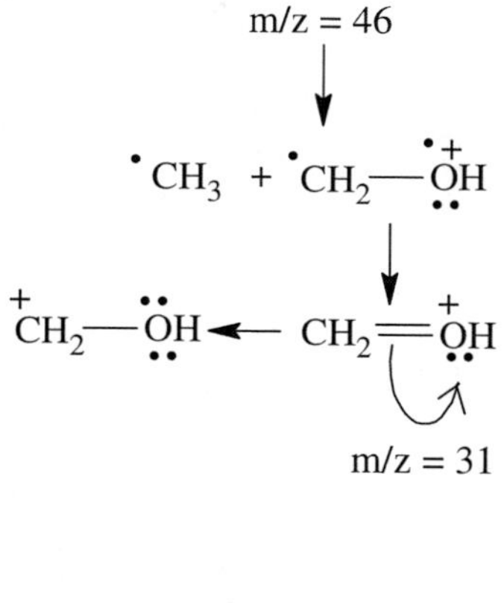

$CH_3—CH_2—\ddot{O}H$

-e

$\dot{C}H_3—CH_2—\dot{O}H^{+}$

m/z = 46

$\cdot CH_3 + \cdot CH_2—\dot{O}H^{+}$

$\overset{+}{C}H_2—\ddot{O}H \leftarrow CH_2=\overset{+}{O}H$

m/z = 31

Fig. 5.23: Fragmentation in ethanol

2-Methyl-2- butanol

-e

$(M)^+$ (m/z = 88)

(Major) $(M-29)^+$ (m/z = 59)

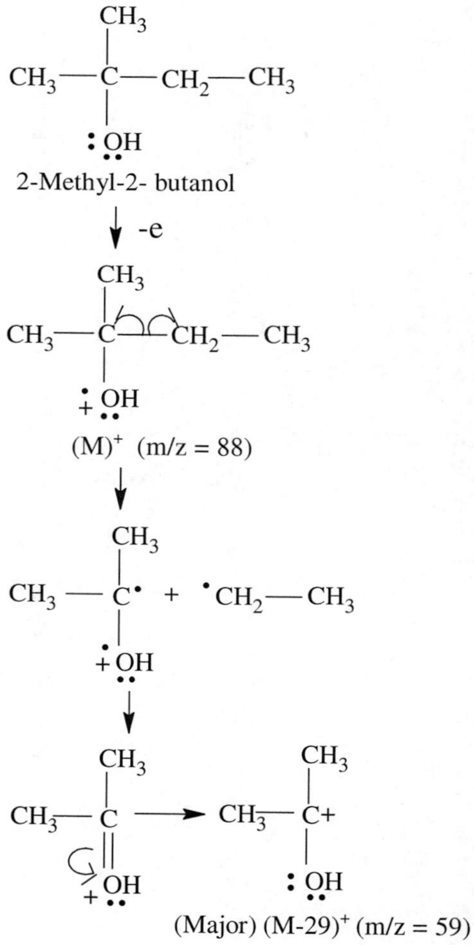

OR

CH_3
$CH_3 — C — CH_2 — CH_3$
$:\ddot{O}H$

2-Methyl-2-butanol

↓ -e

CH_3
$CH_3 — C — CH_2 — CH_3$
$\dot{+}\ddot{O}H$

$(M)^+$ (m/z = 88)

↓

$\dot{C}H_3$ + $\cdot C(CH_3)(\dot{+}\ddot{O}H) — CH_2 — CH_3$

↓

$CH_3 — C(=\overset{+}{O}H) — CH_2 — CH_3$

↓

CH_3
$+C — CH_2 — CH_3$
$:\ddot{O}H$

(Minor) $(M\text{-}15)^+$ (m/z = 73)

Fig. 5.24: Fragmentation in 2-methyl-2-butanol

The elimination of the larger alkyl radical provides the higher stability to the carbocation.

2) Fragmentation by elimination of a water molecule

Another way of fragmentation is by the elimination of water from alcohols. This is seen in case of long chain alcohols or ortho disubstituted aromatic compounds. Dehydration in n-butanol is shown in **Fig. 5.25**. A water molecule and an ethene molecule are eliminated by the combination of a homolytic and a heterolytic cleavage.

In case of o-disubstituted compounds like o-hydroxybenzyl alcohol, H_2O is eliminated by the mechanisms shown in **Fig. 5.26 (i)** and **(ii)**. These are described below.

(i) Electron can be kicked off from the non-bonding electron pair of an electronegative oxygen atom of an alcohol. A water molecule can get eliminated by the heterolytic fission. This mechanism is shown in **Fig 5.26 (i)**.

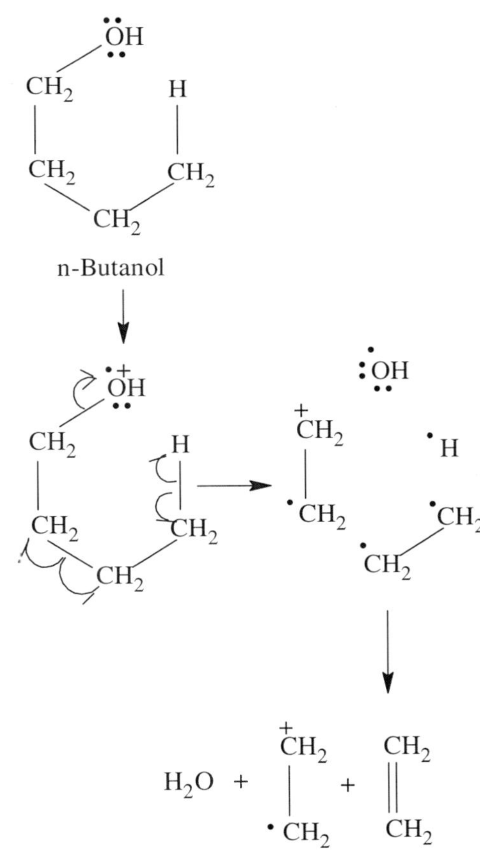

Fig. 5.25: Fragmentation in n-butanol

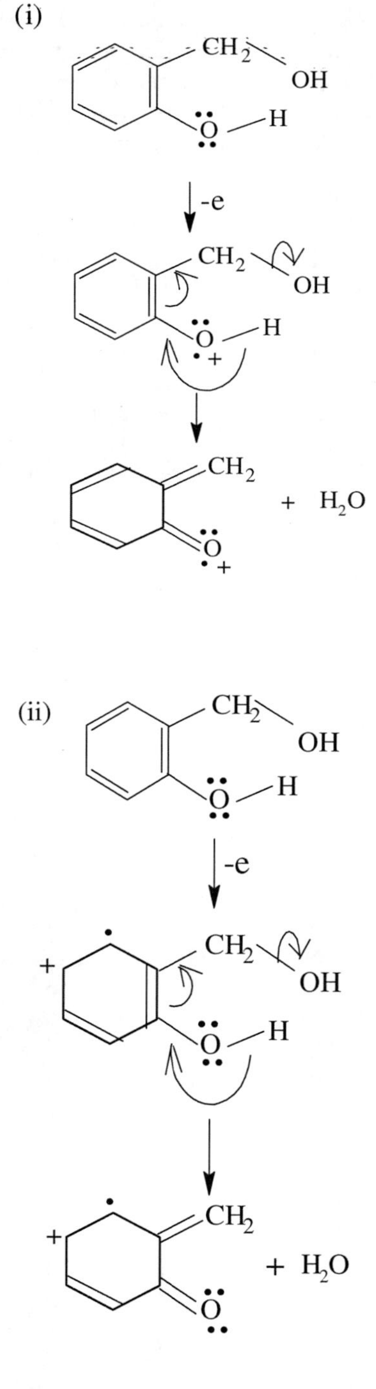

(i)

$\downarrow$ -e

$\downarrow$

$+ H_2O$

(ii)

$\downarrow$ -e

$\downarrow$

$+ H_2O$

Fig. 5.26: Fragmentation in o-hydroxybenzyl alcohol

OR

(ii) Electron can be kicked off from the carbon-carbon double bond of a ring and a water molecule can get eliminated by the heterolytic fission. This mechanism is shown in **Fig. 5.26 (ii)**.

5.12.2.2. Amines

In case of amines, the bombardment of electrons knocks off an electron from the non-bonding electron pair of an electronegative N atom. The α, β- cleavage in n- propylamine, as shown in **Fig. 5.27**, results in the formation of an immonium ion.

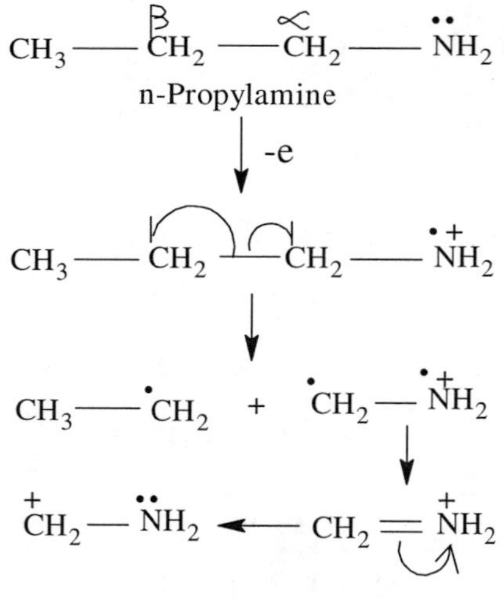

$$CH_3 - \overset{\beta}{C}H_2 - \overset{\alpha}{C}H_2 - \ddot{N}H_2$$

n-Propylamine

$\downarrow$ -e

$$CH_3 - CH_2 - CH_2 - \overset{\bullet +}{N}H_2$$

$\downarrow$

$$CH_3 - \dot{C}H_2 + \dot{C}H_2 - \overset{\bullet +}{N}H_2$$

$\downarrow$

$$\overset{+}{C}H_2 - \ddot{N}H_2 \longleftarrow CH_2 = \overset{+}{N}H_2$$

Fig. 5.27: Fragmentation in n-propylamine

5.12.2.3. Ethers

In ethers, either the bond between the α, β-carbon atoms or between the carbon-oxygen atoms is cleaved, depending upon the stability of the fragment formed. In case of ethers like ethyl methyl ether, the fragmentation occurs as shown in **Fig. 5.28**.

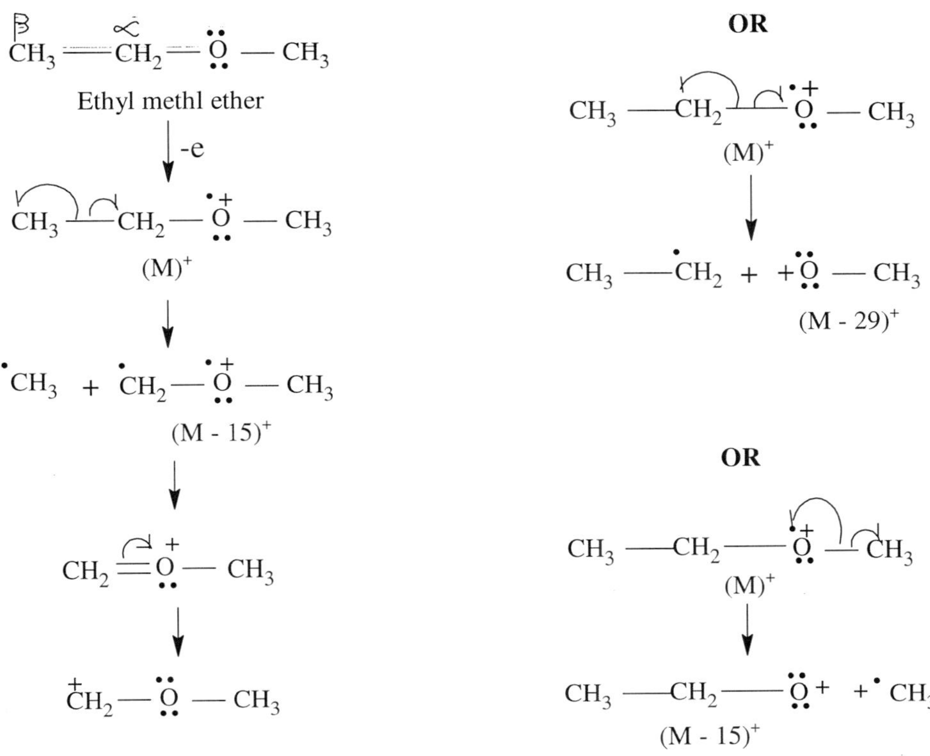

Fig. 5.28: Fragmentation in ethyl methyl ether

5.12.3. Halogenoalkanes or Organic Halides

The halogenoalkanes or organic halides also fragment similar to ethers.

1) In the small chain organic halide, the scission of the bond between the halogen atom and the adjacent carbon atom leads to the formation of a halide and a carbocation, e.g. ethyl chloride gets fragmented into chlorine atom and ethyl carbocation, as shown in **Fig. 5.29**.
2) In the long chain organic halide, the scission of a remote alkyl group results in the formation of a cyclic five membered halonium ion, e.g. in heptyl chloride (**Fig. 5.30**), the loss of a propyl group results in the formation of a cyclic five membered halonium ion.

$CH_3-CH_2-\ddot{Cl}:$

Ethyl chloride

↓ -e

$CH_3-CH_2-\dot{Cl}^{+}:$

$(M)^+$

↓

$CH_3-\overset{+}{C}H_2 + :\dot{Cl}:$

Fig. 5.29: Fragmentation in ethyl chloride

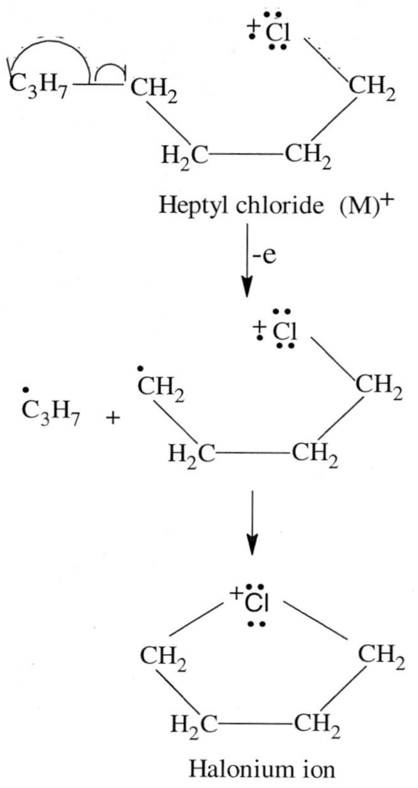

C_3H_7—CH_2, $^+\ddot{Cl}$, CH_2, H_2C—CH_2

Heptyl chloride $(M)^+$

-e

$\dot{C}_3H_7$ + $\dot{C}H_2$, $^+\ddot{Cl}$, CH_2, H_2C—CH_2

CH_2, $^+\ddot{Cl}$, CH_2, H_2C—CH_2

Halonium ion

Fig. 5.30: Fragmentation in heptyl chloride

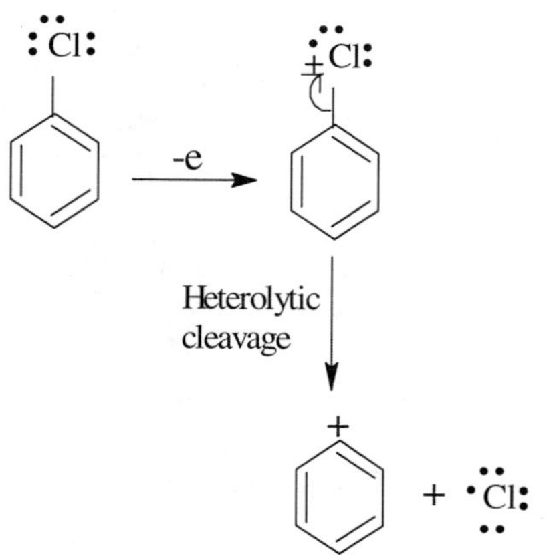

:Cl: -e Heterolytic cleavage + + ·Cl:

Fig. 5.31: Fragmentation in chlorobenzene

3) In the aromatic halides, the cleavage occurs at the bond between the carbon and the halogen atoms, as shown in **Fig. 5.31**.

5.12.4. Carbonyl Compounds

The carbonyl compounds cleave at the C-C bond α to the carbonyl group. An asymmetric ketone, like methyl propyl ketone, undergoes fission in two ways as shown in **Fig. 5.32**. The cleavage occurs at the bonds on either side of a carbonyl group, but the cleavage preferentially occurs at a bond, which favors the elimination of the largest alkyl chain as the neutral fragment. For example, in methyl propyl ketone, the cleavage occurs so as to produce $(CH_3 - C = O^+)$ ion with m/z value 43 abundantly, as compared to $(C_3H_7 - C = O^+)$ ion with m/z value 71.

Ketones can also undergo McLafferty rearrangement as shown in **Fig. 5.33**. Many aldehydes, amides, nitriles and esters also undergo McLafferty rearrangement.

5.12.5. Compounds Containing Two Hetero Atoms

In compounds containing two hetero atoms, the cleavage occurs in such a way so as to retain the charge predominantly on the less electronegative hetero atom. The fragment bearing charge on more electronegative hetero atom is also formed but to a lesser extent. For example, a molecule of aminoethanol undergoes fission in the manner as shown in **Fig. 5.34**.

Thus, mass spectrometry is an important tool in the area of the structure elucidation.

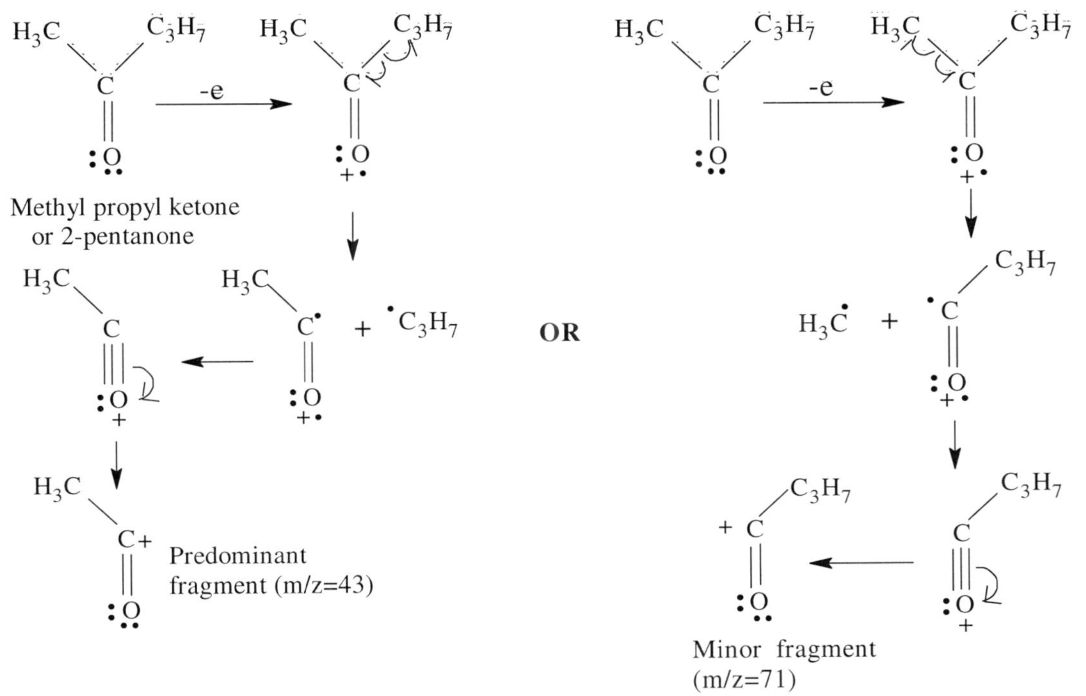

Methyl propyl ketone or 2-pentanone

Predominant fragment (m/z=43)

OR

Minor fragment (m/z=71)

Fig. 5.32: Fragmentation in 2-pentanone

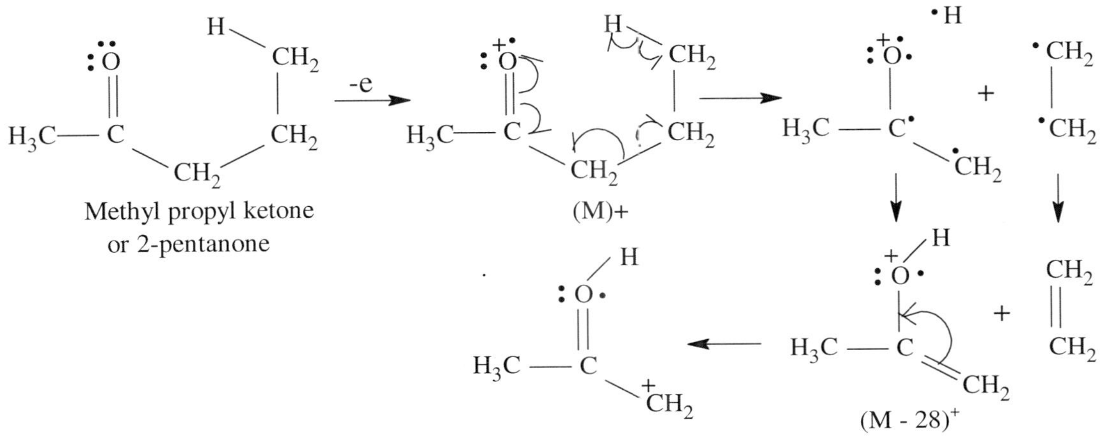

Methyl propyl ketone or 2-pentanone

(M)+

$(M - 28)^+$

Fig. 5.33: McLafferty rearrangement in 2-pentanone

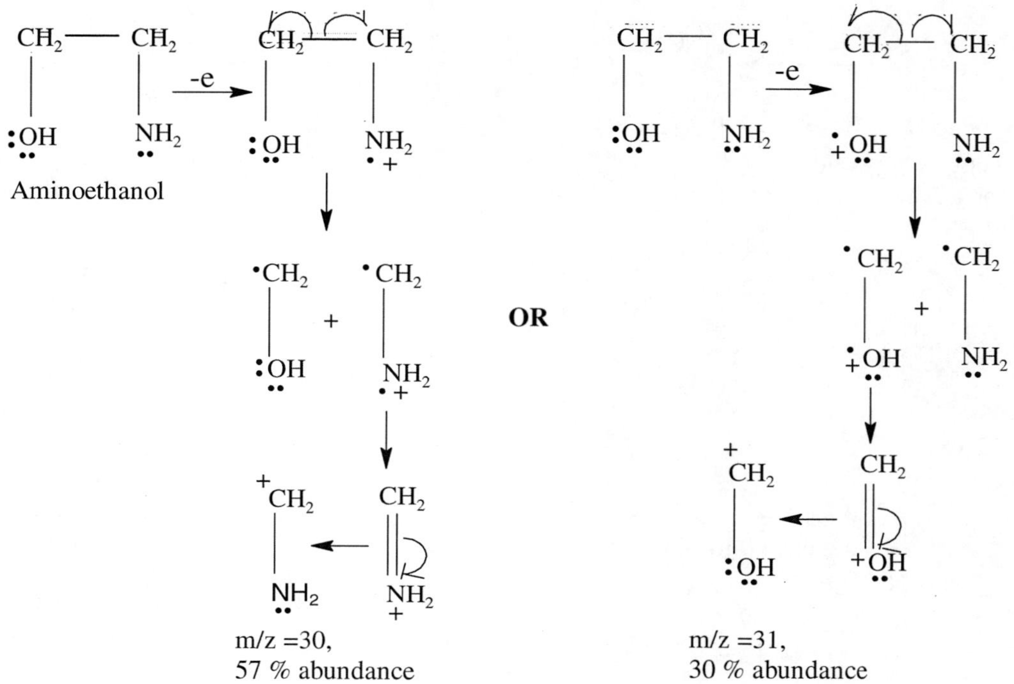

$CH_2—CH_2$ ($:\ddot{O}H$, $\ddot{N}H_2$) Aminoethanol $\xrightarrow{-e}$ $CH_2—CH_2$ ($:\ddot{O}H$, $\ddot{N}H_2^{\bullet +}$) → $^{\bullet}CH_2$–$\ddot{O}H$ + $^{\bullet}CH_2$–$\dot{N}H_2^{+}$ → $CH_2{=}NH_2^{+}$ ← $^{+}CH_2$–$\ddot{N}H_2$

m/z =30,
57 % abundance

OR

$CH_2—CH_2$ ($:\ddot{O}H$, $\ddot{N}H_2$) $\xrightarrow{-e}$ $CH_2—CH_2$ ($\dot{O}H^{+}$, $\ddot{N}H_2$) → $^{\bullet}CH_2$–$\dot{O}H^{+}$ + $^{\bullet}CH_2$–$\ddot{N}H_2$ → $CH_2{=}\ddot{O}H^{+}$ ← $^{+}CH_2$–$:\ddot{O}H$

m/z =31,
30 % abundance

Fig. 5.34: Fragmentation in aminoethanol

CHAPTER 6

FLUORESCENCE AND PHOSPHORESCENCE

Fluorescence and phosphorescence are the luminescent processes. A luminescent process is associated with the absorption of energy in some form and the emission of the absorbed energy in the form of light. The type of energy used for excitation can vary. The luminescent processes are differentiated in the following classes based on the type of energy used for excitation.

6.1. TYPES OF LUMINESCENCE

1) Photoluminescence

In this case, light is produced by exposing the substance to UV radiation.

2) Bioluminescence

In this case, light is produced as a result of biological processes. The light emitted by a glow-worm is because of bioluminescence.

3) Chemiluminescence

The emission of light as a result of chemical reactions is called chemiluminescence. Light sticks producing light as a result of a mixture of chemicals is an example of chemiluminescence.

4) Radioluminescence

The emission of light as a result of interaction of radioactive particles with a compound is called radioluminescence, e.g. luminous paints glow because of the interaction of a compound in it with the radioactive particles, usually provided by tritium (^3H) atoms.

The advantage of using luminescent methods for analysis is that these processes are highly *sensitive* and *selective* in nature. Because they are sensitive, they can be used to analyze concentrations as low as parts per billion (ppb). Since very few molecules are luminescent, the analytical method based on luminescence is highly selective. However, it is less widely applicable than the absorption methods, since relatively few molecules are luminescent in nature.

PHOTOLUMINESCENCE

Photoluminescence includes *fluorescence* and *phosphorescence*. Photoluminescent systems are excited by the absorption of photons and they re-emit energy in the form of radiation of the wavelength which is same or longer than the wavelength used for the excitation. If the wavelength of radiation absorbed and emitted is exactly the same, the phenomenon is termed as the *resonance radiation* or *resonance luminescence*. If the wavelength of emitted radiation is longer than the wavelength of absorption, the phenomenon is called as *Stokes' effect*.

6.2. ELECTRONIC STATES OF A MOLECULE

Two common phenomena of photoluminescence - the fluorescence and the phosphorescence - occur by different mechanisms. To understand these mechanisms, it is necessary to know the meaning of the terms *singlet*, *doublet* and *triplet* electronic states of a molecule.

6.2.1. A Singlet State

In a molecule, if all the electron spins are paired, then the molecular electronic state is called a *singlet state*. The ground state is always a singlet state. In a singlet state, the electric and the magnetic fields produced by the two electrons spinning in the opposite directions are exactly the same in magnitude but opposite in directions. Hence, a system as a whole is associated with only one fixed quantum of energy. When one of the electrons from a pair of electrons in the ground state is excited, either a *singlet* or a *triplet state* results. An excited singlet state results when one of the electrons from the pair is excited to the higher energy level *without the change in its spin.* As a result, two electrons, one in the ground state and another in the excited state, still spin in the opposite directions and cancel the electric and the magnetic fields of each other. As a whole, the system is associated with only one fixed quantum of energy. The only difference between the *ground singlet state* and the *excited singlet state* is that the latter is associated with the higher amount of energy as compared to that of the former. The ground and the excited singlet states of a molecule are shown in **Fig. 6.1(a)**.

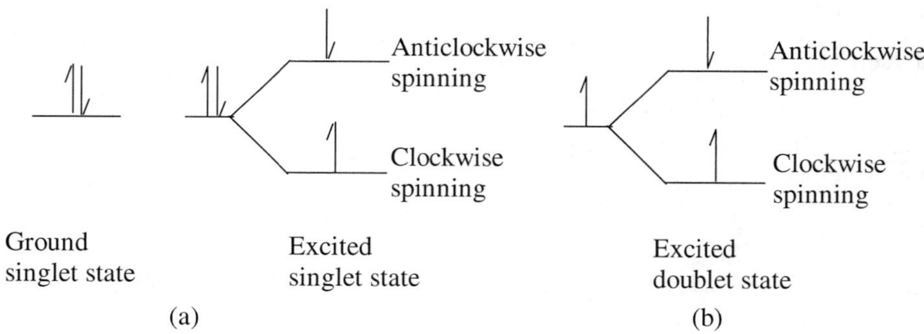

Fig. 6.1: (a) Ground and excited singlet states (b) excited doublet state

6.2.2. A Doublet State

In a molecule containing an odd number of electrons in the outermost shell or a molecule containing an unpaired electron, as in case of a ground state of a free radical, a single electron can spin either clockwise or anticlockwise and can assume two orientations in the magnetic field. This results in the production of the field in two directions, one along the direction of an external magnetic field and another in the direction opposite to the direction of an external magnetic field. Since an unpaired electron assumes two molecular electronic states, the system as a whole is associated with two different quanta of energy. Such a system is termed as a *doublet state* and is shown in **Fig. 6.1(b)**.

6.2.3. A Triplet State

When one of the electrons from a pair of electrons in the ground state is excited and if the excitation of an electron occurs *with the change in the spin*, both the electrons, one in the ground state [1 in **Fig. 6.1(c)**] and another in the excited state [2 in **Fig. 6.1(c)**], spin in the same direction. An electron in the ground state can spin either clockwise or anticlockwise and can assume two orientations [3 and 4 in **Fig. 6.1(c)**, respectively] in the magnetic field. Similarly, an electron in the excited state can spin either clockwise or anticlockwise and can assume two orientations [5 and 6 in **Fig. 6.1(c)**, respectively] in the magnetic field. The energy associated with these energy levels [5 and 6 in **Fig. 6.1(c)**] is higher compared to the energy associated with the energy levels of an electron in the ground state [3 and 4 in **Fig. 6.1(c)**]. As shown in **Fig. 6.1(c)**, the higher energy level of an electron in the ground state [4 in **Fig. 6.1(c)**] usually overlaps with the lower energy level of an electron in the excited state [5 in **Fig. 6.1(c)**], because of almost the same energy content associated with them. Thus, practically, a molecule is associated with only three different quanta of energy when excitation of one of the electrons from the pair occurs with the change in the spin. The electronic state, in which the spins of the electrons are unpaired or parallel, is therefore, called a *triplet state*.

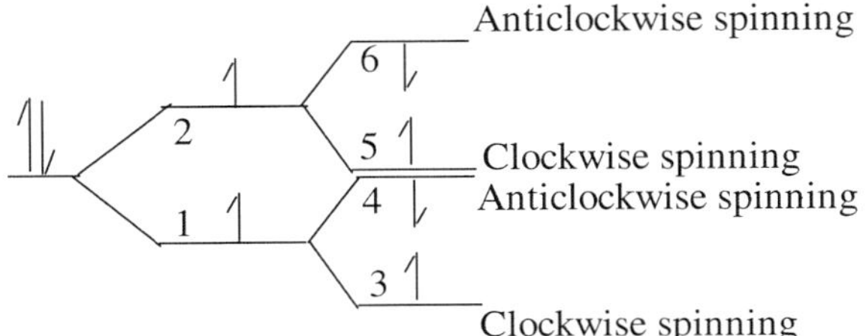

Fig. 6.1 (c): A triplet state

The *excited triplet state* is always less energetic compared to the corresponding *excited singlet state*. In a singlet state, a molecule is diamagnetic whereas in a triplet state, a molecule is paramagnetic. The transition of an electron to an excited singlet state does not involve a change in the spin of an electron but the transition of an electron to an excited triplet state does necessarily involve a change in the spin of an electron. Hence, a singlet to singlet transition is more probable than a singlet to triplet or a triplet to singlet transition. Thus, a singlet-singlet transition occurs faster than a singlet-triplet or a triplet-singlet transition. Secondly, a direct excitation of an electron from a ground singlet state to an excited singlet state is possible but the excitation of an electron, directly from a ground singlet state to an excited triplet state is not possible. An electron can enter the excited triplet state through an excited singlet state only. This is shown in **Figures 6.2** and **6.3**.

6.3. MECHANISM OF FLUORESCENCE AND PHOSPHORESCENCE

The major difference between fluorescence and phosphorescence is that fluorescence involves singlet-singlet transition whereas phosphorescence involves triplet-singlet transition.

In **Fig. 6.2**, out of the two electrons in the ground singlet state (**GSS**), one of the electrons is excited to the higher energy level by supplying energy. If this excitation is not associated with the change in the spin of an electron, the two electrons - one that remains in the ground state and another which occupies an excited state - still spin in the opposite directions. In such a case, an electron is said to be present in an excited singlet state (**ESS**). On the other hand, if the excitation is associated with the change in the spin, both the electrons spin in the same direction and then an electron is said to be present in the excited triplet state (**ETS**).

Fluorescence and phosphorescence are the deactivation processes, in which an excited electron tries to come back to the GSS by giving out the absorbed energy. If an electron has to come back from the ESS to the GSS, it can do so without the change in the spin. Hence, it just emits out the

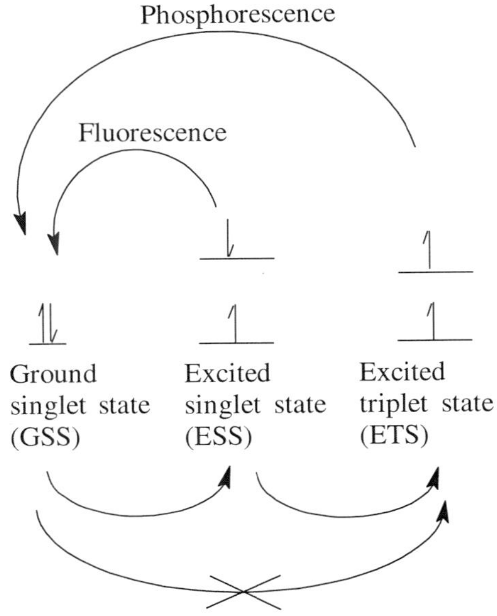

Fig. 6.2: Mechanisms of fluorescence and phosphorescence

absorbed energy and enters the GSS. However, if an electron has to come back from the ETS to the GSS, it has to first change its spin, give out the absorbed energy and then enter the GSS. Since the transition of an electron from the ESS to the GSS does not require change in the spin of an electron, this transition occurs in a short time period, ranging from 10^{-6} to 10^{-9} sec. On the other hand, the transition of an electron from the ETS to the GSS requires comparatively longer time period, ranging from 10^{-4} sec to few seconds or minutes, since this transition is associated with the change in the spin of an electron. Coming back of an electron from the ESS to the GSS, by giving out energy in the form of radiation, is called *fluorescence*, whereas coming back of an electron from the ETS to the GSS, by giving out energy in the form of radiation, is called *phosphorescence*. These mechanisms are shown in **Fig. 6.2**.

The difference between the fluorescence and phosphorescence is indicated in **Table 6.1**.

6.4. DEACTIVATION PROCESSES

Deactivation processes are the processes by which excited electrons give out the absorbed energy and come back to their original position, i.e. to the ground state in most of the cases.

Various deactivation processes, as mentioned and described below, are shown in **Fig. 6.3**.

6.4.1. Vibrational relaxation
6.4.2. Internal conversion
6.4.3. Fluorescence
6.4.4. External conversion
6.4.5. Intersystem crossing
6.4.6. Phosphorescence
6.4.7. Dissociation
6.4.8. Predissociation

Florescence and phosphorescence are the deactivation processes by which a molecule gives out the absorbed energy and returns back to the ground state. In **Fig. 6.3**, the loss of energy by an electron, while coming back from an excited state (S_1) to the ground state (S_o), is shown by two types of arrows. A *wavy arrow* indicates the *radiationless loss* of energy, which is usually in the form of heat. A *straight arrow* indicates the loss of energy, which is usually in the form of radiation. In case of fluorescence and phosphorescence, the loss of energy is in the form

Table 6.1: Difference between fluorescence and phosphorescence

	Fluorescence	Phosphorescence
1	Excitation of an electron occurs without the change in the spin	Excitation of an electron occurs with the change in the spin.
2	Coming back of an electron from the ESS to the GSS is termed as fluorescence	Coming back of an electron from the ETS to the GSS is termed as phosphorescence
3	Fluorescence occurs due to singlet – singlet transition.	Phosphorescence occurs due to triplet - singlet transition.
4	The life-time of an excited state is short, ranging from 10^{-6} -10^{-9} sec.	The life-time of an excited state is as long as 10^{-4} sec to few seconds or minutes.
5	Fluorescence stops immediately as soon as the source of excitation is removed.	Phosphorescence is seen for a sufficiently longer period, even after removing the source of excitation.

of radiation and not in the form of heat.

An excited molecule can return to the ground state (GS) by a combination of deactivation processes. A process, which brings the molecule to the GS faster or which reduces the life time of an excited state, is favored.

In **Fig. 6.3**,

S_o represents the ground singlet state (GSS),

S_1 represents the first excited singlet state (FESS),

S_2 represents the second excited singlet state (SESS),

T_1 represents the first excited triplet state (FETS),

thick lines are the electronic states, and thin lines are the vibrational energy levels.

6.4.1. Vibrational Relaxation

In **Fig. 6.3**, when an electron from the GSS (S_c), is excited using a narrow range of wavelengths, centered around $_1$, it occupies any one of the vibrational energy levels of the first excited singlet state (FESS, S_1). Direct excitation of an electron from the GSS to the first excited triplet state (FETS, T_1) does not occur since it requires a change in the spin of an electron, which is less probable. Deactivation by vibrational relaxation is so fast that the life time of an excited state is only 10^{-12} sec or less. It is characterized by the transition of an electron from the higher vibrational energy level to the lower

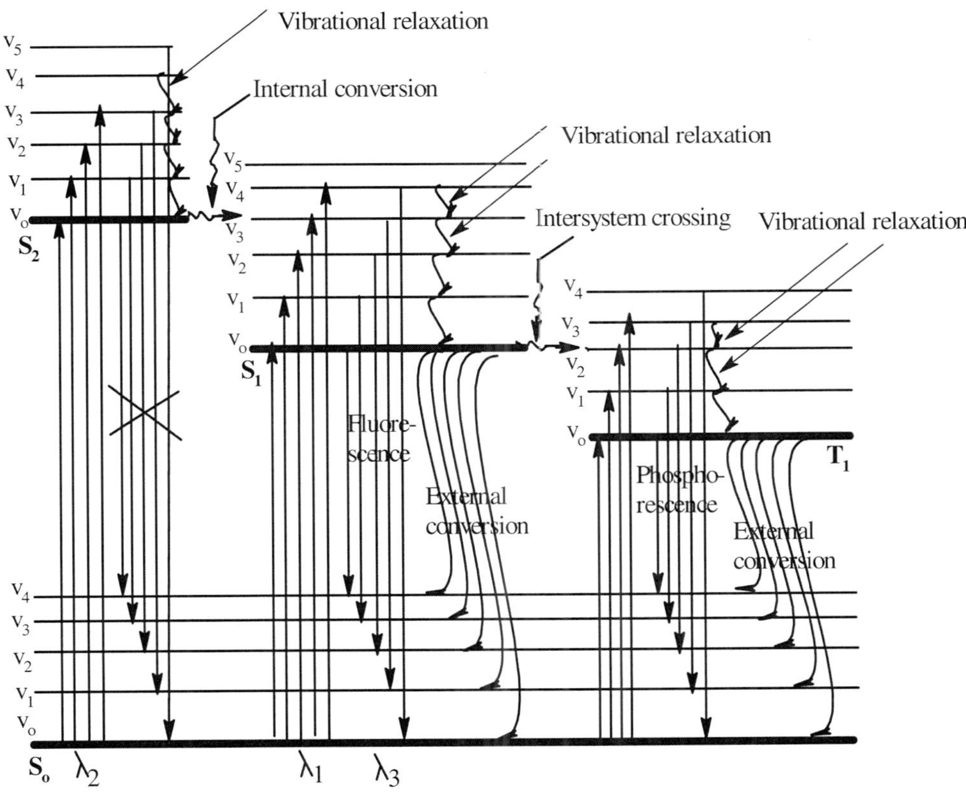

Fig. 6.3: Various deactivation processes

vibrational energy level, within the same electronic state. It also involves radiationless loss of energy, i.e. the loss of energy is in the form of heat and hence, it is indicated by wavy arrows. Since the transition of an electron is within the electronic state, the amount of energy lost in the form of heat, during vibrational relaxation, is less. This results in the nominal increase in the temperature of the surrounding environment (solvent in most of the cases) of a molecule.

By vibrational relaxation, an electron reaches the ground vibrational energy level (v_o) of that electronic state (S_1 in this case). Further deactivation takes place either by fluorescence or external conversion or intersystem crossing, depending on the intrinsic structure of a molecule and its surrounding. These deactivation processes are described below. By these deactivation processes, an electron drops down to any of the vibrational energy levels of the ground state (S_o). Further vibrational relaxations bring down an electron from the higher vibrational energy levels of the GS (S_o) to the ground vibrational energy level (v_o) of the GS (S_o).

6.4.2. Internal Conversion

Instead of excitation of an electron from S_o to S_1, using a wavelength centered around λ_1, if a shorter or a more energetic wavelength centered around λ_2 is used, an electron can get excited to the second excited single state (SESS, S_2). In this electronic state, an electron can enter any of the vibational energy levels of S_2. In order to come back to the GS, the electron chooses the fastest deactivation process, the vibrational relaxation process, by which it comes down from the higher vibrational energy level of S_2 to the ground vibrational energy level (v_o) of S_2. An electron cannot directly fall down from S_2 to any of the vibrational energy levels of S_o by giving out energy in the form of radiation (fluorescence from S_2) because it is a slower process of deactivation compared to the other available deactivation processes. An internal conversion is one such process, which is faster and efficient compared to the fluorescence from S_2.

When one of the vibrational energy levels of the lower excited singlet state (e.g. v_3 of S_1 in **Fig. 6.3**) overlaps with the ground vibrational energy level (v_o) of the higher electronic singlet state (S_2), an electron prefers to deactivate by the process of internal conversion. Since the potential energy of the ground vibrational energy level of the higher electronic state (v_o of S_2) and the overlapping vibrational energy level of the lower electronic state (in this case, v_3 of S_1 in **Fig. 6.3**) is almost same, an electron can easily enter from the higher electronic state (S_2) to the lower electronic state (S_1) without emission of radiation. Once an electron enters the overlapping vibrational energy level of the lower excited singlet state (v_3 of S_1), further deactivation by vibrational relaxation brings down an electron to the ground vibrational energy level (v_o), of S_1 Again, from v_o of S_1, an electron can deactivate by the external conversion or fluorescence or intersystem crossing, as shown in **Fig. 6.3**. Internal conversion through overlapping vibrational energy levels is usually more probable than the loss of energy by fluorescence from a higher excited state (S_2). Because of this, fluorescence usually occurs at a wavelength (λ_3), which is less energetic or longer than the wavelength used for the excitation (λ_1 or λ_2) of an electron.

Thus, a deactivation process involving transition of an electron from a higher singlet state to a lower singlet state, through overlapping vibrational energy levels, without significant loss of energy, is termed as *internal conversion*. The minute loss in energy is in the form of heat, which is a radiationless loss of energy.

6.4.3. External Conversion

Like vibrational relaxation, external conversion is also associated with the radiationless loss of energy, i.e. in this deactivation process, energy is lost by an excited molecule to its surrounding (either to the solvent or the neighboring molecules of the solute itself) in the form of heat. Hence, it is represented by wavy arrows in **Fig. 6.3**. The only difference between the vibrational relaxation process and the external conversion is that the former corresponds to the transition of an excited electron from the higher vibrational energy level to the ground vibrational energy level of the same electronic state, whereas the latter corresponds to the transition of an excited electron from the ground vibrational energy level (v_o) of the higher electronic state to any of the vibrational energy levels of the lower electronic state. Since the transition of an electron is within the electronic state, in case of the vibrational relaxation process, the amount of energy given out in the form of heat is less. Hence, there is slight increase in the temperature of the solvent. In case of external conversion, the transition of an electron is from one electronic state to the other. Hence, the amount of energy given out in the form of heat is much more compared to that produced during vibrational relaxation and therefore, there is a marked increase in the temperature of the solvent.

Usually, external conversion occurs from the lowest excited singlet (S_1) and triplet (T_1) states to the ground state, which is shown in **Fig. 6.3**.

6.4.4. Fluorescence

When an electron is excited using a wavelength λ_2 (**Fig. 6.3**), it occupies any vibrational energy level of the second excited singlet state (S_2). While coming back, it first gets transferred to the ground vibrational energy level (v_o) of the second excited singlet state (S_2) via vibrational relaxation. From v_o of S_2, it does not directly fall down to any of the vibrational energy levels of the ground state, i.e. neither by giving out energy in the form of radiation (fluorescence from S_2) nor by giving out energy in the form of heat (external conversion from S_2). This is because the rate of deactivation by internal conversion, which allows entry of an electron from v_o of S_2 to the overlapping vibrational energy level of S_1, is usually faster compared to the fluorescence or external conversion from S_2. Once the electron enters the vibrational energy level of S_1, it comes down to v_o of S_1 by vibrational relaxation.

From v_o of S_1, it can fall down to any of the vibrational energy levels of the GS (S_o), either by giving out energy in the form of heat (external conversion) or by giving out energy in the form of radiation (fluorescence). The difference between the external conversion and fluorescence is that the former is associated with the radiationless loss of energy (loss of energy in the form of heat), whereas the latter is characterized by the loss of energy in the form of radiation.

The actual deactivation process followed by a molecule depends on the rates of possible deactivation processes. A molecule chooses that particular path, which takes it faster to the ground state. The rates of deactivation processes can explain why fluorescence usually occurs from the lowest excited singlet state, irrespective of whether λ_1 is used for the excitation or λ_2. Hence, fluorescence is usually observed at a wavelength which is longer than the wavelength used for excitation.

6.4.5. Intersystem Crossing

This deactivation process is more or less similar to the internal conversion. In case of internal conversion, an electron is transferred from the higher excited singlet state to the lower singlet state (either excited or ground) without substantial loss of energy. Internal conversion being a singlet-singlet transition does not involve change in the spin of an electron.

Deactivation by intersystem crossing occurs if any of the vibrational energy levels of a triplet excited state (v_2 of T_1 in **Fig. 6.3**) overlaps with the ground vibrational energy level (v_o) of the lowest excited singlet state (S_1). Thus, as shown in **Fig. 6.3**, intersystem crossing involves singlet-triplet transition and hence, it is associated with the change in the spin of an electron. This change in the spin occurs in molecules that contain heavy atoms like I, Br, etc. In heavy atoms, the number of electrons is more. During excitation, an electron occupies a new orbit. If an excited electron interferes with the spin and orbital motion of electrons, which are already there in that orbit, and if the change in the spin of an excited electron reduces the interference with the spin and orbital motion of electrons already existing in that orbit of the heavy atom, then only the excited electron changes its spin. That is how an electron enters from a singlet state into a triplet state. If v_0 of the lowest excited singlet state (S_1) and one of the vibrational energy levels of a triplet state overlap, then the potential energy of the two levels being almost the same, the transfer of an electron from a singlet system to a triplet system takes place without substantial loss of energy. This entry of an electron from a singlet system into a triplet system is called an *intersystem crossing*. Like internal conversion, this deactivation process also involves radiationless loss of energy.

6.4.6. Phosphorescence

By intersystem crossing, an electron enters into any of the vibrational energy levels of the lowest excited triplet system. From there, it drops down to the ground vibrational energy level (v_0) of the lowest excited triplet system (T_1) by vibrational relaxation (**Fig. 6.3**). From v_0 of T_1, it tries to come down to any of the vibrational energy levels of the ground electronic state, either by external conversion (by losing energy in the form of heat) or by phosphorescence (by losing energy in the form of radiation).

Coming back of an electron from the excited singlet state to the ground state by giving out energy in the form of radiation is called *fluorescence*, whereas coming back of an electron from an excited triplet state to the ground state by giving out energy in the form of radiation is called *phosphorescence*. This is clear from **Fig. 6.3**. Thus, both these phenomena occur by different mechanisms. A triplet-singlet transition, involving change in the spin of an electron (**Fig. 6.2**) requires more time as compared to a singlet-singlet transition, which does not involve change in the spin of an electron. Hence, the life time of an excited state is more in case of phosphorescence than that in case of fluorescence. The life time of an excited state in fluorescence is of the order of 10^{-9} - 10^{-7} sec, whereas that in case of phosphorescence is 10^{-4} sec to several seconds or sometimes, to several minutes also. Therefore, fluorescence stops as soon as the source of excitation is removed, while phosphorescence is seen for quite some time, even after the removal of the source of excitation.

External conversion competes so successfully with phosphoresce that the use of very low temperature or a viscous medium that avoids collision of molecules, is required for observing phosphorescence. This is the reason why intensity of phosphorescence is not used for quantitative estimation

6.4.7. Predissociation

When an electron is excited from S_0 to S_2 by a shorter wavelength λ_2, it can undergo deactivation, first by vibrational relaxation and then by the internal conversion. This allows entry of an electron from v_0 of S_2, into any of the vibrational energy levels of the lower excited electronic singlet state (S_1). This internal conversion may sometimes, results in predissociation. In predissociation, an electron enters such a vibrational energy level of the lower electronic singlet state (S_1), whose energy is equivalent to the energy of one of the bonds in a molecule. Hence, as soon as an electron occupies that particular vibrational energy level, it results in the rupture of a particular bond in a molecule. Thus, a part of the absorbed energy is lost in the form of heat (during vibrational relaxation from the higher vibrational energy level of S_2 to v_0 of S_2) and a part of it is used to break a bond in the molecule.

6.4.8. Dissociation

In case of predissociation, the rupture of a bond results as a consequence of the absorption of energy by some chromophore in a molecule, followed by the internal conversion of the electron into the vibrational energy level of the lower excited singlet state, which is associated with the bond energy of one of the bonds in a molecule.

In case of dissociation, the absorption of energy by an electron, directly takes it to that vibrational energy level, whose energy corresponds to one of the bonds in a molecule and results in the rupture of that particular bond.

If the molecules deactivate mainly by fluorescence, i.e. when the rate of deactivation by fluorescence is more, the intensity of fluorescence is also more. If other deactivation processes also compete with fluorescence, the intensity of fluorescence is reduced to some extent. Exactly which particular deactivation process would occur faster would be decided by the intrinsic structure of a molecule and its environment.

6.5. FACTORS AFFECTING INTENSITY OF FLUORESCENCE AND PHOSPHORESCENCE

Two major factors deciding whether a molecule will or will not fluoresce or phosphoresce and if at all it fluoresces or phosphoresces, to what extent it would fluoresce or phosphoresce, are described below.

6.5.1. Intrinsic structure of a molecule and
6.5.2. Environment of a molecule

The extent to which molecules fluoresce or phosphoresce is expressed quantitatively in terms of quantum yield or quantum efficiency, designated by the symbol ϕ (Phi, Gr.).

The quantum efficiency for fluorescence (ϕ_f) is the ratio of the rate of deactivation of molecules by fluorescence to the rates of all the deactivation processes followed by it. In short, it is the ratio of the number of molecules that fluoresce to the total number of excited molecules. The quantum yield of fluorescence can be expressed quantitatively by the following equation.

$$\varphi_f = \frac{K_f}{K_f + K_{ph} + K_{ic} + K_{ec} + K_{is} + K_{pd} + K_d}$$

where, K_f = rate of deactivation by fluorescence,

K_{ph} = rate of deactivation by phosphorescence,

K_{ic} = rate of deactivation by internal conversion,

K_{ec} = rate of deactivation by external conversion,

K_{is} = rate of deactivation by intersystem crossing,

K_{pd} = rate of deactivation by predissociation, and

K_d = rate of deactivation by dissociation.

6.5.1. Intrinsic Structure of a Molecule

The intrinsic structure of a molecule takes into account the following factors.

6.5.1.1. The Type of Electronic Transition Involved

1) Saturated compounds involving σ to σ^* transition

The saturated compounds or the compounds which absorb below 250 nm seldom show fluorescence. This is because the wavelengths shorter than 250 nm are sufficiently energetic to cause rupture of few bonds in a molecule by dissociation or predissociation.

2) Unsaturated compounds involving either π to π^* or n to π^* transitions

In case of unsaturated compounds, the π to π^* transition or n to π^* transition is possible. These transitions are less energetic compared to σ to σ^* transition and hence, such molecules can deactivate very fast by fluorescence. In most cases, π to π^* transition is less energetic compared to n to π^* transition and fluorescence is commonly observed in molecules involving π to π^* transition. The quantum efficiency is greater for molecules involving π to π^* transition compared to those involving n to π^* transition because of the following two reasons.

(i) The molar absorptivity of a π to π^* transition, or the ease with which electrons get excited from π to π^* orbital, is 100-1000 times more than that for n to π^* transition. Hence, a greater number of molecules is present in the $\pi\pi^*$ excited state as compared to that in the $n\pi^*$ excited state. Since the rate of deactivation is directly proportional to the number of molecules present in the excited state, deactivation of molecules from the $\pi\pi^*$ state occurs faster than that from the $n\pi^*$ state. Thus, the lifetime of the $\pi\pi^*$ excited state is shorter, of the order of 10^{-7} to 10^{-9} sec, compared to the lifetime of the $n\pi^*$ excited state, which is of the order of 10^{-5} to 10^{-7} sec. Therefore, quantum efficiency is greater for molecules involving π to π^* transition.

(ii) The second reason for high rate of deactivation by fluorescence in molecules involving ππ* transition state is the larger gap between the singlet (S_1) and the triplet (T_1) energy levels as compared to that for the molecules involving nπ* transition state. This is shown in **Fig. 6.4(a)** and **(b)**. Therefore, the rate constant for intersystem crossing is smaller for ππ* excited state. In case of nπ* excited state, the non-bonding electron can change its spin and enter the triplet state because of the greater overlapping of the triplet vibrational energy levels with the singlet state. Because of the higher rate of intersystem crossing in molecules involving nπ* state, such molecules deactivate by phosphorescence or vibrational relaxation or external conversion, but the rate of fluorescence is reduced in such molecules.

6.5.1.2. Aromatic, Aliphatic and Alicyclic Compounds

The aromatic compounds containing double bonds involve low energy π to π* transition and hence, they show high degree of fluorescence. The most unsubstituted aromatic hydrocarbons fluoresce in solution. The intensity of fluorescence increases with the increase in the number of rings and the degree of condensation of the rings.

In case of aliphatic or alicyclic compounds, one of the vibrational energy levels of the ground state (v_3 of S_o in **Fig. 6.5**) overlaps with the ground vibrational energy level of the first excited singlet state (v_o of S_1). Hence, in these compounds, deactivation is mainly by the internal conversion (singlet-singlet) as shown in **Fig. 6.5**, wherein an electron enters from the v_o of S_1 into any of the vibrational energy levels (v_3 in **Fig. 6.5**) of the ground state (S_o). From there, an electron falls down to v_o of S_o by vibrational relaxation Thus, aliphatic and alicyclic compounds seldom show fluorescence.

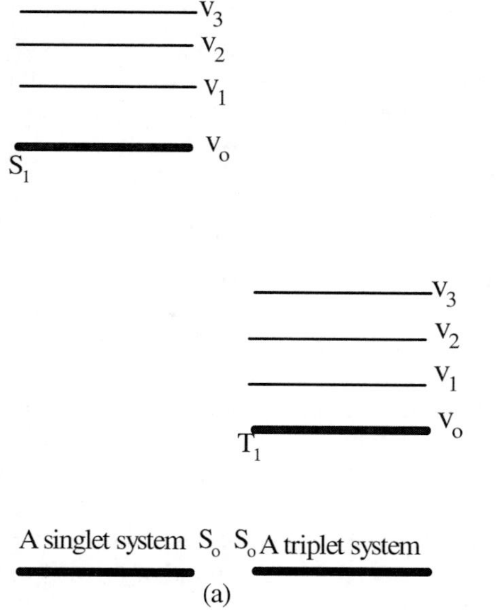

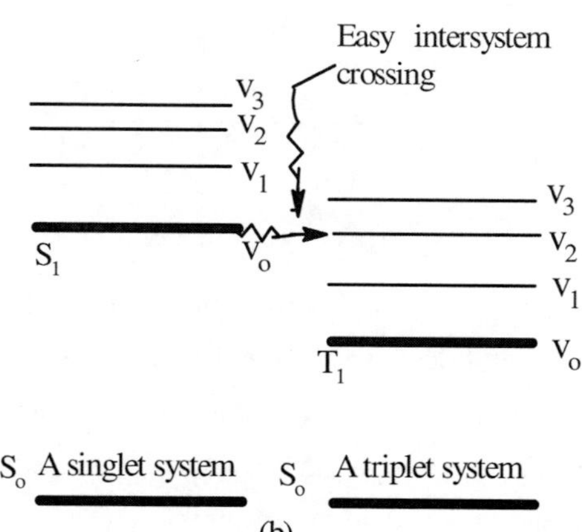

Fig. 6.4: Gap between a ground and a first excited state in a singlet and a triplet system in molecules involving (a) ππ* and (b) nπ* excited states

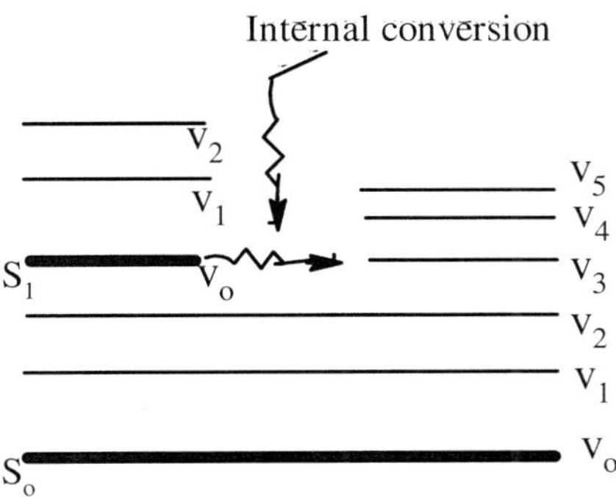

Fig. 6.5: Internal conversion in aliphatic and alicyclic compounds

6.5.1.3. The Heterocyclic Compounds

The heterocyclic compounds like pyridine, imidazole, pyrrole, furan, thiophene, etc., which contain only one heterocyclic ring [**Fig. 6.6(a)**], do not show fluorescence, since the lone pair of electrons on the heteroatom of these compounds has a tendency to enter the triplet system by intersystem crossing.

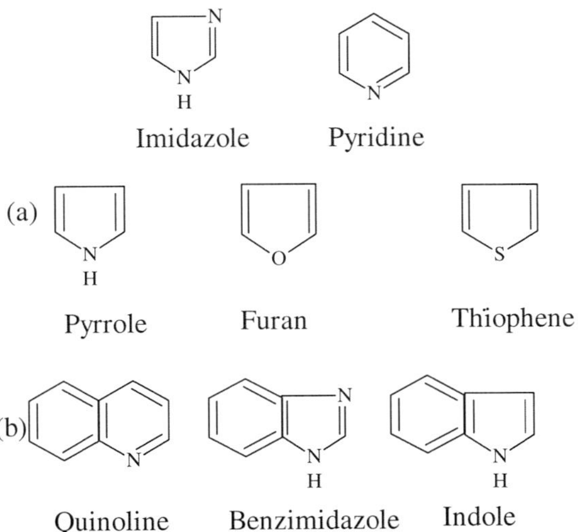

Fig. 6.6: (a) Non-fluorescent and (b) fluorescent heterocyclic compounds

If these single heterocyclic rings are fused with benzene ring [**Fig. 6.6(b)**], as in case of quinoline, isoquinoline, benzimidazole, indole, etc. the compounds become fluorescent in nature. This is because the lone pair of electrons on the heteroatom is delocalized over the extended conjugation provided by the benzene ring. This increases the molar absorptivity of the nð* transition and prevents the entry of electrons into a triplet system.

6.5.1.4. The Presence of Certain Substituents on the Benzene Ring

The presence of certain substituents on the benzene ring can also influence intensity of fluorescence. The halogen atoms containing lone pairs of electrons reduce the rate of deactivation of a molecule by fluorescence, thereby increasing the probability for an intersystem crossing from a singlet state to a triplet state. The reduction in the intensity of fluorescence is increased with the increase in the atomic number of the halogen atoms. In case of iodobenzene and nitrobenzene, deactivation mainly occurs by predissociation. The substituents like carboxylic group (COOH) or a carbonyl group (C=O), reduce the intensity of fluorescence since in these compounds, the energy of the $n\pi^*$ system is less than that of the $\pi\pi^*$ system and the fluorescent yield from the former type of a system is ordinarily low.

6.5.1.5. The Rigidity

The rigid molecules are more fluorescent as compared to the flexible molecules. For example, a fluorene molecule, as shown in **Fig. 6.7**, is more

CH_2

Biphenyl (Flexible) Flourene (Rigid)

Fig. 6.7: Effect of a methylene bridge on the rigidity of a molecule

rigid as compared to biphenyl, since the bridging methylene group in fluorene imparts more rigidity to the molecule.

Another example of increase in the intensity of fluorescence because of the rigidity is the enhanced fluorescence by the fluorescent dyes when they are adsorbed on some solid supports, which provide rigidity to the dyes. Like adsorption of molecules on a solid surface, complexation also results in the enhanced fluorescence. Hence, a zinc complex of 8-hydroxyquinoline shows more intense fluorescence compared to the fluorescence shown by 8-hydroxyquinoline. Both these compounds are shown in **Fig. 6.8**. Lack of rigidity in a molecule probably allows it to deactivate by internal conversion or intersystem crossing and reduces the possibility of deactivation by fluorescence.

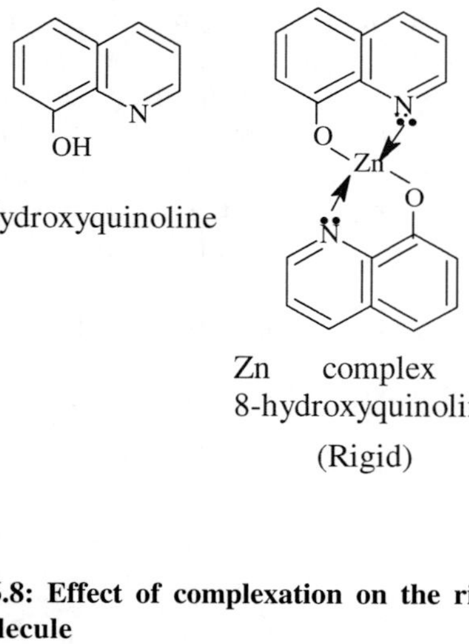

8-Hydroxyquinoline

Zn complex of 8-hydroxyquinoline (Rigid)

Fig. 6.8: Effect of complexation on the rigidity of a molecule

6.5.2. Environment of a Molecule

Environment of a molecule is the solvent in which it is dissolved. Temperature, pH, viscosity and polarity of a solvent and also the impurities dissolved in it, affect the intensity of fluorescence. All these factors are considered in detail below.

6.5.2.1. Temperature of a Solution

Increase in the temperature of the solution results in the increase in the energy of the molecules of the solute as well as of the solvent. This in turn results in the increase in the number of collisions of the molecules. Each collision imparts energy to the neighboring molecules in the form of heat. Hence, hardly any energy is left with the molecules, which can be lost in the form of radiation, i.e. by fluorescence. Therefore, increase in the temperature of the surrounding results in the decrease in the intensity of fluorescence.

6.5.2.2. Viscosity of the Solution

Increase in the viscosity of the solution reduces the number of collisions of the solute as well as the solvent molecules and hence, increases the intensity of fluorescence. Like increase in the temperature of the solvent, the decrease in the viscosity also increases the likelihood of external conversion and leads to the increase in the temperature of the solution and consequently results in the reduction of intensity of fluorescence.

6.5.2.3. Polarity of the Solvent

Fluorescence occurs due to transition of non-bonding (n) or π electrons to π^* orbital. The polar solvents interact with the non-bonding electrons and form hydrogen bond with them, thereby increasing the energy required for their transition. This results in the hypsochromic shift and can reduce the intensity of fluorescence at the wavelength used for the measurement. The π to π^* transition, on the other hand, involves a bathochromic shift, i.e. the shift to the longer wavelength, in the presence of polar solvents. This shift occurs because the polar solvent drags non-bonding electrons on the electronegative atom of the solute and reduces electron density on it, thereby imparting a partial positive charge to the electronegative atom in the solute, leading, in turn, to the reduction in the bond strength and also the bond energy of the π bond between the electronegative element and the carbon atom of a solute. Because of the shift in the wavelength of absorption, the intensity of fluorescence is reduced at the wavelength used for the measurement. The interaction of acetaldehyde (solute) and ethanol (solvent) is shown in **Fig. 6.9**.

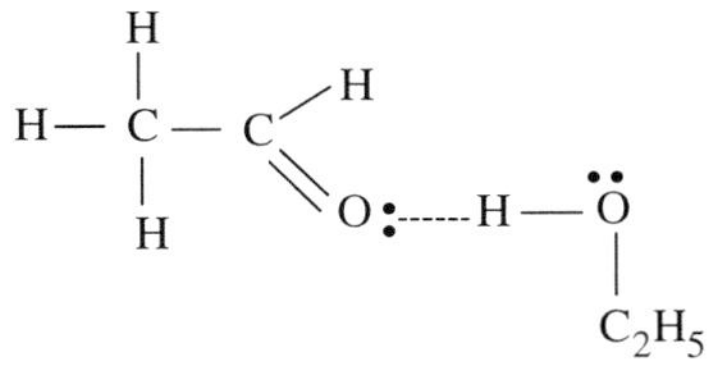

Fig. 6.9: Hydrogen bonding between acetaldehyde (solute) and ethanol (solvent)

6.5.2.4. pH of the solution

Fluorescence of aromatic acids and bases depends on the pH of the solution. The wavelength of absorption or emission and the intensity of fluorescence for the ionized and the non-ionized forms of a compound depend on the pH of the solution. Fluorescence is more favored in polar solvents, e.g. as shown in **Fig. 6.10**, the phenolate anion **(II)**, possesses more electron pairs compared to phenol and therefore, provides more stable π^* system, thereby reducing a gap between π and π^* molecular orbitals. Hence, the phenolate anion **(II)** shows greater fluorescence as compared to phenol **(I)**. Thus, the fluorescence of phenol is recorded in the alkaline medium and not in the acidic medium. Such compounds, which exhibit change in emission with the change in pH of the solution, are used as indicators in acid-base titrations, when the solutions are highly colored and the change in the color produced by the normal acid-base indicators is not distinct.

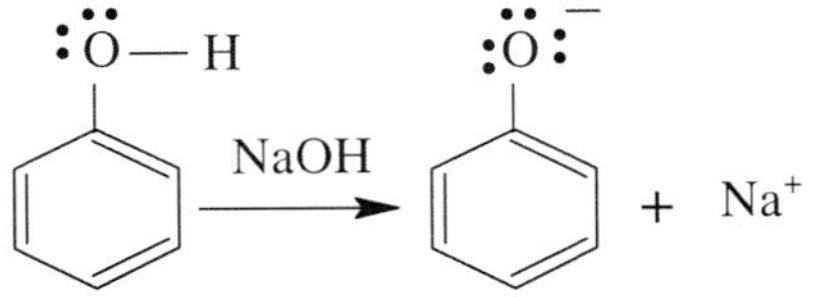

Phenol **(I)** Phenolate anion **(II)**

Fig. 6.10: Phenol and phenolate anion

The compound, 1-naphthol-4-sulfonic acid **(III)**, shown in **Fig. 6.11**, in the non-ionized form, shows fluorescence in the UV region and hence, its fluorescence is not visible. As the alkali in the form of a titrant is added to this acidic medium, the alkaline pH, at the equivalence point, converts 1-naphthol-4-sulfonic acid to the corresponding phenolate anion **(IV)**, and results in the shift of emission peak from UV region to the visible region. Hence, its fluorescence is easily visualized in the alkaline medium. Therefore, such fluorescent compounds can be used as acid-base indicators.

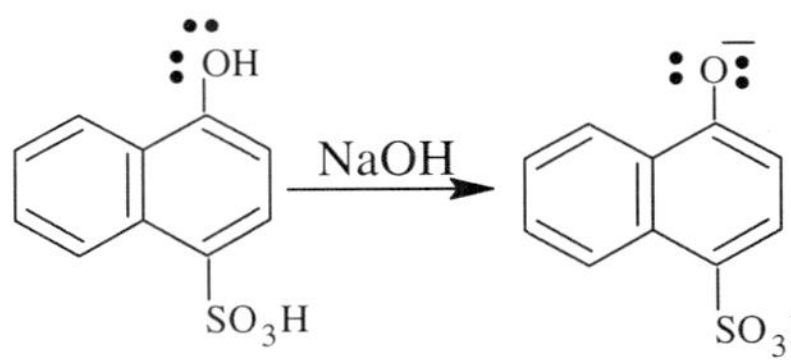

1-Naphthol-4-sulfonic acid **(III)** 1-Naphthol-4-sulfonic acid phenolate anion **(IV)**

Fig. 6.11: 1-Naphthol-4-sulfonic acid and the corresponding phenolate anion

Fluorescein, o-coumaric acid and 3,6-dihydroxyphthalamide are also used as fluorescent indicators.

6.5.2.5. Impurities Present in the Solution

The presence of dissolved oxygen in the solution reduces the intensity of fluorescence. Dissolved oxygen can bring about the photochemical oxidation of the fluorescent species and can convert it to an altogether different species. Secondly, the oxygen molecule is paramagnetic in nature, i.e. it contains unpaired electrons. Any paramagnetic species promotes deactivation by intersystem crossing and consequently, by phosphorescence, instead of by fluorescence. Hence, the intensity of fluorescence is reduced or lost totally in the presence of dissolved oxygen.

Like oxygen molecule, the presence of heavy atoms such as iodine or bromine, or compounds containing heavy atoms, also facilitate the singlet to triplet transition and bring about deactivation of a molecule by intersystem crossing and consequently by phosphorescence.

6.5.2.6. Concentration of the Solution

The concentrated solution contains more particles and hence, there is a greater chance of collisions among them. Hence, up to a particular concentration, the intensity of fluorescence increases as the number of absorbing and energy emitting particles increases, but beyond a particular concentration, the intensity of fluorescence starts declining because of the increased number of collisions of the particles.

6.6. QUENCHING OF FLUORESCENCE

The reduction in or the total loss of intensity of fluorescence is called as *quenching* of fluorescence. Whenever fluorimetry is used for the quantitative estimation of compounds, one should try to achieve higher intensity of fluorescence in order to have the greater accuracy in the measurement. This can be achieved in two ways.

A) By incorporating unsaturation in the compound by chemical derivatization, or

B) By controlling the surrounding environment

It is easy to control the surrounding environment of a molecule, rather than its chemical derivatization. Thus, the factors which affect fluorescence adversely should be controlled in order to avoid quenching of fluorescence.

Environmental factors responsible for quenching of fluorescence are as follows.

1) Temperature of the solution

Increase in the temperature of the solution increases the number of collisions among the neighboring molecules (solute-solute or solute-solvent). This reduces the intensity of fluorescence and brings about quenching of fluorescence.

2) Viscosity of the solution

Decrease in the viscosity of the solution also increases the number of collisions among the neighboring molecules, thereby causing quenching of fluorescence.

3) Polarity and pH of the solution

The polarity and pH of the solution decide the wavelength of maximum absorption of a solute. Any solvent or the change in pH, which brings about the change in the wavelength of maximum absorption of a solute, results in the decrease in the intensity of fluorescence.

4) Presence of any paramagnetic species in the solution

The presence of a paramagnetic species like oxygen or the presence of halides or compounds containing heavy atoms in solution, also decreases the intensity of fluorescence.

5) Concentration of the solution

The use of highly concentrated solution reduces intermolecular distance. This increases the collisions among the molecules. The loss or decrease of fluorescence due to collisions between the excited molecules of a solute is referred to as *self quenching*. The increase in the concentration of a solute increases the extent of self quenching.

6) The Self absorption

The *self absorption* also results in the quenching of fluorescence. The self absorption occurs when the wavelength of emission overlaps the wavelength of absorption, i.e. whatever energy is absorbed by the compound, the same is emitted out by it and is absorbed by the other molecules of the same sample in the solution.

6.7. INSTRUMENTATION

Instruments used for the measurement of fluorescent intensity are either *fluorimeters* or *spectrofluorimeters*. A single beam or a double beam instrument can be used but a double beam instrument is preferred, since it provides more accurate results as it compensates for the voltage fluctuations or the fluctuations in the power or intensity of the source.

The major difference between the spectrometers and spectrofluorimeters is that the former uses only one monochromator while the latter involves the use of two monochromators. The first monochromator is used to isolate the *excitation wavelength*, i.e. the wavelength required for the excitation of a fluorescent molecule. The second monochromator is required to isolate the *emission wavelength*, i.e. the wavelength emitted by the molecule while coming back from an excited state to the ground state.

The second difference between the spectrometers and spectrofluorimeters is in the position of the detector. Except for fluorimetry, in other spectrometric methods, the intensity of the emitted beam is measured along the direction of the path of the incident beam, whereas in case of fluorimetry, the intensity of the emitted beam is measured at an angle between 75° and 135°, preferably at 90°, with respect to the direction of the path of the incident beam. The radiation of fluorescence is emitted in all the directions, but the intensity is usually measured at 90° to the incident beam since along 90°, the intensity of fluorescence is maximum and therefore, the accuracy of the measurement is also maximum. In other directions, the intensity is reduced due to the increased scattering from the solution and also from the walls of the cuvette or sample holder.

Components of the fluorimeter and spectrofluorimeter

1) Source

A fluorimeter makes use of a mercury lamp, whereas a spectrofluorimeter makes use of a xenon lamp as a source of radiation.

Mercury arc lamp produces intense radiation but gives a line spectrum. Under high pressure, lines are obtained at 366, 405, 436, 446, 577, 691 and 773 nm. Under low pressure, the additional line at 254 nm is also obtained.

Xenon arc lamp produces more intense radiation than mercury arc lamp and gives a continuous spectrum between 250 and 660 nm.

2) Filters and monochromators

Fluorimeters make use of two monochromators in the form of filters, a *primary filter*, which selects the wavelength required for the excitation (λ_{exc}) of a molecule and a *secondary filter*, which selects the wavelength of emission (λ_{em}). Either the interference filters or absorption filters can be used.

The spectrofluorimeters make use of two monochromators in the form of gratings.

3) Cuvettes or sample holders

The cuvettes are usually made up of quartz and contain the solution of a sample to be analyzed. Glass or silica cuvettes can also be used but glass absorbs in the range of 120 – 350 nm. Hence, it cannot be used if λ_{exc} falls in the UV region. Since fluorescence is measured at 90° to the incident beam, all the four faces of a cell are polished.

4) Detectors

The intensity of fluorescence is usually low. In order to measure the concentration of a sample accurately, the intensity should be measured accurately. Hence, a large amplification factor is required for its measurement. This necessitates the use of a photomultiplier tube as the detector in fluorimetry and spectrofluorimetry. Detectors are usually placed at right angles to the incident beam.

5) Recorder and a printer

The intensity of fluorescence can be recorded on a recorder and printed out using a printer.

A block diagram for a fluorimeter is shown in **Fig. 6.12**.

substance. The excitation and emission spectra are shown in **Fig. 6.13**.

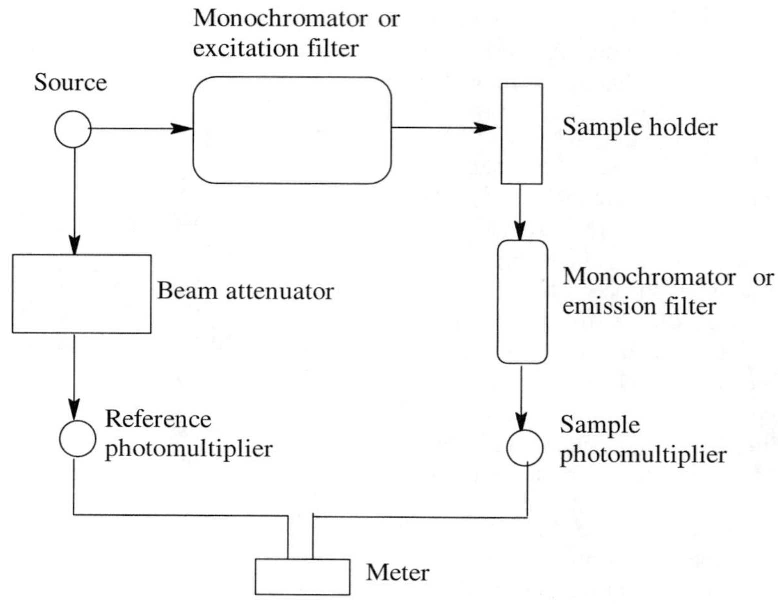

Fig. 6.12: A block diagram for a fluorimeter

6.8. EXCITATION AND EMISSION SPECTRA

For recording absorption or an *excitation spectrum*, the substance is excited by using a number of wavelengths and the emission of radiation is measured at a fixed wavelength. The wavelength at which a substance absorbs the maximum is referred to as *excitation wavelength* (λ_{exc}) and it should be used for the measurement in order to excite the maximum number of molecules and to get the maximum intensity of emission. On the other hand, the fluorescence and phosphorescence spectra, i.e. the *emission spectra* are recorded by exciting the molecules at a fixed wavelength and recording the intensity of emission at varying wavelengths. The wavelength at which the molecules give out maximum energy is referred to as *emission wavelength* (λ_{em}) of that substance. The excitation and emission spectra are shown in **Fig. 6.13**.

Use of proper values of λ_{exc} and λ_{em} during analysis, can make possible the selective measurement of a particular compound from a mixture of compounds, e.g. if a mixture has two compounds A and B, and both of them have the same wavelength of emission, then the selective analysis of the compounds can be carried out based on the adjustment of λ_{exc}. If λ_{exc} of the two compounds is not the same, by choosing λ_{exc} of compound A, the emission can be obtained only from A. Since compound B is not excited at this wavelength, it does not contribute to any intensity of fluorescence. Hence, the measurement of the intensity of fluorescence under this situation corresponds only to compound A.

Similarly, if the two compounds A and B have the same wavelength of excitation (λ_{exc}) but

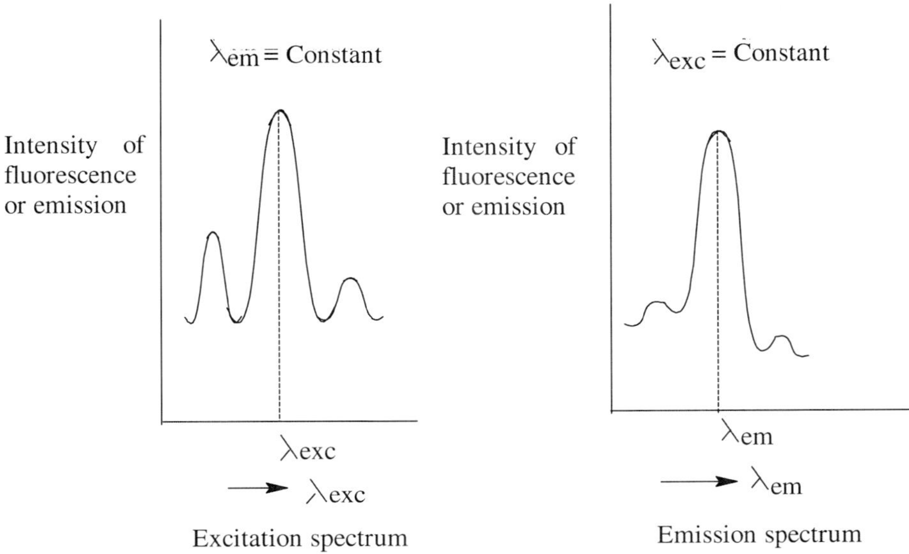

Fig. 6.13: Excitation and emission spectra

different wavelengths of emission, $\lambda_{em(A)}$ and $\lambda_{em(B)}$, then both the substances get excited at the same time by using λ_{exc}, but while measuring the intensity of fluorescence, if the secondary monochromator is adjusted at $\lambda_{em(A)}$, then the intensity of fluorescence of only A is measured. If the secondary monochromator is adjusted at $\lambda_{em(B)}$, then the intensity of fluorescence of only B is measured. However, in this case the accuracy is slightly reduced as compared to that in the first case because the energy provided by the source is absorbed by both the compounds A and B, but the emission is measured only from one compound.

Thus, proper selection of λ_{exc} and λ_{em} helps in the selective analysis of one compound from a mixture of compounds without any need to isolate or purify a compound.

6.9. APPLICATIONS OF SPECTROFLUORIMETRY

The method of spectrofluorimetry is used for the analysis only if the compounds are fluorescent in nature. The fluorescent nature of a compound is associated with its inherent structural characteristics. Compounds containing following characteristics usually show a property of fluorescence.

1) A conjugated π system or
2) Some extent of rigidity or
3) Absence of electron withdrawing groups such as – COOH or NO_2.

Moreover, such compounds can fluoresce only if the environment is conducive. An environment which does not facilitate collisions, i.e. a more viscous solution at low temperature and devoid of any paramagnetic impurities such as O_2, can facilitate fluorescence.

In practice, very few molecules are found to be fluorescent in nature. Hence, the use of spectrofluorimetry is limited as compared to the UV-visible spectrometry, but still it is becoming more popular because of the greater selectivity and sensitivity offered by it.

The UV-visible spectrometry is chosen when the concentration of an analyte is not very low and there is no interference from many substances. On the other hand, the spectrofluorimetry is chosen when an analyte is in low concentration and there are many interfering substances in the sample to be analyzed. Thus, if quinine sulphate is to be estimated from a tablet of 300 mg label claim, the UV spectrometry is preferred, but if the concentration of quinine sulphate is to be found from the biological samples, then spectrofluorimetry is the method of choice.

Spectrofluorimetry, like UV-visible spectrometry, is mainly used for the quantitative analysis. Both these techniques have limited qualitative application. Quantitative analysis in spectrofluorimetry is carried out by setting the excitation wavelength at the maximum absorption and setting the emission wavelength at the maximum intensity of emission.

Weissler and White have listed methods for the determination of over 200 substances, including a wide variety of substances covering organic compounds, enzymes, co-enzymes, medicinal agents like antimalarials, glucocorticoids, sedatives, plant products, steroids, vitamins, etc.

As far as applications are concerned, spectroflourimetric methods for the quantitative analysis can be categorized in the following five classes.

6.9.1. Direct Methods ˘ which are used for the compounds that are naturally fluorescent.

6.9.2. Derivatization Methods ˘ which are used for the compounds that are non-flourescent in nature.

6.9.3. Quenching Methods ˘ which are used for the compounds that are able to quench the intensity of fluorescence of some fluorescent species.

6.9.4. Fluorescence and Chromatography

6.9.5. Fluoroimmunoassays

6.9.1. Direct Methods

Direct methods can be used for inorganic as well as organic species.

6.9.1.1. Inorganic Species

The number of fluorescent inorganic species is limited. The only simple species which are naturally fluorescent in solution are the ions of lanthanides (the rare earth elements) and the actinides (the trans-uranic elements). Most of the elements are fluorescent in solid state, but Samarium (Sm), Europium (Eu), Gadolinium (Gd), Terbium (Tb) and Dysprosium (Dy) are fluorescent in aqueous solution.

Actinides are radioactive and their analysis is usually carried out by radiochemical methods. However, the spectrofluorimetric methods are frequently used for the determination of uranium salts in the field of nuclear research. Uranium salts produce uranyl (VI) ion (UO^{+2}) in aqueous solution and it exhibits green fluorescence, when excited by the blue incident radiation.

6.9.1.2. Organic Species

The range of organic compounds, which can be directly excited in solution to emit fluorescence, is much wider than that in the inorganic field. Many conjugated and rigid organic molecules are naturally fluorescent. The spectrofluorimetric technique is used for the quantitative analysis of the following groups of compounds

1) Polyaromatic hydrocarbons

The analysis of polyaromatic hydrocarbons is especially important for the higher members that are carcinogenic, e.g. anthracene, benzpyrene, etc. Benzpyrenes are present in tar from tobacco smoke and also found in traces in rivers after forest fires, having been washed out of the atmosphere by subsequent rainfall.

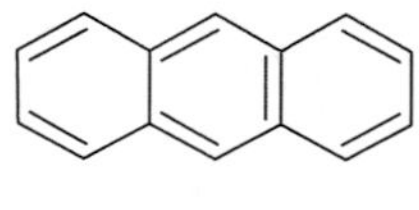

Anthracene 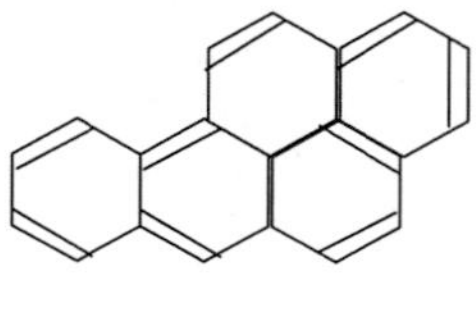 Benzpyrene

2) Vitamins

A number of vitamins are found to be naturally fluorescent, mainly because of the extended π system and the fused ring system.

(i) Vitamin A

Vitamin A containing five conjugated double bonds is naturally fluorescent. Vitamin A, a fat soluble vitamin, is a pale yellow compound and has a blue green fluorescence.

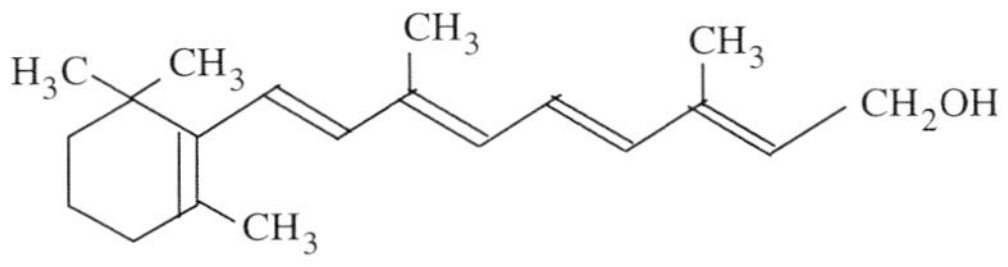

Vitamin A

(λ_{exc} = 325 nm and λ_{em} = 470 nm and the minimum concentration required for the assay, i. e. C_{min} = 0.01 μg/mL)

(ii) Riboflavin (Vitamin B_2)

This vitamin is one of the B complex vitamins and has natural fluorescence. It has yellow to orange yellow crystals. It is more soluble in alkaline solutions than in H_2O but dissolves in H_2O.

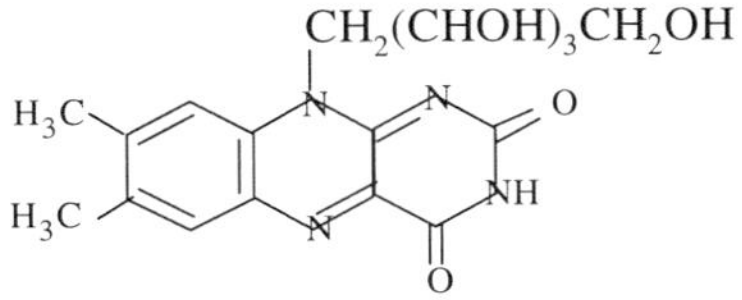

Riboflavin

(λ_{exc} = 444 nm and λ_{em} = 520 nm and the minimum concentration required for the assay, i. e. C_{min} = 0.01 μg/mL)

(iii) Cyanocobalamine (Vitamin B_{12})

Cyanocobalamine is a red colored, water soluble compound. It has a highly complex structure and contains two heterocyclic systems, a benzimidazole and a modified porphyrin nucleus.

(λ_{exc} = 275 nm and λ_{em} = 305 nm and the minimum concentration required for the assay, i. e. C_{min} = 0.003 μg/mL)

(iv) Folic acid

Folic acid is a yellow or yellowish orange crystalline compound, very slightly soluble in H_2O but readily dissolves in dilute alkali and acid.

(λ_{exc} = 365 nm and λ_{em} = 450 nm at pH = 7, and the minimum concentration required for the assay, i. e. C_{min} = 0.01 μg/mL)

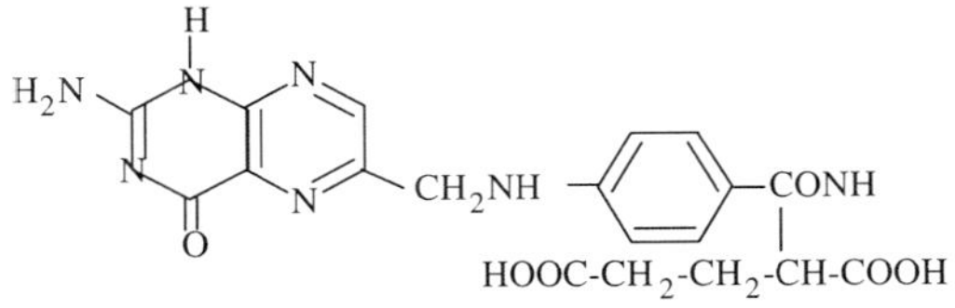

Folic acid

Since the values of λ_{exc} and λ_{em} of all the vitamins mentioned above, are different, analysis of these vitamins from their mixture can be carried out selectively, in presence of each other, without separating them. The specific values of λ_{exc} and λ_{em} of vitamins can be used to analyze them selectively. Thus, simultaneous analysis of vitamins from a multi-vitamin capsule becomes very easy by spectrofluorimetry, just by selecting proper λ_{exc} and λ_{em} values. Whenever two compounds have the same or almost the same values of λ_{exc}, their selective estimation can be carried out by recording intensity of fluorescence at respective emission wavelengths, λ_{em}. If the values of λ_{em} of the two compounds match, then they can be excited by choosing respective values of wavelengths of excitation.

Thiamine (Vitamin B_1) is not naturally fluorescent, but requires oxidation to thiochrome and hence, is not considered here.

3) Alkaloids

Spectrofluorimetry is also useful for quantitative estimation of certain alkaloids like cinchona alkaloids or opium alkaloids.

(i) Cinchona alkaloids

Cinchona alkaloids such as quinine, cinchonine and cinchonidine, from the class of antimalarials, are naturally fluorescent. Their quantitative estimation can be carried out selectively by choosing proper values of either λ_{exc} or λ_{em}. The values of λ_{exc} and λ_{em} for these alkaloids are mentioned below.

Quinine: λ_{exc} = 250, 350, λ_{em} = 450 nm (pH = 1, C_{min} = 0.002 μg/mL)

Cinchonine: λ_{exc} = 320, λ_{em} = 420 nm (pH = 1, C_{min} = 0.01 μg/mL)

Cinchonidine: λ_{exc} = 315, λ_{em} = 445 (pH =1, C_{min} = 0.01 μg/mL)

For quinine and cinchonidine, the values of λ_{em} are very close to each other, i. e. 450 nm and 445 nm, respectively, but if the excitation wavelength equal to 250 or 350 nm is used for the analysis, only quinine molecules would get excited and not the cinchonidine molecules. Thus, even if λ_{em} is adjusted to 445 or 450 nm, only the excited quinine molecules would emit radiation and would contribute to the intensity of fluorescence, if λ_{exc} is selected as 250 or 350 nm. Thus, selective estimation of compounds can be achieved even in the presence of each other. This definitely increases the accuracy of the measurement, since the errors involved during separation of compounds from each other are eliminated.

Spectrofluorimetry is commonly used to determine the concentration of quinine in urine. In this case, urine sample is made alkaline to pH 9-10 with dilute NH_4OH and quinine is extracted in $CHCl_3$. The chloroform layer is made acidic with H_2SO_4 and the fluorescence of an acidic extract is measured by using λ_{exc} = 350 nm and λ_{em} = 450 nm. The blank is carried out using the identical procedure, but without the sample. Quinine is mainly metabolized in liver and the degradation products are eliminated in urine. Its plasma half life is 10 hrs, but it is prolonged in case of hepatic impairment. Only 5 % of the total dose is excreted after 24 hrs. Thus, delayed excretion of quinine in urine indicates hepatic impairment.

Estimation of quinine in tonic water is a routine analysis in the soft drinks industry.

Quinine is readily available in the pure form and its excitation and emission wavelengths fall in the middle of the UV-visible region so that it is often used as a test material to check the performance of the fluorescence instruments or to calibrate them.

(ii) Opium alkaloids

Estimation of opium alkaloids is a very good example to illustrate selectivity of spectrofluorimetry.

Analysis of a mixture of four alkaloids, viz., morphine, codeine, papaverine and narcotine from opium, illustrated the use of natural fluorescence modified by the control of pH and solvent extraction to make the method more specific. These alkaloids are the *drugs of abuse* (because of their narcotic action) and hence, determination of their concentration in blood becomes very important.

Papaverine and narcotine do not interfere with the determination of morphine and codeine because they fluoresce at longer wavelengths. However, both of them absorb at 285 nm at which morphine and codeine also absorb. Thus, their presence reduces the sensitivity of the method. The sensitivity can be increased by extracting papaverine and narcotine from an alkaline aqueous solution (pH = 9) with ethanol free chloroform. In the alkaline solution of these alkaloids, morphine and codeine remain as their sodium salts, whereas papaverine and narcotine remain as bases and can be extracted in chloroform. Thus, morphine and codeine are separated from papaverine and narcotine. In the chloroform layer, papaverine fluoresces strongly at 348 nm. Narcotine fluoresces weakly at much longer wavelength, i.e. at 400 nm. If a small amount of trichloroacetic acid (CCl_3COOH) is added to the mixture of papaverine and narcotine, then the fluorescence of papaverine is considerably suppressed and shifted to a longer wavelength. Thus, the selective analysis of narcotine and papaverine in chloroform is possible.

The alkaline solution containing morphine and codeine is analyzed selectively, with the help of a calibration curve, shown in **Fig. 6.14**.

Calibration curves for morphine and codeine

In the presence of H_2SO_4, both the OH groups in morphine remain unchanged, but in the presence of NaOH, they exist as O^- and Na^+ ions. Similarly, in the presence of H_2SO_4, the OCH_3 and OH groups in codeine remain unchanged and in the presence of NaOH, the OH group exists as O^- and Na^+ ions. The number of unpaired electrons on the oxygen atom increases when OH group is converted to O^- ion. Also, delocalization of electrons over a long chain of atoms is not possible in these compounds. Therefore, the possibility of a molecule going into a triplet state increases. This leads to the decrease in the intensity of fluorescence for morphine and codeine in the alkaline medium as compared to their intensity of fluorescence in the acidic medium. The calibration curves A, B, C and D, shown in **Fig. 6.14**, are

N—CH_3

RO O OH

Morphine, R = - H

Codeine, R = -CH_3

obtained by recording intensity of fluorescence for 100 % pure samples of morphine and codeine in H_2SO_4 and NaOH.

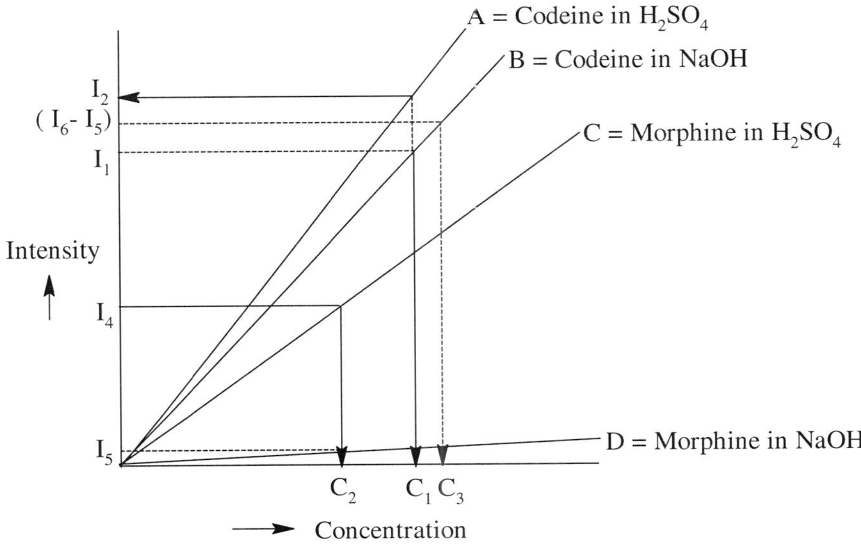

Fig. 6.14: Calibration curves for morphine and codeine

Analysis of morphine and codeine from their mixture using calibration curves

Concentrations of morphine and codeine can be determined independently because both fluoresce strongly at the same wavelength in H_2SO_4. Secondly, morphine has negligible fluorescence in 0.1 M NaOH.

1) When intensity of fluorescence (I_1) of the sample in NaOH is recorded, it corresponds to the concentration of codeine in the sample, since morphine has negligible fluorescence in 0.1 M NaOH. Using curve B, concentration (C_1) of codeine can be obtained.
2) From this concentration (C_1) of codeine, its fluorescent intensity (I_2) in H_2SO_4 is obtained using curve A.
3) When intensity of fluorescence (I_3) for the sample, containing a mixture of morphine and codeine, is recorded in H_2SO_4, it corresponds to both, the concentration of morphine as well as codeine in the sample. The intensity (I_2), of codeine, obtained from curve A, is subtracted from the total intensity (I_3) obtained for the sample in H_2SO_4. This difference in intensities gives the intensity of fluorescence for morphine (I_4) in 0.05 M H_2SO_4. From this intensity of fluorescence for morphine (I_4), the concentration (C_2) of morphine can be calculated using curve C in **Fig. 6.14**.

Thus, we assume that fluorescence intensity of two compounds is additive.

The initial values can be refined, correcting the codeine concentration for the small fluorescence intensity (I_5) of morphine in NaOH, which is not negligible when the morphine concentration is high and codeine concentration is low.

How is this correction made?

a) From the concentration (C_2) of morphine, found from curve C, the intensity (I_5) of fluorescence in NaOH corresponding to this concentration, is found from curve D.
b) When the total fluorescence intensity (I_6) for the sample containing morphine and codeine is found in NaOH, the intensity (I_5) of morphine in NaOH is subtracted from (I_6). This difference in the intensities (I_6-I_5) is extrapolated to the standard curve for codeine in NaOH to find actual concentration (C_3) of codeine in the solution.
c) This concentration (C_3) can be used to find intensity of fluorescence corresponding to codeine in H_2SO_4 using curve A.
d) Subtract this intensity from the total intensity of fluorescence (I_3) for the sample containing morphine and codeine, in H_2SO_4. This gives intensity of fluorescence for morphine in H_2SO_4.
e) This intensity, corresponding to morphine alone in H_2SO_4, can be used to find concentration of morphine accurately at this time using curve C.

4) Steroids

The most important compounds like cholesterol, cortisone (**Fig. 6.15**) or hormones, present in the body fluids, are steroidal in nature and possess natural fluorescence. Steroids like aldosterone, testosterone, progesterone, etc. can be analyzed selectively by fluorimetry. All these compounds contain fused ring systems and therefore, provide rigidity to the molecules, which is essential for the natural fluorescence. Fluorescence of these compounds can be recorded in H_2SO_4. Although this is often described as *natural fluorescence*, it is likely that H_2SO_4 is not merely a solvent but causes condensation reaction between and within these molecules. In fact, the precise nature of the fluorescent species has not been definitely established.

11-Hydroxysteroids (**Fig. 6.15**) such as beclomethasone (topical antinflammatory agent), betamethasone (an effective glucocorticoid) and cortisol (another glucocorticoid) are applied locally in case of certain skin diseases like eczema. Systemically, they are used for acute bronchial asthma and chronic pulmonary diseases. They fluoresce in H_2SO_4. Cholesterol and cholesterol esters are some of the major interfering fluorogens in their assay. Hydrocortisone is used many a times as a standard when these steroids are assayed by fluorimetry.

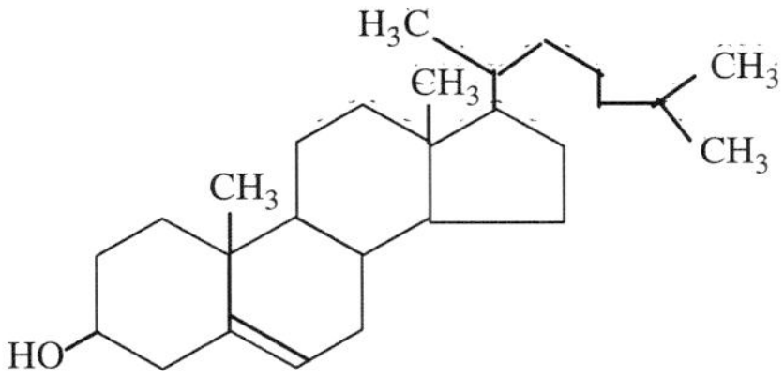

Cholesterol

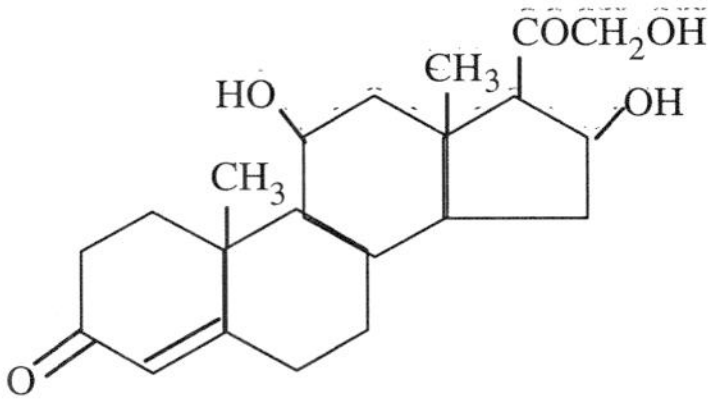

Cortisone

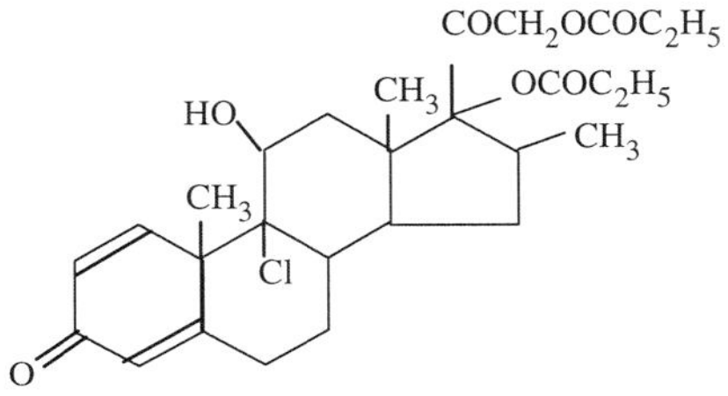

Beclomethasone

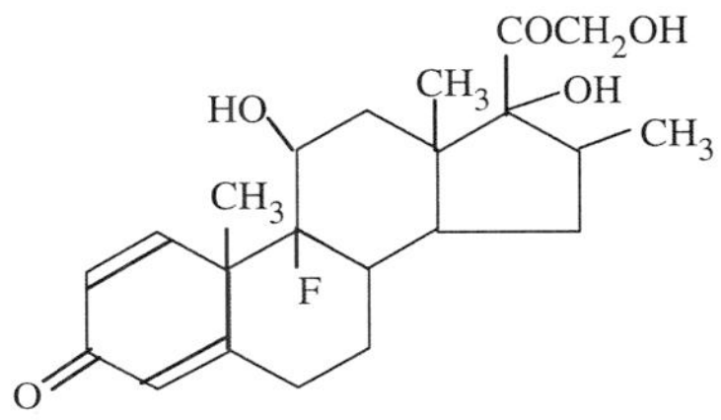

Betamethasone

Fig. 6.15: Structures of steroids that can be analyzed by spectrofluorimetry

5) Medicinal agents

Some of the medicinal agents such as phenobarbitone and pentobarbitone are also naturally fluorescent (**Fig. 6.16**).

6.9.2. Derivatization Methods

Compounds which do not fluoresce naturally can be made to fluoresce by reacting them with some other fluorescent compound. This

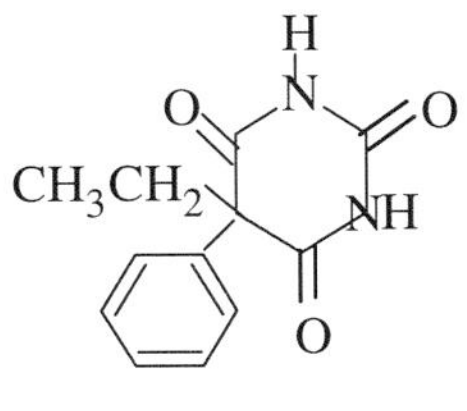

Phenobarbitone

(λ_{exc} = 265, λ_{em} = 440,

pH = 13, C_{min} = 0.1 μg /mL)

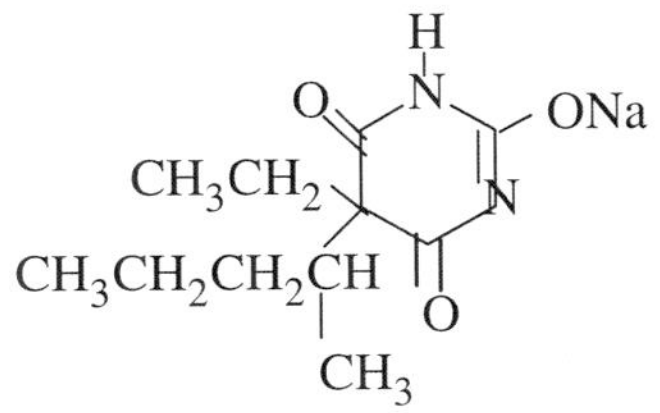

Pentobarbitone

(λ_{exc} = 265, λ_{em} = 440,

pH = 13, C_{min} = 0.5 μg /mL)

Fig. 6.16: Fluorescent medicinal agents

technique is entirely analogous to the formation of colored complexes from the colorless compounds using a coloring agent.

Colorless compound + coloring agent → colored compound

Non - fluorescent compound + fluorescing or a fluorogenic agent → fluorescent compound

The use of fluorescence measurements rather than absorption measurements may be advantageous under the following conditions.

(i) When the analyte concentration is so low that the colorimetry cannot provide the required accuracy in the measurement.

(ii) Also, when there is interference from other compounds, spectrofluorimetry offers more selectivity than spectrophotometry because of the use of two wavelengths, λ_{exc} and λ_{em}, during the measurements.

Derivatization of various species for making a non-fluorescent species a fluorescent one is possible. Derivatization of the following species is discussed.

6.9.2.1. Non-Metals
6.9.2.2. Metals
6.9.2.3. Organic compounds

6.9.2.1. Derivatization of Non-metals

Non-metals and anions do not readily form rigid or fused ring complexes and their analysis by spectrophotometry or spectrofluorimetry is limited only to certain elements.

1) Boron

A compound containing boron (B) is converted to boric acid, which is converted to a fluorescent complex and analyzed. Boric acid is a weak acid and cannot be titrated accurately by acid base titration. Non-aqueous titration requires absolute control on the moisture. Titrimetry cannot provide adequate accuracy if the analyte concentration is low. If concentration of boric acid is low, it can be analyzed accurately by derivative spectofluorimetry. One mole of boric acid when condensed with two moles of benzoin, produces a rigid complex, which is fluorescent. The reaction is shown in **Fig. 6.17**. The intensity of fluorescence

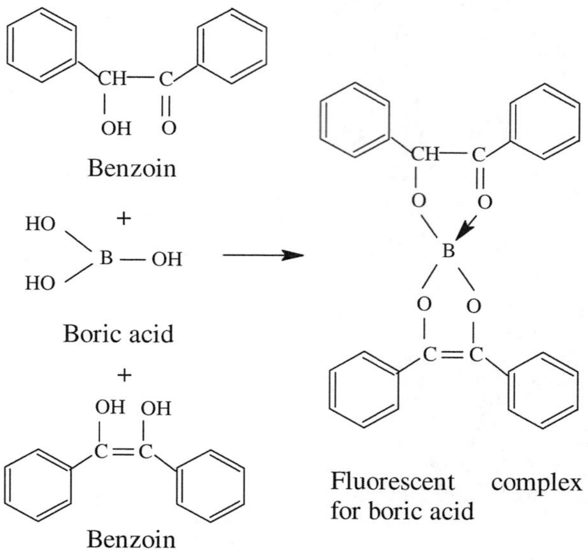

Fig. 6.17: Formation of a fluorescent derivative for boron

of this complex is measured to find its concentration.

2) Sulphur

Sulphur can also be determined by derivative spectrofluorimetry. A molecule containing sulphur is converted to hydrogen sulphide (H_2S) by first preparing sodium fusion extract and then acidifying it. This H_2S is allowed to react with two moles of 1,4-diaminobenzene. A cyclic compound produced by the ring closure with 1,4-diaminobenzene undergoes further rearrangement to form a fluorescent compound, as shown in **Fig. 6.18**.

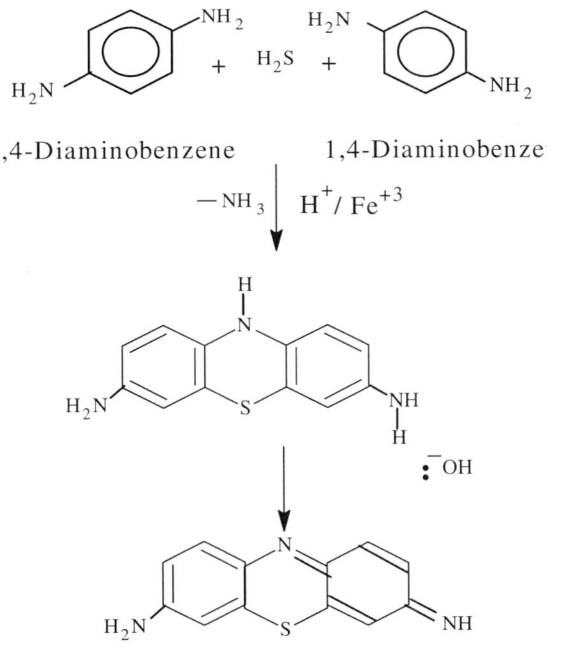

1,4-Diaminobenzene + H_2S + 1,4-Diaminobenze

$-NH_3$ H^+/Fe^{+3}

A flourescent derivative for sulphur

Fig. 6.18: Formation of a fluorescent derivative for sulphur

3) Nitrogen

Nitrogen in the analyte can be converted to a cyanide ion by preparing sodium fusion extract. Cyanide ion can then be determined by reacting it with benzoquinone so as to obtain 2,3-dicyanohydroquinone, as shown in **Fig. 6.19**.

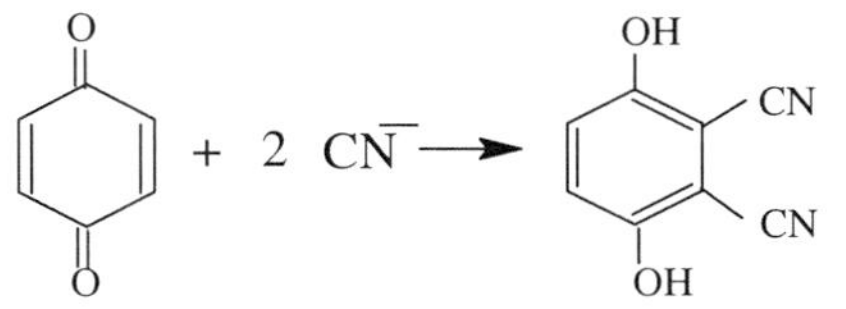

Benzoquinone + 2 CN^- → 2,3-Dicyanohydroquinone

Fig. 6.19: Formation of a fluorescent derivative for nitrogen

6.9.2.2. Derivatization of Metals

The simplest example of a fluorescent derivative is the complex formed between a metal ion and a donor organic molecule. Ideally, both of these components should be non-fluorescent so that when the fluorescent complex is formed, its fluorescence can be observed easily. In practice, any natural fluorescence of the components can be tolerated, provided that it is weak and occurs at a wavelength, which is far from that of the complex.

Complex formation can be used in two ways.

(i) To determine either the metal (analyte) species where the organic molecule is the reagent, or

(ii) To determine the organic compound (analyte) where the metal ion is the reagent.

Usually, the metal species are analyzed by using organic molecules as reagents, but currently, much research interest is in the use of metals, particularly the lanthanides, as *probes* to determine organic species in quite complex matrices. When the metal is used for the determination of organic molecules, it is called as a *probe*. The complex formed must have characteristic properties so that it can be identified and measured easily even when the sample produces a high fluorescent background.

Europium (Eu) and terbium (Tb) are found to form useful complexes with proteins and other compounds of biological interest, as shown in **Fig. 6.20**.

Proteine - 1 Complex 1
Proteine - 2 + Tb → Complex 2
Proteine - 3 Complex 3

Fig. 6.20: Formation of fluorescent complexes of terbium with proteins

This derivatization method is of particular significance in the analysis of biological samples which usually contain many other substances as impurities and face a lot of interference in their assay.

This technique suffers from one drawback. All the complexes of Tb or lanthanides have almost the same wavelength of emission as the free ion (terbium ion or a europium ion). Therefore, if more than one protein is present in the mixture, many complexes, having the same wavelength of emission, would be formed in the mixture. Hence, it will not be possible to discriminate between them based on the wavelength of emission, but still they can be estimated selectively, without their separation because of the following facts.

(i) The lifetime of an excited state of complexes is distinctly larger than that of free ions. Hence, the fluorescence from free ions is seen for a very short time period, whereas the fluorescence from the complexes is seen for a longer time period. If the fluorescence of complexes is measured after the fluorescence of free ions is ceased, then the complexes need not be separated from the free ions.

(ii) Secondly, the intensity of fluorescence of complexes is considerably higher (10^5 times more) than that of the free ions.

(iii) The excitation wavelength of complexes is a characteristic of the organic part of the molecules in their structures. If there is sufficient difference between λ_{exc} of different organic compounds, then the intensity at λ_{em} can be measured by using different values of λ_{exc}. For emission of energy, the compound should first absorb radiation, i.e. fluorescence would be observed only if a compound gets excited. Thus, complexes need not be separated from each other.

Fluorimetric Reagents for Metals

One way to achieve selective analysis of metals is to form stable complexes, which can show fluorescence when metals are reacted with fluorimetric reagents. For this purpose, the fluorimetric reagents should have two functional groups, one containing an acidic, replaceable hydrogen atom and another containing an atom carrying a lone pair of electrons. For stable complexes to be formed, the complex or a chelate between the metal ion and the fluorimetric reagent should result in the formation of a 5- or 8-membered ring. The common reagent used for this purpose is salicylaldehyde (**Fig. 6.21.**).

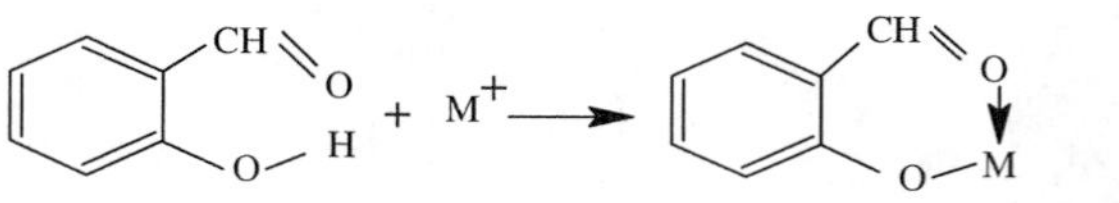

Fig. 6.21: Complex formation with salicylaldehyde

Another very well-known complexing agent, which forms complexes with a large number of metals, is 8-hydroxyquinoline (oxine). This reagent is used in gravimetry, colorimetry and in fluorimetry because it can form solid complexes quantitatively, as shown in **Fig. 6.22** and also because it can form colored or fluorescent complexes. The sulfonic acid group (SO_3H) is often incorporated at the 5-position of 8-hydroxyquinoline to facilitate the use of this reagent in aqueous solution. The neutral complexes can be extracted into an organic solvent such as ether or chloroform. Since oxine forms

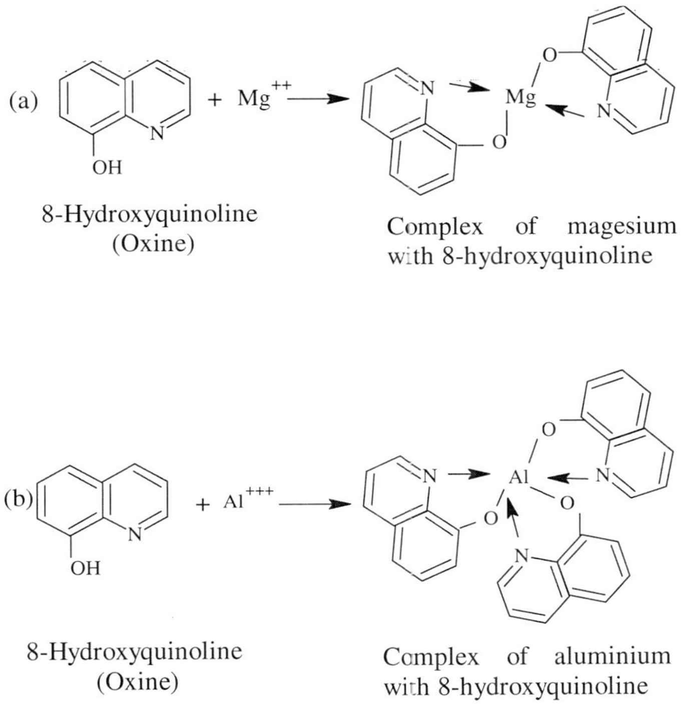

(a) 8-Hydroxyquinoline (Oxine) + Mg^{++} ⟶ Complex of magesium with 8-hydroxyquinoline

(b) 8-Hydroxyquinoline (Oxine) + Al^{+++} ⟶ Complex of aluminium with 8-hydroxyquinoline

Fig. 6.22: Complexes of 8-hydroxyquinoline (oxine) with (a) magnesium and (b) aluminium

neutral complexes, they can be easily separated from the charged complexes of other metals and ions.

Various reagents which are specific for a particular metal or a group of metals are mentioned in **Table 6.2**.

Table 6.2: Fluorescing agents for specific metals

Metal	Reagent	λ_{exc} (nm)	λ_{em} (nm)	Limit of detection (mg/lL)
Al	Alizarin garnet red	470	580	0.007
Be	Morin	420	525	0.01
Mg	8-Hydroxyquinoline	420	530	0.01
Mn	Carminic acid	467	556	0.9
Sn	3-Hydroxyflavone	415	495	0.004
Zn	8-Quinolinol or	375	517	0.5
	Rhodamine B	366	580	0.5

6.9.2.3. Derivatization of Organic Compounds

If any organic compound is contaminated with a number of impurities, then derivative spectrofluorimetry is preferred for its quantitative estimation. In the presence of many interfering impurities, derivatization of an organic molecule using another organic compound, helps in the formation of a compound which can fluoresce at a wavelength longer than the excitation or emission wavelengths corresponding to the individual compounds. This method is useful for the samples that contain impurities which are naturally fluorescent but fluoresce at shorter wavelengths or for samples containing non-fluorescent impurities.

Although inorganic probes are being developed for some classes of organic analytes, most organic derivatizations involve the use of pure organic reagents. Two organic compounds result in the formation of a compound containing an enlarged π system as compared to the analyte so that it absorbs and emits at longer wavelengths or the combination may result in the formation of a more rigid structure. Some of the fluorogenic reagents are mentioned below.

1) 5-Dimethylaminonaphthalene-1-sulfonyl chloride (Dansyl chloride DNS-Cl)

This reagent reacts with phenols and primary or secondary amines under slightly basic conditions to form sulfonate esters or sulfonamides, respectively, as shown in **Fig. 6.23**. The derivatives are highly fluorescent, whereas the reagent itself is not.

Use – This reagent is used to detect amino acids, polyamines, biogenic amines, estrogen, serotonin, alkaloids, barbiturates, insecticides, ureas, organophosphates, etc.

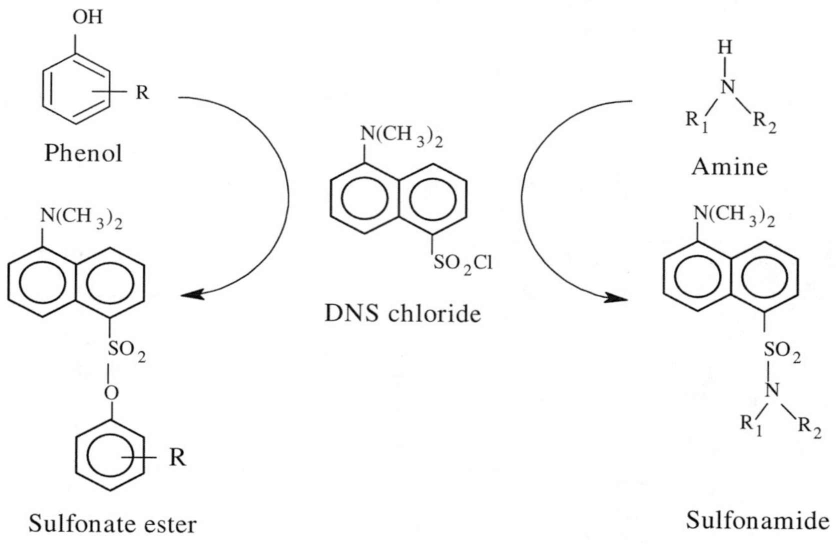

Fig. 6.23: Derivatization using dansyl chloride

2) 4 Chloro 7 nitrobenz 2,1,3 oxadiazole (NBD chloride)

This reagent reacts with primary amines to form highly fluorescent derivatives, but it is specific only for aliphatic amines. Its reaction with secondary amines is illustrated in **Fig. 6.24**.

Use – It is used in the analysis of amino acids, biogenic amines, amphetamines, methylcarbamate, insecticides, alkaloids, antithyroids, thiols, nitrosamines, etc.

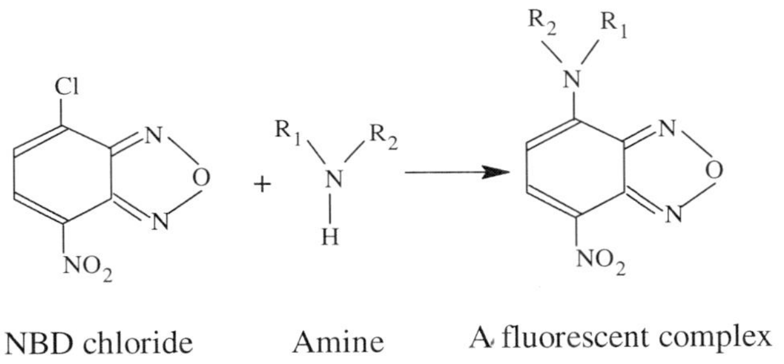

NBD chloride   Amine   A fluorescent complex

Fig. 6.24: Derivatization using NBD chloride

3) Fluoresamine [4-Phenyl-spiro (furan -2-(3H)-1′-phthalan-3, 3′- dione)]

It is a selective reagent for primary amines. The reaction of a primary amine with this reagent is given in **Fig. 6.25**.

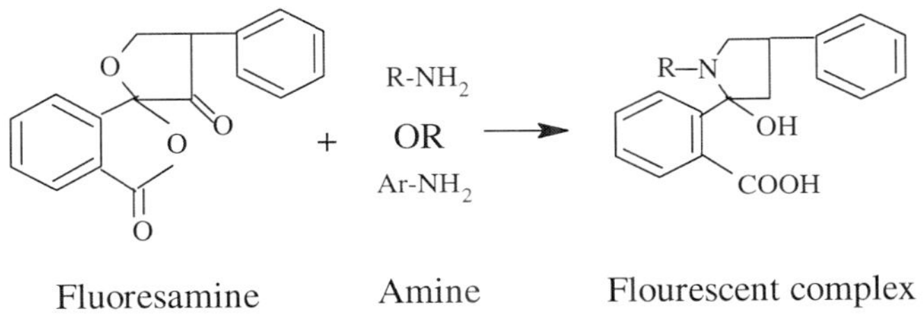

Fluoresamine   Amine   Flourescent complex

Fig. 6.25: Derivatization using fluoresamine

Use – Fluresamine is used for prechromatographic derivatization of polyamines, catecholamines and aminoacids.

4) Diphenylindenonesulfonyl chloride (Disyl chloride)

Disyl chloride reacts with amines and phenols, as shown in **Fig. 6.26**. The products however, require treatment with sodium ethoxide to induce fluorescence.

Use – Disyl chloride is used to determine amino acids, amino sugars, vitamin B_6 (pyridoxine) and tetrahydrocannabinols.

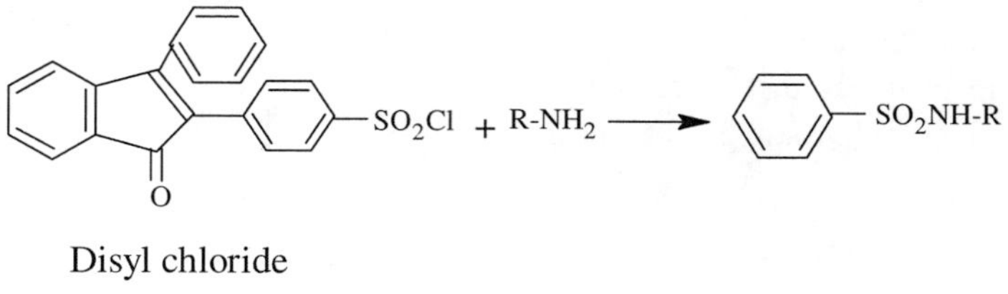

SO_2Cl + $R\text{-}NH_2$ ⟶ $SO_2NH\text{-}R$

Disyl chloride

Fig. 6.26: Derivatization using disyl chloride

5) o-Phthalaldehyde (OPA)

o-Phthalaldehyde is also used for the analysis of biogenic amines, amino acids, catecholamines and histamines. The reaction of o-phthalaldehyde with amino acid is shown in **Fig. 6.27**.

6) 4-Bromomethyl-7-methoxycoumarin (Br-MMC)

This reagent reacts with monocarboxylic acids in acetone in the presence of solid K_2CO_3 to form highly fluorescent derivatives. Its reaction with carboxylic acid is shown in **Fig. 6.28**.

Use –It is used to detect fatty acids and acidic herbicides.

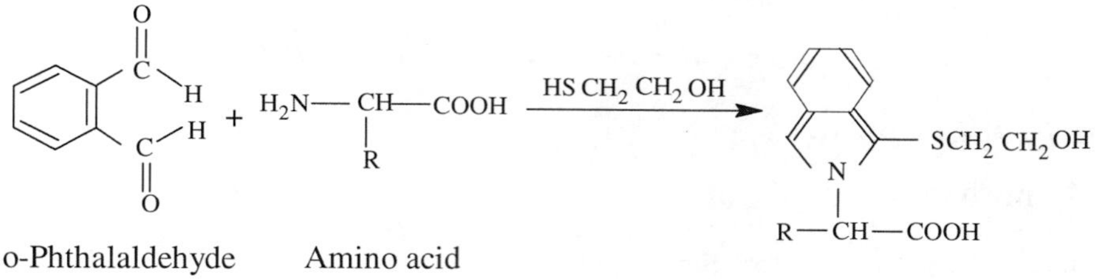

o-Phthalaldehyde + $H_2N—CH(R)—COOH$ (Amino acid) $\xrightarrow{HS\,CH_2\,CH_2\,OH}$ product with $SCH_2\,CH_2\,OH$ and $R—CH—COOH$ on N

o-Phthalaldehyde Amino acid

Fig. 6.27: Derivatization using o-phthalaldehyde

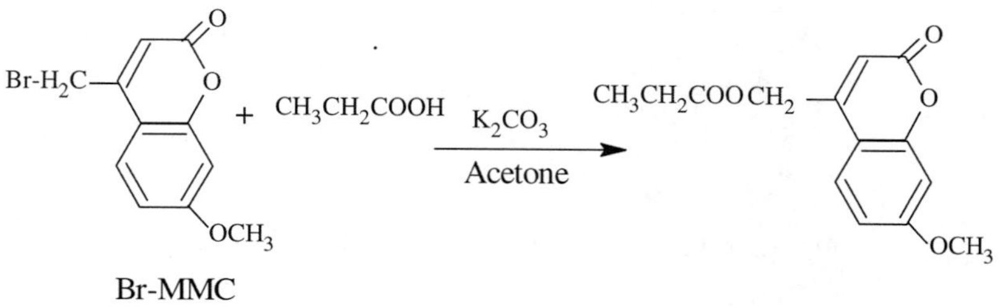

$Br\text{-}H_2C$– ... OCH_3 (Br-MMC) + CH_3CH_2COOH $\xrightarrow[\text{Acetone}]{K_2CO_3}$ $CH_3CH_2COO\,CH_2$– ... OCH_3

Br-MMC

Fig. 6.28: Derivatization using 4-bromomethyl-7-methoxycoumarin

7) 5-Dimethylaminonaphthalene-1 sulfonyl hydrazine (Dansyl hydrazine)

This reagent has been used to form fluorescent hydrazones of aldehydes and ketones including ketosteroids, glycoproteins and reducing sugars. The reaction of this reagent with ketone is shown in **Fig. 6.29**.

Choice of a proper complexing or a derivatizing agent for the analytes is required because sometimes, a reagent cannot react with an analyte if too much of steric hindrance is present.

Fluorescent Indicators

For many substances, the intensity and the color of fluorescence depends upon the pH of a solution. These compounds are termed as *fluorescent indicators*. They are mainly used in acid-base titrations. Some of the fluorescent indicators are mentioned in **Table 6.3**.

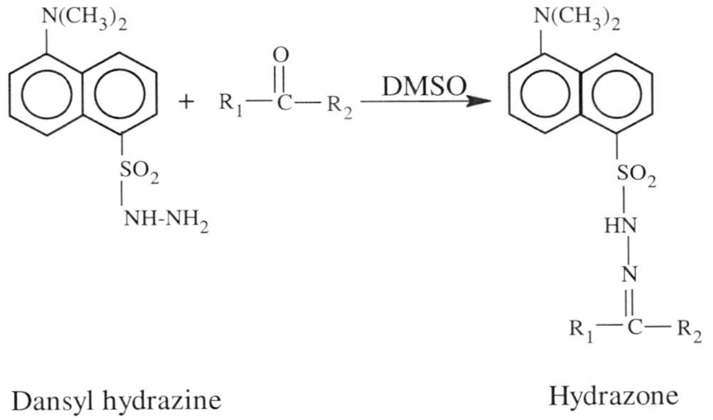

Fig. 6.29: Derivatization using dansyl hydrazine

Sometimes, simple reactions like oxidation, as shown in **Fig. 6.30**, make the molecule fluorescent, e.g. thiamine can be oxidized with potassium ferricyanide to thiochrome.

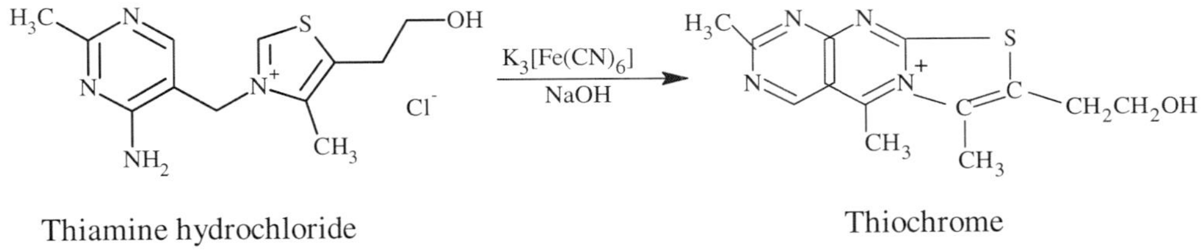

Fig. 6.30: Oxidation of thiamine by potassium ferricyanide

Table 6.3: Fluorescent indicators and pH range for color change

Name of indicator	Approximate pH range	Color change
Fosin	3.0-4.0	Colorless to green
Quinine sulphate	3.0 -5.0	Blue to violet
Fluoresceine	4.0-6.0	Colorless to green
2-Naphthaquin one	4.0-6.3	Blue to colorless
Acridine	5.2-6.6	Green to violet blue
2-Hydroxycinnamic acid	7.2-9.0	Colorless to green

6.9.3. Quenching Method

In this case, an analyte 'Q' is not fluorescent but it is able to quench the fluorescence of a fluorescent compound A*. The fluorescence intensity falls as the concentration of an analyte increases and hence, this method can be used for quantitative analysis.

Mechanism

1) An analyte Q collides with a fluorescent molecule A*, gets excited to Q* and thus, reduces the fluorescence of an original fluorescent compound A*.
2) Instead of collision of an analyte Q with a fluorescent molecule A*, a chemical reaction can take place between them so as to form an

$$A^* + Q$$

Fluorescent compound   Quencher or Analyte

↓ Collision

$$A + Q^*$$

Excited Analyte

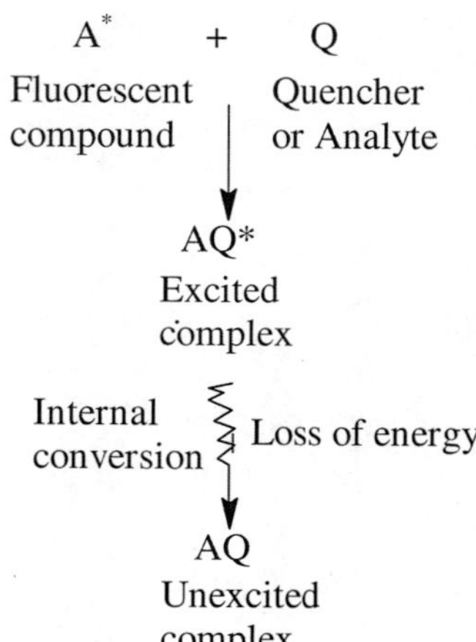

excited complex AQ*, which can deactivate by internal conversion to produce an unexcited complex AQ.

The phenomenon of quenching suffers from the following two drawbacks.

1) It is totally non-specific, i.e. apart from an analyte, some of the impurities like halides may also quench the fluorescence. Therefore, decrease in the fluorescence intensity cannot be totally related to the concentration of a quencher.
2) Fluorescence intensity decreases as concentration of a quencher increases and the calibration is also non-linear. This is shown in **Fig. 6.31**.

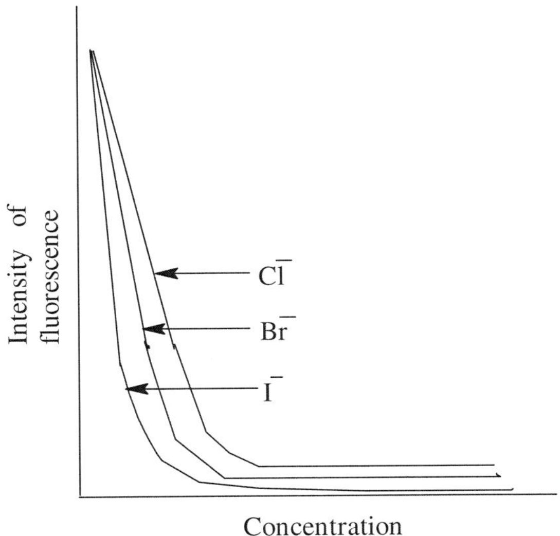

Fig. 6.31: Quenching by halides

A quenching method is used only when an analyte is known to be the only species capable of quenching the fluorescence. This is a very severe limitation of this method. A quenching method is used to find out the presence or the absence of halide impurities in the samples like quinine. The greater the slope of the curve, the more is the reduction in the intensity with small change in the concentration of an analyte, i.e. the loss of energy is more by collision and less by fluorescence. Therefore, the greater the slope of the curve, the more is the lifetime of an excited species, which allows enough time for collision, required for the formation of Q* or AQ*.

The most important application of quenching is in the determination of O_2, which is a well known quencher, being paramagnetic in nature. This can be used to detect the absence of O_2 in N_2 when O_2 free N_2 or inert gas is required to provide a suitable atmosphere for certain reactions. Fluorescence quenching provides a possible method for monitoring low levels of O_2 in such a situation. The sensitivity of this method is directly proportional to the lifetime of a fluorescent species.

Another indirect fluorimetric method, often referred to as quenching incorrectly, is one in which the ligands in a fluorescent complex are replaced by an analyte species to give a complex which is not fluorescent. An example of this is breaking of Al-oxine, a fluorescent complex, by fluoride ions (analyte). Three moles of 8-hydroxyquinoline form a stable complex with one mole of aluminium ions. When excess of sodium fluoride solution is added to the solution of this complex, fluoride ions precipitate Al^{+3} ions from the complex and form insoluble aluminium fluoride. Chemical reaction between aluminium oxine and fluoride is shown in **Fig. 6.32**. Thus, the intensity of fluorescence decreases, not because of quenching but because of the reduction in concentration of the fluorescent complex, Al-oxine. Its concentration is reduced because of its destruction due to the chemical reaction with fluoride. Hence, it is incorrect to call this analytical method as a quenching method. In a true quenching method, the fluorescent species is deactivated and not destroyed. Hence, in a true quenching method, concentration of an analyte remains fixed throughout.

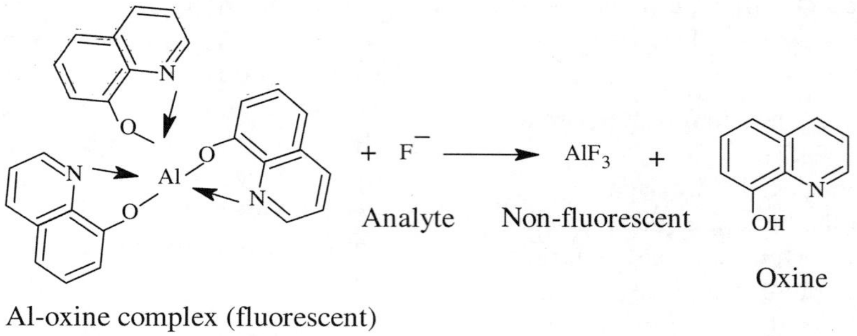

+ F^- ⟶ AlF_3 +

Analyte Non-fluorescent OH

Oxine

Al-oxine complex (fluorescent)

Fig. 6.32: A chemical reaction between aluminium oxine and fluoride

6.9.4. Fluorescence and Chromatography

6.9.4.1. Fluorescence and Planar Chromatography

Apart from the above mentioned applications, fluorescence is more applied in chromatography today.

For qualitative analysis of compounds by planar chromatography, it is essential to know the R_f values of compounds separated by chromatographic techniques. For quantitative analysis of compounds by thin layer chromatography, it is essential to scrape off the stationary phase from the place where compounds are concentrated on it. Hence, for qualitative as well as quantitative analysis of compounds, it is essential to locate the position of the separated compounds on the stationary phase. Fluorescence has been used for many years as a means of locating the components of a mixture separated by paper or thin layer chromatography.

(i) If the separated compounds are naturally fluorescent in nature, their fluorescence can be detected in the visible region. The compound is located on the plate or on the paper in the region where fluorescence is seen.

(ii) If the compounds are not fluorescent in nature, their positions on the stationary phase can be located by the following two methods.

(a) After the separation of compounds on the plate, a plate can be sprayed with a fluorescent material to prepare fluorescent derivatives of the separated components. More than one reagent can be sprayed on the same plate to prepare fluorescent derivatives of the separated compounds.

(b) In some cases, a fluorescent compound is introduced throughout the stationary phase used for the TLC or paper chromatography. After the separation of compounds on the plate, the place where a non-fluorescent compound is concentrated, shows a dark spot. This dark spot helps in locating the compound on the fluorescent background in the chromatogram. Manganese activated zinc silicate absorbs at 254 nm and emits strongly in the visible region. Hence, this material is used as a background for the location of compounds by this method.

This is a non-specific method because the presence of other impurities can also produce black spots on the plate.

6.9.4.2. Fluorescence and Column Chromatography

In case of HPLC, detection of components which are eluted from the column is very crucial because they are eluted out along with a large volume of a mobile phase. Thus, the eluted component is in the diluted form and a detector should be highly sensitive to detect low concentrations (up to 1 μg) of the material. The success of HPLC is therefore, critically dependent on the efficiency of the detector. The fluorescence detector is 2–3 times more sensitive than the UV detector and hence, it is more advantageous, but it is less widely applicable because very few compounds are naturally fluorescent. In order to make use of fluorescent detectors more widely, the components which are non-fluorescent can be derivatized either before they are introduced into the column (pre-column derivatization) or after the components are eluted out from the column (post–column derivatization). These pre-column or post–column derivatization techniques have widened the scope of fluorescent detectors.

1) Pre-column derivatization

In this case, the derivatives of all the species present or as many as are of interest, are formed by adding the reagent/s to the sample before it is injected into the column. This technique is particularly useful when the derivatization of components is complicated and requires addition of several derivatizing reagents. It is also useful when derivatization requires heating of the mixture and also when it requires a longer time for the completion of a reaction.

Drawback of this technique is that it modifies the chemical structure of the components getting separated and therefore, changes the chemical properties of the analytes. This results in the change in the R_f values of the components. This makes the separation less satisfactory, most of the times. When this problem is acute, it is necessary to turn to the post–column derivatization.

2) Post–column derivatization

In this case, a derivatizing agent is injected continuously in the eluate from the column. Usually, the derivatizing agent is used in excess in order to complete the reaction. It may be necessary to insert heating coils or *delay coils* in the path between the column and the detector to ensure that the derivatization is complete before the components reach the detector. This technique suffers from the following two drawbacks.

(i) The reagent, which is used for derivatization, itself may contribute to a background fluorescence and can reduce the sensitivity of the method, since the reagent is used in much higher concentration than the analyte, to ensure efficient and complete formation of the derivative.

(ii) The additional path length between the column and the detector can bring about diffusion and spreading of components in the eluate and impair the resolution of the separation.

Many times, pre-column derivatization is the method of choice though the range of suitable reagents is limited. This is because all the reaction conditions can be maintained so as to achieve the complete conversion of a non-fluorescent compound to a fluorescent one. All the reagents used in the standard fluorimetric procedure can be adapted for the HPLC work. However, since their effect on the separation can be critical, several new reagents have been developed, specifically for this purpose, e.g. 4 –bromomethyl–7–methoxycoumarin, 7–chloro–4–nitrobenzyl–2–oxa–1,3–diazole (NBD–chloride), dansyl chloride, dansyl hydrazine, etc.

6.9.5. Fluoroimmunoassays

A fluoroimmunoassay is one more example of a derivatization technique. It is of great importance in analytical chemistry and in biological field. It is specifically used to study antigen-antibody reaction from which the cause of infection or a disease can be diagnosed.

Antigen is a protein which can induce the synthesis of antibodies. Antibodies produced by the immune system of our body are typically very large protein molecules, which circulate in the blood stream. They form a complex with antigens, which is safely eliminated from the system.

Principle of radioimmunoassays (RIA) is applied to fluoroimmunoassays (FIA). In case of RIA, antigen (Ag), i.e. an analyte, and a known weight of a radioactively labeled version of the same antigen (Ag*) are mixed with the limited amount of the appropriate antibody (Ab) so that the total antigen (Ag + Ag*) is in excess. Both Ag and Ag* compete equally for the antibody and form complexes with it, which are insoluble in the reaction medium.

$$2\,Ag + 2\,Ag^* + 2\,Ab$$
$$\downarrow$$
$$(Ag - Ab + Ag^* - Ab) + (Ag + Ag^*)$$

Bound antigens (Insoluble complex) — Free or unbound antigens

Insoluble complexes can be separated from the reaction medium by centrifuging or filtering the reaction mixture. After the separation, some radioactivity is present in the precipitate and some in the filtrate. Distribution of the radioactivity between the complex, i.e. the precipitate, and the filtrate, is measured, and this ratio is used to determine the concentration of non-labeled antigen (Ag). In the following equation, the ratio of the intensities of the bound to the unbound antigens is known. From this ratio, the concentration of Ag –Ab can be calculated, since the fixed amounts of Ag* and Ab are used. Therefore, the amount of the Ab linked with an Ag can be calculated and hence, the amount of Ag in the complex can also be found out.

$$\frac{\text{Intensity of bound antigen}}{\text{Intensity of unbound antigen}} = \frac{[Ag^* - Ab]}{[Ag^*]}$$

One should note that -

$$\frac{[Ag^* - Ab]}{[Ag^*]} \neq \frac{[Ag - Ab]}{[Ag]}$$

Let us assume that initially, there is no antigen (Ag) present in the sample. When there is no non-labeled antigen (Ag) present, all the complex is in the radioactive form, i.e. Ag* -Ab and the amount of free Ag* is less. Therefore, the ratio of the radioactivity of the bound to the unbound antigens is high. As the concentration of a non-labeled antigen increases, it replaces some of the labeled antigen (Ag*) in the complex and so the concentration of Ag* - Ab, and hence, the radioactivity of the complex decreases, while the activity of the filtrate increases because the concentration of Ag* increases. Hence, the ratio of the radioactivity of the bound to unbound decreases. Thus, the increase in the concentration of an antigen (Ag) is correlated with the decrease in the ratio of the bound to unbound radioactivity. Thus, the concentration of an analyte can be readily calculated from the algebraic relationships derived from the equilibrium equations.

In case of fluoroimmunoassays, the same principle is used but instead of a radioactive label, a fluorescent label is used, i.e. Ag is an analyte, which is not fluorescent and Ag* is an analyte reacted with a fluorescing agent so as to make it fluorescent.

$$\underset{\text{Non-fluorescent antigen}}{2\,Ag} + \underset{\text{Fluorescent antigen}}{2\,Ag^*} + \underset{\text{Antibody}}{2\,Ab}$$
$$\downarrow$$
$$\underset{\text{Bound antigen}}{(Ag - Ab + Ag^* - Ab)} + \underset{\text{Free or unbound excess antigen}}{(Ag + Ag^*)}$$

Advantages of fluoroimmunoassays

1) If Ag* - Ab has different fluorescence characteristics than the free fluorescent antigen (Ag*), then there is no need to separate these two species from their mixture. Under this condition, the assay is termed as a *homogeneous assay* and is much more rapid and

convenient than the *heterogeneous radioimmunoassay*, involving the separation of the radioactive complex and radioactive antigen.

2) Handling of radioactive isotopes is not involved.
3) Cost of the radioactive isotopes is saved and cost of measuring the radioactivity is also saved.
4) Provision of a safe and secluded environment is not essential.
5) Shelf life a of fluorescing agents is much more than the shelf life of radioisotopes.

The materials used as fluorescent labels need to emit and absorb at the longer wavelengths to avoid the interference from the natural fluorescence present in the biological samples at the shorter wavelength.

Advantages of radioimmunoassays

In case of radioactive labeling, an atom in the antigen molecule is replaced with its radioisotope. This does not alter chemical or physical properties of an antigen. However, a fluorescent label is often a sizeable molecule and therefore, adding it to the antigen molecule is quite likely to affect the properties of the antigen.

CHAPTER 7

ATOMIC SPECTROMETRY

The ultraviolet-visible (UV-visible) spectrometry, infrared (IR) spectrometry and nuclear magnetic resonance (NMR) spectrometry deal with the molecular samples, whereas the atomic spectrometry deals with the atomic samples. Hence, it is essential to decompose a molecule into its constituent atoms and then vaporize them. This process is termed as *atomization*. The accuracy of the quantitative estimation by this method depends on the efficiency of atomization.

Unlike the broad bands obtained in the UV-visible, IR or NMR molecular spectra, the atomic spectra consist of relatively limited number of discrete lines because of the presence of only electronic energy levels and the absence of the vibrational and the rotational energy levels in atoms.

The atomic spectrometry is usually carried out in the UV-visible and X-ray regions. It is a highly *specific* and *sensitive* method for the qualitative as well as quantitative analysis of inorganic salts. The metals can be detected accurately to the ppm (parts per million) or ppb (parts per billion) levels.

The sources used for the atomization of a sample in the atomic spectrometry are of two types.

1) Low temperature sources like flames, obtained by the combustion of gases
2) High temperature sources like an electric arc, spark and argon plasma

When flame is used for atomization, the technique is called as *flame spectrometry*.

FLAME SPECTROMETRY

7.1. PRINCIPLE

In flame spectrometry, an aqueous solution of inorganic salts is aspirated into the hot flame or a burner. Inside the flame, the solvent is evaporated and the molecules are dissociated into ions. The ions of the metal extract electrons from the flame and get reduced to the elemental state. Due to high temperature of the flame, these atoms are in the vapor form. In case of inefficient atomization, the process of dissociation of a molecule into its constituent ions or the reduction of the constituent ions into atoms, remains incomplete. This results in the mixture of vapor of atoms, ions and molecules, in the flame. The gaseous solution or a homogeneous mixture of vapor of different species, which is present within the flame, is termed as *plasma*. It usually contains a significant concentration of the elementary particles, i.e. atoms. The atoms formed after atomization of the sample, may absorb energy from the flame. Thus, energy of the flame or any other excitation source can excite electrons of an atomic sample. The intensity of emission, absorption or fluorescence, can then be measured for quantitative analysis.

7.2. FLAME SPECTRA

The flame spectra are recorded by using the following three techniques.

7.2.1. Flame Emission Spectrometry

In flame emission spectrometry, a sample is introduced in the flame and is excited. An exited sample emits radiation, which is passed through a collimator to a monochromator. A monochromator or a filter separates the wavelength of emission of an atomic sample from the wavelength of emission of the flame. The intensity of emission is measured at the wavelength of emission of the sample. The set-up for the flame emission spectrometry is shown in **Fig. 7.1**.

When the chopper is used to chop the beam from the source before it reaches the flame, detector receives output from the flame only. The detector circuitry is designed to reject the DC output from the flame emission and measure the AC absorption

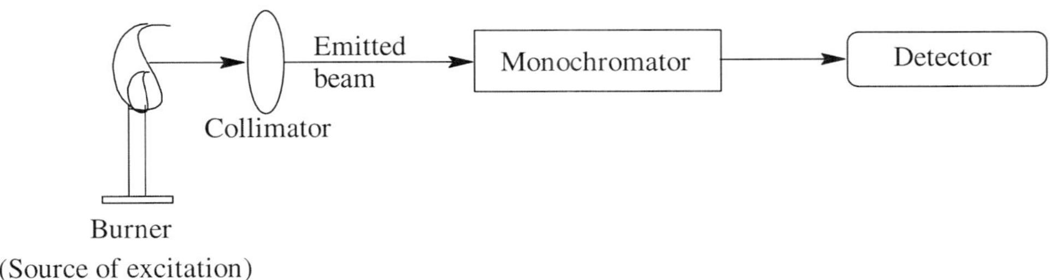

Fig. 7.1: Set-up for flame emission spectrometry

signal from the source and the sample. The difference between P_o (the incident power) and P (the transmitted power) is the measure of the concentration of an analyte in the sample. The set-up for the flame absorption spectrometry is shown in **Fig. 7.2**.

7.2.2. Flame Absorption Spectrometry

In flame absorption spectrometry also, the flame of the burner acts as a sample holder or a cuvette, since the vapor of the sample is present within the flame. The sample present in the flame is then exposed to a suitable source of radiation. A part of the energy of radiation is absorbed by the sample and the remaining is transmitted out. The monochromator allows measurement of the intensity of absorption at the wavelength of absorption of a sample. A chopper is introduced between the source and the flame. When the beam from the source is not chopped, detector receives the output from the flame as well as the source.

7.2.3. Flame Fluorescence Spectrometry

In this case also, flame serves as a sample holder as in case of flame absorption and emission spectrometry. The sample is excited using a source of radiation. When the sample absorbs incident radiation of intensity (P_o), it gets excited and starts fluorescing. The intensity of fluorescence (P) is

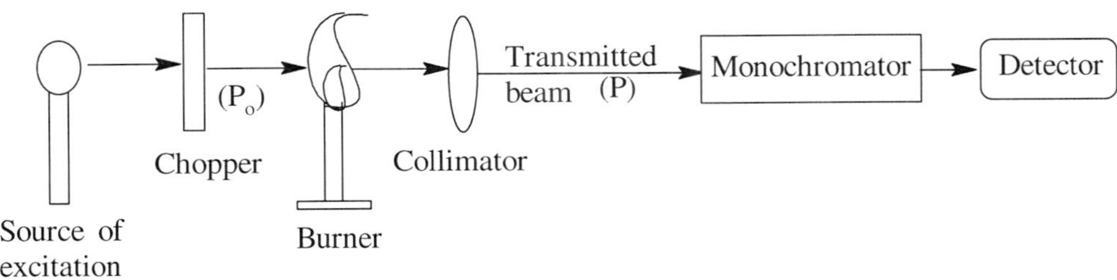

Fig. 7.2: Set-up for flame absorption spectrometry

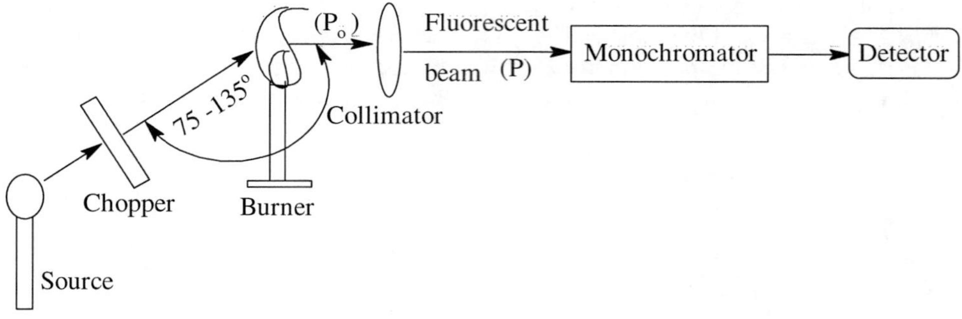

Fig. 7.3: Set-up for flame fluorescence spectrometry

measured at an angle of 90° or at any angle between 75° and135°, for higher accuracy. The measurement of the intensity of fluorescence in other directions involves great loss of energy and results in the reduction of accuracy. The set-up for flame fluorescence spectrometry is shown in **Fig. 7.3**.

The emission, absorption and fluorescence spectra for atoms consist of well defined narrow lines in the UV-visible region. These lines arise from the electronic transitions of the outermost electrons. The type of spectrum obtained depends on the energy level pattern of an element.

In the energy level diagrams (**Figures 7.4** and **7.5**) for any atom containing one electron in its outermost shell, the p-orbitals are split into two levels that differ slightly in energy. This can be explained on the basis of the magnetic fields produced by the moving electrons. Any electron spins about its own axis. It is also associated with the orbital motion. Both these motions produce magnetic fields in some direction. If the direction of the spin and the orbital motion are same, a force of repulsion is generated. On the other hand, if these two motions produce magnetic fields in opposite directions, a force of attraction is generated. The energy of an electron, whose spin motion is in the opposite direction of its orbital motion, is slightly lesser than the energy of an electron spinning in the same direction as its orbital motion. Hence, the p-orbitals are associated with two energy levels (a *doublet* state) and are shown as two separate lines in the energy level diagrams (**Figures 7.4** and **7.5**). For d- and f- orbitals also, the similar differences in the energies exist, but the difference in the energy is usually so small that it can be neglected. Hence, they are shown by a single line only.

The splitting of the p-, d- and f- orbitals into two states is a characteristic of all the species containing one valence electron, e.g., Na atom (11 = 2, 8, 1), Mg^{+1} ion (Mg = 12, Mg^{+1} = 11) and Al^{+2} ion (Al = 13, Al^{+2} = 11). Therefore, the energy level diagram and hence, the nature of the atomic spectra

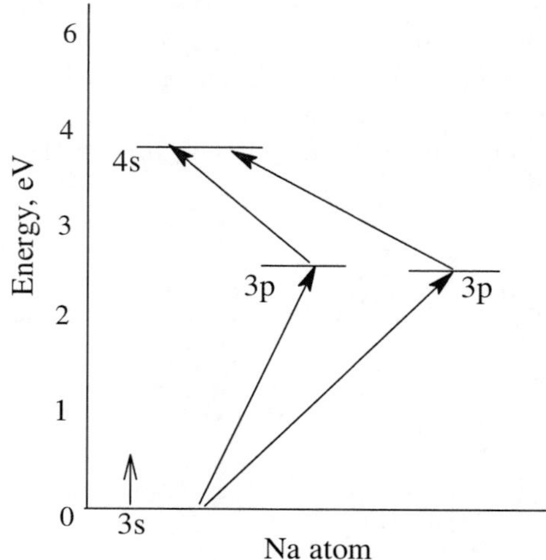

Fig. 7.4: Energy level diagram for Na atom

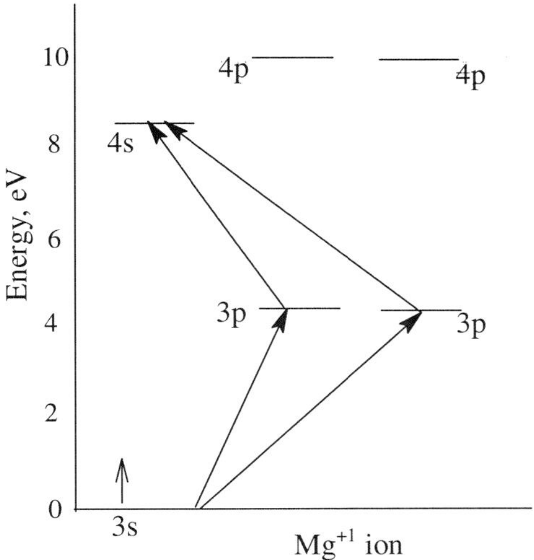

Fig. 7.5: Energy level diagram for Mg^{+1} ion

for all these species is more or less same, except for the energy gaps between different energy levels. For example, the energy difference between the 3s and 3p orbitals of Mg^{+1} ion is approximately twice as compared to that for Na atom. This is because of the larger nuclear charge in case of Mg^{+1} ion compared to that for Na atom. **Figures 7.4** and **7.5** indicate the energy level diagrams for Na atom and Mg^{+1} ion, respectively.

For a species containing two electrons (A and B, **Fig. 7.6**) in the outermost shell, such as Mg atom or Al^{+1} ion, an excitation of one of the electrons in the 3s atomic orbital [Mg = 12 = 2, 8, 2 ($3s^2$)] results either in a *singlet* state or a *triplet* state (**Fig. 7.6**). A singlet state results when an excitation of an electron from the lower energy level to the higher one results without the change in its spin. Since there is no change in the spin of electrons, the electric and the magnetic fields produced by both the electrons are of equal magnitude but opposite in direction. Hence, they cancel each other. Thus, only one single energy level is associated with such a system. The system, in which an excitation of one of the electrons from the lower energy level to the higher energy level occurs without the change in the spin, is called a *singlet* system.

On the contrary, a *triplet* state results when an excitation of an electron from the lower energy level to the higher one, occurs with the change of spin of one of the electrons from the pair. When both the electrons spin in the same direction, their electric and magnetic fields interact in such a way so as to produce three energy levels for a system, as shown in **Fig. 7.6**. Hence, such a system in which an excitation of one of the electrons from the lower energy level to the higher one, occurs with the change in the spin, is known as a *triplet* system. This is well explained in **Chapter 6** with the help of **Fig. 6.1(c)**.

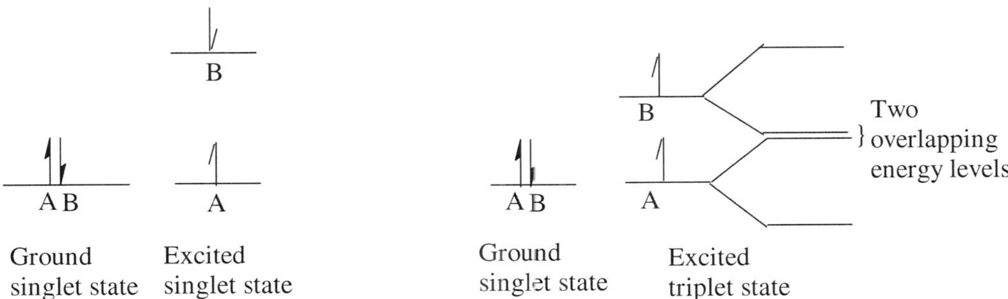

Fig. 7.6: Singlet and triplet states of atoms

The presence of a singlet and/or a triplet system is a characteristic of all the species containing a pair of electrons in the outermost shell, e.g. aluminium ion (Al^{+1}) and beryllium atom (Be = 4 = 2, 2). The singlet and the triplet systems in magnesium atom are shown in **Figures 7.7(a) and (b)**, respectively.

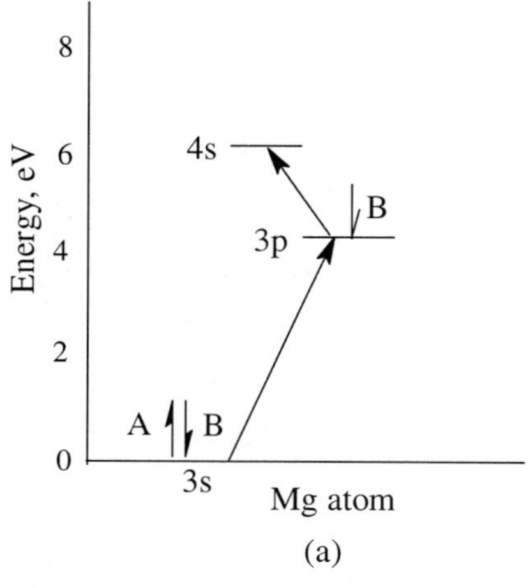

A singlet system

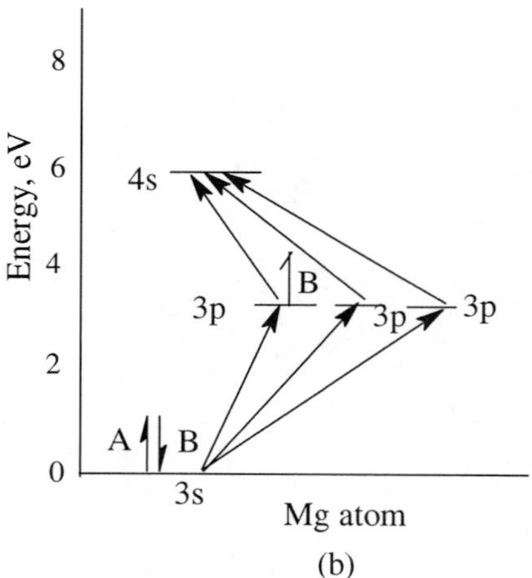

A triplet system

Fig. 7.7: (a) A singlet and (b) a triplet system in Mg atom

As the number of electrons in the outermost shell increases, the energy level diagram becomes more and more complex. With three outer electrons, splitting of energy levels into two and four states occurs. With four outer electrons, singlet, triplet and quintet states occur. Hence, for elements with higher atomic numbers, the atomic spectra are complex and therefore, their identification becomes a difficult task.

7.3. FLAME CHARACTERISTICS

In order to get a proper or a characteristic flame spectrum of any species, that species should be exposed to a particular portion of the flame that provides a constant temperature. Hence, it is required to select the appropriate mixture of a fuel and an oxidant, which provides the

Table 7.1: A list of fuels, oxidants and the temperature obtained by their combustion

Sr. No.	Fuel	Oxidant	Temperature (°C)
1	Natural gas	Air	1700-1900
2	Natural gas	O_2	2500-2700
3	Hydrogen	Air	2000-2700
4	Hydrogen	O_2	2500-2700
5	Acetylene	Air	2100-2500
6	Acetylene	O_2	3000-3200
7	Acetylene	Nitrous oxide	2600-2800
8	Cyanogen (C_2N_2)	O_2	4500

temperature required for the complete atomization and excitation of an analyte. Depending on the temperature required for analysis, different fuels and oxidants are used. **Table 7.1** gives a list of fuels, oxidants and the temperature obtained by their combustion.

The lower temperatures provided by the flame are useful in case of alkali and alkaline earth metals, which require lower excitation energies. Flames which provide higher temperatures are useful to excite metals with higher excitation energy.

7.4. TEMPERATURE PROFILES

A temperature profile shows variation in the temperature in different portions of the flame. **Figure 7.8** shows the temperature profile of a flame obtained by using a mixture of natural gas and air.

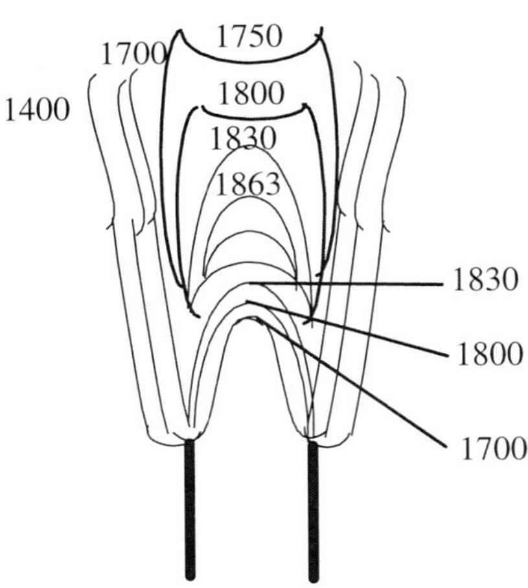

Fig. 7.8: Temperature profile of a flame obtained by burning natural gas and air

The flame is divided into four different portions as shown in **Fig. 7.9**.

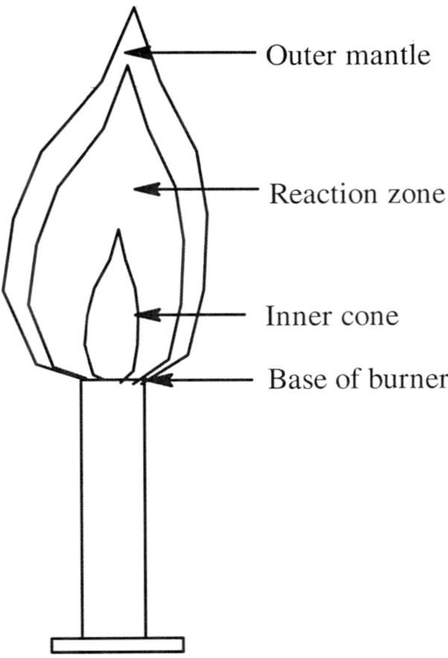

Fig. 7.9: Different portions of the flame

1) Base

The sample enters the base of the flame in the form of minute droplets. Within this region, water evaporates and a substantial fraction of the droplets gets converted to solid particles.

2) Inner Cone

In this region, most of the sample enters as solid particles. Solid molecules dissociate into the corresponding ions, which in turn get reduced to atomic states. Atomization of the sample, thus, occurs in this region. The dissociation and atomization of calcium chloride is shown by **reactions (7.1) and (7.2)**, respectively. Vaporization of the atomic sample, absorption of energy and excitation to higher energy level also commence in the inner cone itself. The sample then passes to the reaction zone.

$$CaCl_2 \rightleftharpoons Ca^{+2} + 2\,Cl^- \quad \ldots (7.1)$$

$$Ca^{+2} + 2\,e^- \longrightarrow Ca \quad \ldots (7.2)$$

3) Reaction zone

In the reaction zone, the sample reacts with an oxidant, either air or O_2 used along with the fuel to get the flame, and gets converted to the corresponding oxide, e.g. calcium gets converted to calcium oxide, as shown by **reaction (7.3)**.

$$2\ Ca + O_2 \longrightarrow 2\ CaO \quad ...\ (7.3)$$

4) Outer Mantle

The oxide formed in the reaction zone gets ejected out of the flame from this region.

The actual number of droplets that evaporate and the actual amount of the sample that is atomized and further vaporized, depends on the droplet size, the flow rate of the sample and also on the temperature of the flame. At the higher flow rate, a significant portion of the sample passes through the flame unaltered. This can bring down the temperature of the flame, thereby reducing the extent of atomization or the degree of excitation of the sample in the flame.

The maximum temperature of the flame is obtained somewhat above the inner cone of the flame. There is a decrease in the temperature of the flame, both the length wise and the breadth wise, as we move on the outer side of the flame.

7.5. EFFECT OF TEMPERATURE VARIATION ON FLAME SPECTRUM

The variation in the temperature of the flame affects the flame spectra of samples in many ways, as described below.

7.5.1. Variation in the temperature of the flame changes the *nature of the flame spectrum*, i.e. the number of lines in the spectrum and their position.

7.5.2. Temperature variation also changes the *intensity of lines* in the spectrum.

7.5.3. Temperature also decides the *sensitivity* of a particular method, i.e. of absorption or emission spectrometry.

7.5.1. Effect of Temperature on the Nature of the Flame Spectrum

The temperature of the flame decides the nature of the emission, absorption or fluorescence spectrum. This can be explained with the help of the sample of a magnesium salt. A sample of magnesium, when introduced into a low temperature flame (2000-2540 °C), is completely atomized. Thus, the plasma contains a homogeneous mixture of gaseous fuel, gaseous oxidant and Mg atoms in the vapor form. Hence, at the lower temperature, a spectrum corresponding to a singlet and a triplet state of Mg atoms is obtained as explained before [**Figures 7.7(a)** and **(b)**]. On the other hand, at the higher temperature of 4500 °C, provided by the cyanogen gas, some of the Mg atoms that are formed, again lose electrons and get converted to Mg^{+1} ions. Thus, a mixture of Mg atoms and Mg^{+1} ions is present in the plasma. Hence, at the higher temperature, the flame spectrum is a mixture of spectrum for Mg atoms [**Figures 7.7(a)** and **(b)**] and the Mg^{+1} ions (**Fig. 7.5**), both of which are discussed before.

7.5.2. Effect of Temperature on the Intensity of the Flame Spectrum

The temperature of the flame decides the degree of atomization of the sample. At low temperatures, atomization is incomplete. At very high temperatures, the atoms which are formed get ionized, forming the ions again. The total number of atoms available for the excitation decides the number of atoms that can occupy an excided state. The higher degree of atomization makes available the greater number of atoms in the ground state for the purpose of excitation. This leads to the excitation of more atoms to the excited state. If the degree of atomization is low, the number of atoms in the ground state, available for excitation, is less. Subsequently, the number of atoms in the excited state is also automatically reduced. The number of atoms getting excited to the higher energy level decides the amount of energy absorbed or amount of energy emitted by them. If more atoms absorb energy, then the intensity of lines in their atomic spectrum is more. Similarly, if more atoms are present in the excited state, a larger amount of energy is given out by them, while returning back to the ground state. Thus, the degree of atomization of the sample affects the intensity of lines in the absorption, emission as well as fluorescence spectrometry.

The ratio of the number of atoms in the excited state (N_j) to the number of atoms in ground state (N_o) is given by Boltzmann **equation (7.4)** as follows.

$$\frac{N_j}{N_o} = \frac{P_j}{P_o} e^{-\frac{E_j}{kT}} \quad \cdots (7.4)$$

where, k = Boltzmann constant = 1.38×10^{-16} erg/deg,

T = Temperature in °K,

E_j = Difference in the energies of the excited and the ground state of atoms, and

P_j and P_o are the statistical factors that are determined by the number of states having equal energy at each quantum level.

The temperature fluctuation results in a change in the number of excited atoms. This leads to the corresponding change in the intensity of the emitted beam.

Absorption and fluorescence spectrometry are comparatively less affected by the temperature changes in the flame as compared to the emission spectrometry. This is because absorption and fluorescence spectrometry depend on the total number of atoms available for the excitation, whereas emission spectrometry depends on the number of atoms excited to the higher energy level as well as on the number of atoms available for the excitation. Thus, an emission method is based upon a small fraction of the analyte that is excited, whereas absorption and fluorescence methods depend on a great portion of the atoms that remains in the ground state, even after the excitation. Hence, emission spectrometry requires a close control on the temperature of the flame.

7.5.3. Effect of Temperature on the Type of Spectrum or on the Sensitivity of the Method

Temperature of the flame decides the sensitivity of emission, absorption and fluorescence spectrometry.

In atomic absorption and fluorescence spectrometry, the intensity or the power of the beam before interaction with the matter (P_o) and after interaction with the matter (P) is measured. The difference between the two, (P_o – P), is a measure of the amount of analyte present in the sample. If an analyte concentration is more, its interaction with the beam of radiation is more and the value of P is considerably low. If the value of P is very small, there would be error in its measurement and then the accurate value of (P_o – P) cannot be obtained. On the contrary, when the analyte concentration is less, its interaction with the radiation is also less and the value of P is sufficiently large or close to the value of P_o. In this case, the difference between P_o and P is so small that a small error in the measurement of the difference between P_o and P gets magnified at the end, during the calculation of the concentration of an analyte. Hence, for absorption and fluorescence spectrometry, medium interaction of the sample with radiation, which would give a measurable magnitude of P as well as of the difference between P_o and P, is desirable.

For emission spectrometry, the intensity of the lines depends on the number of atoms which give out energy while coming back from the higher energy level to the lower energy level. The more the number of atoms in the excited state the more is the intensity of emission and the higher is the sensitivity of the method.

At lower temperatures of the flame, few atoms are available for the excitation, because the degree of atomization is low. Hence, only few atoms are excited to the higher energy level and a greater number of atoms remains in the ground state. This increases the sensitivity of absorption and fluorescence spectrometry over emission spectrometry. At higher temperatures of the flame, the degree of atomization is higher and more atoms are available for the excitation. The excitation of more atoms to the higher energy level results in the emission of more energy, when atoms come back from the higher energy level to the lower one. This contributes to the higher intensity of emission and increases the sensitivity of emission spectrometry. When more atoms are excited to the higher energy level, the number of atoms remaining in the lower energy level is reduced considerably and the intensity of the transmitted beam (P) cannot be measured accurately. This reduces the sensitivity of absorption and fluorescence spectrometry.

7.6. FLAME PROFILES

The flame profiles provide useful information about the processes that occur in different portions of the flame when the sample is introduced in it. From the nature of the flame profile, the portion of the flame, which is to be focused on the sample to get the maximum sensitivity, can be selected. The flame profiles are of two types.

7.6.1. Flame absorption profile

7.6.2. Flame emission profile

7.6.1. Flame Absorption Profile

In order to explain different kinds of flame absorption profiles, three elements, magnesium (Mg), silver (Ag) and chromium (Cr) are selected. These three elements provide different kinds of absorption profiles because of the difference in their capacity to get oxidized. Magnesium gets oxidized slowly, silver resists oxidation and chromium gets oxidized very easily.

When the magnesium salt solution is introduced in the flame, the number of magnesium atoms goes on increasing as the temperature increases from the base of the flame to the inner cone and hence, the absorbance also increases from the base of the flame to the inner cone (**Fig. 7.10**). Beyond the inner cone, however, in the reaction zone, magnesium atoms react with O_2 in the flame and get converted to the non-absorbing magnesium oxide particles. These are then ejected

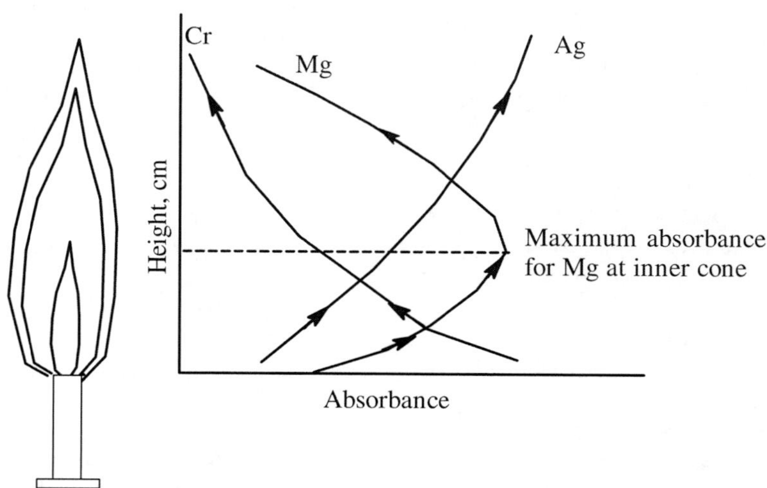

Fig. 7.10: Atomic absorption profiles of magnesium, silver and chromium

out of the flame from the outer mantle. The changes in the absorbance of magnesium, silver and chromium atoms with the flame height are shown in **Fig. 7.10**.

In case of silver salts, Ag atoms which resist oxidation are formed in the flame. Hence, the number of Ag atoms goes on increasing from the base of the flame to the outer mantle. Thus, a continuous increase in the absorbance is seen, in case of silver sample from the base of the flame to the outer mantle.

Chromium, in contrast, undergoes oxidation right from the base of the flame and forms a stable oxide, which is non-absorbing. Thus, it shows a continuous decrease in the absorbance from the base of the flame to the tip of the flame.

7.6.2. Flame Emission Profile

Flame emission profile for calcium salts is produced due to the presence of Ca^{+1} ions in the flame. The three dimensional figure (**Fig. 7.11)** illustrates the intensity of emission by Ca^{+1} ions

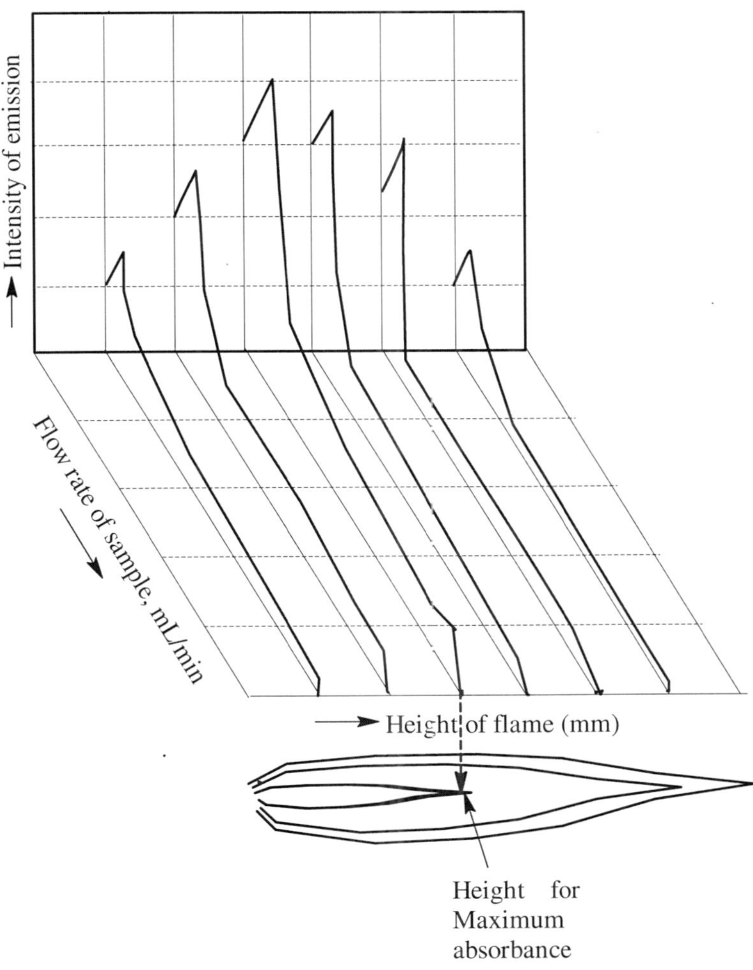

Fig. 7.11: Flame emission profile of Ca^{+1} ions

with respect to the temperature of the flame and also with respect to the flow rate of the sample solution into the flame. In this figure, flame height is expressed in millimeters along X-axis, sample flow rate, expressed in milliliter per minute, is plotted along Y-axis and the intensity of emission is plotted along Z-axis.

With the increase in the temperature of the flame, the number of Ca^{+1} ions increases and therefore, the intensity of emission also increases. The intensity of emission also increases with the increase in the sample flow rate, since more of Ca^{+1} ions are formed from more of the sample entering into the flame, but beyond a particular flow rate, a significant portion of the sample just flows through the flame without undergoing evaporation, atomization and excitation. This reduces the number of Ca^{+1} ions in the flame, thereby reducing the intensity of emission. Moreover, the presence of water in the sample reduces the flame temperature and lowers down the extent of atomization, which ultimately reduces the intensity of emission.

Thus, the temperature of the flame and the flow rate of the sample, both affect the intensity of emission of the spectral lines.

7.7. ATOMIZERS FOR ATOMIC SPECTROMETRY

Atomizers are used to convert a molecular sample into an atomic one. The atomizers used in atomic spectrometry are of two types.

7.7.1. Flame atomizers and
7.7.2. Non-flame atomizers

7.7.1. Flame Atomizers

Flame atomizers consist of the following components.

1) A nebulizer
2) A burner

A nebulizer produces a fine spay or an aerosol of the liquid sample. Thus, it helps in introducing the sample solution in the form of fine droplets near the base of the flame. Burners produce flame by burning of the fuel in the presence of O_2 or air. Burners are of two types.

1) Total consumption burners or turbulent flow burners
2) Premixed burners or laminar flow burners

1) Total consumption burners or turbulent flow burners

As shown in **Fig. 7.12**, in turbulent flow burners, fuel is passed through one tubing and O_2 or air is passed through another tubing. Fuel and O_2 pass through these tubings and undergo sudden expansion (venturi action) at the tip of the burner, where they are burnt so as to get the flame. The sample solution is drawn up the capillary and nebulized by the venturi action.

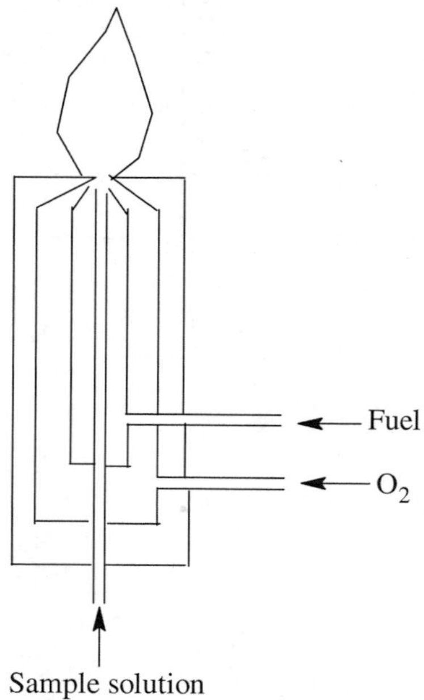

Fig. 7.12: A turbulent flow burner

Advantages of turbulent flow burners

(i) In turbulent flow burners, there is no hindrance to the flow of sample solution. Hence, a relatively large and representative sample reaches the flame so as to provide adequate sensitivity to the method.

(ii) Because of the higher pressure of gases inside the burner and because of the flow of fuel and oxidant through separate tubings, there is no risk of explosion of the gases.

Disadvantages of turbulent flow burners

(i) Nebulization of the sample is because of the venturi action of gases. Since the gases expand suddenly, the sample deposits at the tip of the burner, thereby clogging it.

(ii) Because of sudden expansion of gases, they spread in the periphery and produce a broad flame instead of a long flame. Hence, the path length provided by these burners is short.

(iii) Turbulent flow burners produce a lot of auditory and electronic noise.

2) Premixed or laminar flow burners

In laminar flow burners, as shown in **Fig. 7.13**, the sample solution is nebulized because of the venturi action of O_2 gas. The aerosol or the fine droplets of the sample solution are then mixed with the fuel in a mixing chamber. A mixture of sample droplets, O_2 and fuel is then made to pass through a series of baffles or parallel slots. Hence, the majority of the sample gets collected at the bottom of the mixing chamber. Only a smaller fraction of the sample then passes through parallel slots, into the flame. The slots provide a laminar flow of the mixture of O_2 and fuel.

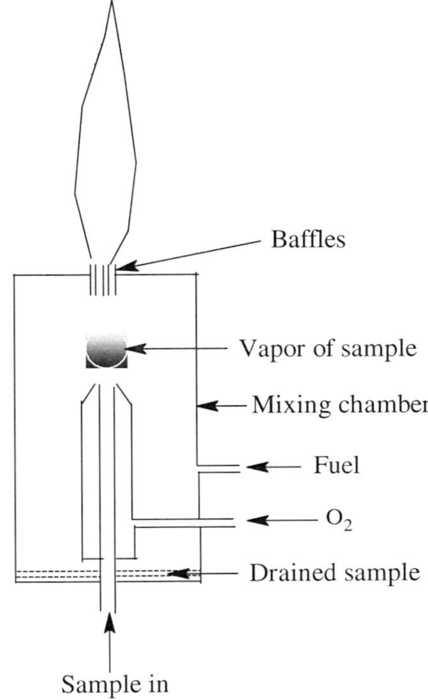

Fig. 7.13: A laminar flow burner

Advantages of laminar flow burners

(i) Because of the parallel slots, a definite direction is given to the flow of gases. This produces a longer flame in these burners rather than a broader flame as in case of turbulent flow burners.

(ii) Laminar flow burners are not noisy from the auditory and electronic point of view.

(iii) Clogging of the tip of the burner does not occur commonly because of the absence of venturi action.

Disadvantages of laminar flow burners

(i) In these burners, a majority of the sample is drained out. Hence, the representative sample does not reach the flame.

(ii) Fuel and O_2 are present together in a mixing chamber. This increases the risk of explosion.

In spite of the advantages and disadvantages of both the burners, they are comparable to each other in sensitivity and reproducibility. This is because the laminar flow burner does not allow representative sample to reach the flame but provides a longer flame or a longer path length to the sample. On the other hand, the turbulent flow burner allows representative sample to reach the flame but provides a shorter flame or a shorter path length.

The comparison between the turbulent flow burners and the laminar flow burners is given in **Table 7.2**.

7.7.2. Non-flame Atomizers

The non-flame atomizers are electrothermal

atomizers. In this case, the atomization of the sample occurs due to the heat produced by the passage of current through a graphite cylinder, which is 3-5 cm in length and 0.5-1 cm in breadth. A small amount of the sample is kept at the centre of the cylinder. Due to the heat of the cylinder, the sample vaporizes and gets atomized in the vicinity of the cylinder. The source of excitation is kept in line with the area of atomization. The amount of energy absorbed or emitted by the atomic sample is then measured for the quantitative estimation. A non-flame atomizer is shown in **Fig. 7.14**.

Advantages of non-flame atomizers

(i) The efficiency of atomization of the non-flame atomizers is very high. Hence, a very small amount of the sample is required for analysis.

(ii) The sensitivity of these atomizers is very high and hence, even the trace amounts can be analyzed accurately.

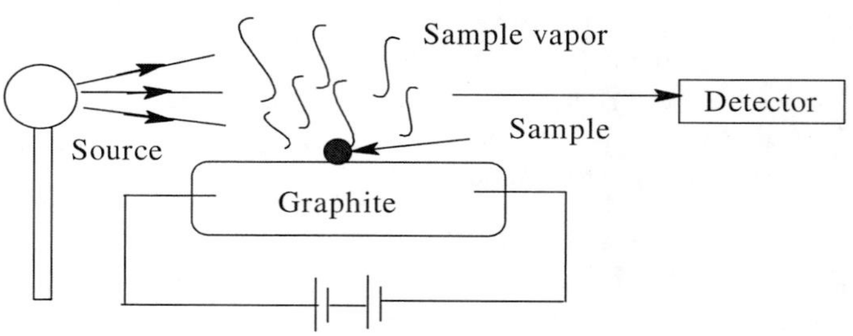

Fig. 7.14: A non-flame atomizer

Table 7.2: Comparison between turbulent flow burners and laminar flow burners

	Turbulent flow burner	Laminar flow burner
1	It produces a shorter and a broader flame.	It produces a longer and a narrower flame.
2	Representative sample reaches the flame.	Most of the sample is drained out at the bottom of the chamber.
3	There is a possibility of clogging of the tip of the burner.	Clogging of the tip of the burner does not occur.
4	There is no risk of explosion.	Explosion can occur in the mixing chamber.
5	This burner is a noisy burner from the auditory as well as electronic point of view.	This burner produces a silent flame.

CHAPTER 8

X-RAY DIFFRACTION CRYSTALLOGRAPHY

8.1. INTRODUCTION

In the electromagnetic spectrum, γ (gamma, Gr.) radiation is the shortest radiation covering a range of waves corresponding to a length of 10^{-11} to 10^{-8} cm (0.001 to 1.0 A°). X-radiation has longer waves compared to γ-radiation and shorter waves compared to UV radiation. They cover a range of waves

Wavelength of γ-radiation	Wavelength of X-rays
0.001-1.0 A°	0.1 - 100 A°
10^{-11} - 10^{-8} cm	10^{-9} - 10^{-6} cm

$1A° = 10^{-10}$ m $= 10^{-8}$ cm
1 nm $=10^{-9}$ m $= 10^{-7}$ cm
$1\mu m = 10^{-6}$ m $=10^{-4}$ cm

corresponding to a length of 10^{-9} to 10^{-6} cm (0.1 to 100 A°). X-ray crystallography, however, makes use of waves in the range of 0.1 to 25 A°.

X-ray crystallography is also called as *optical spectroscopy*. X-radiation being very short, is highly energetic, and interacts with the matter so as to cause the transition of electrons present in the inner orbitals of atoms, which are near the nucleus.

8.2. PRINCIPLE OF X-RAY DIFFRACTION CRYSTALLOGRAPHY

The principle behind X-ray diffraction crystallography is based upon *Bragg's equation*. In case of many crystals, the distance between the atomic centers is of the same order of magnitude as the wavelength of X-radiation. Consider an X-ray beam incident on the surface of a crystal at an angle θ (Theta, Gr.). A part of the radiation is scattered from the surface of a crystal and a part of it is transmitted to the second layer of atoms, where again a fraction is scattered and the remainder is transmitted to the third layer (**Fig. 8.1**).

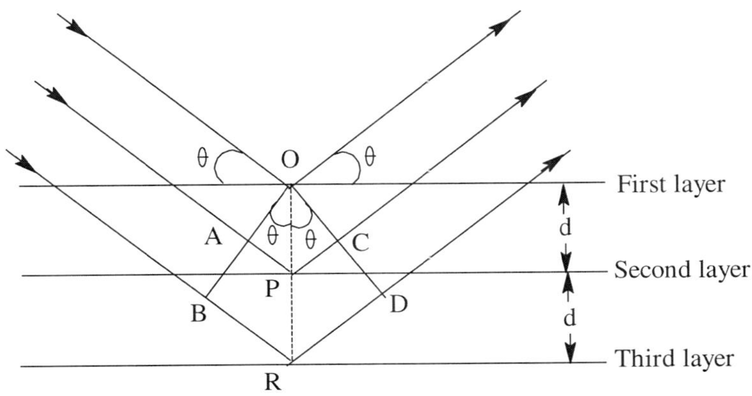

Fig. 8.1: Diffraction of X-rays by a crystal

X-ray diffraction from any crystal is more intense under two conditions.

1) When different layers of atoms in the crystal are equally spaced and the spacing between the layers is of the same order as the wavelength of the radiation.
2) Secondly, the atoms, which are the scattering centers, are present in a highly ordered manner in a solid.

In **Fig. 8.1**, the X-rays which are scattered from the atoms at O, P and R undergo either *constructive* or *destructive* interference. Wavelengths which undergo constructive interference are made available for studies. Wavelengths undergoing destructive interference are not available after scattering.

How is crystal identified using X-ray diffraction?

Bragg studied X-ray diffraction by using a number of crystals.

X-rays scattered from an atom P (**Fig. 8.1**), would be in phase with X-rays scattered from an atom O if the following condition, mentioned in **equation (8.1)**, is satisfied.

$$AP + PC = n\lambda \dots (8.1)$$

where, `n' is an integer or order of the spectrum and λ is the wavelength of X-radiation falling on the crystal. When this happens, the radiation scattered from an atom P and the radiation scattered from an atom O, undergo constructive interference.

Similarly, X-rays scattered from an atom R would be in a phase with X-rays scattered from an atom P if the following condition, mentioned in **equation (8.2)**, is satisfied.

$$BR + RD = n\lambda \dots (8.2)$$

This would result in the constructive interference between the radiation scattered from atoms R and P. In **equation (8.1)**, AP = PC = d sin θ, where `d' is the distance between the two consecutive layers of atoms in a crystal. Thus, the constructive interference of the two beams would occur if -

$$AP + PC = d \sin\theta + d \sin\theta$$

$$= 2d \sin\theta = n\lambda$$

$$\therefore \quad \boxed{n\lambda = 2d \sin\theta} \quad \dots (8.3)$$

Equation (8.3) is called the *Bragg's equation*. Thus, for any angle of incidence (θ), there would be a constructive interference of only those wavelengths which satisfy Bragg's equation. Since, the distance between the layers of atoms in a crystal is characteristic, every crystal diffracts X-rays of definite wavelength only. Hence, X-ray diffraction crystallography is used for qualitative analysis, i.e. for the identification of crystals.

Note: Reflection of X-rays from the crystals is seen only if the angle of incidence (θ) satisfies the condition that -

$$\boxed{\sin\theta = n\lambda / 2d}$$

At all other angles, destructive interference occurs.

8.3. INSTRUMENTATION

The instrument used in X-ray diffraction crystallography consists of the following components.

8.3.1. A source
8.3.2. A wavelength selector
8.3.3. A sample holder
8.3.4. A detector
8.3.5. A recorder

8.3.1. A Source

Two major sources used to obtain X-radiation are as follows.

8.3.1.1. X-ray tube
8.3.1.2. Radioisotopes

8.3.1.1. Production of X-rays Using an X-ray Tube

The X-ray tube, also called as a *Coolidge tube*, is the most common source of X-radiation. As shown in **Fig. 8.2**, it consists of an evacuated tube made up of glass, fitted with a cathode and an anode.

The cathode is a tungsten filament which is heated by using a high voltage. An anode is a heavy block of copper which is coated with a target material (which emits X-rays) such as tungsten, copper, molybdenum, rhodium, silver, iron or cobalt. Cold water can be circulated in some areas of anode to avoid its excessive heating.

The cathode in the form of a heated tungsten filament emits electrons, which are accelerated towards anode due to its positive potential. Accelerated electrons hit the metallic target, used in the form of an anode. When the electrons hit the target material, X-rays are emitted out. The voltage applied for heating the cathode decides the number of electrons emitted by the cathode and hence, the intensity of the emitted X-rays. The higher the voltage applied to the cathode, the greater is the number of electrons emitted out and the higher is the intensity of X-rays. The accelerating potential (i.e. the positive potential applied to anode) determines the force with which the emitted electrons hit the target metal and therefore, decides the energy or the wavelength of the emitted X-rays. The greater the accelerating force, the higher is the energy of X-rays and the shorter is their wavelength. The emitted X-rays come out of a beryllium window, fitted on one side of a Coolidge tube.

A disadvantage of producing X-rays by bombarding a beam of high energy electrons on a metal is the poor output efficiency. Hardly 5 % of the electric power is converted to the radiant power for producing X-rays by using a Coolidge tube.

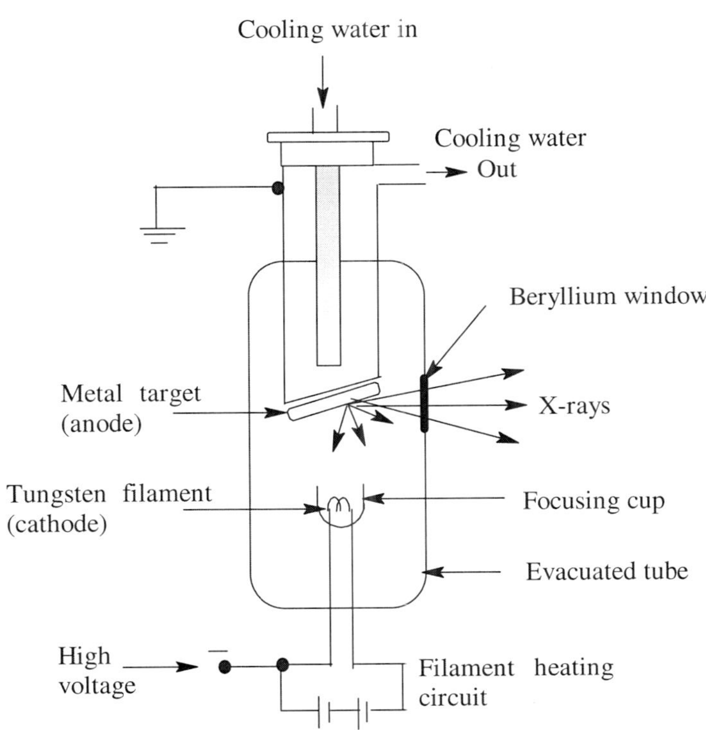

Fig. 8.2: X-ray tube or a Coolidge tube

The majority of the electric power gets converted to heat, which results in unnecessary heating of the anode. This necessitates the water cooling of the anode. To overcome this disadvantage, the modern X-ray spectroscopes make use of highly sensitive X-ray detectors, which can measure the intensity of less intense or less powerful X-rays also and allow the production of X-rays of low power. The use of low voltage at cathode to emit few electrons, which on hitting the anode produce X-rays of low intensity or power, is thus possible.

The advantage of an electron bombardment on some target material like molybdenum or tungsten is that it produces a continuous spectrum in the X-ray region.

8.3.1.2. Production of X-rays Using Radioisotopes

Certain radioactive substances produce X-rays as a result of their radioactive decay process and can act as a source for X-rays. The elements such as ${}_{26}Fe^{55}$, ${}_{27}Co^{57}$, ${}_{48}Cd^{109}$ and ${}_{53}I^{125}$ produce X-rays by electron capture or K-capture*. Tritium

$$_{26}Fe^{55} \longrightarrow {}_{25}Mn^{55} + h\nu$$

$$_{27}Co^{57} \longrightarrow {}_{26}Fe^{57} + h\nu$$

$$_{48}Cd^{109} \longrightarrow {}_{47}Ag^{109} + h\nu$$

$$_{53}I^{125} \longrightarrow {}_{52}Te^{125} + h\nu$$

(${}_{1}H^{3}$) and lead (${}_{82}Pb^{210}$) produce X-rays by β-emission process.

8.3.2. A Wavelength Selector

Many a times, for practical purposes, X-ray beam of the restricted wavelength range is required. The isolation of a narrow range of wavelengths (monochromatic X-rays) from the full range can be achieved by using following devices.

8.3.2.1. Filters

8.3.2.2. Monochromators

The instruments which make use of filters are called as *X-ray photometers* and those using monochromators are called as *X-ray spectrophotometers*. Isolation of a narrow range of X-rays can also be done electronically. Some electronic devices isolate a part of the X-rays based on the energy of radiation, rather than their wavelengths. Hence, the spectra can be resolved based on either the energy of X-rays or wavelength of X-rays. Accordingly, the instruments are called as *energy-dispersive instruments* and *wavelength-dispersive instruments*, respectively.

8.3.2.1. Filters

X-ray filters are specific materials of definite thickness or they are thin metallic strips. A molybdenum target produces a continuous spectrum in the range of 0.4 to 0.6 A°. It also produces two lines (K_β and K_α) at around 0.62A° and 0.75 A°. If X-rays from this target are allowed to pass through a thin strip (0.01cm thickness) of zirconium (a zirconium filter), it absorbs K_β line and

***K-Capture**

When the high energy electrons from the cathode are bombarded on some target material like molybdenum or tungsten, they remove electrons from the orbitals, which are nearest to the nucleus of the target material. This results in the formation of excited ions. The electrons from the outer orbitals then occupy the vacated inner orbitals and emit X-rays during this transition. When the electron from the K-shell is removed, the outer electrons are transferred to the K-shell. This produces X-rays in the *K-series* and corresponds to a line spectrum. Similarly, *L- series* of lines is produced when an electron is lost from the second principal quantum level or from the L shell, either because of a direct hit of electrons from the cathode or because of the transition of an L electron to the K Level. Radioactive isotopes thus produce line spectra and not the continuous spectra.

most of the continuous radiation from it. Thus, a pure K_α line is isolated by this filter.

A number of filters can be used against specific targets, which allow isolation of intense lines of target element. Since, the number of target–filter combinations is limited, the number of wavelengths available by this technique, is also limited.

Thin metallic strips can also be used as filters to isolate a narrow band from the continuous radiation from the X-ray tube.

8.3.2.2. Monochromators

X-ray monochromators are nothing but the crystals which can diffract X-rays according to their wavelengths. The useful wavelength range from a crystal is determined by its lattice spacing (d). A crystal is placed on a rotating table or a *goniometer. A* crystal monochromator works on the principle of Bragg's equation, described by **equation (8.3)**.

$$n\lambda = 2d \sin \theta \quad \dots (8.3)$$

For a particular crystal, the lattice spacing (d) is constant. The angle of incidence (θ) of radiation can be changed in order to collect X-rays of definite wavelengths. A particular wavelength (λ) would be collected at an angle of 2θ.

Construction of a crystal monochromator

A crystal monochromator is shown in **Fig. 8.3**.

1) The crystal monochromator consists of a source of X-rays. The X-rays coming out of a source are allowed to pass through a

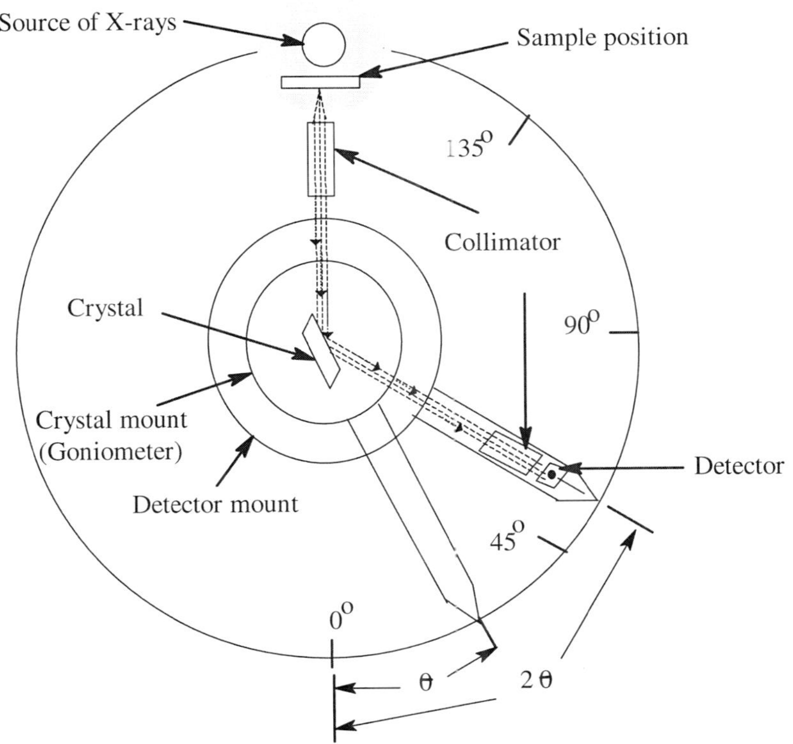

Fig. 8.3: A crystal monochromator

collimator, which makes the beams parallel.

2) The parallel beams fall on a single crystal which is mounted on a goniometer or a rotating table.
3) The rotating table can permit variation and precise determination of the angle of incidence (θ) between the crystal face and the collimated incident beam.
4) From Bragg's equation ($n\lambda = 2d \sin \theta$), it is clear that for a particular crystal, the distance between the two layers of atoms (d) remains constant. Thus, the rays of different wavelengths (λ) can be collect only if the angle θ is varied.
5) In order to derive a spectrum, the beam coming out of the crystal is allowed to pass through a second collimator which is placed on another rotator or a goniometer. Detector is also placed on this goniometer. This goniometer is rotated at twice the rate of the first one, i.e. as the crystal on the first goniometer rotates through an angle θ, the detector moves through an angle 2θ.

Limitations of crystal monochromators

1) When a flat crystal is used as a monochromator, as much as 99 % of the radiation is diverted in different directions. These diverted beams pass through the collimator. The collimator is nothing but the closely spaced metal plates or tubes that absorb all but parallel beams of radiation. Thus, most of the diverted beams are absorbed by the collimator. This leads to a considerable loss in the intensity of the beam reaching the detector. This limitation, however, can be overcome by using a curved crystal surface, which can diffract as well as focus the divergent beam from the source onto the exit collimator.
2) Analytically important X-rays fall in the range of 0.1 to 25 A°. The range of wavelengths available from a particular crystal is determined by its lattice spacing (d). No single crystal satisfactorily disperses radiation over the entire range of 0.1 to 25 A°. Hence, the use of two or more crystals is essential. The crystals commonly used to isolate X-rays of different wavelengths are listed in **Table 8.1**.

Table 8.1: Diffracting crystals and their properties

Name of crystal	Lattice spacing (d) (A°)	Wavelength range isolated (A°)
NaCl	2.820	0.49 - 5.55
LiF	2.014	0.35 – 3.97
Topaz	5.325	0.93 – 10.50

The crystals, such as topaz, lithium fluoride (LiF), sodium chloride (NaCl), ethylene diamine ditartrate (EDDT) or ammonium dihydrogen phosphate (ADP), are commonly used to obtain X-rays in different wavelength regions.

The crystals with large lattice spacing, as in topaz, provide a wider range of wavelengths as compared to the crystals with smaller lattice spacing (d). However, with the increasing values of lattice spacing, the extent of dispersion is reduced. This can be deduced by taking the first derivative of Bragg's equation as follows.

$$n\lambda = 2d \sin \theta$$

$$n.d\lambda = 2d \cos\theta \, d\theta$$

$$\therefore \frac{d\theta}{d\lambda} = \frac{n}{2\,d\cos\theta}$$

where, $d\theta$ is a measure of dispersion, which is inversely proportional to the grating spacing (d). The crystals with higher value of 'd' are therefore, not suitable in the region of short wavelengths. Crystals like topaz or lithium fluoride can be used in this region.

3) The atmospheric gases absorb X-rays which are longer than 2 A°. Hence, the sample compartment and the monochromator area should be either evacuated or air in those areas should be replaced by a continuous flow of helium.
4) At certain angles of θ or 2θ, detection of radiation becomes problematic (e.g., when 2θ

approaches zero or 180°). When 2θ is less than 10° (i.e. θ <5°), the scattering of a polychromatic radiation is very high. When 2θ > 160°, the intensity of the diffracted beam cannot be measured, since the location of the source unit prohibits the positioning of the detector at such an angle.

8.3.3. A Sample Holder

The sample holder is nothing but a rotating table called as a *crystal mount*. A crystal (i.e. a sample) is placed at the centre of a crystal mount, which is kept rotating at a particular speed.

8.3.4. X-ray Detectors

Three types of detectors are used for X-ray detection.

8.3.4.1. Gas filled detectors
8.3.4.2. Scintillation counters
8.3.4.3. Semiconductor detectors

8.3.4.1. Gas Filled Detectors

As shown in **Fig. 8.4**, a gas filled detector consists of a metal tube filled with an inert gas such as argon, xenon or krypton. The tube is provided with two transparent windows on its opposite sides. Windows are made up of mica, beryllium, aluminum or Mylar. The tube contains a centrally placed anode in the form of a wire. The lower side of the tube is negatively charged and acts as a cathode. X-rays are passed through one of the windows into the gas. The interaction of X-rays with the atoms of an inert gas results in their excitation and the loss of one of the outer electrons.

This results in the production of a large number of positive gaseous ions and electrons, i.e. ion-pairs are formed in the metal tube. One X-ray photon gives rise to one ion-pair. An electron, which is ejected out from one atom, knocks off electrons from other atoms and thus, brings about ionization of many more atoms of the gas inside the tube. At the end, the shower of electrons is attracted by the centrally placed anode. The cations being heavier compared to the electrons, move towards the cylindrical metal cathode, but slowly, as compared to the electrons. All the ejected electrons do not reach anode. The number of electrons reaching the anode for each entering X-ray photon depends on the potential applied to anode and is described below.

(i) Potential of anode less than 200 volts

If the potential applied to the centrally placed anode is less than 200 volts, the force of attraction exerted by the electrodes (cathode and anode) on the oppositely charged ions is less and hence, the accelerating force on the ion pairs is also less. Hence, the rate at which the positive and the negative ions are separated is also low. This can lead to the partial recombination of the oppositely

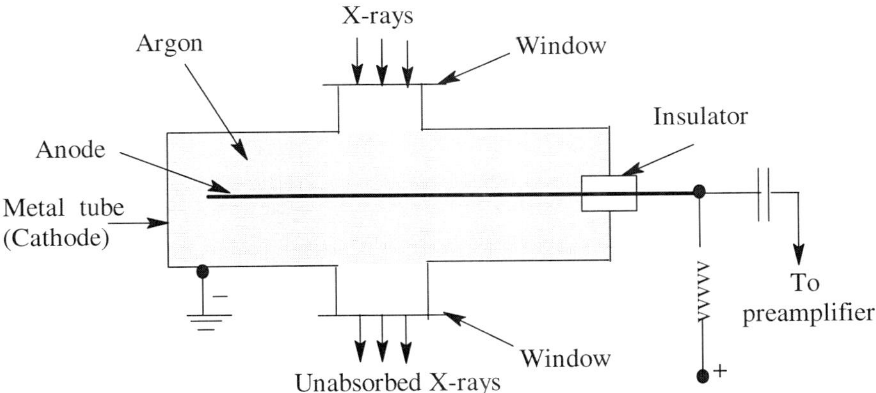

Fig. 8.4: A gas filled detector

charged ions. Hence, the number of ions reaching anode is smaller than the number of ions produced by the incoming X-rays.

(ii) Potential between 200 – 400 volts (Ionization chamber region)

When the potential of anode is kept between 200 – 400 volts, the accelerating force on the ion pairs is adequate to separate the positive and the negative species. Hence, there is no recombination of ions. Thus, the number of electrons reaching the anode is almost constant and represents the total number of ions formed by a single photon. The current produced being very small (10^{-13} -10^{-16} amperes) in this region, the gas filled tube lacks the sensitivity and hence, is not used at such a low voltage or in the ionization chamber region.

(iii) Potential between 800 – 1100 volts (Proportionate counter region)

When the potential as high as 800-1100 volts is applied to anode, the electrons produced by the X-ray photon are accelerated so highly that they in turn ionize other gaseous atoms in the tube, thus producing secondary ion pairs. Since, the number of electrons produced in this region is amplified, the ion current is also amplified. The intensity of the response, i.e. the pulse height, depends upon the energy or the frequency of the incoming X-radiation. Since, the pulse height is sufficiently large in this region, this region is widely used for X-ray detection.

(iv) Potential between 1100 – 1600 volts (Geiger counter region)

In this range of potential, the degree of amplification of electric pulse is very high. Each photon is capable of producing enormous number of electrons and cations, giving the amplification factor as high as 10^9. This results in very large values of current which can be very easily measured.

8.3.4.2. Scintillation Counters / Detectors

Principle

When X-rays strike a fluorescent or a phosphorescent substance, they excite an electron in that material to the higher energy level. The excited electron, while coming back to its original energy level, gives out luminescence or some energy in the form of fluorescence or phosphorescence, resulting in the production of *scintillations* or shiny spots or flashes on the fluorescent substance on the plate. In olden days, these spots or flashes were actually counted, which made the detection process tedious and inaccurate. To overcome this difficulty, the gas filled detectors were very popularly used. With the advent of a photomultiplier tube and better luminescent substances, scintillation counters again became popular.

Construction

Scintillation counter consists of a transparent, cylindrical crystal of sodium iodide (NaI), 3-4 inch in length and breadth. Thallium iodide is added to sodium iodide in 0.2 % quantity for the purpose of ease of activation of electrons in the crystal.

Working

When X-rays strike the crystal, the electrons in the crystal are excited. When the electrons come back to their original position, they give out photons and produce scintillations on the fluorescent material. A large number of electrons are produced in the photomultiplier tube, which results in the production of a large number of photons, which are collected ultimately at one electrode. The amount of energy released by the electrons while coming back from the excited state is called *scintillation energy*. This energy is converted to an electric energy to get the equivalent current, the value of which depends on the intensity of X-rays striking the surface.

8.3.4.3. Semiconductor Detectors

Semiconductor detectors find major application in X-ray crystallography. These are called as –

1) Lithium drifted silicon detectors-Si (Li)
2) Lithium drifted germanium detectors-Ge (Li)

1) Lithium drifted silicon detectors

As shown in **Fig. 8.5**, lithium drifted silicon detector consists of the following three layers –

(i) p-type semi-conducting layer
(ii) central intrinsic layer
(iii) n-type semi-conducting layer

An outer layer of p-type semiconductor is coated on its outer side with a thin layer of gold for electric contact, which in turn is covered with a thin beryllium window. This window is transparent to X-rays. On the other side of the p-type semi-conductor is present an intrinsic layer of lithium drifted silicon. At the end of this intrinsic layer is present n-type of semi-conductor, which is coated externally with a thin layer of aluminum for the electric contact. This aluminum sheet is connected to a preamplifier, which in turn is connected to an amplifier and a recorder.

The middle layer of lithium drifted silicon is formed by mixing lithium and p-doped silicon crystal together and then heating this mixture to about 400 – 500 °C. On heating, lithium diffuses into p-type silicon crystal and loses electrons. This results in the production of positive holes in this crystal. If a DC voltage is applied across the crystal, at still higher temperature, then the electrons released from lithium are attracted towards the electrode at the positive potential and the positive holes in the p-type silicon crystal move towards the electrode at negative potential. The current across the 'np' junction requires migration or drifting of lithium ions into the p-layer, where lithium ions replace the holes lost by the conduction. On cooling, this intrinsic layer provides resistance to the flow of current, since lithium ions are less mobile compared to the holes.

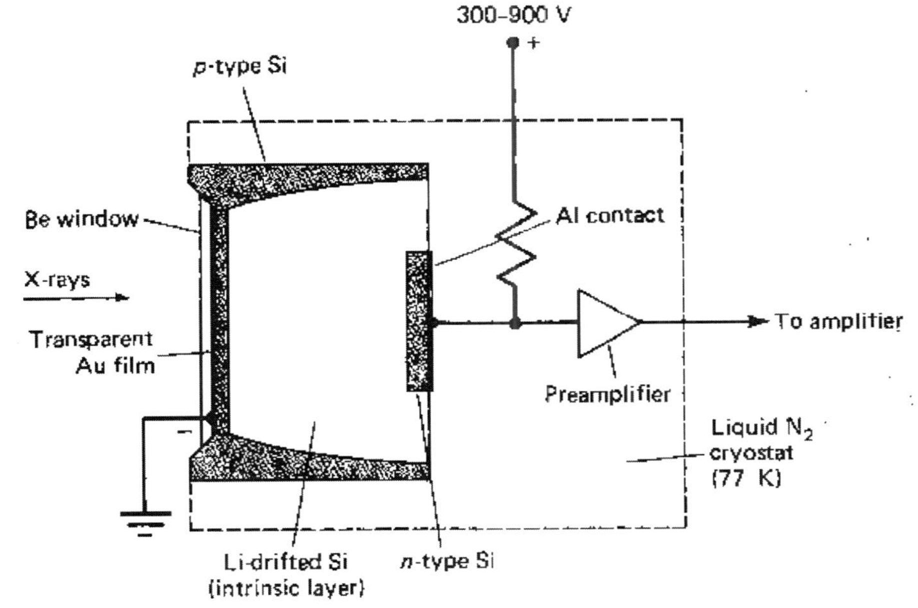

Fig. 8.5: Lithium drifted silicon detector

2) Lithium drifted germanium detectors

These detectors are exactly same as the lithium drifted silicon detectors, but in this case, instead of silicon as a semi-conductor, germanium is used. These detectors are mainly used to detect X-radiation shorter than 0.3 A°.

8.4. APPLICATIONS OF X-RAY DIFFRACTION CRYSTALLOGRAPHY

1) The arrangement and the spacing of atoms in crystalline materials can be deduced by this technique.
2) Physical properties of metals, polymeric materials and other solids can be studied.
3) Rigid compounds diffract X-rays in a particular fashion. The compounds containing a number of rings in their structure can therefore be analyzed very easily by this technique. Thus, with the help of X-ray diffraction crystallography, the structures of complex compounds such as steroids, vitamins, antibiotics, etc. can be elucidated.
4) It is a qualitative as well as a quantitative tool of estimation of compounds in the solid form.
5) X-ray diffraction pattern is unique for each crystalline compound. Hence, from the intensity of diffracted X-rays, the crystals (e.g. KBr, NaCl etc.) in a solid mixture can be identified. Various polymorphs can also be identified by X-ray crystallography.

CHAPTER 9

LIQUID CHROMATOGRAPHY

The common methods for accomplishing the separation of compounds from their mixture include distillation, crystallization, solvent extraction and chemical or electrolytic separation. Chromatography is also an effective tool for the separation of structurally and chemically closely related compounds of a complex mixture. The term chromatography cannot be defined precisely, since it includes a variety of separation techniques. However, all the techniques in the chromatography necessarily employ a stationary phase and a mobile phase. The compounds in the mixture are carried through the stationary phase by the flow of the mobile phase. The compounds get partitioned between a mobile phase (a gas or a liquid) and a stationary phase (a liquid or a solid). The separation of compounds occurs based on their difference in the rates of migration in two phases.

9.1. TYPES OF CHROMATOGRAPHY

The chromatographic techniques are divided into two main classes depending on the type of the mobile phase used for the separation.

9.1.1. Liquid Chromatography (LC)

In liquid chromatography, liquid is used as a mobile phase.

9.1.2. Gas Chromatography (GC)

In gas chromatography, gas is used as a mobile phase.

Depending on the type of the stationary phase used during the separation, the chromatographic techniques are further sub-classified as follows.

9.1. 1. Liquid Chromatography

9.1.1.1. If the stationary phase used is solid, then the LC is called as *liquid-solid chromatography* (**LSC**).

9.1.1.2. If the stationary phase used is liquid, then the LC is called as *liquid-liquid chromatography* (**LLC**).

9.1.1.3. If the stationary phase used is an ion exchange resin, then the LC is called as *ion exchange chromatography* (**IEC**).

9.1.1.4. If the stationary phase used is molecular sieves or a non-ionic gel, then the LC is called as *gel chromatography or exclusion chromatography* (**EC**).

9.1. 2. Gas Chromatography (GC)

9.1. 2.1. If the stationary phase is solid, then the GC is called as *gas-solid chromatography* (**GSC**).

9.1.2.2. If the stationary phase is liquid, then the GC is called as *gas-liquid chromatography* (**GLC**).

This chapter deals with the principles of chromatography and various techniques under liquid chromatography. A gas chromatographic technique is discussed in detail in **Chapter 10**.

Table 9.1 enlists different kinds of chromatographic techniques and the stationary and the mobile phases used for the same.

In chromatography, the compounds to be separated must be soluble in the mobile phase. They must also be capable of interacting with the stationary phase, either by dissolving in it or by getting adsorbed on it or by reacting with it chemically. Therefore, there is a distribution of compounds between the phases.

Table 9.1: Types of chromatography based on the mobile and the stationary phases used

Mobile phase	Stationary phase	Type of chromatography
Gas	Solid	Gas-solid chromatography
Gas	Liquid	Gas-liquid chromatography
Liquid	Solid	Liquid-solid chromatography
Liquid	Liquid	Liquid-liquid chromatography
Liquid	Ion exchange resins	Ion exchange chromatography
Liquid	Molecular sieves	Exclusion chromatography

9.1.1.1. Liquid Solid Chromatography (LSC)

In case of LSC, the mobile phase is a liquid, whereas the stationary phase is a finely divided solid. The type of interaction of a solute with the stationary phase is its adsorption on the stationary phase. Hence, the LSC is termed as *adsorption chromatography*. The difference in the degree of adsorption of two solutes on the stationary phase decides the cleanness of their separation from each other.

The adsorbents used as the stationary phase are silica gel, alumina, celite, diatomaceous earth, porous glass and so on. The adsorbent may be packed in a column or can be applied on a planar surface in the form of a thin film, depending on which the chromatographic techniques are referred to as either *column chromatography* or *planar chromatography*.

In column chromatography, the mobile phase is forced through the stationary phase under pressure (*High Pressure Liquid Chromatography, HPLC*) or allowed to percolate through it by the gravity (*Classical chromatography*). In the planar chromatography, the stationary phase may be a finely ground solid that has been spread in the form of a thin layer on a glass plate (*Thin Layer Chromatography, TLC*) or it may be present on a porous paper (*Paper Chromatography, PC*). In these techniques, the mobile phase passes through the solid either by capillary action or under the influence of the gravity.

9.1.1.2. Liquid Liquid Chromatography (LLC)

In case of LLC, the mobile as well as the stationary phases are liquid in nature. Two solutes get partitioned between two liquid phases. Hence, LLC is also called as the *partition chromatography*. The difference in the degree of partitioning of the two solutes in two liquid phases determines the cleanness of the separation of solutes from each other. The stationary phase is a liquid, which is immobilized using some support. This liquid should be immiscible with the liquid used as the mobile phase. Several procedures are employed to fix the liquid used as a stationary phase on some support, e.g. a finely divided solid, coated with a thin layer of liquid, may be held in a glass or a metal tube, through which the mobile phase flows or percolates. Ordinarily, the solid plays no direct part in the separation, but helps only to hold the stationary liquid phase in place by adsorption. Alternatively, the inner walls of the capillary tube can be coated with a thin layer of a liquid. This is useful when a gaseous mobile phase is to be used to flow through the tube. Finally, the stationary liquid phase can be held in the interstices of a paper or on the surface of finely ground particles held on a glass plate.

9.1.1.3. Ion Exchange Chromatography (IEC)

The ion exchange chromatography uses zeolites and synthetic organic and inorganic resins as the stationary phase to perform chromatographic separation by an exchange of ions between the sample and the resin. The compounds which have ions with different affinities for the resin can be separated using this technique. The most common use of an ion-exchange chromatography is for the separation of amino acids as well as many inorganic metallic compounds.

9.1.1.4. Exclusion Chromatography (EC)

In the exclusion chromatography, uniform and highly porous, non-ionic gel is used as a stationary phase, which separates solutes according to their molecular size. The smaller molecules can enter into the polymeric network of the stationary phase and are retarded, whereas the larger molecules cannot enter the polymeric network and come out or elute out from the column faster. The order in which the solutes come out of the column in this technique is therefore, the bigger molecules first, followed by the medium size particles and finally, the smallest molecules. Exclusion chromatography is of two types.

1) Gel filtration chromatography
2) Gel permeation chromatography

The *gel filtration chromatography* is generally applied to the use of polymers, which swell in water, e. g. Sephadex, a polysucrose or dextran, as a sieving agent. The *gel permeation chromatography* makes use of polymers which swell in organic solvents. In both the types, exclusion process is the same.

9.2. LINEAR CHROMATOGRAPHY

All the chromatographic separations are based upon the difference in the extent to which the solutes are partitioned between the mobile and the stationary phases. The equilibrium involved between the concentration of a solute in the stationary phase (C_S) and in the mobile phase (C_M) can be described quantitatively by means of a temperature-dependent constant, the partition coefficient [K, **equation (9.1)**].

$$K = \frac{C_S}{C_M} \quad \ldots (9.1)$$

In the ideal case, the partition coefficient is constant over a wide range of solute concentration, i.e. C_S is linearly related to C_M ($C_S \propto C_M$). However, in most

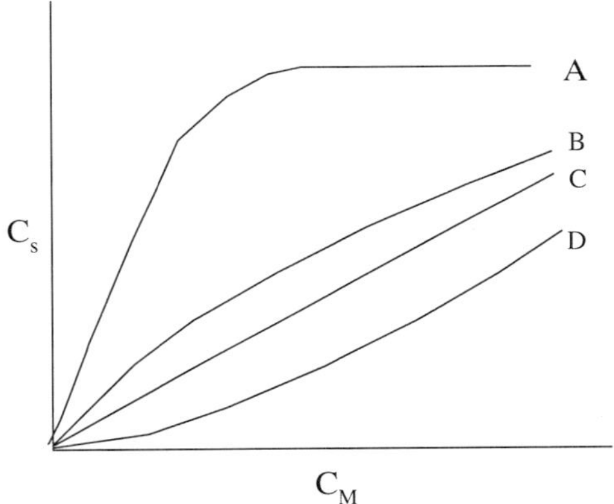

Fig. 9.1: A graph of C_S vs. C_M

of the cases, a non-linear relationship occurs between C_S and C_M. The curve C in **Fig. 9.1** is an ideal curve which is obtained only if distribution equilibrium between the phases occurs without association or dissociation of a solute in either phases. In case of association or dissociation of a solute in the stationary or mobile phase, the curves B or D are obtained. For example, a weak organic acid like benzoic acid, dissociates as benzoate anion and H^+ ion in polar solvents. Only the undissociated acid is soluble in benzene. In the aqueous solution or the polar solvents, however, appreciable amounts of both the undissociated acid and its conjugate base are present. If water represents the stationary phase

$$C_6H_5COOH \rightleftharpoons C_6H_5COO^- + H^+$$

Undissociated benzoic acid | Dissociated benzoic acid

and benzene represents the mobile phase for benzoic acid, then a curve of the type B is observed. Since the stationary phase is able to dissolve dissociated as well as undissociated forms of benzoic acid in it, $C_S > C_M$. Hence, the partition ratio, ($K = C_S / C_M$) would be higher in this case. On the other hand, if water represents the mobile phase, and benzene represents the stationary phase, then the dissociated and undissociated forms of benzoic acid would be present in the mobile phase. In this case, the concentration of benzoic acid would be more in the mobile phase ($C_M > C_S$) and hence, a curve of the type D would be expected. Though the concentration of species is more in aqueous phase always, the actual ratio, C_S / C_M, is concentration dependent. Hence, instead of a straight line, curves are obtained.

The curve A is a typical adsorption isotherm, which relates the amount of solute adsorbed on the surface of a solid (stationary phase) to the solute concentration in the solution (mobile phase) from which the solute is made available for the adsorption on a solid. When the solute concentration in the solution is increased slowly, the extent of adsorption is also increased and hence, a steeply rising portion of the curve A is obtained. When the solute concentration in the solution is increased further, all the adsorption sites on the solid surface are occupied and no more active sites are available on the solid. Further increase in the concentration of a solute in the solution, does not result in the increase in the concentration of the solute on the solid, since all the active sites are already occupied by the solute. The extent of adsorption then becomes independent of the solute concentration. The curves of this type are described by the **equation (9.2)**.

$$C_S = K\, C_M^n \quad ...(9.2)$$

where, K, i.e. the partition coefficient of a solute and 'n' are constants.

In all the chromatographic techniques, while deriving and applying various equations, it is assumed that the partition coefficient (K) for a solute remains constant throughout the separation. The curves B and C, which are common for solutes in chromatography, suggest that at lower concentrations, the partition coefficient remains almost constant, but at higher concentrations, because of the curvature, C_S is not directly proportional to C_M and hence, the partition coefficient does not remain constant. Therefore, chromatographic separations are always carried out using lower concentrations. Thus, in chromatographic techniques, the separation of compounds cannot be carried out on a large scale. Chromatography carried out under the condition such that K remains constant throughout the separation, is called *linear chromatography*. This chapter deals with all the linear chromatographic techniques.

9.3. LINEAR ELUTION CHROMATOGRAPHY

In column chromatography, a glass column or a burette is filled with a suitable stationary phase. A mixture to be isolated is dissolved in the mobile phase and is introduced carefully on the top of the stationary phase (**Fig. 9.2**). Under the force of gravity, this sample solution passes down the stationary phase. In this portion of the stationary phase, the compounds to be separated interact with the fresh surface of the stationary phase. The compounds in the mixture distribute themselves between two phases. Thus, the compounds are present on the stationary phase as well as in the mobile phase. When the additional mobile phase is allowed to pass through the stationary phase, it forces the mobile phase containing a part of the sample down the column, where the mobile phase encounters the fresh portion of the stationary phase. The compounds are adsorbed on the fresh stationary phase. Simultaneously, the compounds adsorbed on the stationary phase in the previous zone of the column, encounter the fresh mobile phase. In this portion, the compounds are desorbed from the stationary phase into the mobile phase. The continued addition of the mobile phase helps in the stepwise movement of solute molecules down the column in a continuous series of transitions. The movement of a solute down the column is mainly because of the movement of the mobile phase. However, the average rate at which a solute migrates down the column depends upon the time spent by a solute in the mobile phase. The solutes having more affinity for the mobile phase spend more time in it and travel down the column faster. Such solutes are eluted out of the column first. The solutes with high partition ratios (C_S/C_M) have more affinity for the stationary phase and hence, they spend more time in the stationary phase. Such solutes are retained in the column for a longer time and hence, are eluted out late from the column. Thus, a solute having higher partition ratio lags behind a solute having smaller partition ratio. The difference in the partition ratios of different solutes leads to different rates of migration down the column. The difference in the rates of migration causes the compounds in a mixture to separate into bands, located along the length of the column. The isolation can then be accomplished by passing a sufficient quantity of the mobile phase through the column to cause elution of various bands out of the column, where they are collected in different receivers. The process whereby the solute is washed off through the column by the addition of fresh solvent is called *elution*. If a detector that responds to the solute concentration is placed at the end of the column and its signal is plotted as a function of time, or the volume of the mobile phase required for the elution of a particular compound, or the distance migrated by a compound, then a series of symmetric peaks is obtained. Such a plot is called a *chromatogram* (**Fig. 9.3**) and is useful

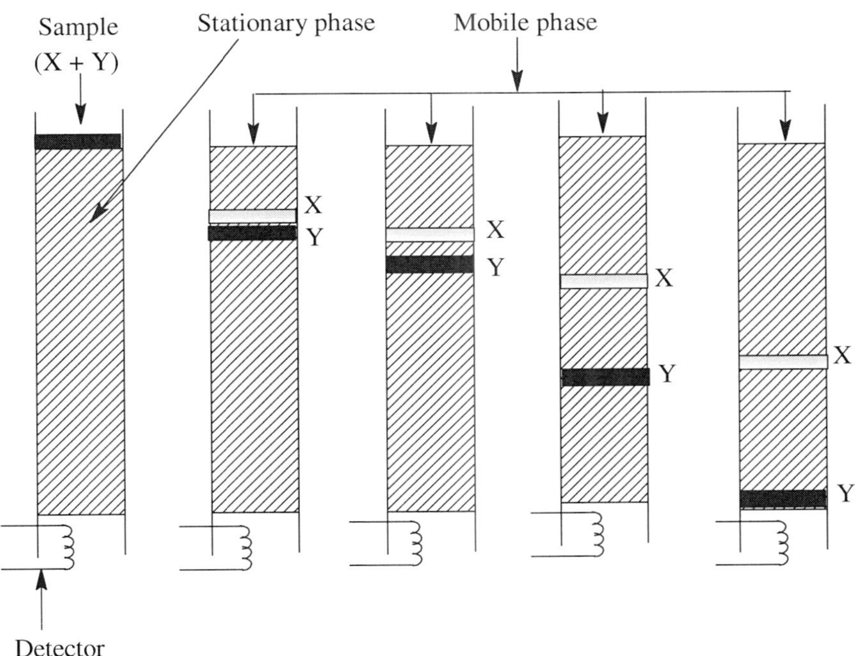

Fig. 9.2: Separation of two compounds by linear elution chromatography

for both qualitative and quantitative analysis. The position of the peaks may serve to identify the compounds of the sample and the area under the peaks can be related to their concentrations. The whole set of apparatus used to carry out chromatography is called a *chromatograph*. The separation of two compounds (X and Y) by *linear elution chromatography* is shown in **Fig. 9.2**.

9.4. THEORIES OF ELUTION CHROMATOGRAPHY

Figure 9.3 describes the difference in the chromatograms for two compounds X and Y with respect to the distance traveled by them inside the column. Compound X lags behind compound Y since the partition coefficient of compound X is larger as compared to that of compound Y (**Stage 1**). As the compounds move down the column, the distance between the two peaks increases. At the same time, however, broadening of both the peaks also takes place (**Stage 2**). If this peak broadening (also called as band or zone broadening) is not controlled, the separated peaks would keep on broadening, and at one point, they would merge with each other (**Stage 3**). This merging lowers the efficiency of the column as a separating device. Zone broadening is unavoidable. Fortunately, however, it occurs more slowly than the zone separation. Thus, compounds X and Y can be separated from each other if the column is sufficiently long.

The cleanness of separation of two compounds from each other is equally dependent upon the following two rates.

1) The rate of migration of solutes down the column
2) The rate of zone broadening during migration.

The original theory of chromatography, called the *plate theory*, is able to describe the rates of migration of solutes in quantitative terms. Unfortunately, however, its utility was limited because it could not explain the effect of different variables on zone broadening. As a consequence, another theory, known as *kinetic theory* or *rate theory*, which is capable of accounting for these variables (particle size, rate of diffusion, flow rate, temperature and other basic column parameters), was developed.

9.4.1. The Plate Theory of Chromatography

The plate theory was developed by Martin and Synge in 1941. According to this theory, a chromatographic column is considered to be composed of a series of discrete, but continuous, narrow and horizontal layers called *theoretical*

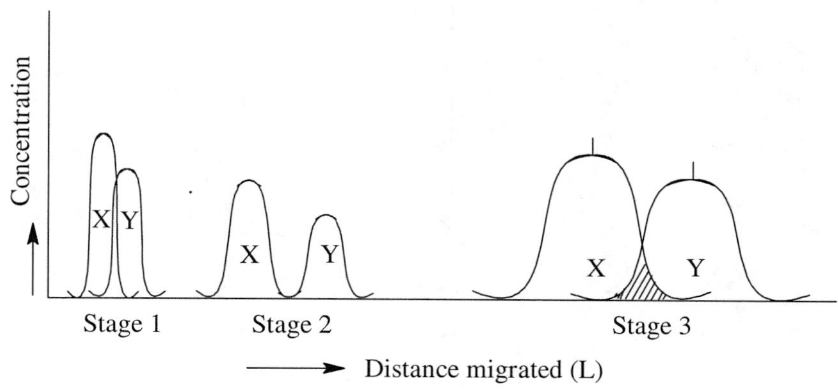

Fig. 9.3: A chromatogram for two compounds X and Y

plates. It should be noted that a plate as a physical entity does not exist in a column. It is totally an imaginary concept. At each plate, equilibrium of the solute between the mobile phase and the stationary phase is assumed to take place. The movement of a solute and a solvent is thus viewed as a series of stepwise transfer from one plate to the next.

The efficiency of a chromatographic column as a separation device improves as the number of theoretical plates (N) in the column is increased. This is because the partitioning of a solute between the phases takes place at each theoretical plate and with the increase in the number of theoretical plates, the number of equilibrations or exchanges also increases. The more the number of equilibrations, the more is the degree of separation of compounds from each other. Thus, the number of exchanges or the number of theoretical plates in the column is used as a measure of efficiency of the column to separate the compounds from each other. The height of one theoretical plate is referred to as the '*Height Equivalent of a Theoretical Plate* (HETP). As shown in **Fig. 9.4**, if the height of one plate is less, then more number of plates can be accommodated in the same space of the column as compared to when the plate height is more. Thus, by reducing the HETP value, more number of exchanges and therefore, a clear separation of compounds, can be achieved. Hence, HETP value is also used as the measure of column efficiency. The relation between the total number of plates (N), in the column and the HETP (H) value is given by **equation (9.3)**.

$$N = \frac{L}{H} \quad ...(9.3)$$

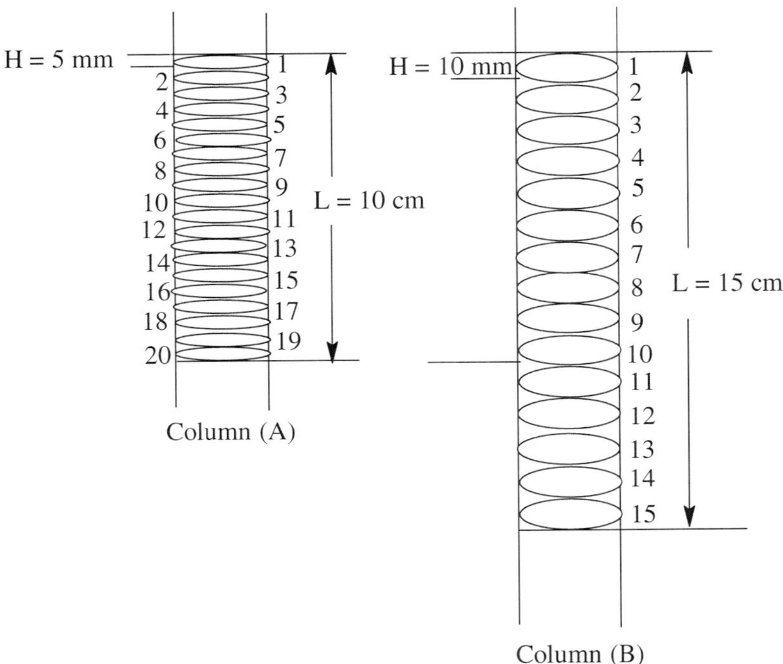

Fig. 9.4: Comparison between columns of different lengths

where, L is the length of the column packing. The total number of plates (N) and the plate height (H) or HETP value should be viewed as criteria for the column efficiency. The increase in the number of plates (N) or a decrease in the plate height (H) results in the increase in the efficiency of the column to separate compounds from each other. However, HETP value is the preferred parameter for expressing the column efficiency, since it allows comparison of columns of different lengths. As HETP value reduces, the number of equilibrations that occur in a given length of the column increases. As shown in **Fig. 9.4**, a longer column (B) of 15 cm has higher HETP value (H = 10 mm) because it is not packed properly. Hence, the number of equilibrations taking place in this longer column is 15. A shorter column (A) of 10 cm has smaller HETP value (H = 5 mm) because it is packed properly or uniformly. Hence, the number of equilibrations taking place in this shorter column is more, i.e. 20. Thus, though column A is shorter, the number of exchanges taking place in it is more than the number of exchanges that take place in a longer column B. Hence, without increasing the column length more exchanges or a better separation can be achieved if the value of H is controlled properly. This can be achieved by selecting the stationary phase of uniform particle size and also by packing the column uniformly so as to reduce the gaps between the particles. A good contact of the particles of the stationary phase avoids large intermolecular gaps and allows the mobile phase to remain close to the stationary phase. This facilitates an easy exchange of a solute from one phase to the other, thereby increasing the number of exchanges of the solute over a shorter length of the column. This increases efficiency of the column for separating solutes from each other. In case of large intermolecular gaps, a solute takes more time to reach from the mobile phase to the stationary phase, thereby reducing the efficiency of an exchange of a solute from one phase to the other. Hence, a longer column is required for the clear separation of solutes from each other in this case. Both the parameters, H and N, are still retained as efficiency parameters in the rate theory. The increase in the number of plates by increasing the length of the stationary phase in the column increases the time of elution of compounds and subsequently, the time of isolation of compounds. Hence, the decrease in the value of H, leading to an increase in number of plates, without increasing the length of the column, is a better solution to increase the column efficiency. This avoids unnecessary increase in the elution time of compounds of a mixture. High performance columns have plate heights of 0.03 to 1.0 mm.

9.4.2. The Rate Theory of Chromatography

The rate theory of chromatography was developed by Lepidus and Amundsen in 1952. It describes the effect of variables which affect the width of an elution band as well as its time of appearance at the end of a column, i.e. its time of elution. Since the efficiency of a column for the clear separation of compounds from each other depends on the sharpness of the peaks, a proper control on the peak widths is essential. Hence, it is absolutely essential to control the parameters responsible for band broadening. If these parameters are not controlled properly, the separated compounds or peaks would spread and merge together, as shown by the shaded portion in **Fig. 9.5(b)**.

9.5. IMPORTANT PARAMETERS IN CHROMATOGRAPHY

9.5.1. Column Resolution

The extent to which the peaks are separated from each other is termed as *resolution* of peaks. The capacity of a column to separate two or more compounds from their mixture is called the *resolving power* of that column. The resolution (R_s) between the two compounds (X and Y) is given by **equation (9.4)**. It can be calculated from the chromatogram shown in **Fig. 9.6**.

$$R_S = \frac{t_{R2} - t_{R1}}{\frac{W_2 + W_1}{2}} = \frac{2\,\Delta t}{W_2 + W_1} \quad \ldots (9.4)$$

where, t_{R2} and t_{R1} are the retention times of the

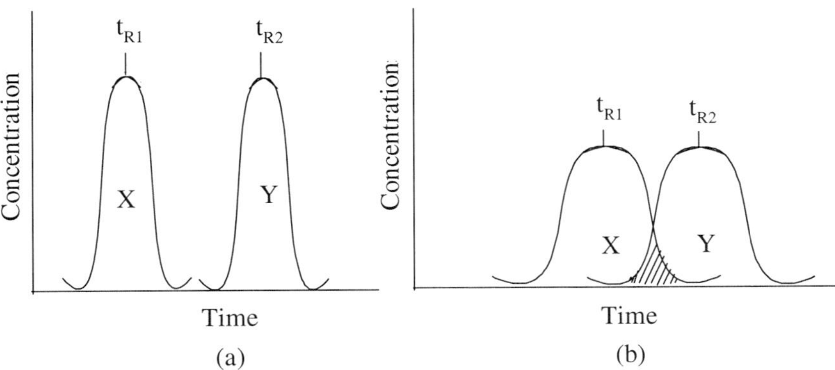

Fig. 9.5: (a) Clear separation of peaks (b) merging of peaks due to band broadening

compound Y and X , respectively, measured from the injection to the peak maximum, and w_2 and w_1 are their peak widths in units of time, measured at the base. For two close peaks, if $w_1 = w_2 = w$, then $w_1 + w_2 = 2w$. Thus, the resolution (R_S) can be expressed quantitatively by **equation (9.5)**.

$$R_S = \frac{2\,\Delta t}{2\,w} = \frac{\Delta t}{w} \quad \cdots (9.5)$$

$\Delta t \leftarrow$ depends on column selectivity

$w \leftarrow$ depends on column efficiency

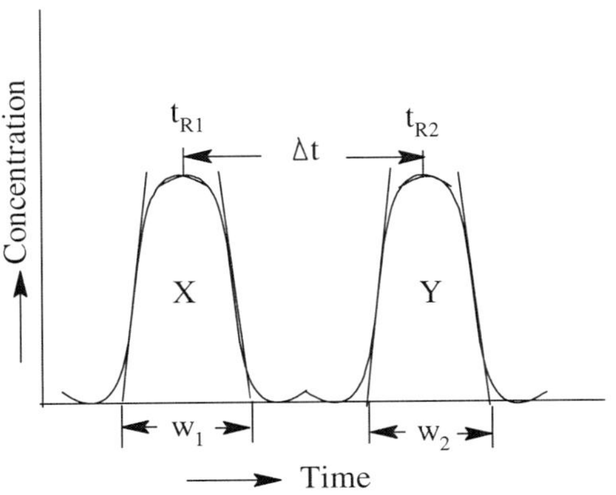

Fig. 9.6: Resolution of peaks for compounds X and Y

From **Fig. 9.7**, it is clear that resolution (R_S) of 1.5 gives an initially complete separation of X and Y, whereas a resolution of 0.75 contains about 4 % of Y.

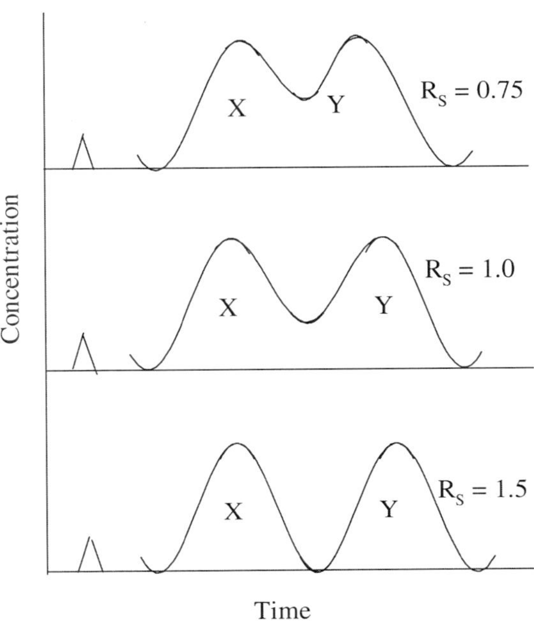

Fig. 9.7: Separation of two compounds (X and Y) at different values of resolution

9.5.1.1. Relation between Resolution, Column Selectivity, Column Efficiency and Capacity Factor

Resolution of peaks from each other depends upon the following three factors –

1) The distance (Δt) between the peak maxima, i.e. zone separation or peak separation

Since the difference between the retention times t_{R2} and t_{R1} (**Fig. 9.6**) is decided by the nature of the stationary and the mobile phases, the 1st factor, i.e. the peak separation, is a function of *column selectivity.*

2) The narrowness of the peaks or the zone width (w)

The second factor, i.e. the zone width or the peak width or zone spreading, depends on the *column efficiency*, which is a function of column parameters such as length of the column, diameter of the column, flow rate of the mobile phase, particle size of the stationary phase, etc. An efficient column does not allow zones to spread.

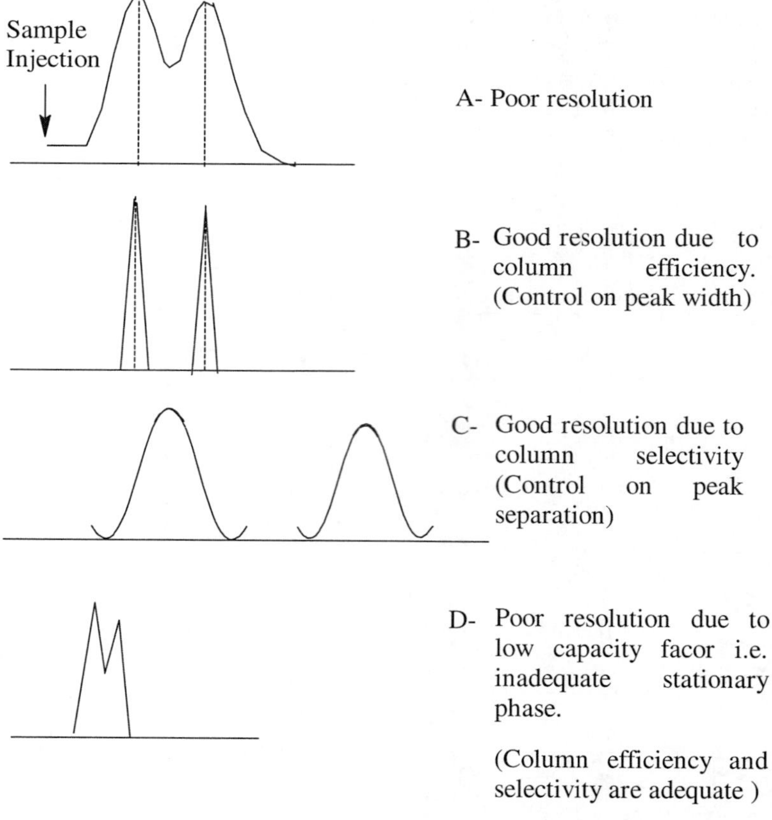

Fig. 9.8: Relation between resolution, column efficiency, column selectivity and capacity factor

3) The relative amounts of the stationary and the mobile phases

The elution time of a particular compound, i.e. the time taken by that compound to come out of the column, is determined by the relative amounts of the stationary and the mobile phases and the effective utilization of the stationary phase, i.e. the *capacity factor*. The capacity factor provides the information about the capacity of the stationary phase to accommodate a particular compound on it.

Poor resolution results when the compounds on the stationary phase elute close to each other. In order to have good resolution of compounds, the values of parameters, viz. column selectivity, column efficiency and capacity factor, need to be adjusted. The information about the parameter to be adjusted to achieve good resolution is obtained from the nature of the chromatogram recorded after injecting the sample into the column for the first time. The relation between the resolution, column efficiency, column selectivity and capacity factor is shown in **Fig. 9.8**

9.5.2. Column Efficiency and Zone Spreading

The column efficiency is expressed quantitatively by the number of theoretical plates (N) and is represented by **equation (9.6)**. The parameters w, t_R and σ are indicated in **Fig. 9.9**.

$$N = \left(\frac{t_R}{\sigma}\right)^2 \quad \ldots (9.6)$$

where, σ is the peak standard deviation and $4\sigma = w$. **Equaion (9.7)** is obtained by substituting the value of σ in **equation (9.6)**.

$$N = 16\left(\frac{t_R}{w}\right)^2 \quad \ldots (9.7)$$

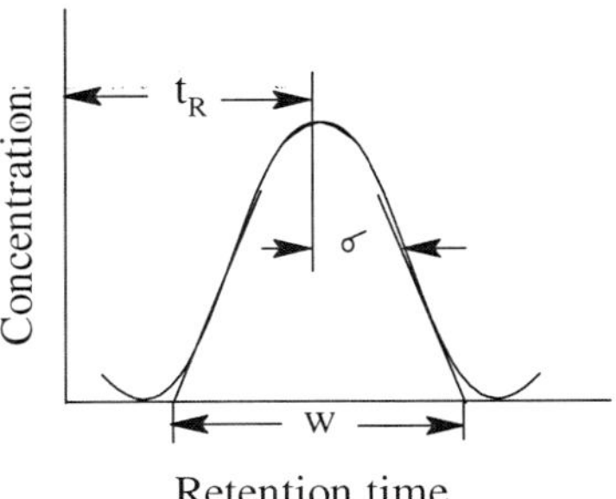

Fig. 9.9: A chromatogram showing peak width and retention time of a component

Basically, **equation (9.7)** compares the width of the peak (w) to the length of time (t_R), for which the component is retained in the column. Many scientists have given several theoretical explanations for the zone spreading in chromatography.

9.5.2.1. Factors Responsible for Zone Spreading in Chromatography

It is now established that the column zone spreading originates from three main sources.

1) **M**ultiple paths (Eddy diffusion)
2) **M**olecular diffusion (Longitudinal diffusion)
3) **M**ass transfer under non-equilibrium conditions

A number of equations have been developed that relate the efficiency of a chromatographic column to the extent to which these three processes occur. The earliest and the simplest of these, which is known as the *Van Deemter equation*, was derived for GLC. It provides an approximate relationship between the flow rate (u) and the plate height (H), expressed by **equation (9.8)**.

$$H = A + \frac{B}{u} + Cu \quad \ldots (9.8)$$

Factor 'A' is associated with the eddy diffusion,

Factor 'B' is associated with the longitudinal

diffusion, and

Factor 'C' is associated with the mass transfer under non-equilibrium conditions

If the magnitudes of A, B/u or Cu are large, the value of H is also high and hence, the column efficiency is low.

1) Multiple paths or eddy diffusion

The zone broadening from eddy diffusion arises mainly because of the availability of multiple paths for different molecules of the same solute while passing through a packed column. The availability of multiple pathways for different molecules of the same solute in the column occurs mainly due to the following two reasons.

(i) Non-uniform particle size of the stationary phase in the column, and

(ii) Non-uniform packing (tight or loose) of the column

Eddy diffusion due to these two factors is shown in **Fig. 9.10(b)** and **(c)**. In order to understand how broadening of the peak occurs due to eddy diffusion, consider that the column is loaded with only one solute (X)

As shown in **Fig. 9.10(a)**, the column is packed uniformly with the uniform particles size of the stationary phase. When such a column is loaded with a solute X dissolved in the mobile phase, all the molecules of X travel with the same velocity inside the column and reach the detector simultaneously. This results in the production of a sharp peak for X in the chromatogram and avoids band broadening.

Column with uniform particle size of stationary phase and uniform packing

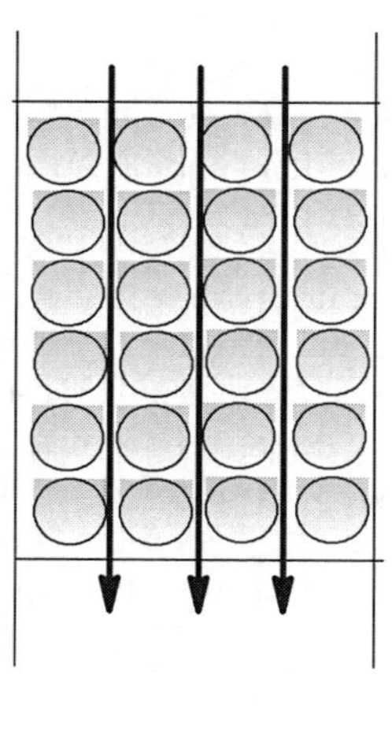

(a)

Column with Non-uniform particle size of stationary phase

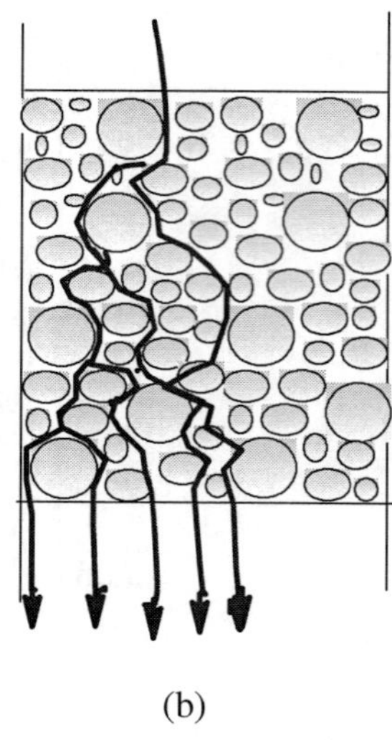

(b)

Column with uniform particle size of stationary phase but non-uniform packing

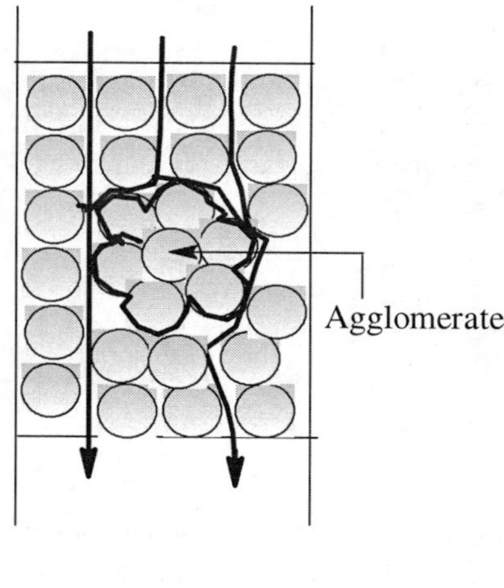

(c)

Fig. 9.10: (a) Flow of mobile phase involving no eddy diffusion (b) eddy diffusion due to non-uniform particle size of stationary phase and (c) eddy diffusion due to non-uniform packing of the column

In **Fig. 9.10(b)**, column consists of a stationary phase containing particles of non-uniform size. A few particles are bigger in size and a few others are smaller in size. When the solution of X is introduced on the top of the stationary phase of such a column, different molecules of solute X follow different paths inside the column due to the obstruction to their flow by the bigger particles of the stationary phase. The molecules, which come across the bigger particles of the stationary phase, have to change their linear path (eddy diffusion) in order to flow down the column. The molecules, which do not come across the bigger particles in their path, move down the column without undergoing eddy diffusion The molecules undergoing eddy diffusion have to travel little longer distance in changing their linear path, whereas the molecules, which do not undergo eddy diffusion, travel comparatively a shorter distance in the column in order to reach the other end of the column. Since the lengths of these pathways differ, the residence time in the column, for different molecules of the same species (X) also varies. The solute molecules then reach the end of the column over a wider time interval that tends to broaden the elution band. Because of the hindrance provided by the bigger particles of the stationary phase to the flow of certain molecules of solute X, their velocity through a column is reduced as compared to the velocity of the particles that do not come across the bigger particles in their path. Thus, some molecules travel more rapidly by following open pathways (channeling), while the others diffuse into the restricted areas (eddy diffusion) and lag behind. The average velocity of all the particles of solute X determines their retention time, but the differing velocities, i.e. the velocities of the individual particles of solute X, decide the extent of band broadening.

The same phenomenon occurs when the molecules of X travel through a column containing uniform particle size of the stationary phase but which is not packed uniformly. As shown in **Fig. 9.10(c)**, the agglomerates can be seen in some parts of the column when the stationary phase is packed very tightly. Similarly, a loose packing of the stationary phase leaves gaps or voids in the column. The molecules of X, moving through a part of the column, where the stationary phase is loosely packed, do not experience any hindrance to their flow. Hence, they come down the column faster and reach the detector, kept at the other end of the column, earlier than the other molecules, thereby producing an early signal in the chromatogram. The molecules of X, moving through a part of the column, where the stationary phase is tightly packed, experience hindrance to their flow due to the presence of an agglomerate in their path. The particles coming in the path of an agglomerate undergo eddy diffusion. Hence, these particles of solute X come down the column at a slower rate compared to the molecules which pass through a loosely packed part of the column, and reach the detector quite late. These molecules produce signal later than that produced by the molecules reaching the detector earlier. Since all the molecules of solute X do not elute out at the same time, they do not get recorded at the same time in the chromatogram and therefore, they do not produce a sharp peak. Instead, they get eluted out over a longer time period and therefore, produce a broad peak. This band broadening due to eddy diffusion is represented by the quantity 'A' in Van Deemter equation. The factor 'A' describes the effect of eddy diffusion on column efficiency (H) and can be related to the particle size and geometry of the stationary phase, and also to the tightness of the packing of the stationary phase. The value of 'A' is independent of the flow rate (u) and is given by **equation (9.9)**.

$$A = \lambda\, d_R \quad \dots (9.9)$$

where, λ is the *packing factor*, and d_R is the average particle diameter of the particles of the stationary phase.

The value of the packing factor (λ) depends on the range of the particle size in the stationary phase and also on how the column is packed. The value of λ should be low to keep the value of H small, i.e. to get higher column efficiency. For a narrow range of particles with 20 to 40 # size, $\lambda = 1$. For a broad range of particles with 200 to 400 # size, $\lambda = 8$. Thus, the value of λ is more for the bigger particles and for the particles lying in a broad range of sizes.

Band broadening due to eddy diffusion is minimized by the careful packing of a column with small spherical particles (d_R) possessing a limited range of sizes. The care should be taken, particularly to avoid the open channels or the formation of agglomerates in the stationary phase.

2) Molecular diffusion or longitudinal diffusion

The molecular diffusion or the longitudinal diffusion results from the tendency of molecules to migrate from the concentrated part of a band towards more dilute regions on either side. This is shown in **Fig. 9.11**. This type of diffusion can occur in the mobile phase as well as in the stationary phase but since the movement or diffusion of solute particles is hindered by the obstruction provided by the particles of the

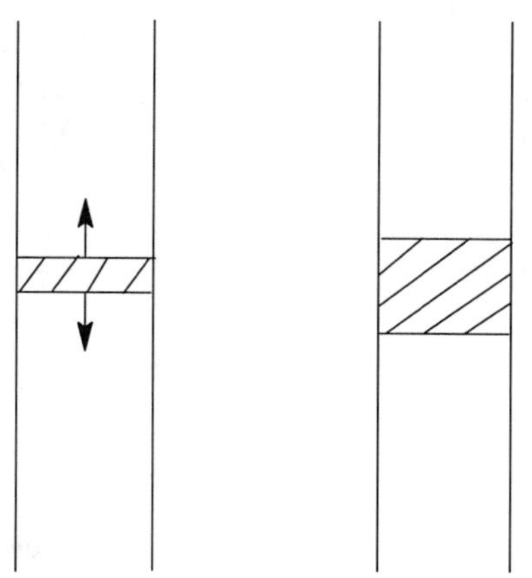

Fig. 9.11: Longitudinal diffusion of a solute in the column

stationary phase, band broadening due to longitudinal diffusion in the stationary phase can be ignored. The longitudinal diffusion is most important when the mobile phase is a gas, because the diffusion rates in the gas phase are several orders of magnitude greater than those in the liquid. The amount of diffusion increases with time. The extent of broadening increases as the flow rate of the mobile phase decreases, since the solute molecules get enough time to diffuse on either side of the band.

The second term 'B', the contribution of the longitudinal diffusion to the column efficiency, in Van Deemter equation ($H = A + B/u + Cu$), is inversely proportional to the flow rate (u) of the mobile phase. When the mobile phase is moving fast through the column, the solute does not get enough time to diffuse in the mobile phase. At the higher flow rates (u), the value of B/u is small. Hence, 'H' is also small and the column efficiency is high. On the other hand, when the mobile phase is moving slowly through the column, the solute gets enough time to diffuse in the mobile phase. At the lower flow rates, the value of B/u is large. Hence, the value of H is also large and column efficiency is low. Since, the slow movement of the mobile phase through the column allows easy diffusion of a solute, it results in a broader band of a solute in the column, as shown in **Fig. 9.11**. When a broad band is produced, the solute reaches the detector over a longer time span. This results in the production of a broad peak in its chromatogram. On the contrary, the fast movement of the mobile phase through the column restricts easy diffusion of a solute and results in a narrow band of a solute in the column. When a narrow band reaches the detector, the solute is detected in a short time span. This results in the production of a sharp peak in its chromatogram. The contribution of factor 'B' to 'H' is given quantitatively by the mathematical **equation (9.10)**.

$$B = 2\,\psi\,D_M \quad \text{... (9.10)}$$

where, ψ is the *obstruction factor* or a *tortuosity*

factor, which is a measure of the hindrance to the free molecular diffusion caused by the presence of particles of the stationary phase and D_M is the diffusion coefficient of a solute in the mobile phase. The value of ψ typically ranges from 0.5 – 0.9, depending upon the type of the packing of the stationary phase. If the stationary phase is packed tightly and uniformly, then a lot of obstruction is provided to the diffusing particles. This helps in reducing the band width and in increasing the column efficiency. A loose packing, on the other hand, provides less obstruction to the diffusing particles and hence, allows band broadening. This results in the decrease in the column efficiency. Broadening due to longitudinal diffusion can be reduced by decreasing the temperature and by increasing the flow rate (u) of the mobile phase. This is because the reduction in the temperature reduces diffusion coefficient (D_M) of a solute in the mobile phase.

3) Mass transfer under non-equilibrium conditions

In order to achieve chromatographic separation within a reasonable time period, the mobile phase should be passed rapidly through the column. Under this condition, the exchange of a solute from one phase to the other does not occur under equilibrium condition. This mass transfer under non-equilibrium condition is responsible for band broadening. This can be explained as follows.

At the front of the zone, where the mobile phase encounters the fresh stationary phase, the equilibrium is not instantly achieved, i.e. the mobile phase containing a solute is not able to transfer the required amount of the solute from it to the fresh stationary phase as expected to be transferred under the equilibrium condition. Because of this, excess quantity of the solute is carried somewhat farther down the column by the mobile phase onto the fresh stationary phase, than would be expected under true equilibrium condition. This leads to band broadening in the front zone of the band. Similarly, at the top end of the zone, a solute in the stationary phase encounters the fresh mobile phase. Again, the transfer of a solute from the stationary phase into the mobile phase is not instantaneous and hence, the required quantity of a solute, as expected to be desorbed from the stationary phase under equilibrium condition, is not desorbed from it into the mobile phase. Hence, the residual solute remains at the top end of the zone, which causes band broadening at the top end of the band. Thus, the tail of the zone is more drawn out on either side of the band than it would be if time existed for equilibrium to occur. The net effect is broadening of a band at both the ends.

The effect of mass transfer under non-equilibrium condition becomes smaller as the flow rate is decreased. At lower flow rates, enough time is available for the mass transfer of a solute to occur under equilibrium condition. Furthermore, a true equilibrium can be approached if the space between the particles of the stationary phase through which the mobile phase flows is narrowed down so that the solute molecules do not have to diffuse far in order to reach the stationary phase. For this purpose, the column should be packed tightly with small spherical particles of the stationary phase. In case of an immobilized liquid as the stationary phase, its layer on the solid support should be as thin as possible. The mobile phase which facilitates the faster diffusion of a solute to the stationary phase should be used. (This is just the opposite effect that diffusivity has on the longitudinal molecular diffusion). Under these conditions, the mass transfer can approach near equilibrium.

The rapid mass transfer depends on the factors originating from the stationary phase as well as the mobile phase and hence, there are two terms to account for the zone dispersion - the stationary phase contribution to the plate height (C_S) and the mobile phase contribution to the plate height (C_M). The term 'C' in Van Deemter equation is therefore, the sum of C_S and C_M. The stationary phase contribution (C_S) to the plate height H, due to the mass transfer under non-equilibrium condition, is given by **equation (9.11)**.

$$Cs = \frac{q\,r\,d^2}{Ds} \quad \dots (9.11)$$

where, q = configuration factor, which depends on the shape of the pool of the stationary phase (uniform film, rod. sphere, etc.),

r = a constant dependent upon the relative rate of migration of a solute and the mobile phase,

d = thickness of the stationary phase, and

D_s = diffusion coefficient of a solute in the stationary phase.

The mobile phase contribution (C_M) to the plate height H, due to the mass transfer under non-equilibrium condition, is given by **equation (9.12)**.

$$C_M = \frac{\omega\, d_R^2}{D_M} \quad \text{... (9.12)}$$

where, ω = column coefficient, determined by the packing structure, column diameter and column shape,

d_R = diameter of the stationary phase particle, and

D_M = diffusion coefficient of a solute in the mobile phase

In Van Deemter equation (H = A+ B/u + Cu), the magnitude of H decreases when the magnitude of all the terms involved in it decreases. The first term (A) is independent of the flow rate of the mobile phase. The second term (B/u) decreases when the flow rate (u) of the mobile phase is increased, i.e. when the mobile phase is passed rapidly through the column. When the mobile phase is passed rapidly, it leads to the increase in the magnitude of the third term (Cu). This leads to the increase in the magnitude of H and decrease in the column efficiency. Thus, increasing the flow rate of the mobile phase is desirable to avoid the longitudinal diffusion (B/u), but is undesirable, since it leads to the mass transfer under non- equilibrium condition and causes band broadening or decreases the column efficiency. Thus, there should be some optimum value of the flow rate (u) of the mobile phase to get the minimum value of H.

For a particular system, i.e. for a column of a definite length and diameter, having a definite type of a packing with a definite particle size and using a particular mobile phase for the separation, the values of B and C can be calculated. From the values of B and C, the magnitudes of B/u and Cu can be calculated for the increasing values of u, and the curves as shown in **Fig. 9.12** can be plotted. The dotted lines show the effect of flow rate on the individual factors, A, B/u and Cu. The term A is unaffected by the changes in the flow rate of the mobile phase and hence, produces a line parallel to X-axis. The term B/u decreases drastically in the beginning with the increase in the flow rate of the mobile phase. Increase in the flow rate beyond a particular value, leads to a slow decrease in the value of B/u. A continuous increase in the term Cu is observed with the increase in the flow rate of the mobile phase. The solid curve shows the effect of the change in the flow rate of the mobile phase on the combination of all the three factors. Thus, the maximum column efficiency (H_{min}) is realized at a flow rate (u_{opt}), corresponding to the minimum in the solid curve.

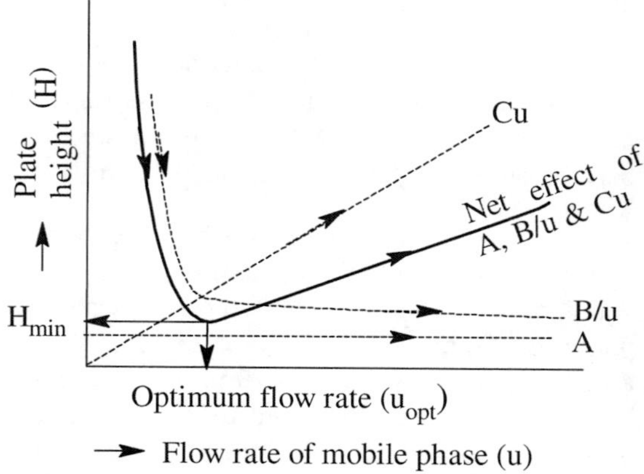

Fig. 9.12: Effect of flow rate of mobile phase on factors in Van Deemter equation

Thus, by manipulating the values of A, B/u and Cu, the band width (w) can be controlled in order to achieve the higher column efficiency or higher resolution.

Another term in **equation (9.5)**, $R = \frac{\Delta t}{w}$, which decides the clear separation of the compounds from each other, is the difference in the retention times (Δt) of the solutes to be separated. The retention time (t_R) of a solute is given by **equation (9.13)**.

$$t_R = t_M\,(1+k') = t_M\left(1+K\frac{V_S}{V_M}\right) \quad \text{... (9.13)}$$

where, t_M is the retention time of the species that is not retained by the column packing, and is taken as the retention time for the mobile phase or air (**Fig. 9.13**),

k' = capacity factor for a solute, which is related to the partition coefficient as-

$$k' = K\frac{V_S}{V_M}, \text{ where,}$$

K = partition coefficient of a solute,

V_S = volume of the stationary phase, and

V_M = volume of the mobile phase

Thus, the retention time of a solute increases with the increase in its partition coefficient ($K = C_S/C_M$).

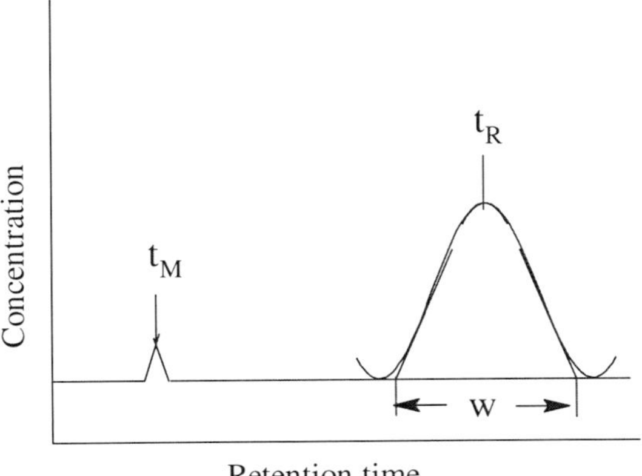

Fig. 9.13: Chromatogram for the compounds not retained and retained on the column

Similarly, if the volume of the stationary phase is more with reference to the volume of the mobile phase, it leads to the increase in the retention time of a solute. The rearrangement of **equation (9.13)** gives **equation (9.14)**.

$$k' = \frac{t_R - t_M}{t_M} \quad \text{... (9.14)}$$

This equation permits the calculation of k' for a solute from the experimental parameters, t_R and t_M. The adjustment of k' allows the solute to elute out with a reasonable retention time (t_R) and provides the required resolving power ($R_S = 1.5$) for the separation.

9.6. OPTIMIZATION OF COLUMN PERFORMANCE

For the optimization of a column, the conditions which are able to provide good resolution (R_S) with suitable retention time values (t_R) for the compounds, are required to be considered. **Equation (9.15)** expresses the resolution (R_S) of compounds quantitatively, in terms of column efficiency, column selectivity and the capacity factor .

$$R_S = \frac{\sqrt{N}}{4}\,\frac{(\alpha-1)}{\alpha}\,\frac{k'_Y}{1+k'_Y} \quad \cdots (9.15)$$

where, α = selectivity factor, and

$$\alpha = \frac{(t_R)_Y - t_M}{(t_R)_X - t_M} = \frac{(t_R)_Y}{(t_R)_X}$$

$$= \frac{k'_Y}{k'_X} = \frac{\text{Capacity factor for Y}}{\text{Capacity factor for X}}$$

$$= \frac{K_Y\,\frac{V_S}{V_M}}{K_X\,\frac{V_S}{V_M}} = \frac{\left(\frac{C_S}{C_M}\right)_Y \frac{V_S}{V_M}}{\left(\frac{C_S}{C_M}\right)_X \frac{V_S}{V_M}}$$

Since, the ratio of the volume of the stationary phase to that of the mobile phase is same for both the solutes, X and Y,

$$\alpha = \text{Selectivity factor} = \frac{\left(\frac{C_S}{C_M}\right)_Y}{\left(\frac{C_S}{C_M}\right)_X}$$

$$= \frac{K_Y}{K_X} = \frac{\text{Partition coeff. for Y}}{\text{Partition coeff. for X}}$$

Rearranging **equation (9.15)**, **equation (9.16)**, for the number of theoretical plates (N) in the column, is obtained.

$$N = 16\, R_S^2 \left(\frac{\alpha}{\alpha - 1}\right)^2 \left(\frac{1 + k'_Y}{k'_Y}\right)^2 \quad \cdots (9.16)$$

Another equation is for the retention time of compound Y. The retention time $(t_R)_Y$ for the compound Y is expressed by **equation (9.17)**.

$$(t_R)_Y = \frac{N.H.(1 + k'_Y)}{u} \quad \cdots (9.17)$$

where, H is the height equivalent to one theorerical plate and 'u' is the flow rate of the mobile phase. Substituting the value of N from **equation (9.16)** in **equation (9.17)**, **equation (9.18)** is obtained.

$$(t_R)_Y = \frac{16\, R_S^2\, H}{u} \left(\frac{\alpha}{\alpha - 1}\right)^2 \frac{(1 + k'_Y)^3}{k_Y'^2} \quad \cdots (9.18)$$

Equations (9.15) and **(9.18)** are considered to be important in column chromatography, because they help in selecting parameters that lead to a desired degree of resolution with a reasonable retention time. In both the equations, the first term is the *efficiency of the column*, which is expressed in terms of N or H. The second term, which is the quotient containing α, is the *selectivity term* and it depends solely on the properties of two solutes. The third term is the *capacity factor* term, which is the quotient containing k', and depends upon the properties of the solute and the column.

9.6.1. Optimization of Column Efficiency

From **equation (9.15)** it is evident that the resolution (R_s) is proportional to the square root of the number of plates (N) in the column. Hence, with the increase in the number of plates in the column, the resolution also increases. Thus, the two compounds can be separated clearly from each other by increasing the number of plates in the column. However, as seen from **equation (9.17)**, since the retention time of a compound is also directly proportional to the number of theoretical plates (N), the increase in the number of plates beyond a certain value, to achieve clear separation of solutes from their mixture, also increases the retention time of a compound in the column. Thus, the time required for the elution of a compound is increased with the increase in the number of plates. In order to avoid this, usually, the increase in the number of plates for the same length of the column is accomplished by reducing the plate height (H). The first term in **equation (9.17)** includes both the terms, the total number of theoretical plates (N) and the height equivalent to one theoretical plate (H), the parameters indicating the column efficiency. Increase in the number of theoretical plates, not by increasing the length of the column, but by packing the column uniformly, using the stationary phase of small and uniform particle size, automatically reduces the value of H. This keeps the product of N and H constant in **equation (9.17)**. This helps in achieving high resolution without unnecessary increase in the length of the column and the retention time of solutes in the column. In order to get the maximum column efficiency (i.e. minimum value of H), the contribution of the three factors (multiple paths, molecular diffusion and mass transfer under non-equilibrium condition) involved in Van

Deemter equation should be made minimum by controlling various parameters which decide their magnitude. Thus, the higher column efficiency leads to the higher resolution or clear separation of compounds within a reasonable time period. The number of theoretical plates for getting good column efficiency should be in terms of few thousands and the HETP value should be in the range of 0.03 – 1.0 mm.

9.6.2. Optimization of Column Selectivity

The second term in **equations (9.15)** and **(9.18)** includes the selectivity factor (α.). From **equation (9.15)**, it is clear that as the selectivity factor increases, the resolution also increases. By keeping other terms constant in **equation (9.15)**, if the values of α are substituted as 2, 3, 4 and so on, the quotient [(α -1)/α] turns out to be 1/2, 2/3, 3/4 and so on, respectively. Since the value of the quotient increases, the resolution (R_S) also increases. Similarly, the quotient [α/ (α -1)] in **equation (9.18)** turns out to be 2/1, 3/2, 4/3 and so on, respectively. As the quotient increases, the retention time (t_R) also increases. When α approaches one, the quotient (α -1)/α, in **equation (9.15)**, turns out to be zero and the resolution is lost, i.e. the separation of compounds from each other is not possible. Similarly, when á approaches one, the quotient, α/ (α -1) in **equation (9.18)**, turns out to be infinity, i.e. an infinite time would be required to separate the compounds clearly from each other. This is as good as no resolution of compounds from each other. Therefore, in order to get the maximum resolution in the minimum time period, the value of α is kept in the range of 2-5.

9.6.3. Optimization of Capacity Factor

To get the required value of R_S, the capacity factor k' for a solute, can be varied over a wider range by altering the composition of the mobile phase or by altering the stationary phase. Generally, it is difficult to change the stationary phase, since the columns are expensive, whereas it is easier to change the mobile phase because of easy availability of a variety of solvents, comparatively at a much cheaper rate. Hence, a mobile phase is often changed to achieve good separation. Since, $k' = K\,(V_S/V_M)$, the increase or decrease in the value of k' can be achieved by changing the ratio of the volume of the stationary phase to that of the mobile phase. The particle size of the stationary phase can also be reduced since it results in the increase in the surface area of the stationary phase and consequently, in the increase in V_S. The increase in V_S increases k'. The increase in k', to increase the resolution, is also possible by increasing the partition coefficient K of solutes [**equation (9.13)**]. Increase in the partition coefficient is because of the increase in the concentration of a solute on the stationary phase. This automatically increases the retention time of a solute in the column. The increase in the resolution R_S as well as the elution time or the retention time (t_R) of a solute with the increase in k' is clear from **equations (9.15)** and **(9.18)**. In order to achieve the maximum resolution R_S, by keeping the retention time to the minimum possible, the optimum value of k' should be selected. To find the optimum value of k', consider the values of all the parameters, except for k'_Y in **equations (9.15)** and **(9.18)**, to be constant. When this is done, **equations (9.15)** and **(9.18)** can be expressed as **equations (9.19)** and **(9.20)**, respectively.

$$R_S = \frac{\sqrt{N}}{4}\,\frac{(\alpha-1)}{\alpha}\,\frac{k'_Y}{1+k'_Y} \cdots (9.15)$$

Let Q be equal to $\frac{\sqrt{N}}{4}\,\frac{(\alpha-1)}{\alpha}$

$$\therefore\ R_S = Q\,\frac{k'_Y}{1+k'_Y}$$

$$\therefore\ \frac{R_S}{Q} = \frac{k'_Y}{1+k'_Y} \cdots (9.19)$$

Similarly,

$$(t_R)_Y = \frac{16\,R_S^2\,H}{u}\left(\frac{\alpha}{\alpha-1}\right)^2 \frac{(1+k'_Y)^3}{k'^2_Y} \cdots (9.18)$$

Let Q' be equal to $\dfrac{16 R_S^2 H}{u}\left(\dfrac{\alpha}{\alpha - 1}\right)^2$

$$\therefore (t_R)_Y = Q' \frac{(1+k'_Y)^3}{k'^2_Y}$$

$$\therefore \frac{(t_R)_Y}{Q'} = \frac{(1+k'_Y)^3}{k'^2_Y} \quad \cdots (9.20)$$

If the terms Q and Q' are assumed to remain approximately constant and if the graphs of R_S/Q and $(t_R)_Y / Q'$, vs. k'_Y are plotted, then the curves as shown in **Fig. 9.14** are obtained. In **equation (9.19)**, as k'_Y increases, R_S/Q also increases.

Beyond a particular value of k'_Y, there is a slow increase in R_S/Q. Hence, in the graph, after a sharp increase in R_S/Q, a plateau is obtained. For the term $(t_R)_Y / Q'$, an initial decrease and then a sharp increase in its value is observed, with the increase in k'_Y. This is because initially, when k'_Y is increased, R_S increases. When R_S increases, Q' also increases, since Q' involves the term R_S in it. When the denominator (Q') in **equation (9.20)** increases, the value of $(t_R)_Y / Q'$ decreases. Beyond a particular value of k'_Y, when R_S remains almost constant (a plateau region in **Fig. 9.14**), Q' also remains almost constant. Hence, $(t_R)_Y / Q'$ increases with the increase in k'_Y in the plateau region for R_S/Q. This gives a sharply increasing portion in the curve for $(t_R)_Y / Q'$ vs. k'_Y. Thus, from this graph, it is clear that the values of k'_Y greater than about 10 are to be avoided because in this region, there is a sharp increase in the retention time of a compound and no substantial increase in the resolution. Hence, the optimal value of k'_Y lies in the range of 2 - 5.

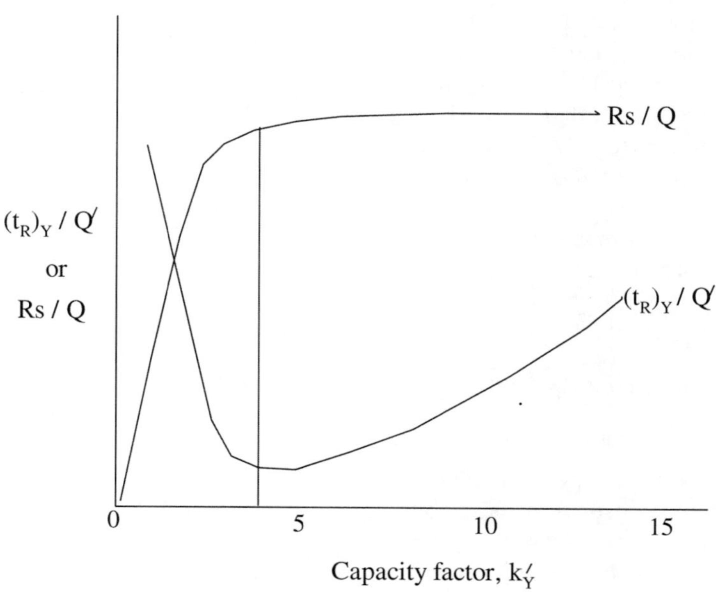

Fig. 9.14: Effect of capacity factor on resolution and retention time

9.7. QUALITATIVE AND QUANTITATIVE ANALYSIS BY CHROMATOGRAPHY

Chromatography is mainly used as a tool to separate closely related chemical species but it can also be used for qualitative as well as quantitative estimation of the separated species.

9.7.1. Qualitative Analysis by Chromatography

Identification of solutes which are separated by the chromatographic technique is the main purpose of qualitative analysis. Retention time (t_R) of a solute or its position on the stationary phase after a certain elution period (for e.g. distance traveled by it in the column), can be used as parameters for the identification of solutes by chromatography. A chromatographic technique is used for identifying only a limited number of species, whose identities are known but confirmation of identity always requires spectral or chemical investigation of the isolated compounds.

9.7.2. Quantitative Analysis by Chromatography

The quantitative estimation by chromatography involves determination of the quantity of the separated fractions. In order to get the accuracy in quantification, the eluted compounds should be detected accurately. The choice of a detector in chromatography is thus, extremely important. The sensitivity, linearity and specificity of a detector play a major role in quantitative estimation by chromatography. For solutes getting separated in smaller concentrations, amplification of the response obtained from the detector is important in getting higher accuracy. Another important parameter for getting higher accuracy in quantification by chromatography is the amount of sample used for loading the column. This is mainly limited by the range of linearity of the detector for different solutes. The specificity of the detector may cause certain peaks to be missed in the quantification process. Similarly, the flow rate of the mobile phase and the temperature of the column and detector also determine accuracy of quantification, e.g. differential refractive index detector requires good control on temperature, while the UV detector is less critical in this respect.

Quantitative analysis involves the following steps.

1) The generation of the signal for each compound in the mixture by the detector after chromatographic separation so as to produce different peaks in a chromatogram.
2) The measurement of some parameters for the peaks obtained in a chromatogram.
3) The calculation of concentration of the separated compounds from the measured parameters.

9.7.2.1. Measurement of Peak Parameters in Chromatography

Various methods used to measure different parameters for the separated compounds in the chromatogram are mentioned below.

1) Analysis based on peak height

As shown in **Fig. 9.15**, the measurement of the height of a peak is a common method of quantification. The height of a peak is measured by drawing a base line on either side of a peak and then dropping a perpendicular on this base line from the top centre of the peak. The measurement of this perpendicular distance for the reference standard (h_1) as well as for the separated compound (h_2) helps in finding the actual concentration of the separated compound.

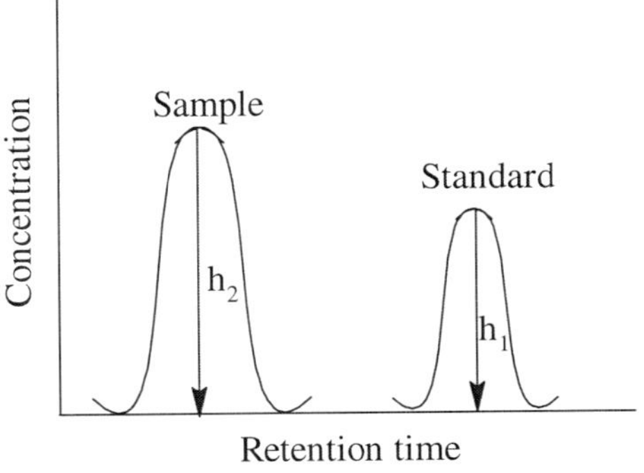

Fig. 9.15: Measurement of peak height in chromatography

Advantages

(i) The measurement of the peak height gives accurate results, provided the widths during the period required to obtain chromatograms for a sample and a standard, the column temperature, the flow rate of the mobile phase and the rate of sample injection, are controlled properly.

(ii) The peak heights are measured more easily and more accurately if the peaks are narrow.

Disadvantage

If the column temperature, the flow rate of the mobile phase and the rate of sample injection are not controlled properly, the variation in the peaks widths is observed. As shown in **Fig. 9.16**, the change in the peak width results in the change in the peak height, leading to an inaccuracy in the measurement.

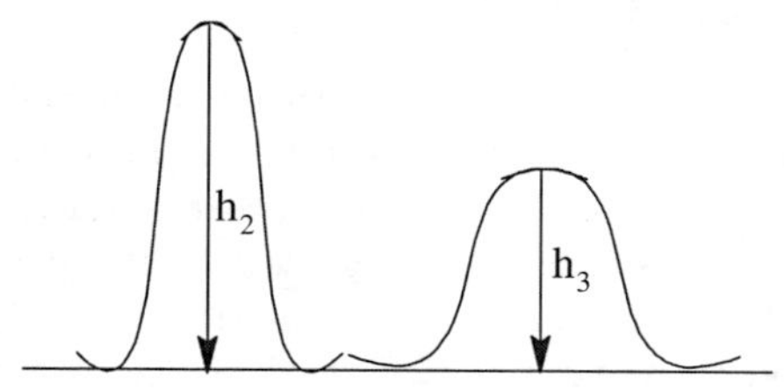

Fig. 9.16: Change in peak height with the change in peak width

2) Analysis based on peak areas

In order to avoid the variation in the measurement of the peak height with the change in the peak width, another parameter, the peak area, is used for quantification. The peak area or area under the curve is independent of the peak width. Thus, broadening of the peaks, due to improper control on parameters involved in Van Deemter equation, does not affect the accuracy of the quantification process. Hence, the measurement of peak areas is preferred over the measurement of peak heights.

A comparison of area under the peak for a standard and a sample is made to find the concentration of each compound in the mixture.

Advantages

(i) The measurement of peak area is independent of the band broadening and hence, offers the advantage of reproducibility. This is because if a band is sharp, its height is increased and if the same band is broadened, its height is reduced. This is shown in **Fig. 9.16**.

(ii) The peak area measurement is the preferred parameter for the asymmetric or skewed peaks.

Disadvantage

The measurement of peak areas is not as easy as the measurement of peak heights. The area determination is carried out either by performing calculation from height and width of the peak or by using some special device.

Measurement of peak areas

The chromatographic instruments are equipped with ball and disc or electronic integrators, which permit the precise estimation of peak areas. If such equipment is not available, a manual estimate must be made. The peak areas are measured using different methods mentioned below.

(a) Area measurement by triangulation technique

Most of the times, the chromatographic peaks are triangular in shape and hence, area under the triangular peaks is obtained by applying the formula for the area of a triangle, as per the **equation (9.21)**.

$$A = \tfrac{1}{2} \times w \times h \quad \dots (9.21)$$

where, 'w' is the width of a peak and 'h' is the height of a peak. In the presence of band broadening, the peak width cannot be measured accurately. Hence, as shown in **Fig. 9.17**, the tangents are drawn along the sides of a triangle. The width of a peak (w) is taken as a distance between the two points of intersection (A and B) of tangents with a base line. The height is measured from the base line to the intersection of the two tangents at point C.

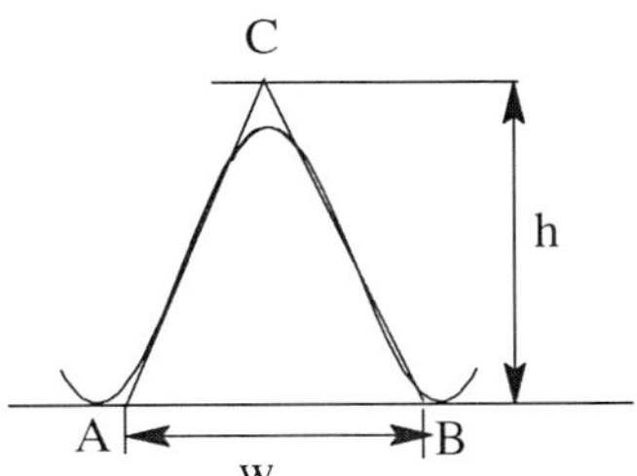

Fig. 9.17: Measurement of width and height of a peak in triangulation technique

Advantage

It makes use of a simple formula for the calculation of area under the curve.

Disadvantages

(i) The triangulation technique is useful only for symmetrical peaks.

(ii) It involves a tedious job of putting tangents along the sides of a triangle.

(iii) Drawing tangents on the sides of a triangle involves operator skill. There can be different values of height and width and therefore, of area of a triangle, depending on the actual position of tangents. A slight error in drawing tangents can have a profound effect on the height measurement.

(b) Area measurement by width at half the height method (h x $w_{0.5}$)

To reduce the errors involved in measuring the width and the height of a peak in the triangulation technique, another more accurate method is used, wherein instead of measuring the width at the baseline, the width at half the height of a peak is measured. This is shown in **Fig. 9.18**. Height to width at half the height ratio of approximately 1-10 is considered to be the best. Area under the curve is calculated as the product of height and width at half the height.

$$A = h \times w_{0.5}$$

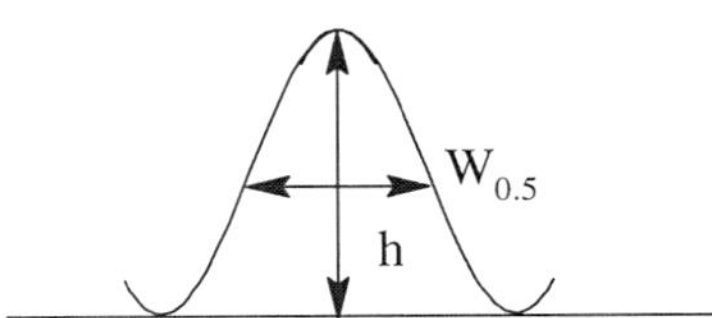

Fig. 9.18: Measurement of width at half the height

Advantages

(i) This method reduces the errors due to tailing, in the measurement of area. Hence, it is more accurate as compared to a triangulation technique.

(ii) This technique does not require drawing tangents along the sides of a triangle and hence, it is a rapid and a simpler method compared to a triangulation technique.

Disadvantage

Like a triangulation technique, this technique is also useful only for symmetrical peaks.

(c) Area measurement by planimetry

Planimetry makes use of a device called a *planimeter* to measure the peak areas. As shown in **Fig. 9.19**, a planimeter consists of a *pivot* in order to keep it fixed at one point. A pivot is connected through a *movable shaft* to a *dial* which provides a digital display of the peak area during the measurement. This dial is in turn connected to another *arm* which can move along the perimeter of a peak. Hence, it is a *perimetry* technique.

Advantages

(i) The technique of planimetry does not provide precise measurements of peak areas.

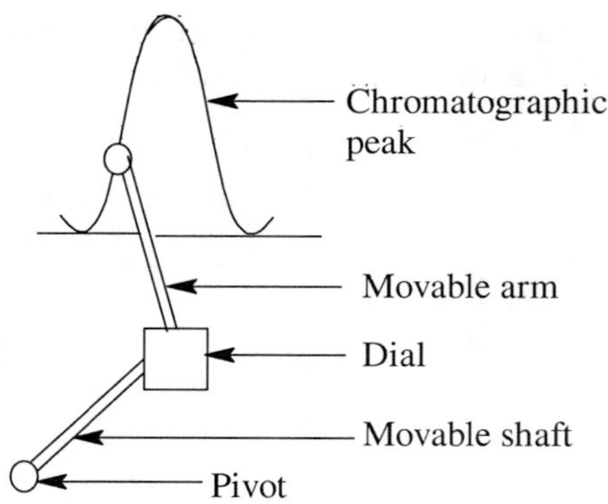

Fig. 9.19: Measurement of peak area by planimetry

Nevertheless, it is more accurate than the triangulation technique.

(ii) It finds wide application in determining the areas, particularly when the peaks are skewed and not symmetrical, because the true peak areas are measured.

Disadvantages

(i) The precision and accuracy of this method are dependent on the skill of an operator.

(ii) The precision in the measurement can be improved by tracing each peak either from its inner or an outer side, continuously. Also, the same peak is traced several times and the average of all the values is calculated.

(iii) Because planimetry requires considerable operator skill and several measurements for the same peak, it is a tedious method.

(iv) It is a time consuming technique.

(d) Area measurement by cut and weigh method

Like planimetry, this is also a perimetry technique. In this technique, the chromatographic peaks for the reference compound and the separated compounds from a sample are recorded on a high quality chart paper. This paper is cut along the perimeter of the peaks corresponding to a reference compound and the separated compounds. These cut outs are then weighed using an analytical balance. The comparison of the weights for the standard and the sample is made to find the concentration of each compound in the mixture.

Advantages

(i) This method is found to be superior to the triangulation techniques.

(ii) It is more useful for the asymmetric or skewed peaks.

Disadvantages

(i) Accuracy of the method depends on the accuracy of cutting the chart paper. The inaccuracy in the cutting procedure can be minimized by keeping the ratio of the height to width at half the height of a peak in the range of 1-10.

(ii) A very high quality chart paper is essential in order to get reproducibility in the measurement. This requires the use of a homogeneous and uniformly porous paper so as to get the constant weight per unit volume of the paper. The control on the moisture content of the paper is also required.

(iii) This method is time consuming.

(e) Area measurement using a ball and disc integrator

A *ball and disc integrator* is the most widely used device for measuring the area under the curve in chromatography. This device is present as a built-in device in the chromatograph.

Advantages

(i) This integrator provides the higher degree of automation and relatively higher accuracy as compared to other techniques discussed so far.

(ii) This technique can be used for the skewed peaks also.

Other more modern methods used for the quantification are the digital or electronic integrators and computers.

Table 9.2 lists the standard deviation for various area measurement techniques.

Table 9.2: Standard deviation for various area measurement techniques

Name of technique	Standard deviation
Electronic integration	0.44
Ball and disc integration	1.3
Cut and weigh	1.7
h x W (at ½ the height)	2.6
Planimetry	4.4

9.7.2.2. Conversion of Numerical Data to Composition

The numerical data obtained in terms of height, area or weight, corresponding to the peak for the reference compound and that for the separated compounds, is required to be converted to the concentration of different compounds in the mixture.

Three important and commonly used methods to relate the digital data obtained from a chromatogram to the composition of the sample are discussed below.

1) Normalization technique
2) Internal standardization technique
3) External standardization technique or calibration

1) Normalization technique

Consider a chromatogram shown in **Fig. 9.20**. It shows elution of three compounds, X, Y and Z from their mixture. Let A_X, A_Y and A_Z be the area under the curves for three compounds, X, Y and Z, respectively. By using this method, percentage of each component in their mixture is calculated by using the formulae.

From the formulae given below, it is clear that in order to calculate the percentage of any one compound, it is essential to know the area under

$$\% \text{ of } X = \frac{A_X}{A_X + A_Y + A_Z}$$

$$\% \text{ of } Y = \frac{A_Y}{A_X + A_Y + A_Z}$$

$$\% \text{ of } Z = \frac{A_Z}{A_X + A_Y + A_Z}$$

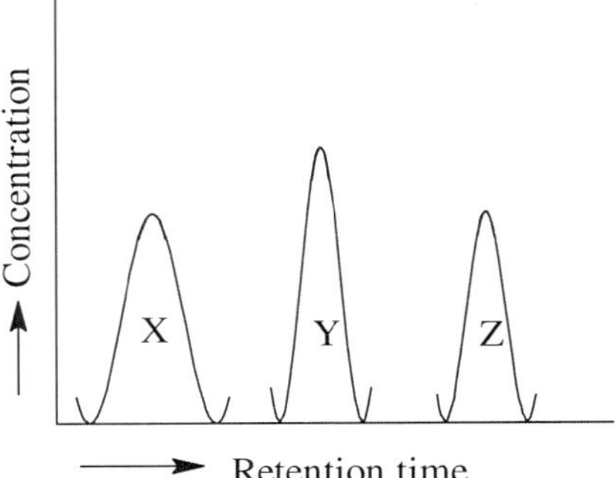

Fig. 9.20: A chromatogram showing three separated compounds

the curves for all the three compounds present in a mixture. Thus, complete elution of a sample is required even if one is interested in finding the amount of the compound getting eluted out first. This unnecessarily adds up to the time and cost of analysis. The normalization technique is used commonly when the separations are carried out by gas chromatography because gas chromatography is much faster than liquid chromatography and all the compounds are eluted out faster as compared to that in liquid chromatography.

Advantages

(i) This is a simple technique to calculate the percentage of compounds when limited number of compounds is present in a mixture.

(ii) It does not require reference standard for finding concentration of compounds.

Disadvantages

(i) Elution of all the compounds in the sample is required even when the percentage of only one compound is to be determined.

(ii) This method is not used when the number of compounds is more, since the elution of a large number of compounds requires more time.

2) Internal standard method

In this method, the amount of each compound in the mixture is calculated by using a reference standard. A reference standard is altogether a different compound than the compounds to be separated. Hence, the elution time of this reference compound is different from the elution time of any of the compounds getting separated from their mixture. The reference compound is mixed along with the mixture to be separated and this mixture is injected in the column. Hence, the reference compound is called as an *internal standard.* The choice of an internal standard is made based on the following criteria.

a) It must have completely different retention time than that for the compounds to be separated.
b) It must not elute out far away from the compounds of interest, i.e. it must elute out near the peaks of interest.
c) It must be similar in concentration to the compounds of interest.
d) It must be chemically inert.
e) It must be absent in the sample.

The internal standard and the compounds in the mixture separate depending on their retention time values. From the height or the area of the peaks for the reference standard and the eluted compounds, the concentration of each compound in the mixture can be found out as follows. Consider that the concentration of an internal standard is 10 µg/ml and it produces a peak corresponding to a height of 10 mm. As shown in **Fig. 9.21**, one of the compounds, X, separated from the sample, produces a peak corresponding to the height of 20 mm. Hence, the concentration of X in the sample is 20 µg/ml. Thus, the height of a peak for an internal standard and its concentration, help in finding the concentration of the compounds present in the sample. The general formula, $h_{std} \cdot C_{std} = h_{sample} \cdot C_{sample}$, can be used to find the concentration of the sample, where, h_{std} and h_{sample} are the heights of the peaks for the standard and the sample, respectively, and C_{std} and C_{sample} are the concentrations of the standard and the sample, respectively.

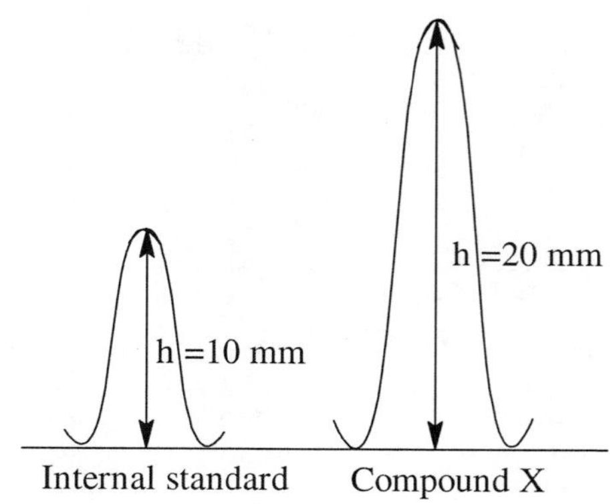

Fig. 9.21: Comparison of peaks for internal standard and an eluted compound

Quantification using an internal standard provides distinct advantages as mentioned below and hence, its use is preferred over an external standard.

Advantages of using an internal standard

(i) Instead of preparing separate solutions of an internal standard and the sample, if a single solution is prepared by mixing an internal standard along with the sample to be separated, higher accuracy is achieved in determining the concentration of the separated compounds, since the error involved during dilution while preparing a common solution, remains same for both. Thus, an internal standard, which is added before the chromatographic process, compensates for the errors during the preparation of the sample.

(ii) Other errors associated with the apparatus (e.g. change in the temperature of the column) and with the procedure (e.g. error during injecting the sample into the column), can also be eliminated by the use of an internal standard.

Thus, the higher accuracy in the measurement is provided by using an internal standard.

Disadvantages of using an internal standard

(i) Sometimes, it is difficult to get a suitable internal standard. An internal standard may not elute out near the compounds of interest.

(ii) An internal standard may not be soluble in the solvent, in the concentration range corresponding to the compounds to be separated.

(iii) It may not be chemically inert.

In case of non-availability of an internal standard, an external standard can be used for quantification.

3) External standard method

As the name suggests, an external standard is used externally, i.e. it is not mixed along with the sample to be separated. Thus, whenever an external standard is used, it is essential to prepare two separate solutions, one of an external standard and another of a sample to be separated. This is because, for a mixture containing compounds X and Y, either X or Y can be used as an external standard. Thus, an external standard is one of the compounds of the sample itself and not an altogether different chemical. This external standard should be 100 % pure (AR grade) or it should be of known purity. Since the retention time of an external standard (either X or Y) and one of the compounds of a mixture match with each other, the standard and the sample cannot be mixed together. Hence, the solutions of an external standard and the sample are injected separately in the column. This produces two separate chromatograms, one for the standard and another for the sample. The height of the peaks for the compounds X and Y is then compared with the height of the peak for a standard and their concentrations are determined.

Advantage of using an external standard

There is no need to find a suitable chemical as a standard since one of the compounds of the sample is used as an external standard.

Disadvantages of using an external standard

(i) Errors occurring during weighing the standard and the sample and also during diluting their solutions, make this process less accurate as compared to that carried out by using an internal standard.

(ii) This method requires precise control on the analytical techniques, particularly while injecting the solution in the column. If an operator makes an error while injecting two solutions (standard and sample) to the column, the final calculation can involve error. For example, if the pressure applied on the piston of a syringe while injecting the solution of an external standard is less, it may leave few drops of solution in the syringe, thereby injecting less than the required amount of the standard solution in the column. However, while injecting the sample solution, if correct pressure is applied on the piston then the sample solution is injected accurately in the column. If an accurate injection of a standard solution, whose concentration is 10 μg/ml, produces a peak of 10 mm height, then the same solution, when injected inaccurately, would produce a peak of less than 10 mm height (say 8 mm). Without realizing the error made during injection of a standard, an operator would correlate the height of 8 mm with 10 μg/ml concentration of the standard. This would give incorrect concentration values for the separated compounds.

(iii) Whenever an external standard is used, two chromatograms are required to be recorded as against one in case of a method involving an internal standard.

Thus, this process is more time consuming as compared to the internal standard method.

4) Preparation of Calibration Curves

The calculation of the concentration of the separated compounds using an external standard is done many times by direct comparison of the height or area of an external standard with that of the separated compounds. However, sometimes, the concentration is determined by preparing the *calibration curves* for the standard.

In order to construct the calibration curves, the standard solutions of the compounds of interest (S_1 for compound X and S_2 for compound Y) are prepared and equal volume of solutions is injected into a chromatograph. A chromatogram for S_1 and S_2 is shown in **Fig. 9.22(a)**. A separate chromatogram for the compounds X and Y from the sample is also recorded **Fig. 9.22(b)**. The area under the curves for S_1 and S_2 is measured and the concentration is plotted against the area as shown in **Fig. 9.23**. The unknown concentration of X and

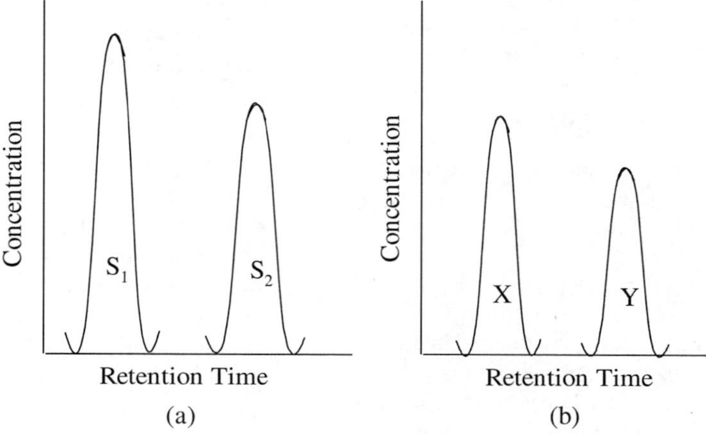

Fig. 9.22: A chromatogram for (a) S_1 and S_2 and (b) X and Y from the sample

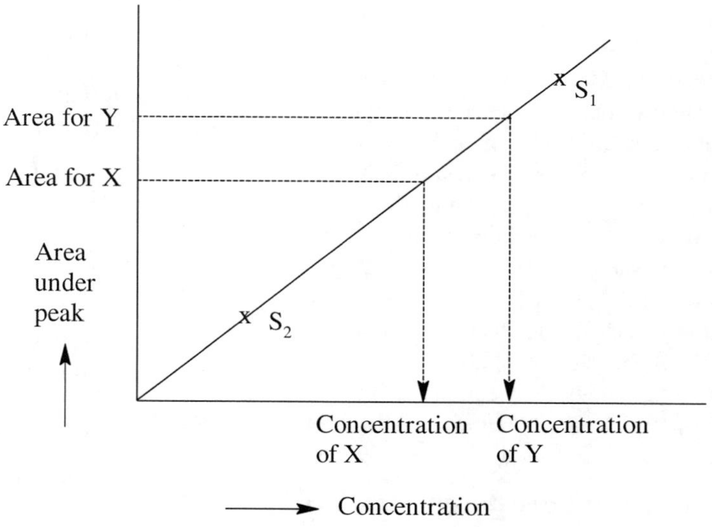

Fig. 9.23: Calibration curve for compounds X and Y

Y from the sample can be obtained by measuring area under their peaks and then dropping a perpendicular on the concentration axis.

Another technique is to prepare the calibration curve by injecting varying amounts of the same standard solution (either S_1 or S_2) and then plotting their areas against concentration. However, this method is less accurate due to the injection errors. This method is usually used to analyze single compound or simple mixtures.

9.8. DIFFERENT TECHNIQUES UNDER LIQUID CHROMATOGRAPHY

In liquid chromatography, liquid is used as a mobile phase. Various techniques under liquid chromatography, based on the kind of stationary phase used, are listed in **Table 9.3**.

In adsorption, partition, gel and ion exchange chromatography, the stationary phase is filled in a tubular column, made up of either glass or metal. Hence, this type of chromatography is termed as *column chromatography*. In thin layer and paper chromatography, the stationary phase is present in one plane, either a glass plate or a paper. This kind of a chromatographic technique is termed as *planar chromatography*.

9.9. COLUMN CHROMATOGRAPHY

In column chromatography, the stationary phase in the form of silica gel, alumina, celite or diatomaceous earth, is filled in a glass column or a stainless steel column of uniform diameter. The normal length of the column (length of stationary phase) is 50 - 500 cm and diameter of the column is 1 - 5 cm. The particle size of the stationary phase is in the range of 150 - 200 μm. The mobile phase used is either a single solvent or a mixture of solvents. A chromatographic technique carried out by using a polar stationary phase and a less polar or a non-polar mobile phase is termed as *normal phase chromatography*. On the other hand, if the

Table 9.3: Various techniques under liquid chromatography

Sr. No.	Type of chromatography	Mobile phase	Stationary phase
1	Adsorption chromatography	Liquid	Solid (Held in a tubular column)
2	Partition chromatography	Liquid	Liquid (Adsorbed on a porous support in a tubular column)
3	Thin layer chromatography	Liquid	Liquid/Solid (Liquid adsorbed on a solid support / solid held on a glass plate)
4	Paper chromatography	Liquid	Liquid (Held in pores of a paper)
5	Gel chromatography	Liquid	Liquid (Held in the interstices of a polymeric gel)
6	Ion exchange chromatography	Liquid	Solid (Resin held in a tubular column)
7	Ion-pair chromatography	Liquid	Solid (Held in a tubular column)

stationary phase is less polar or non-polar compared to the mobile phase, the technique is called as r*everse phase chromatography*. For the reverse phase chromatography, instead of a direct use of silica gel, its modified surface is made use of. The surface modification is carried out by forming a covalent bond between silica gel and a reagent like chlorooctadecylsilane. The chemical reaction between these two is shown in **Fig. 9.24**. In the modified surface of silica gel, 'R' represents the octadecyl group, i.e. $C_{18}H_{37}$ alkyl chain. A chemical reaction between silica gel and chlorooctadecylsilane, converts a polar surface of silica gel (because of the exposed –OH group) into a non-polar one (because of the exposed –R group instead of an –OH group). The columns, which make use of such bonded stationary phases, are

```
                      R
                      |
Si - OH    +    Cl - Si - R
                      |
                      R
Silica gel  Chlorooctadecylsilane
                 |
                 v
           R
           |
Si - O - Si - R
           |
           R
Modified surface of
silica gel
```

Fig. 9.24: Surface modification of silica gel

referred to as *Bondapack columns. The c*olumns with octadecylsilane as stationary phase are referred to as C_{18} columns. Instead of using chlorooctadecylsilane, if chlorooctylsilane (R = C_8H_{17}) is used, then the column is referred to as C_8 column, which is more polar compared to C_{18} column but is less polar compared to a silica gel column. Thus, the surface of silica gel can be modified so as to provide the required polarity to the stationary phase.

In the *normal phase chromatography,* since the stationary phase is more polar, polar solutes interact more with it and they are retained for a longer time in the column, whereas the less polar or non-polar solutes interact more with the mobile phase and move down the column faster along with it. Thus, the order of elution of solutes is, non-polar solutes first, then the solutes of intermediate polarity and at the end, the solutes which are more polar in nature. In the *reverse phase chromatography*, however, since the stationary phase is less polar, polar solutes interact more with the mobile phase and move down the column faster along with it, whereas the less polar or non-polar solutes interact more with the stationary phase and are retained for a longer time in the column. Therefore, the order of elution of solutes is exactly reverse as compared to that in the normal phase chromatography. Thus, the order of elution in the reverse phase chromatography is, more polar solutes first, then the solutes of intermediate polarity and at the end, the solutes which are less polar or non-polar in nature.

Ordinarily, the mobile phase is passed through a column under the force of gravity. Chromatography carried out under normal pressure is called *classical chromatography*. However, many a times, because of few distinct advantages, a mobile phase is passed under pressure through a column. In such a case, the technique is termed as *High Pressure Liquid Chromatography* (HPLC).

9.10. HIGH PRESSURE LIQUID CHROMATOGRAPHY

9.10.1. Need for High Pressure in Liquid Chromatography

In classical liquid chromatography, to assure a reasonable flow rate of the mobile phase, the particle size of the stationary phase is kept larger, i.e. in the range of 150-200 ìm. The bigger particle size of the stationary phase offers less resistance to the flow of mobile phase. In spite of this, the flow rate less than an ml/min or few drops/ min is achieved. Thus, in classical chromatography, the time required for the separation of solutes is long. This can lead to an undesirable phenomenon of band broadening, thereby leading to the less efficient separation.

In order to reduce the time of analysis, it is essential to increase the flow rate of the mobile phase. The flow rate of the mobile phase is increased either by passing the mobile phase under pressure from the top of the column or by applying vacuum at the lower end of the column. However, increase in the flow rate of the mobile phase to complete analysis at a faster rate, leads to the decrease in the column efficiency (increased value of H). This is clear from the solid curve shown in **Fig. 9.25**. In order to achieve faster separation, without compensating for the column efficiency, the parameters other than the flow rate of the mobile phase, involved in Van Deemter equation, can be modified. In Van Deemter equation, the terms 'A' **(equation 9.9)** and C_M **(equation 9.12)** involve the parameter d_R, representing the average diameter of the particles of the stationary phase. Thus, by selecting the stationary phase consisting of smaller particle size, the magnitude of A and C ($C = C_S + C_M$) can be reduced. This in turn, reduces the value of H ($H = A + B/u + Cu$). From **Fig. 9.25**, it is clear that the value of H decreases with the decrease in the particle size of the stationary phase.

Thus, the loss in the column efficiency due to increase in the flow rate of the mobile phase can be compensated by reducing the particle size of the stationary phase, but the columns in which the stationary phase of smaller particle size (≈ 10 ìm) is used, pose the difficulty of high resistance to the flow of mobile phase through a column. Thus, in order to reduce the time of analysis, the flow rate of the mobile phase has to be kept high and to avoid the loss in the column efficiency with the increase in the flow rate of the mobile phase, the particle size of the stationary phase has to be reduced. In order to achieve all this, it is essential to pass the mobile phase under high pressure so that the resistance offered by the stationary phase is overcome. The chromatographic technique, in which the mobile phase is passed under pressure, is known as *High Pressure Liquid Chromatography* (HPLC). Since it provides higher efficiency for the separation of compounds, it is also termed as *High Performance Liquid Chromatography*. This technique requires sophisticated instrumentation as compared to that used in the classical liquid chromatography. This leads to the increased cost of instrumentation and hence, the method becomes *High Price Liquid Chromatography*.

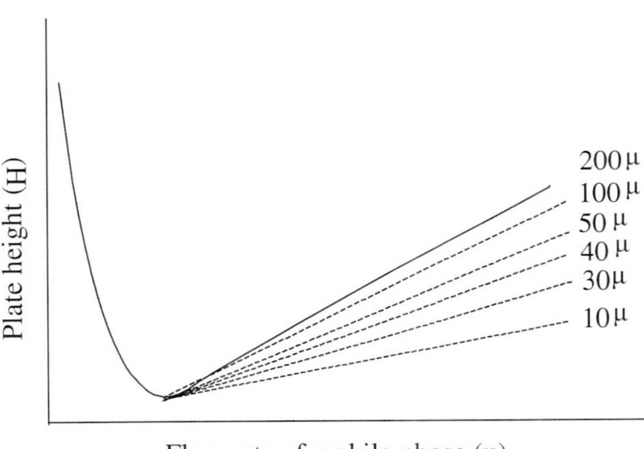

Fig. 9.25: Effect of flow rate of mobile phase and particle size of stationary phase on column efficiency

9.10.2. Instrumentation in HPLC

The components of High Pressure Liquid Chromatograph are as follows.

9.10.2.1. Solvent reservoir and degassing system
9.10.2.2. Pumps
9.10.2.3. Precolumns
9.10.2.4. Sample injection system
9.10.2.5. Columns
9.10.2.6. Temperature controller (Thermostat)
9.10.2.7. Detectors

9.10.2.1. Solvent Reservoir and Degassing System

High pressure liquid chromatography makes use of a single solvent or a mixture of solvents as a mobile phase, which is contained in a reservoir. The elution of solutes from their mixture, when carried out by using a single mobile phase of constant composition, is termed as *isocratic elution*. When a mixture contains solutes of extreme polarities - one polar and another non-polar - separation cannot be carried out within a reasonable time period by using a single mobile phase. If a non-polar mobile phase is used throughout the separation of such a mixture, a non-polar solute would get eluted out faster but a very long time would be required for the elution of a polar compound. In order to elute out a polar compound also within a reasonable time period, another mobile phase, which is polar in nature, is required to be used for such samples. When the elution is carried out by using two (sometimes more) mobile phases that differ significantly in polarity, it is termed as *gradient elution*. The modern HPLC equipments have two or more reservoirs from which different solvents can be introduced into a chamber at the rates which can be varied so as to adjust the polarity of the mobile phase.

A solvent reservoir should be inert to a variety of solvents like water, methanol, acetonotrile, etc. which are commonly used in HPLC. Hence, usually, glass and stainless steel reservoirs of 500 – 1000 ml capacity are used. The HPLC column is very sensitive to impurities and therefore, the solvents used as mobile phase, require special treatment. The special HPLC grade solvents are available in the market, which take care of the impurities in these solvents.

Degassing of these solvents should be done so as to remove air or oxygen dissolved in them, which if present in the mobile phase, can rupture the packing of the column or can produce unwanted peaks in the chromatogram. Degassing of the mobile phase can be done by four methods.

1) By filtration under vacuum

Filtration of the mobile phase using vacuum, removes all dissolved air or oxygen from the mobile phase. Millipore filters are commonly used for the filtration of the mobile phase.

2) By distillation of the mobile phase

When the required mobile phase is distilled under vacuum, the distillate becomes free of dissolved air or oxygen.

3) By ultrasonication

Sonication is the act of applying sound energy to agitate particles in a sample for various purposes. *Ultrasonication* is the sonication using ultrasound, i.e. a sound with the frequency greater than the upper limit of human hearing (approximately 20 KHz). In the laboratory, ultrasonication is usually achieved by using an *ultrasonic bath* or an *ultrasonic probe*, colloquially known as a *sonicator*. If a container bearing the mobile phase is kept in an ultrasonic bath, the mobile phase becomes free of dissolved air or oxygen. This is an alternative to the sparging method.

4) By sparging an inert gas of low solubility

Sparging, also known as gas flushing, is a technique which involves bubbling a chemically inert gas of low solubility such as argon or helium through the mobile phase. This can be used to remove dissolved O_2 and N_2 that interfere by forming bubbles in the column.

Along with a degassing system, HPLC chromatograph also contains a means of filtering dust and particulate matter from the mobile phase.

9.10.2.2. Pumps

Once a suitable mobile phase is selected, it is to be passed under pressure to the column with the help of a pump. The most HPLC pumps have outputs of at least 1000 psi and preferably 4000-6000 psi (pounds per square inch), with a flow delivery rate of at least 3 ml/min. The pumps used in HPLC should satisfy the following conditions.

a) They should generate pressure in the range of 4000-6000 psi.
b) They should provide a continuous or a pulse free flow of the mobile phase.
c) They should produce the flow rate ranging from 0.1 to 10 ml/min.
d) They should provide the flow control and flow reproducibility of 0.5 % or better.
e) They should have corrosion-resistant components made up of stainless steel or Teflon or sapphire.

The high pressure generated by HPLC pumps does not constitute an explosion hazard, because liquids are not very compressible. Thus, the rupture of a component of the system results only in the solvent leakage. Such a leakage may constitute a fire hazard.

Three types of pumps are commonly employed in HPLC. They are described below.

1) Reciprocating pumps
2) Syringe or displacement type of pumps
3) Pneumatic or constant pressure pumps

1) Reciprocating pumps

Construction

The majority of the commercially available HPLC systems make use of the reciprocating pumps. As shown in **Fig. 9.26**, this pump consists of a piston provided in a syringe type of a chamber. The chamber is connected to two *ball check valves* on two ends. The check valves open and close alternately. The solvent is in direct contact with the piston.

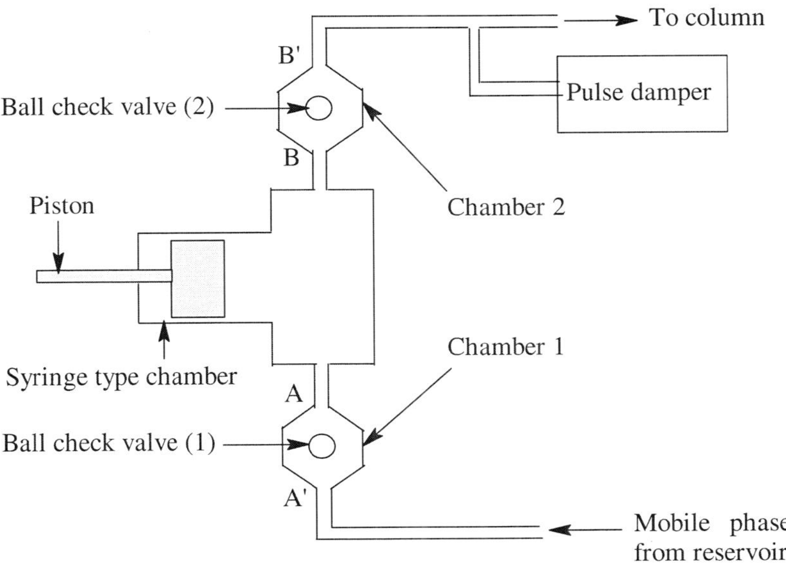

Fig. 9.26: A reciprocating pump

Working

When the piston is drawn at the back, the ball check valves (1) and (2), occupy the positions A and B, respectively. The mobile phase flows from the solvent reservoir into chamber (1) but not in chamber (2). When the piston direction is reversed, the check valves occupy the positions A' and B', respectively. At this stage, the mobile phase from chamber (1) enters chamber (2). The volume of the mobile phase discharged from the pump per unit time can be changed by altering the distance that the piston travels. When the piston is withdrawn, again the fresh mobile phase enters chamber (1), the valve (2) comes at the position B but still the mobile phase from chamber (2) does not enter the column, since there is no force to push it. Again, when the piston direction is reversed, the mobile phase from chamber (1) enters into chamber (2), which pushes the mobile phase already present in chamber (2) to the column. Thus, when the mobile phase enters chamber (1), there is no mobile phase going out in the column. When the mobile phase is entering the column, chamber (1) is empty. This is the reason for the *pulsed flow* of the mobile phase in the reciprocating pumps.

This drawback can be overcome in two ways. The first solution is to reduce the time of filling. This reduces the dead time between the cycles. Another way is to provide a dual piston pump. With this arrangement, when one piston of the pump is moving back, another piston moves in the forward direction. This reduces the pulsation in the flow, since one head is *filling* while the other is *discharging*. The use of a dual piston pump, in combination with a rapid filling phase, almost eliminates the pulsation.

Advantages

(i) The internal volume of the reciprocating pumps is small (35 - 400 μL). This is of importance, especially in case of gradient elution, which requires removal of one mobile phase from the pump before the introduction of another one. Because of the *small internal volume*, the changeover from one mobile phase to the other can be achieved fast.

(ii) The reciprocating pumps provide high output pressure (up to 10,000 psi).

(iii) They provide a constant flow rate of the mobile phase, which is independent of the column back pressure and solvent viscosity.

Disadvantage

The reciprocating pumps produce a pulsed flow, if proper measures are not taken. The pulsed flow from these pumps is not considered to be a major drawback, since a pulsed flow can be easily converted to a pulse-free flow, as described above.

2) Syringe type or displacement type of pumps

Construction

As shown in **Fig. 9.27**, in displacement type of pumps, a piston or a plunger inside the chamber can move *to and fro* with the help of a screw-feed drive, connected to a stepping motor.

Working

In displacement type of pumps, all the mobile phase is contained within the chamber of a pump. The electric supply to the stepping motor allows a continuous and a uniform movement of a screw,

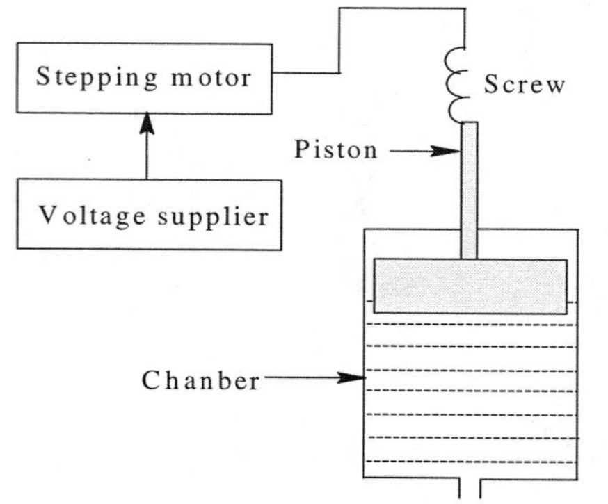

Voltage supplier

Fig. 9.27: A syringe type or a displacement type of a pump

which brings about uniform movement of a piston inside the chamber. This makes possible, delivery of a definite volume of the mobile phase to the pump. The flow rate of the mobile phase or the volume displaced by the pump per unit time depends on the voltage applied to the stepping motor.

Advantages

(i) Displacement pumps produce a pulse free flow since the continuous and uniform movement of the stepping motor with the help of a screw, delivers the mobile phase continuously to the column.

(ii) In these pumps, the flow rate is independent of the back pressure in the column and viscosity of the mobile phase.

Disadvantage

The internal volume of this pump is sufficiently high so as to replace it by another solvent. Hence, this pump is not suitable for gradient elution.

3) Pneumatic pumps

Construction

As shown in **Fig. 9.28**, a pneumatic pump

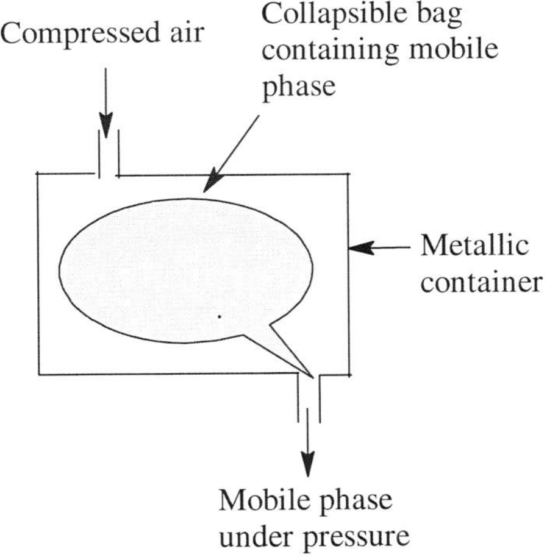

Fig. 9.28: A pneumatic pump

consists of a collapsible bag containing a mobile phase, housed in a metallic container, which can withstand high pressure.

Working

A compressed gas is passed from the inlet into the metallic container. This squeezes the collapsible container and allows the mobile phase to come out from the outlet.

Advantages

(i) Pneumatic pumps are very simple in construction and hence, they are cheap.

(ii) They provide pulse-free flow of the mobile phase.

Disadvantages

(i) In these pumps, the flow of the mobile phase depends on its viscosity and also on the back pressure in the column.

(ii) The pressure provided by these pumps is less than 2000 psi.

(iii)They are not useful for gradient elution.

9.10.2.3. Precolumns

Many HPLC columns possess precolumns. Precolumn is broader than the analytical column. It is filled with the stationary phase, which is chemically identical to the stationary phase in an analytical column (a column which is used for the separation of compounds), but the particle size of the stationary phase in the precolumn is bigger as compared to that in an analytical column. Precolumn is placed between the pump and the sample injection system. Thus, only the mobile phase is passed through the precolumn. Precolumn is used mainly for the following two reasons.

(i) Any impurities, if present in the mobile phase, get adsorbed on the stationary phase present in the precolumn. Thus, these impurities do not pass in an analytical column and do not contaminate it. Hence, these impurities do not interfere with the separation of the sample compounds from an analytical column.

(ii) Another reason for introducing precolumn is that the mobile phase becomes saturated with the stationary phase when it is passed through a precolumn. Hence, when this mobile phase passes through an analytical column, it does not strip off the stationary phase from it and helps in keeping the column packing intact. Thus, it protects or guards the structure of an analytical column. Because of this reason, a precolumn is also called as a *guard column*.

9.10.2.4. Sample Injection System

The sensitivity of an HPLC technique is very high. Hence, it is absolutely essential to introduce an accurate quantity of a sample in the column, which can provide reproducibility in the results. The sample injection system is used to introduce a fixed volume of the sample solution into the mobile phase, while injecting the sample into the column.

Two types of valves are most common in HPLC, which enable the introduction of a fixed volume of the sample accurately in the column.

1) Rotary sampling valve
2) Slider valve

1) Rotary sampling valve

The functioning of a rotary valve can be explained with the help of **Figures 9.29(a)** and **(b)**.

The vertical line in **Fig. 9.29(a)** indicates the original position of a valve. When the valve is in this position, the sample solution is filled in it. This is the *filling mode* of a rotary valve. When the knob in the valve is rotated by an angle of 45°, as indicated in **Fig. 9.29(b)**, the sample enters an analytical column. This is the *loading mode* of a rotary valve.

In the filling mode of the valve [**Fig. 9.29(a)**], a sample solution is introduced from one end. The excess solution drains out from the other end. The loop ABDC thus contains a definite volume of the sample solution. Another loop EF contains mobile phase, which passes through the column. Thus, in the filling mode, the sample solution and the mobile phase are passing through two separate loops.

The valve is then rotated by 45°. This makes changes in the internal connections, thereby connecting points A and C, D and F and points E and B. These connections, which are shown in **Fig. 9.29(b)**, result into two new loops EBDF and AC. The formation of a new loop (EBDF) makes possible the mixing of the stream of the sample with the mobile phase and disconnects the original circuit. The excess sample solution is now present

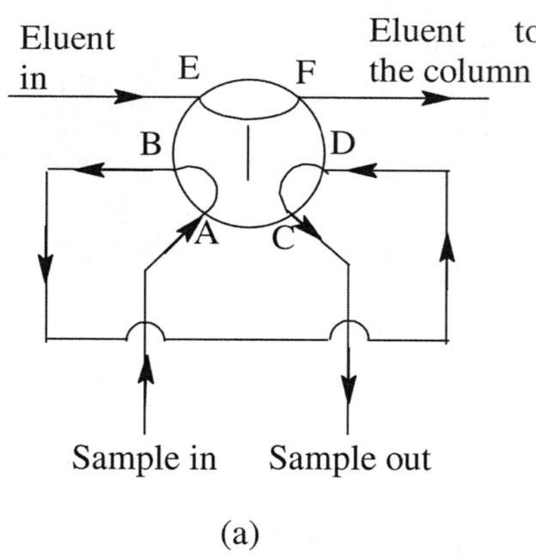

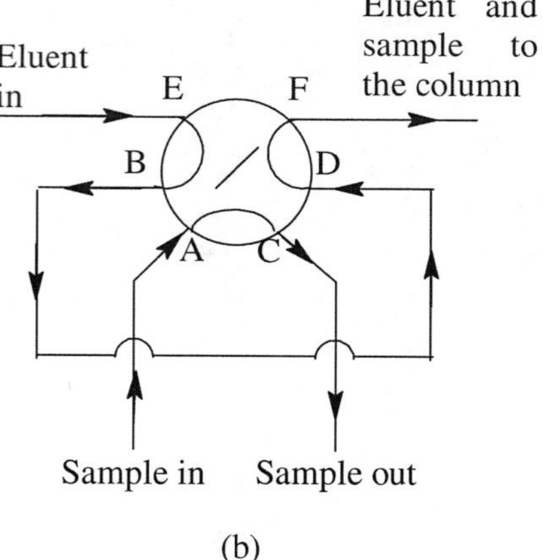

Fig. 9.29: A rotary valve in (a) filling mode and (b) loading mode

in the loop AC, which is separated from another loop. Thus, a fixed and reproducible volume of the sample is introduced in the mobile phase which goes to the column.

2) Slider valve

Construction

As shown in **Fig. 9.30**, a slider valve consists of two vertical chambers A and B, enclosed in a container. The chamber A for the sample solution is connected on one side to the sample reservoir and on the other side to a pump, which draws sample solution into the sample chamber A. The chamber for the sample solution has a small aperture on its right side, which opens up only if pressure is applied on it. Another chamber B is for the mobile phase. It is connected on one side to a mobile phase reservoir and on the other side to an analytical column. The chamber for the mobile phase has a small aperture on its left side.

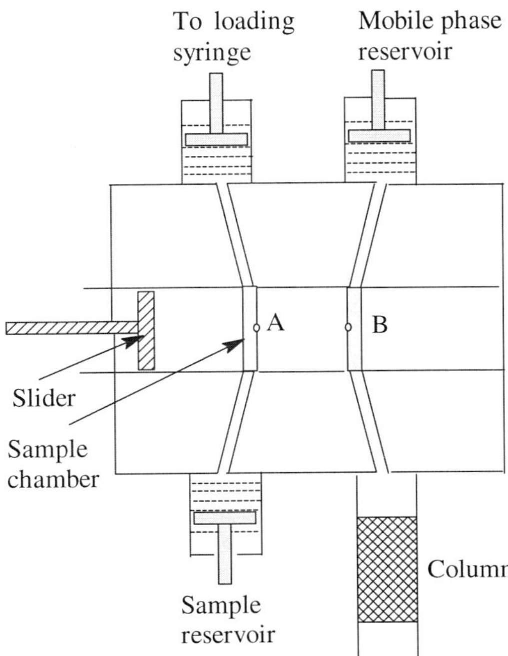

Fig. 9.30: A slider valve

This aperture is closed under normal conditions, but opens up only if the pressure is applied on it. The chamber A containing the sample solution can be pushed towards chamber B containing the mobile phase, with the help of a slider.

Working

The main use of a slider valve is to introduce a fixed and reproducible volume of the sample solution into the column. The sample is drawn in chamber A by means of a syringe. The mobile phase is continuously passing through chamber B .When the slider is moved from left to right, a sample chamber A is pushed on the chamber B containing the mobile phase. Due to the pressure put by chamber A on chamber B, the temperature of the diaphragms of both the chambers increases, which results in the expansion of apertures on both the chambers. This allows entry of sample from chamber A into chamber B. A fixed volume of the sample is thus mixed with the mobile phase, which enters an analytical column for the separation. The slider is then moved towards left so that the sample chambers A moves away from chamber B. When pressure on the apertures is released, they reseal and get closed. Thus, a definite volume of the sample, which is accommodated by chamber A, is introduced into the column. The valves holding volumes from 2-100 μL are available.

9.10.2.5. Columns

The HPLC column is made up of glass or special quality stainless steel. Glass columns can bear low pressures, maximum up to 1000 psi. Stainless steel columns can work at higher pressures, ranging between 2000 and 6000 psi. The length of the column ranges from 15-150 cm and the inner diameter is about 2-3 mm. The inner diameter of the column is controlled precisely, throughout the length of the column. The longer columns are prepared by joining small portions together.

The HPLC columns are usually packed with finely divided silica gel, but occasionally, alumina and celite (a diatomaceous earth) are also employed. The particle size of the stationary phase is in the range of 5-10 μm. Sometimes, *pellicular packings*, which consist of small glass beads of about 40 μm, coated with a 1-3 μm layer (the parameter 'd' in equation for C_S, given below) of a porous material such as silica gel, alumina or an ion exchange resin, is also employed in HPLC. The advantage in using this packing is the higher rate of mass transfer from one phase to the other because of a thin layer of the stationary phase, which results in the higher column efficiency. In Van Deemter equation, the 3rd term is Cu where, C is the sum of C_S and C_M. The term C_S is expressed quantitatively as -

$$C_S = \frac{q\,r\,d^2}{D_S}$$

where, 'd' is the thickness of the stationary phase on the solid support. In the above equation, if 'd' increases, C_S also increases. This results in the decrease in the column efficiency. One drawback of pellicular packings is that they occupy lot of space in the column and hence, reduce the loading capacity of the column, i.e. a limited quantity of the sample can be loaded in the column (roughly 1/10th that of the porous packing).

For reverse phase chromatography, C_{18} columns are commonly used (refer to **Section 9.9** for details).

9.10.2.6. Thermostats

Most of the times, HPLC is performed at room temperature and without using a thermostat. However, if a solute takes longer time for its elution from the column, the separation can be carried out at higher temperatures. Water jacketed columns are available commercially when a precise temperature control is desired. Increase in the temperature of the column decreases the retention time of a compound in the column.

9.10.2.7. Detectors

Once the solutes are separated from their mixture using a chromatographic technique, their presence in the eluate should be detected. In order to detect the compounds of a mixture, different kinds of detectors are used depending upon the nature of a substance. Various detectors used in chromatography work on the basis of the following methods.

(i) Ultraviolet absorption (ii) Infrared absorption (iii) Fluorimetry (iv) Refractive index determination (v) Conductimetry (vi) Mass spectrophotometry (vii) Polarography (viii) Radioactivity

An ideal detector should satisfy the following conditions.

1) An ideal detector should produce *linear response*, i.e. it should produce higher response for more concentrated solutions and lower response for the less concentrated solutions.
2) It should be *sensitive*, i.e. a detector should be able to detect very low concentrations of solutes.
3) It should be *selective*, i.e. it should be able to detect specific substances only.
4) It should be *non-destructive*, i.e. it should not destroy the sample during its detection.

Few detectors are described below.

1) Ultraviolet - visible (UV - visible) detector

The most common detectors for HPLC are based upon the absorption of UV or visible radiation. For this purpose, the spectrophotometers and photometers are made use of. The spectrophotometric detectors are considerably more versatile than the photometric detectors because the radiation corresponding to all the wavelengths of interest, i.e. corresponding to the absorption peaks of the sample components, can be used in this, whereas the photometric detectors make use of a limited number of wavelengths. The photometers employ the wavelengths of 254 and 280 nm from the mercury source, at which most of the organic compounds show absorption.

Construction

As shown in **Fig. 9.31**, UV-visible detector consists of a chamber, which is made up of two compartments having quartz windows, in order to allow the passage of UV radiation through them. A source for UV-visible radiation is placed in front of this chamber. A monochromator and two phototubes are placed in the path of the transmitted beams for the measurement of the signal produced by the blank and an eluted solute. The signals from the two phototubes are fed to one more phototube to get the net signal. An amplifier, for the amplification of the signal produced and a recorder for recording a chromatogram, are provided in the circuitry.

Working

Plane mobile phase is allowed to pass through one compartment and an eluate coming out from the column is continuously passed through another compartment. Ultraviolet or visible radiation is passed through the quartz windows, in both the compartments. When there is no solute present in the eluate, both the compartments contain the plane mobile phase. Hence, the absorption of UV or visible radiation by the solutions in two compartments is same. This produces some current in the circuit, which can be adjusted to a zero value. In presence of some solute in the eluate, because of the absorption of UV or visible radiation by an organic compound in the eluate, the net signal produced differs. This difference in the signal is due to the presence of an organic compound in the eluate. The magnitude of this difference depends on the actual concentration of a compound in the eluate. The detector is calibrated so as to provide a linear response over a broad concentration range. The signal is then amplified and recorded to provide the chromatogram.

Advantages

(i) The UV-visible detector is an universal detector, if wavelengths such as 254 and 280 nm, at which most of the organic compounds show absorbance, are used. Thus, it can be used for

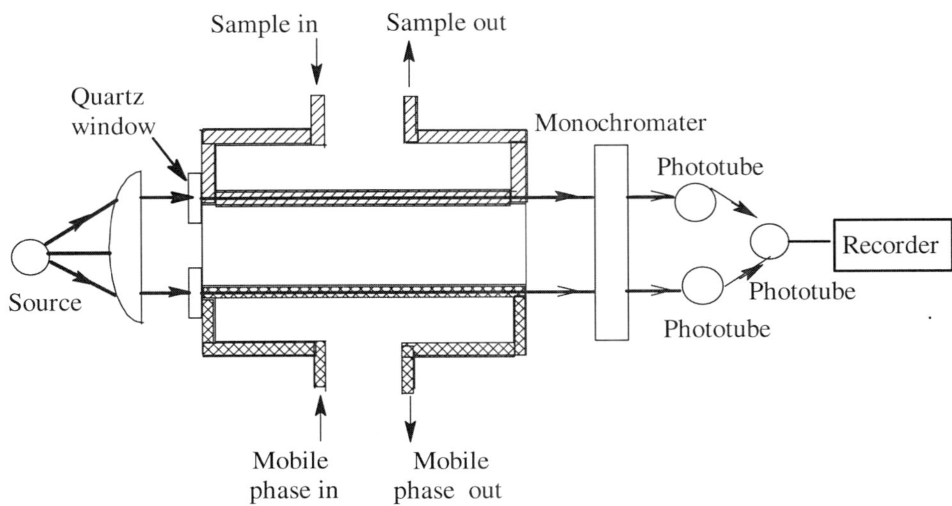

Fig. 9.31: UV-visible detector

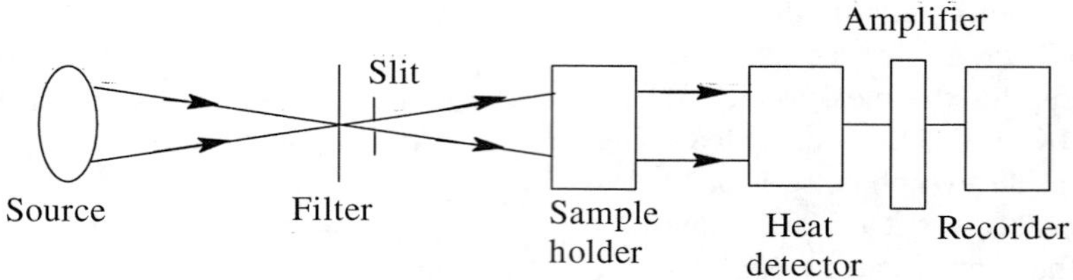

Fig. 9.32: IR detector

the detection of many organic compounds.

(ii) Fabrication of this detector is very easy.

(iii)It can be made selective so as to detect the presence of specific organic compounds, if the wavelength of maximum absorption (λ_{max}) of that compound is used for the detection.

Disadvantage

Since it is an universal detector, the presence of certain impurities in the eluate may also contribute to the signal of an analyte.

2) Infrared (IR) detector

Like UV-visible radiation, IR radiation can also be used for detecting various organic compounds. The IR detector is similar in construction to the UV-visible detector and is shown in **Fig. 9.32**.

3) Differential refractive index detector (DRID)

Construction

As shown in **Fig. 9.33**, differential refractive index detector consists of a light source, a slit and a lens to make the beams coming out from the source parallel. A glass chamber, which is divided into two compartments by a glass plate mounted at an angle, is kept in the path of radiation. A plane mirror is kept beyond the glass chamber for reflecting the beam of radiation

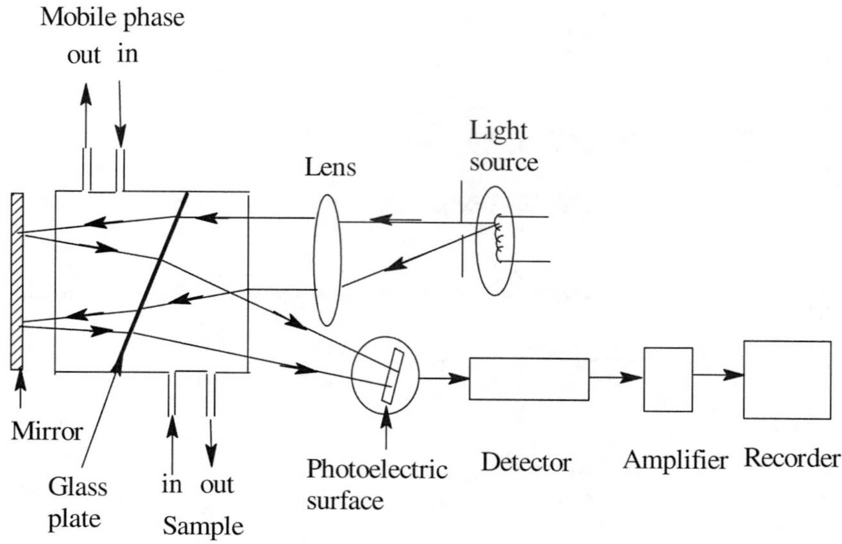

Fig. 9.33: Differential refractive index detector

passing through the glass chamber. A photosensitive surface is used to collect the reflected beam, which liberates electrons and generates current, so as to produce the quantitative signal.

Working

The plane mobile phase is continuously passed through one compartment of a glass chamber. An eluate coming out from the column is passed through another compartment of a glass chamber. If no fraction gets eluted out from the column, the eluate is simply the plane mobile phase and hence, both the compartments of a glass chamber contain the same solution. Since there is no difference in the refractive index of solutions in two compartments, both the refracted beams bend to the same extent and fall at the same point on the photosensitive surface. This generates the standing current in the circuit, which can be taken as a reference value. When some solute is eluted out from the column, one compartment in the glass chamber contains plane mobile phase and another compartment contains mobile phase along with an eluted solute. These two solutions differ in refractive indices. Under this situation, the bending of the refracted beams from the plane mobile phase and the eluate, occurs to a different extent and hence, they do not fall at the same point on the photoelectric surface. As a consequence, the output signal varies. The difference in the output signals is because of the presence of a solute in the eluate and it depends on the actual concentration of a solute in the eluate. The electric signal is then amplified and recorded to provide a chromatogram. The refractive index of a solution depends on the concentration of a solute in it. The higher the concentration of a solute the higher is the refractive index of a solution and the greater is the response from the detector.

Advantages

(i) Refractive index detector is very easy to fabricate.

(ii) It is an universal detector, which can be used for the detection of any kind of a solute.

Disadvantages

(i) Refractive index detector is general rather than selective and hence, responds to the presence of all the compounds, including impurities present in the eluate.

(ii) It is less sensitive compared to the other detectors used in HPLC.

4) Flame ionization detector [FID]

Construction

As the name suggests, flame ionization detector makes use of an oven, wherein a flame is produced by burning hydrogen gas in presence of oxygen or air. A continuously moving wire loop is provided to transport a portion of the eluate in the furnace. As shown in **Fig. 9.34**, two electrodes, anode (A) and cathode (C), are placed on either side of a flame. A definite potential difference is maintained across the two electrodes with the help of a series of batteries. An amplifier and a recorder are included in the circuitry for recording chromatograms.

Working

A continuously moving wire loop transports a portion of the eluate coming out from the column into the furnace, where the solvent is evaporated first. Most organic compounds get pyrolyzed at the temperature provided by H_2–air or H_2–O_2 flame. Certain compounds are able to form ions after pyrolysis. These ions are attracted, either towards an anode or towards a cathode, depending on the charge present on them. The attraction of ions by the electrode results in the change in the potential difference across the electrodes, which in turn results in the change in the current in the circuit. The electrical resistance of a flame is very high (as high as $10^{12}\ \Omega$) and the resulting current is therefore, minuscule. In order to measure small magnitude of current accurately, an *electrometer* must be employed.

The volatile products, which are able to form ions after pyrolysis, are detected by the ionization detector. Ionization of carbon compounds is poorly understood, although it is known that the number of ions produced is roughly proportional to the number of reduced carbon atoms in the flame. The

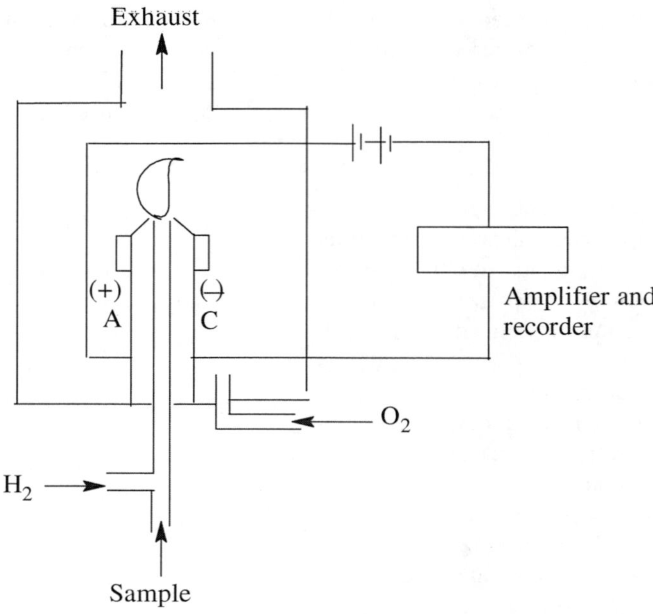

Fig. 9.34: Flame ionization detector

functional groups such as carbonyl, hydroxyl and amino, produce fewer ions or none at all during pyrolysis and therefore, the change in the current is not much when these species are introduced in the flame. Hence, their detection by flame ionization detector is difficult.

Advantages

(i) Flame ionization detector can detect minute quantities of solutes and hence, it is the most sensitive and one of the most popular detectors.

(ii) It produces linear response over a wide range of concentration.

Disadvantages

(i) Hydrogen flame ionization detector is more complicated and more expensive than other detectors.

(ii) The biggest disadvantage of this detector is that it is destructive of the sample.

5) Detector based on mass spectrometry

A mass spectrometer has also been employed as a sensitive and a specific detector in chromatography. A stainless steel or a polyamide belt is used to pass the eluate in an IR evaporator to remove most of the solvent. The vapor of the solvent is sucked by using vacuum. Then the solute in the solid state is allowed to pass through the ion source of a mass spectrometer. Here, the sample is flash vaporized and ionized. The ions are then identified in the mass spectrum based on their m/z values. The intensity of the peaks in the mass spectrum provides idea about the concentration of solutes in the eluate and the m/z values help in the identification of fractions.

Advantage

It is a very sensitive and specific detector. Detection limits with this detector are as low as 0.2-1 ng.

Disadvantage

This is an expensive method for the detection of solutes.

9.11. DETAILED DISCUSSION OF CHROMATOGRAPHIC TECHNIQUES

9.11.1. Column Chromatography

9.11.1.1. Adsorption chromatography
9.11.1.2. Partition chromatography
9.11.1.3. Ion-exchange chromatography
9.11.1.4. Gel chromatography
9.11.1.5. Ion-pair chromatography
9.11.1.6. Chiral chromatography
9.11.1.7. Affinity chromatography

9.11.2. Planar Chromatography

9.11.2.1. Thin layer chromatography (TLC)
9.11.2.2. Paper chromatography (PC)
9.11.2.3. High pressure thin layer chromatography (HPTLC)

9.11.1.1. Adsorption Chromatography

1) Principle

This is a liquid-solid chromatography, in which liquid is used as a mobile phase and solid is used as a stationary phase. In adsorption chromatography, the type of interaction of a solute with the stationary phase is *adsorption*. The separation of solutes is based on the difference in the distribution coefficients of solutes X and Y, which can be expressed as follows.

$$K_X = \frac{(C_S)_X}{(C_M)_X}$$

$$\text{Similarly}, K_Y = \frac{(C_S)_Y}{(C_M)_Y}$$

where, K_X and K_Y are distribution coefficients for solutes X and Y, respectively, $(C_S)_X$ and $(C_S)_Y$ are the concentrations of solutes X and Y, respectively, in the stationary phase and $(C_M)_X$ and $(C_M)_Y$ are the concentrations of solutes X and Y, respectively, in the mobile phase. The two solutes X and Y can be separated from each other, only if K_X and K_Y are different. If K_X and K_Y are not same, their degree of adsorption on the stationary phase varies. A solute having greater distribution coefficient, possesses a greater degree of adsorption on the stationary phase and is retained for a longer time in the column as compared to a solute having smaller distribution coefficient and a smaller degree of adsorption.

2) Stationary phase

In adsorption chromatography, the stationary phase is a finely divided solid silica gel or alumina. Ideally, distribution of a solute between a mobile phase and an adsorbing solid is described by an adsorption isotherm, as shown in **Fig. 9.35**. The curve is nearly a straight line at low concentrations. Beyond a particular concentration of a solute in the mobile phase, there is no corresponding increase in its concentration in the stationary phase, even if its concentration in the mobile phase is increased, as indicated by a plateau in **Fig. 9.35**.

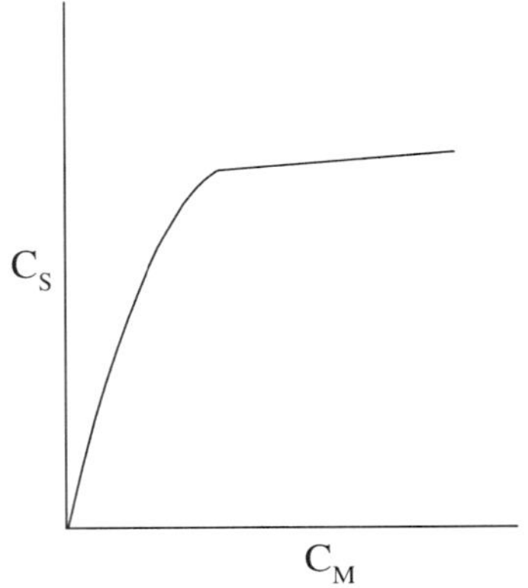

Fig. 9.35: Adsorption isotherm in adsorption chromatography

3) Mobile phase

The change in the stationary phase of a column is not easy since, columns are expensive. Hence, the choice of a mobile phase is very important in the clear separation of solutes from each other. By varying mobile phase, the selectivity factor (α) and the capacity factor (k') for a solute can be varied until they fall in the range of 2-5. The effect of a given solvent on k' depends upon its eluent strength ε^o, which can be measured relative to some reference solvent. Thus, for a solute X, it has been shown that -

$$\log \frac{(K_X)_1}{(K_X)_2} = A_X \left(\varepsilon_2^o - \varepsilon_1^o\right) ... \text{(9.21)}$$

where, $(K_X)_1$ and $(K_X)_2$ are the partition coefficients of solute X in two mobile phases 1 and 2, respectively, A_X is the molecular size of solute X and $\varepsilon_1{}^o$ and $\varepsilon_2{}^o$ are the eluent strengths of two mobile phases 1 and 2, respectively. The eluent strength of a reference is taken as zero. A solvent with the higher eluent strength elutes an adsorbed species more rapidly than one with the lower value. The ε^o values for silica gel are equal to about 0.77 that for alumina.

4) Applications

Adsorption chromatography is mainly used for the separation or identification of compounds with different functional groups. The tendency of a solute to get adsorbed on a polar stationary phase (normal phase chromatography) decreases in the following order -

Acid > Alcohol > Carbonyl > Ester >Hydrocarbon

9.11.1.2. Partition Chromatography

1) Principle

Partition chromatography is a liquid-liquid chromatography, which makes use of a liquid as a stationary phase. Another liquid, which is immiscible with the liquid used as a stationary phase, is immobilized on some solid support and is used as a mobile phase. In partition chromatography, a solute gets partitioned between the stationary and the mobile phases. The separation of solutes is based on the difference in the partition coefficients of solutes X and Y, which are expressed as -

$$K_X = \frac{(C_S)_X}{(C_M)_X} \text{ and } K_Y = \frac{(C_S)_Y}{(C_M)_Y}$$

Here, K_X and K_Y are the partition coefficients for solutes X and Y, respectively, $(C_S)_X$ and $(C_S)_Y$ are the concentrations of solutes X and Y, respectively, in the stationary phase and $(C_M)_X$ and $(C_M)_Y$ are the concentrations of solutes X and Y, respectively, in the mobile phase. Two solutes X and Y can be separated from each other, only if K_X and K_Y are different, since their degree of partitioning between the phases varies. A solute having higher solubility in the stationary phase is retained in the column for a longer time as compared to a solute having lower solubility in the stationary phase.

2) Solid supports

The most widely used solid support for partition chromatography is silica gel. In case of a requirement of a non-polar liquid as the stationary phase, other support media like alumina, diatomaceous earth, starch, cellulose and powdered glass can also be made use of.

3) Stationary phase

Whenever silica gel is used as a solid support, because of its polar nature, it often adsorbs atmospheric moisture and hence, the stationary phase is aqueous as a consequence. For the same reason, in some separations, buffers or other polar liquids like strong acids or bases in water, aliphatic alcohols, glycols, or nitromethane alone or mixed with H_2O are used as stationary phases.

4) Mobile phase

The mobile phase in partition chromatography may be a pure solvent or a mixture of solvents, but it should be immiscible with the liquid used as a stationary phase. If the stationary phase is more polar and the mobile phase is less polar in nature then the technique is termed as *normal phase chromatography.* If the stationary phase is less polar and the mobile phase is more polar in nature then the technique is termed as *reverse phase chromatography.*

5) Applications

Partition chromatography has become a powerful tool for the separation of closely related substances, e.g. separation of numerous amino acids formed in the hydrolysis of a protein can be separated using partition chromatography. Similarly, the separation and analysis of closely related aliphatic alcohols and of sugar derivatives is also carried out successfully by using a technique of partition chromatography.

9.11.1.3. Ion-Exchange Chromatography

1) Principle

It is a liquid-solid chromatography. Ion-exchange chromatography involves the exchange of ions of like sign between a solution of a solute and an ion-exchange resin in contact with the solution. This technique finds special application in the separation of compounds existing in the form of ions. Two ions can be separated from each other if they have different degree of affinity for the stationary phase in the form of an ion-exchange resin. An ion possessing greater affinity for the ion-exchange resin lags behind an ion having lesser affinity.

2) Stationary Phase

An ion-exchange resin acts as a stationary phase in this technique. Following two types of ion-exchange resins are commonly in use.

(A) Natural ion-exchange resins ˘ The ion-exchange resins like *clays and zeolites* are commonly used as the stationary phase in case of ion-exchange chromatography.

(B) Synthetic ion-exchange resins ˘ These resins are high molecular weight polymeric materials, containing a large number of ionic functional groups per molecule. These ionic functional groups may be cationic or anionic in nature, i.e. they involve exchange of either cations or anions of solutes with cations or anions of an ion exchange resin. Accordingly, resins are categorized as follows.

a) Cation exchange resins
b) Anion exchange resins

a) Cation exchange resins

The cation exchange resins contain acidic groups. They are sub-classified as follows.

(i) Strongly acidic resins, which consist of sulfonic acids ($R.SO_3^-$ H^+)
(ii) Weakly acidic resins, which consist of carboxylic acids (R.COOH)

The strongly acidic resins are used widely.

b) Anion exchange resins

The anion exchange resins contain basic groups. They are sub-classified as follows.

(i) Strongly basic resins, which consist of quaternary amines
(ii) Weakly basic resins, which consist of secondary or tertiary amines

For a particular solute MA, dissociating into M^+ and A^- ions in aqueous solution, following reactions take place on the cationic and the anionic resins in the column.

$$MA \rightarrow M^+ + A^-$$

$RSO_3^-H^+$ + M^+
Cationic resin   Cation in solution

↓

$RSO_3^-M^+$ + H^+
Cation on resin   Ion released from resin

Similarly,

$RN^+(CH_3)_3OH^-$ + A^-
Anionic resin   Anion in solution

↓

$[RN^+(CH_3)_3]A^-$ + OH^-
Anion on resin   Ion released from resin

$$H^+ + OH^- \rightarrow H_2O$$

3) Mobile Phase

In contrast to the other chromatographic methods, the mobile phase is generally water or aqueous solution.

4) Applications

In case of ion-exchange chromatography, the species to be separated are ionic in nature. Hence, this technique finds wide use in inorganic chemistry. The polyvalent ions are much more strongly held than the singly charged species within a given charge group. However, affinity of ions for the stationary phase is related to the size of the hydrated ions as well as to the other properties. Thus, for a typical sulfonated cation exchange resin, the distribution coefficient (K_D) for different ions is in the following order.

$Cs^+ > Rb^+ > K^+ > NH_4^+ > Na^+ > H^+ > Li^+$

For divalent cations, the order is as follows.

$Ba^{+2} > Pb^{+2} > Sr^{+2} > Ca^{+2} > Cd^{+2} > Cu^{+2} > Zn^{+2} > Mg^{+2}$

Ion-exchange chromatography also finds extensive use in the separation of amino acids and other organic acids and bases.

In order to show that the general principles of chromatography can be applied to the separation carried out by using an ion-exchange resin as the stationary phase, consider that a cation B^+ is interacting with an ion exchange resin (RH). The following equilibrium is established between the concentration of a solute in the stationary phase and that in the mobile phase.

$$RH + B^+ \rightleftarrows RB + H^+$$

$$\therefore K = \frac{[RB][H^+]}{[RH][B^+]} \cdots (9.22)$$

where, K is the equilibrium constant for an ion exchange reaction between the solute and the resin, [RB] is the concentration of an analyte on the cationic resin and [RH] is the concentration of hydrogen ions on the resin. This also represents the availability of the active sites on the resin. The term $[B^+]$ represents the concentration of an analyte in the mobile phase and the term $[H^+]$ represents the concentration of hydrogen ions in the mobile phase. Rearranging the terms in **equation (9.22)**, **equation (9.23)** is obtained.

$$\frac{[RB]}{[B^+]} = \frac{K[RH]}{[H^+]} = K_D \cdots (9.23)$$

where, K_D is the distribution coefficient of a solute. Once the cation is taken up by the resin, it is to be slowly eluted out of the column by the addition of an acid like HCl. Thus, B^+ ions are released from the resin into the mobile phase. With the addition of enough hydrochloric acid, complete elution of B^+ ions occurs from the column.

In **equation 9.23**, the term on the left side, i.e. the ratio of [RB] to $[B^+]$, represents the ratio of the concentration of a solute on the stationary phase (C_S) to its concentration in the mobile phase (C_M). Similarly, the term on the right hand side, i.e. the ratio of [RH] to $[H^+]$, represents the ratio of the total number of active sites on the resin to the concentration of H^+ ions in the mobile phase. Thus, **equation 9.23** can be written as follows.

$$\frac{[C_S]}{[C_M]} = \frac{K[RH]}{[H^+]} = K_D \cdots (9.24)$$

In order to apply principles of chromatographic separations to ion-exchange chromatography, the ratio on the left hand side of **equation 9.24** should remain constant. On the right hand side, the parameter K, the equilibrium constant, is a constant term. The term [RH] can be assumed to remain constant even when certain sites on the resin are occupied by the cations (B^+) of a solute. This is because the number of available active sites on the resin is too large as compared to the number of active sites occupied by the cations of a solute. To make it simple, let us assume that the available active sites on the resin are 1 lakh and the solute occupies only 100 sites on it. Since the concentration of a solute is low, the number of ions (B^+) of a solute is considerably smaller than the number of H^+ ions available on the resin. Hence, the exchange of H^+ ions of the resin with few B^+ ions of a solute does not lead to a substantial decrease in the number of active sites available on the stationary phase. Therefore, [RH] is considered to be unaltered and hence, it represents another constant term on the right hand side of equation **9.24**. Similarly, the term [H^+] represents the third constant term on the right hand side of **equation 9.24**. This is because the concentration of H^+ ions is due to the passage of HCl as the mobile phase. The number of H^+ ions present in the mobile phase is very large. When the B^+ cations of the solute occupy some sites on the resin, it results in the liberation of H^+ ions from the resin into the mobile phase, but since the amount of solute loaded on the column is very small, the number of H^+ ions liberated by it is also very small as compared to the number of H^+ ions present in the mobile phase. Thus, all the three terms on the right hand side of **equation 9.24** are constant. Hence, the left hand side of **equation 9.24** should also be constant. Since the ratio of C_S to C_M remains constant, all the principles of chromatographic separation can be very well applied to the separation carried out by using ion-exchange resins.

9.11.1.4. Gel Chromatography

Gel chromatography is also known as *gel permeation chromatography* or *exclusion chromatography* or *molecular sieve chromatography*.

1) Principle

In gel chromatography, the fractionation is based mainly upon the molecular size and partly upon the shape of the species in the sample and sometimes, upon their tendency to be adsorbed on the gel. When solute molecules of different sizes are introduced in the column containing a polymeric gel as a stationary phase, the smaller molecules enter into the polymeric network (interstices) of the gel, whereas the bigger molecules are unable to enter the interstices **(Fig 9.36)**. Because of this, the bigger molecules escape through the space between the particles of the stationary phase and experience less hindrance to their motion. The smaller molecules are retarded, since they experience more hindrance to their motion and hence, take a longer time for their elution as compared to the bigger molecules. The degree of retardation depends upon the extent to which the solute molecules or ions can penetrate the interstices or the pores of the polymeric network. The molecules or ions larger than the pores of the gel are completely excluded from the interior, while smaller species are more or less free to enter these regions. This provides the difference in the time of elution of the compounds

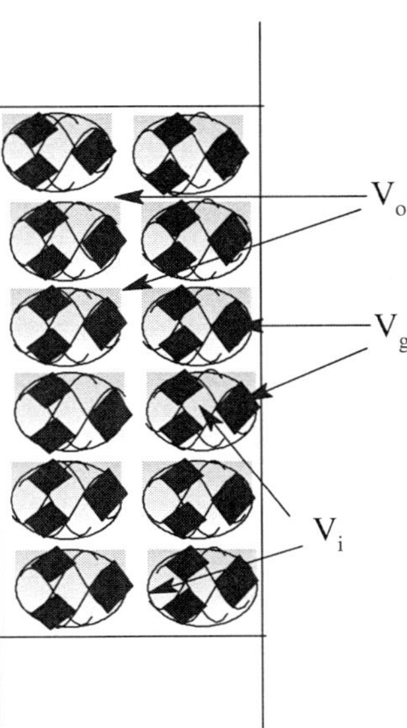

Fig. 9.36: Polymeric network in gel chromatography

from their mixture and allows clear separation of compounds of different sizes.

2) Stationary phase

The stationary phase in gel chromatography is a liquid held in the interstices of the beads of the porous polymeric material. The polymeric gel is soaked in water or some other solvent, which is to be used as the stationary phase. Gel readily absorbs water or a solvent, which is held in the interstices of the polymeric network. The average size of the resulting pores or the interstices in the gel is directly related to the quantity of the solvent absorbed, which in turn is determined by the degree of cross-linking in the polymer molecules. When a polymer swells by absorbing water, the technique is called as *gel filtration chromatography* and when a polymer swells by absorbing non-polar organic solvent, the technique is called as *gel permeation chromatography*. The former technique makes use of hydrophilic polymer packing whereas the latter technique makes use of hydrophobic polymer packing.

One of the most widely used polymers is prepared by cross-linking the polysaccharide *dextran* with *epichlorhydrin*. By varying the amount of the latter, a series of resins with differing pore size is obtained. These gels sell under the trade name of *Sephadex*. Another group of commercial resins consists of *polyacrylamide* cross-linked with *methylene-bis-acrylamide*.

3) Mobile phase

The mobile phase can be either a polar or a non-polar liquid. Unlike other chromatographic techniques, the separation of solids by gel chromatography is not by the interaction of solutes with the mobile phase, but depends on the degree of retardation of solutes in the gel. The role of the mobile phase is just to push the solutes down the column.

4) Applications

(i) Tightly cross-linked gels with small pores, such as *Sephadex G-25* and *G-50,* have found wide applications in effective separation of amino acids like cysteine, glycine, phenylalanine, etc. from polypeptides or low molecular weight proteins like trypsin, pepsin, and so on.

(ii) *Sephadex G-25* and *G-50* are also useful in the separation of low molecular weight proteins from the medium molecular weight proteins like nucleic acids, polysaccharides, ribonuclease, cytoctrome C, etc.

(iii) More porous gels like *Sephadex G-75*, have found wide applications for the separation of the medium molecular weight proteins from the high molecular weight proteins such as serum albumin, hemoglobin and fibrinogen.

(iv) Gel chromatography is also used by polymer chemists and biochemists to estimate molecular weights of compounds.

5) Theory of gel chromatography

As shown in **Fig. 9.36**, the total volume of a column packed with a gel that has been swelled by H_2O (or other solvent) is given by **equation 9.25**.

$$V_t = V_g + V_i + V_o \quad \dots (9.25)$$

where, V_g is the volume occupied by the solid matrix of the gel, V_i is the volume of the solvent held in the interstices of the gel and V_o is the volume of the space outside the gel particles. Assuming that all the particles of a bigger solute remain in the space between the particles of the gel, throughout the length of the stationary phase and no particles enter the interstices of the polymeric network, V_o also represents the volume of the solvent required to carry through the column, those compounds too large to enter the pores of the gel. However, in practice, some mixing and diffusion does occur and as a consequence, the compounds appear in a Gaussian shaped band with a concentration maximum at V_o. The solutes which are smaller in size enter freely into the interstices of the gel. The band maxima for small molecules appear at the end of the column because of the higher degree of retardation, at an elution volume corresponding to ($V_i + V_o$). The molecules which are of the intermediate size and are able to enter the interstices of the gel in some fraction k_d, require the elution volume V_e, which is expressed by **equation (9.26).**

$$V_e = V_o + k_d V_i \; ... \; (9.26)$$

This **equation (9.26)** describes the behavior of a gel column with reference to all the solutes, which get eluted out from the column. For molecules too large to enter the interstices of the gel, $k_d = 0$ and $V_e = V_o$. For molecules that can enter the pores unhindered, $k_d = 1$ and $V_e = (V_o + V_i)$. **Equation (9.26)** is derived by assuming that there is no interaction between the solute molecules and the gel surface (Adsorption). If such an interaction does occur, the amount of interstitially held solute increases. For interacting solutes that can freely enter the pores, k_d will be greater than unity.

9.11.1.5. Ion-Pair Chromatography or Soap Chromatography

1) Principle

Ion-pair chromatography is a type of reverse phase partition chromatography that is used for the separation and determination of ionic species. In reverse phase chromatography, the stationary phase is non-polar or less polar as compared to the mobile phase. In ion-pair chromatography, the sample is introduced in the form of ions. The mobile phase is aqueous in nature and is mixed with *a pairing agent*. A pairing agent is ionic in nature and interacts with the solutes to be separated. When it is loaded on the column, either the cations or the anions of the pairing agent, pair up with the oppositely charged ions of the solutes in the sample and form undissociated neutral species called *ion-pairs*. An ion-pair being undissociated, interacts more with a less polar or a non-polar stationary phase in the column as compared to the more polar mobile phase. Thus, in ion-pair chromatography, a pairing agent converts an ionic compound into an undissociated ion-pair. For different solutes, different ion-pairs are formed.

2) Stationary phase

The stationary phase used in the reverse phase chromatography is non-polar or less polar compared to the mobile phase. The bonded packing in the form of chlorooctadecylisilane (C_{18}) is used as the stationary phase.

3) Mobile phase

The mobile phase in the ion-pair chromatography consists of an aqueous buffer containing an organic solvent such as methanol or acetonitrile and an ionic compound (a pairing agent) containing a *counter ion* (an ion bearing charge opposite to that of an analyte ion). A counter ion combines with the analyte ion to form an ion-pair which is retained by the reverse phase packing.

4) Pairing agents

The pairing agents provide either cations or anions for the interaction with the oppositely charged ions of an analyte. For the formation of an ion-pair, a substance to be analyzed is dissolved in aqueous solution (acid, base or buffer). Amines ($R\text{-}NH_2$) are dissolved in acid and therefore, exist as $R\text{-}(NH_3)^+$ in acids. For this positively charged species, a pairing agent is the perchlorate (ClO_4^-) anion. Thus, the positively charged species from an analyte and the negatively charged species from a pairing agent form an ion-pair, $[R\text{-}(NH_3)]^+ [ClO_4]^-$. This species remains undissociated and hence, interacts more with the non-polar stationary phase. The carboxylic acids exist as $RCOO^-$ and the sulfonic acids exist as RSO_3^-, when dissolved in a base. For these anions, the pairing agent is the tetrabutylammonium $[(C_4H_9)_4 N^+]$ cation. Thus, the pairing agents, most frequently used to provide anion to the cation of an analyte are – the long chain alkylsulfates, usually 4-8 carbon alkylsulfates. The pairing agents, most frequently used to provide cation to the anion of an analyte are – the long chain alkylammonium salts, i. e. tetramethyl, tetraethyl, tetrapropyl or tetrabutylammonium salts. As the chain length of the pairing agent increases, the retention time of an ion-pair on the stationary phase also increases. The concentration of the pairing ion also affects the retention time of an ion-pair. Increasing the pairing ion concentration increases the retention time but the effect is less dramatic than that seen with the increase in the chain length. Increasing the concentration of the pairing agent is limited by the solubility of the pairing ions. The effect of pH on the retention time of an ion-pair is determined by the type of ion being analyzed. The pH of the mobile phase is usually adjusted so that the analyte exists entirely in the desired ionic form.

5) Applications

(i) Applications of ion-pair chromatography frequently overlap those of an ion-exchange chromatography. Ion-exchange chromatography is usually performed for the separation of small inorganic and organic ions. Ion-exchange chromatography cannot be used for the separation of ions which are bigger in size. Hence, for the separation of ions like chlorate and nitrate, ion-pair method is preferred to ion-exchange chromatography. With large ions, the resolution by ion-exchange chromatography is often impaired because ion-exchange resins have tight internal networks that slow the mass transfer process with a consequent loss of efficiency.

(ii) Ion-pair chromatography is preferred when the species to be separated have a high affinity for ion-exchangers, which make their elution difficult. For the same reason, the surfactants are not separated using ion-exchange chromatography but the ion-pair chromatography is the preferred method for them. Moreover, because of the bigger size of the surfactant ions, ion-pair chromatography becomes the method of choice for their separation. Since ion-pair chromatography is commonly used for surfactants, the method is also termed as *soap chromatography.*

9.11.1.6. Chiral Chromatography

Resolution of enantiomers by liquid chromatography is called as *chiral chromatography*. Many drugs such as β-blockers (propranolol, metropolol), calcium channel blockers (captopril, enalapril) etc. are chiral in nature. The two enantiomers usually exhibit different physiological properties. Sometimes, one enantiomer is therapeutically useful and another enantiomer produces untoward effects, e.g. the R-isomer of thalidomide is found to be an effective sedative, whereas the S-isomer is teratogenic in nature and causes fetal abnormalities. Similarly, (S,S) ethambutol is tuberculostatic and (R,R) isomer causes optical neuritis or blindness. The therapeutic effect of â-blockers like propranolol and atenolol is due to S-enantiomer and R-enantiomer just contributes to the *isomeric ballast* (an effect contributing only to the side effects of the drug and not to its therapeutic activity). Hence, there is a need of separation of enantiomers from their mixture. The general method to separate enantiomers is to convert them to diastereomers by reacting them with another chiral substance. This is explained with the help of the formation of an epoxide in **Fig. 9.37**.

Enantiomers have the same physicochemical properties but they differ in the rate of reaction with another chiral reagent. Diastereomers have the same chemical properties but different physical properties. Hence, diastereomers have different densities, solubilities, melting points, affinity for the stationary phase, etc. They can therefore, be separated from each other by fractional crystallization method. Separation of enantiomers, based on the difference in their physical properties, is not 100 % in most of the racemic mixtures. The traditional methods like optical rotation measurement or the fractional crystallization of diasteromers, for determining the composition of enantiomers in the racemic mixture, are insensitive and inaccurate. Chiral chromatography provides an accurate,

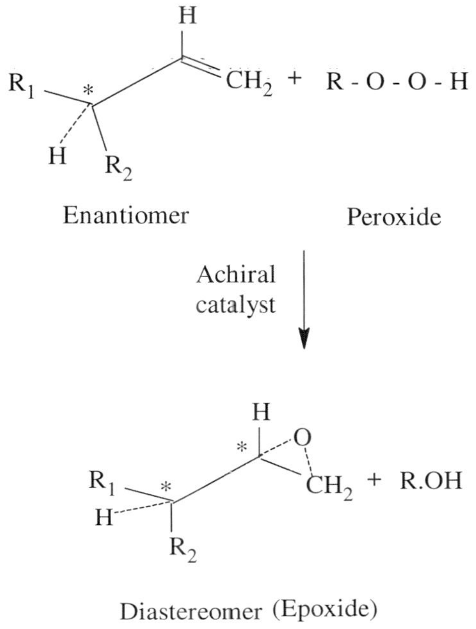

$$R_1\text{-}\overset{*}{C}H(R_2)\text{-}CH{=}CH_2 + R\text{-}O\text{-}O\text{-}H$$

Enantiomer Peroxide

Achiral catalyst ↓

$$R_1\text{-}\overset{*}{C}H(R_2)\text{-}\overset{*}{C}H(O)CH_2 + R.OH$$

Diastereomer (Epoxide)

Fig. 9.37: Formation of a diastereomer from an enantiomer

reproducible, sensitive, specific and rapid method for determination of an enantiomeric composition.

Chiral Chromatography can be carried out in three different ways for the separation of enantiomers.

1) Indirect liquid chromatographic resolution of enantiomers via precolumn derivatization
2) Direct resolution of enantiomers on an achiral stationary phase
3) Direct resolution of enantiomers using selective chiral stationary phases

1) Indirect liquid chromatographic resolution of enantiomers via precolumn derivatization

Principle

In precolumn derivatization, enantiomers are converted into diastereomers, before they are fed to the column. Because of the difference in the affinity for the stationary phase, diastereomers can be easily separated by chromatography. In this case, enantiomers are reacted with a chiral substance to get diastereomers. For example, a mixture of S and R isomers of ibuprofen (IBP), when reacted with R- proline, produces two diastereomers as shown in **Fig. 9.38**.

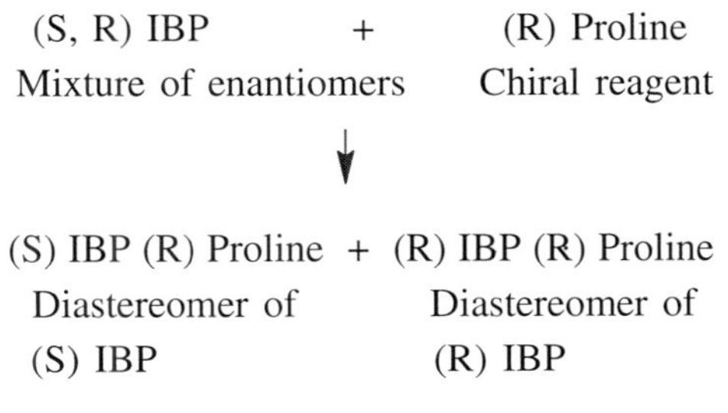

(S, R) IBP + (R) Proline
Mixture of enantiomers Chiral reagent

↓

(S) IBP (R) Proline + (R) IBP (R) Proline
Diastereomer of (S) IBP Diastereomer of (R) IBP

Fig. 9.38: Formation of diastereomers from enantiomers of ibuprofen

The chiral reagent used for converting enantiomers to diastereomers should react quantitatively with enantiomers for accurate determination of enantiomeric composition. Different types of chiral derivatizing agents are used for drugs with different functional groups. For drugs containing amino group, e.g. in many non-steroidal anti-inflammatory drugs (NSAIDS), the chiral reagents like acyl chlorides or acids, or the reagents possessing isocyanate or isothiocyanate group, can be used for getting diastereomers.

Two diastereomers, though chiral in nature, differ in their affinity towards an achiral stationary phase and hence, can be separated on an achiral stationary phase using an achiral mobile phase. Achiral stationary phases, like silica gel, alumina, celite, etc. can be used for their separation. Similarly, the mobile phases consisting of methanol, acetonitrile, water, etc. can be used for the separation of diastereomers.

2) Direct resolution of enantiomers on an achiral stationary phase

Principle

This technique does not require derivatization of enantiomers using chiral reagent. It does not require chiral stationary phase also, but it requires a mobile phase containing *chiral additives*. A suitable chiral reagent is added to the mobile phase. The chiral enantiomers from the racemic mixture react with the chiral additive in the mobile phase and form diasteromers, which can be separated by reverse phase chromatography. A diastereomer, which is adsorbed strongly on the stationary phase, is retained for a longer time on the column and a diasteromer, which has more affinity for the mobile phase, is eluted out first.

Based on the type of chiral additives and the mechanism under which enantioselectivity is achieved, this technique is classified as –

(i) Ligand exchange chromatography
(ii) Chiral ion–pair chromatography
(iii)Chromatography using mobile phases containing macromolecular aggregates

(i) Ligand exchange chromatography

This method is commonly used for the resolution of enantiomers of amino acids. Here, the stationary phase consists of a *polymeric resin*, bonded to transition metal ions such as Cu^{+2} ions. The cupric (Cu^{+2}) ions are the most frequently used transition metal ions because of their strong chelating ability, so that they react quantitatively with amino acids. The amino group of amino acids possesses a lone pair of electrons and hence, acts as a *ligand*. A lone pair of electrons can be donated to the transition meal ion (Cu^{+2} ion), which acts as an *acceptor*. The reaction between a ligand and an acceptor results in the formation of a *complex* or a *chelate*. Each amino acid has different affinity for an acceptor (Cu^{+2} ions) on the stationary phase. Hence, the stationary phase has the enantioselectivity for amino acids to be resolved. The affinity of different amino acids towards an acceptor on the stationary phase, the stability of a complex between the ligand and an acceptor, and the affinity of the complex or a chelate formed on the stationary phase towards the mobile phase, decide the retention time of amino acids in the column. Thus, two enantiomers of an optically active amino acid can be separated. This kind of a stationary phase cannot be used under high pressure. Hence, a number of acceptors were then bonded to silica gel in place of a polymeric resin. This could be used under high pressure and hence, can be used for the separation of enantiomers of amino acids using HPLC. The elution of amino acids from the column is brought about by using optically pure amino acid or its derivative.

(ii) Chiral ion-pair chromatography

Principle

In ion-pair chromatography, ionic compounds are reacted with counter ions added to the mobile phase and are converted into non-polar compounds, which can then be separated by reverse phase chromatography. If the counter ion is chiral then the ionic chiral enantiomers can form *diastereomeric ion-pairs*. The mobile phases of low polarity are normally used to allow the satisfactory degree of ion-pair formation. The stereo-selectivity of the separation is dependent on the structure of the counter-ion added. Usually, the enantioselectivity of the separation is high when the counter-ion containing binding groups having a rigid ring system with bulky groups, is in the vicinity of the chiral centre. The commonly used chiral counter ion is quinine, camphor sulfonate or tartaric acid ester. These can be used to separate carboxylic acids or amines. The stationary phase used for the chiral ion-pair chromatography is normally non-polar in nature, as in case of a C_{18} column.

(iii) Chromatography using mobile phases containing macromolecular aggregates

Proteins and cyclodextrins are the natural macromolecules, which bind stereoselectively with low molecular weight molecules. Hence, if macromolecules are used as mobile phase additives, they can bind selectively with low molecular weight molecules. Cyclodextrin is available in different molecular sizes because it is produced by partial degradation of starch followed by the enzymatic coupling of the glucose units. Thus, cyclodextrins are chiral structures. β-Cyclodextrin has 35 stereogenic centres. Cyclodextrins, which are bound chemically to silica gel, are available in market under the trade name of *Cyclobond*. Apart from α, β and γ cyclodextrins, human serum albumin can also be used as a chiral mobile phase additive. The stationary phase used for the separation of enantiomers in both the cases is tetraoctadecylsilane (C_{18} column).

3) Direct resolution of enantiomers using selective chiral stationary phases

Chiral compounds can also be separated using chiral stationary phase. Chiral molecules react with another chiral moiety at a definite rate. Difference in the rate of reaction of chiral solutes with chiral stationary phase is made use of in the separation of enantiomers from their mixture. Commercially used chiral stationary phases are columns having chiral molecules bonded to the support. Examples of chiral molecules, which can be bonded to the stationary phase in the column are – R-phenylglycine, R- or S-leucine, R- or S-naphthylamine, α, β and γ cyclodextrins, etc.

9.11.1.7. Affinity Chromatography

1) Principle

Unlike most of the chromatographic methods, affinity chromatography is a *non-partition chromatography*, wherein solutes to be separated do not get partitioned between the stationary and the mobile phases. The major application of affinity columns is in the purification of proteins by HPLC. Only one solute can be separated from a multi-component mixture, using this technique. Hence, this technique provides very high specificity.

In affinity chromatography, specific types of molecules are bound to the column. These molecules are called as *recognizers*. The compound to be separated or purified is called as a *target compound*. The recognizer forms a tight complex with one and only one site on the compound to be purified. Such a column must be used for the separation of a particular compound or a particular class of compounds, wherein the structures are closely related to each other, because the recognizer attached to the column cannot be removed and used for the separation of other compounds.

The principle used in the affinity separation is analogous to the reaction between a substrate and a receptor site or a substrate and an enzyme, which fit with each other similar to a lock and key. The recognizer on the affinity column is the lock and the target site on the compound to be separated is the key. When a solution containing the target compound is loaded on the affinity column, only one compound is taken up by the recognizer on the column and other compounds escape freely, out of the column. The target compound bound to the recognizer on the column can be eluted out with a change in pH or with the use of a concentrated salt solution or by using a molecule similar to the recognizer.

2) Stationary phase

The column used is usually broad and short with a large surface area of the stationary phase. A suitable recognizer is bound chemically to the stationary phase, which provides specificity for the compound or a target to be separated. Then the slurry of this stationary phase is packed into the column. The column packing can be modified in a number of ways for different applications. By knowing the 'key' characteristics of the substrates, the 'locks' or the molecules, into which this key can be exactly fitted, can be synthesized or isolated from some sources. These molecules are then attached to the column and act as recognizers on affinity supports. These molecules are often bound to a 6-carbon spacer so that they protrude farther away from the packing surface towards the mobile phase and are therefore, more available for the sample solution. The recognizers can be used to separate only one compound selectively or a range or a class of compounds. For the separation of metal ions, ligands are chemically bound to the stationary phase. For the separation of immunoglobulin (IgG) or any antibody, antigen columns are used, which are microporous and cross-linked polymers.

3) Mobile phase

The elution of a solute from the column can be made using concentrated salt solution or by changing the pH of the mobile phase, to break the complex between the recognizer and a target. For a very tightly bound material, the natural substrate, which can form a very tightly bound complex with the target and breaks a complex of a target with the recognizer on the stationary phase, is required to be added. Thus, a natural substrate results into a tighter fit and serves as a displacer for the solute on the stationary phase. For example, the metal ions can be eluted out from the affinity column, by using a strong metal chelator such as EDTA as a mobile phase, which helps in breaking the binding between the metal ion and the stationary phase. Similarly, elution of IgG can be achieved using buffers with different pH values.

4) Applications

(i) Affinity chromatography is commonly used for the separation of proteins. The stationary phase, in this case, contains enzyme recognition sites as recognizers.

(ii) Affinity chromatography is also used for the separation of antibodies, where antigens are bound chemically to the stationary phase. Antibodies have a specific three dimensional shapes and specific distribution of an electrical charge. Because of this, these substrates interact with only specific molecules.

(iii) Analysis of enzymes can also be carried out by using affinity chromatography. For the separation of enzymes, called hydrogenases, certain natural and synthetic dyes have been used to build affinity columns. Many enzymes require vitamins or metal ions as cofactors for their activity and therefore, they are used as recognizers for building affinity columns. These recognizers can also be used for purification of enzymes from other impurities.

(iv) Affinity chromatography can also be used for the separation of optical isomers, since one optical isomer of the isomeric pair can approach and bind the chiral compound better and faster than the other, leading to their separation.

Advantage

Because of very high specificity, affinity chromatography provides 100 % pure compounds from a very complex mixture in a single run.

Disadvantages

(i) It suffers from the major drawback of finding the specific recognizer for a particular target and binding it to the column. Developing optimum eluting conditions for the target is also difficult.

(ii) It requires separate column for each new separation. It is more commonly used at low pressure.

9.11.2. Planar Chromatography

In planar chromatography, the stationary phase is present in one plane. The planar chromatography is classified as follows.

9.11.2.1. Thin layer chromatography (TLC)
9.11.2.2. Paper chromatography (PC)
9.11.2.3. High pressure thin layer chromatography (HPTLC)

Though a technique of TLC was developed after paper chromatographic technique, it has acquired a lot of popularity because of its consistency in qualitative and semi-quantitative applications. In TLC, the separation takes place on a thin layer of a finely divided solid that is fixed on a flat surface. In paper chromatography, a sheet or a strip of a good quality and a homogeneous filter paper, serves as the separatory medium.

Advantages of planar chromatography

(i) Both paper and thin layer chromatographic techniques provide remarkably simple and inexpensive means for separating and identifying the compounds of complex inorganic, organic and biochemical substances.
(ii) Both the methods, particularly TLC, permit reasonably accurate determination of the concentration of the compounds in their mixture.
(iv) A number of samples can be analyzed at a time.
(v) The sample is required in very small amount.

General Considerations

Most of the times, planar chromatography is classified as a liquid-liquid chromatography (partition chromatography). In case of thin layer chromatography, when silica gel is used as a support on the plane surface of a glass plate, it adsorbs moisture from atmosphere and this water layer on silica gel acts as a stationary phase. Thus, usually, the stationary phase is H_2O or some other polar liquid. In paper chromatography, liquid entrapped in the pores of the paper, acts as the stationary phase. Planar chromatography can also be used as liquid-solid chromatography (adsorption chromatography) when other solids like alumina or celite are used as stationary phases. Ion-exchange resin can also be used as the stationary phase in planar chromatography. Nowadays, modified surfaces which can provide non-polar surface as the stationary phase, are also encountered. This makes possible the separation of compounds by reverse phase chromatography.

In planar chromatography, a drop of a solution containing the sample is introduced with the help of a capillary, at some point on the planar surface of the stationary phase. The solvent is evaporated from this spot and the planar stationary phase is placed in the container having a mobile phase (the developer). The mobile phase moves across the surface of the stationary phase by the capillary action. The movement of the mobile phase causes solutes in the sample to partition between the stationary phase and the mobile phase and brings about their separation.

The general principles developed earlier for column chromatography, appear to apply equally well to planar chromatography also. Within thin layer and paper as media, the repeated transfers of a solute between the stationary and the mobile phases occur. The rate of movement of a solute depends upon its partition coefficient for the pair of phases. It is customary to describe the travel of a particular solute in terms of its *radiation factor* (R_F), which is defined as the movement of a solute *relative to the solvent front.*

$$R_F = \frac{\text{Distance traveled by the solute}}{\text{Distance traveled by the mobile phase}}$$

To compensate for uncontrolled variables, the distance traveled by a solute is frequently compared with that for a standard substance under identical conditions. The ratio of these distances is designated as R_{std} for a standard substance.

9.11.2.1. Thin Layer Chromatography (TLC)

1) Stationary phase

The most widely used solid support in thin layer chromatography is silica gel, which often functions as a support for water or other polar solvents such as acids, bases, buffers or glycols. If however, the silica layer is oven dried after the preparation of the plate, much of the moisture is lost and the surface becomes predominantly a solid one that serves as an adsorbent for liquid-solid separation. In this latter mode, care must be taken to avoid exposing the surface to the atmosphere, since water adsorption from air occurs in a few moments and the surface then reverts back to the support for a liquid. Ordinarily, particle size of silica gel is 150-250 μm.

2) Mobile Phase

The choice of a mobile phase used in thin layer chromatography is made based on the nature of the solutes to be separated. Either a single solvent or a mixture of solvents can be used. Solvents such as methanol, water, acetic acid, ammonia, etc. can be used.

3) Preparation of plates

A thin layer plate can be prepared by spreading an aqueous slurry of the finely ground solid onto the clean surface of a glass or Mylar plate or a microscope slide. For analyzing many compounds simultaneously, a 20 x 20 cm square glass plate is used. A slurry of silica gel G (silica gel mixed with gypsum) or silica gel GF (silica gel mixed with gypsum and a fluorescent material) is used commonly. Gypsum is used as a binder along with silica gel and is incorporated into the slurry to enhance the adhesion of the solid particles to glass and to each other. Slurry is prepared either in water, methanol or benzene. It should be easily pourable. With the help of an *applicator*, the slurry is spread uniformly on the plate so as to get a constant thickness of the stationary phase. A narrow range of particle size and the uniformity of the thickness of the stationary phase on the plate decide the cleanness of separation on the thin layer. The plate is then allowed to stand in air until the layer has set up and adheres tightly to the surface. Sometimes, plates may be dried in an oven for several hours, in order to activate the surface of the stationary phase. For example, when reverse phase thin layer chromatography is to be carried out, a layer of silica gel can be coated with n-octanol in order to have a less polar stationary phase for the reverse phase chromatography. Silica gel plates are activated by putting them in oven, at least for two hrs. Then the plates are put in the chamber containing n-octanol, which is allowed to rise up the plate through silica gel. In place of n-octanol, any other suitable material can be used for coating silica gel surface. Nowadays, ready made plates for the normal phase and the reverse phase chromatography are available commercially.

4) Plate Development

A drop of sample solutions to be analyzed is introduced, with the help of a capillary or a micro syringe, at some point on the planar surface of the stationary phase on a glass plate or on an aluminum foil. Solvent is evaporated from the spots and the plate is placed in the chamber containing a mobile phase (the developer).

The chamber is kept tightly closed so that it becomes saturated with the vapor of the mobile phase. In order to achieve effective saturation of the chamber, a filter paper is kept immersed in the chamber, throughout its length, as shown in **Fig. 9.39**. The mobile phase rises up through the filter paper and constantly keeps it wet. Evaporation of the solvent from the paper helps to keep the

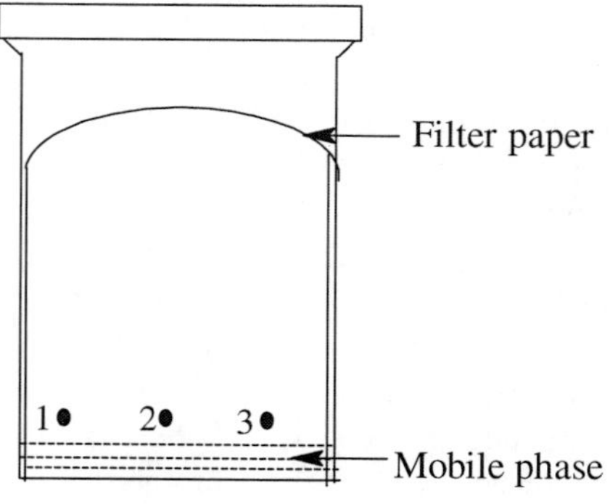

Fig. 9.39: Chamber used for development of the plate (1, 2, and 3 are the spots for analytes)

chamber saturated with vapor of the mobile phase. If the chamber is not saturated, the mobile phase rising through the plate evaporates and then it is not available to the solutes on the plate for the separation purpose. Thus, the proper separation of compounds is not achieved if the chamber is not saturated with the vapor of the mobile phase.

The mobile phase can be passed through the stationary phase on the plate in different ways. The typical arrangements for the development of thin layer plates are discussed below.

(i) Ascending development

In ascending development, the motion of the mobile phase is in upward direction. As shown in **Fig. 9.40(a)**, the plate is introduced in a closed chamber containing mobile phase in such a way that the spot of the sample is above the level of the mobile phase in the chamber. In ascending development, the mobile phase is moving slowly, since its flow is against the force of gravity. Hence, this type of a technique is used when there is a little difference in the R_F values of solutes getting separated on the plate. A plate developed by using this technique is shown in **Fig. 9.40(b)**.

(ii) Descending development

In descending development, the plate is placed on a solid support. A sample is spotted on the top of the plate. As shown in **Fig. 9.41**, the

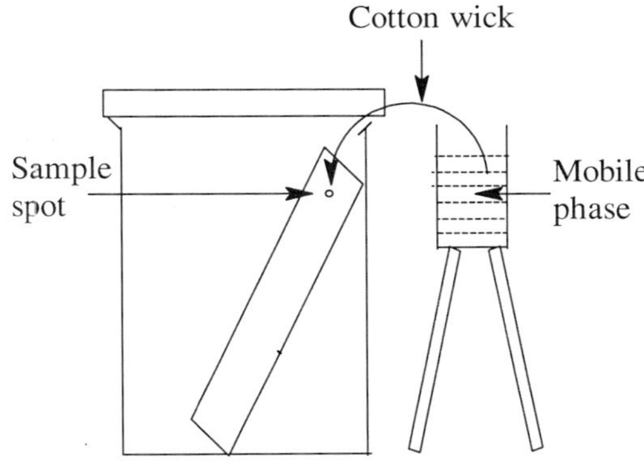

Fig. 9.41: Descending development

mobile phase is kept in a reservoir, which is placed at a height. The mobile phase from the reservoir is passed on to the upper end of the plate, with the help of a cotton wick. The motion of the mobile

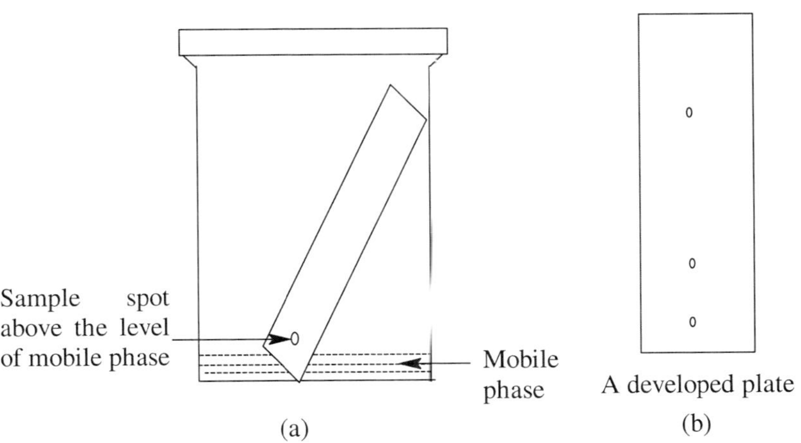

Fig. 9.40: Ascending development of a plate

phase is downward, wherein the gravitational force contributes to the solvent flow. Hence, this type of a technique is used when there is sufficient difference in the R_F values of solutes getting separated on the plate.

(iii) Radial development

In radial development, the sample is spotted at the center of a plate. The mobile phase is dropped at the center, with the help of a cotton wick, directly at the point where the sample is spotted. The motion of the mobile phase is outward from a central spot. As a result, different solutes are separated in the form of rings, as shown in **Fig. 9.42**, and not in the form of spots.

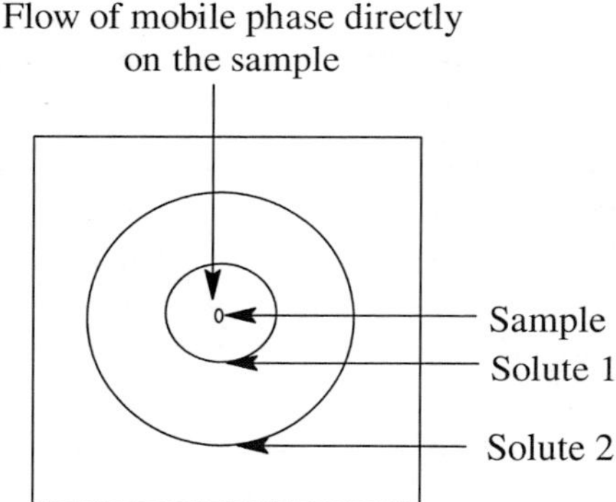

Fig. 9.42: Radial development

(iv) Horizontal development

As shown in **Fig. 9.43**, in horizontal development, the sample is spotted at one end of a plate. The mobile phase is dropped, with the help of a cotton wick, directly at the end of the plate, where the sample is spotted. The motion of the mobile phase is in the horizontal direction. The mobile phase is collected at the other end of the plate.

After the developer has traversed the length of the plate, the latter is removed, dried and the position of the compounds determined. This method is used when there is sufficient difference in the R_F values of the compounds of the sample.

(v) Two dimensional development

Development in two dimensions is undertaken when a sample contains a large number of compounds in it. In this type, the sample is spotted at one corner of a square plate, as shown in **Fig. 9.44**, and the mobile phase is passed in the ascending direction along the side AD of the plate. The separation of solutes takes place along the direction AD. Since the number of compounds is large, each separated spot may contain more than a single compound in it. After the development, the plate is removed from the chamber containing the mobile phase. The solvent is then removed by evaporation and the plate is rotated anticlockwise by 90°. Now, the mobile phase is passed in the direction along the side DC

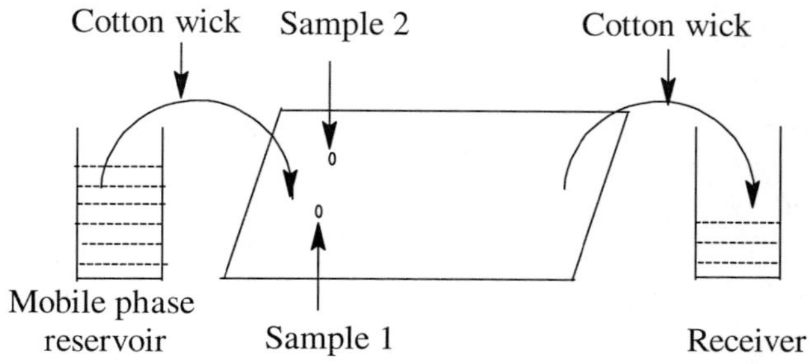

Fig. 9.43: Horizontal development

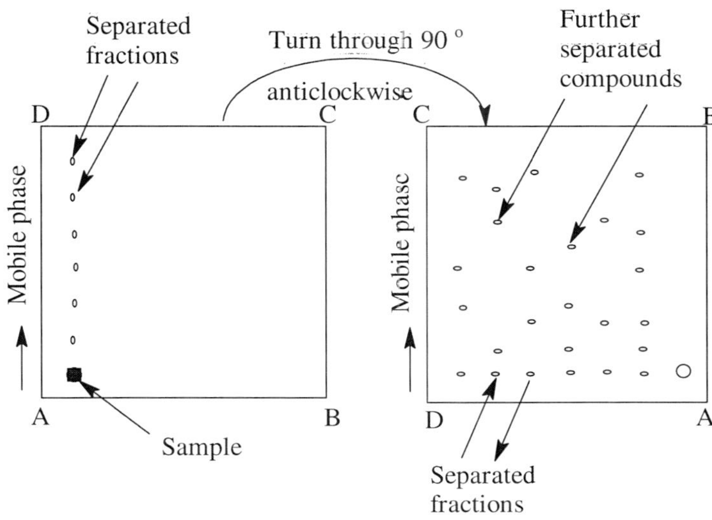

Fig. 9.44: Two dimensional development

so that further separation of compounds in each spot takes place on the stationary phase. Thus, the ascending development with mobile phase in two directions of the plate results in the complete separation of compounds from each other. This development technique is specially used for the separation of amino acids from protein hydrolysate (the mass obtained after hydrolysis of proteins).

5) Methods to locate the position of the separated spots on the plate

Several methods are employed to locate the position of the isolated compounds of the sample on the plate after its development.

(i) By using concentrated H_2SO_4

After the separation of compounds on the plate, the mobile phase is evaporated from it and the plate is sprayed using concentrated H_2SO_4. Most of the organic compounds get charred in presence of concentrated H_2SO_4 and form dark brown to black spots on the plate. The distance of these isolated spots, from the base line, where they were spotted on the plate before the separation, is measured. Similarly, the distance traveled by the mobile phase is also measured. From these two distances, the R_F value of the separated compounds is calculated by using the formula mentioned before.

(ii) By using iodine chamber

Many a times, after the development of the plate, it is kept in an iodine chamber. Few crystals of solid iodine are put in an enclosed chamber. Iodine being volatile in nature, saturates the chamber with its vapor. When the plate is kept in this chamber, most of the organic compounds absorb iodine vapor and develop yellow to brown colored spots on the plate. This helps in identifying the position of the separated compounds on the plate.

(iii) Use of specific reagents

Sometimes, some specific reagents can also be used for locating separated species, e.g. amino acids, separated on the plate, become visible (pink) when a *nihydrin* reagent is sprayed on the plate.

(iv) Use of fluorescent property

If the separated compounds are fluorescent in nature, they can be detected by using UV cabinet. Fluorescent compounds absorb UV radiation and start fluorescing, thereby helping to locate of the spots on the plate. Alternatively, if the separated compounds are not fluorescent, then a fluorescent material is incorporated into the stationary phase. After the development of the plate, when it is placed in the UV cabinet, the whole plate fluoresces except at the place, where non-fluorescing sample compounds are present, thereby locating the position of the compounds on the plate.

6) Quantitative Analysis

A semi-quantitative estimate or the approximate amount of the separated compounds present on the plate can be obtained by comparing the area under the curves for the compounds in the separated spots with that of a standard. Area under the curve for a particular spot can be obtained by scraping off the stationary phase from the plate where the spot is separated, extracting the analyte from it in a solvent, filtering the solution to remove the stationary phase, evaporating the solvent from it and then analyzing it by any suitable analytical method.

9.11.2.2. Paper Chromatography (PC)

Paper chromatography is also a planar chromatographic technique. It is an example of liquid-liquid chromatography, wherein the stationary as well as the mobile phases are liquid in nature and the solute is partitioned between them. Hence, PC is an example of partition chromatography.

1) Stationary phase

In paper chromatography, paper does not act as the stationary phase but acts as a support for the stationary phase. A good quality paper, which is highly purified and is uniform with respect to weight, thickness and porosity, so as to provide reproducibility in the results, is used. Paper is kept immersed in a chamber containing a liquid, which is used as a stationary phase. The liquid rises up through the paper and occupies the interstices or the pores of the paper. For normal phase chromatography, a polar liquid like water, glycols or buffers, can be used as a stationary phase. Instead of polar liquids, if a non-polar liquid like silicone oil or paraffin oil is used as a stationary phase, then paper chromatography can be used as reverse phase chromatography. Also, special papers containing an adsorbent or an ion-exchange resin, can also be used so as to permit *adsorption paper chromatography* and *ion-exchange paper chromatography* in place of liquid-liquid chromatography.

2) Mobile phase

Liquid used as a mobile phase should be immiscible with that of the stationary phase. For normal phase chromatography, a non-polar or a less polar liquid is used as a mobile phase and for reverse phase chromatography, a polar liquid is used as a mobile phase.

9.11.2.3. High Pressure Thin Layer Chromatography (HPTLC)

Thin layer chromatography (TLC) is very widely used for the analysis of complex mixtures of natural origin. Though it is cheap and simple, it suffered from certain drawbacks, which are as follows.

1) Major drawbacks of TLC

(i) Its surface cannot be modified easily, i.e. the polarity of the stationary phase cannot be modulated.

(ii) It is a semi-quantitative technique. It can be made quantitative but the method is tedious and may involve some errors in it.

For the purpose of quantification, HPLC is therefore, more commonly used as compared to TLC. However, HPLC is also not found to be suitable under certain conditions.

2) Drawbacks of HPLC

(i) HPLC is not convenient when a sample contains a large number of compounds, since it requires a large number of mobile phases for their separation and becomes inconvenient and costly. Thin layer chromatography is specifically used under this situation. In TLC, this type of analysis can be carried out at a reasonably fare cost by providing a large number of solvent tanks.

(ii)In HPLC, a solute is eluted out along with a solvent, thereby causing an interference with the detection of a solute. In TLC, solvent is evaporated before the detection and hence, there is no interference from the solvent.

(iii)Columns in HPLC are costly, whereas plates used in TLC are available cheaply.

(iv)Very slow eluting compounds can spoil the costly columns in HPLC. There is no such danger in TLC.

To overcome drawbacks of TLC and HPLC, a new technique called High Pressure Thin Layer Chromatography (HPTLC), involving combination of the two techniques, HPLC and TLC, is developed.

The comparison between HPLC and TLC is condensed in **Table 9.4**.

3) Comparison of TLC with HPTLC

Taking into account the drawbacks of TLC, scientists have provided improved support materials or sorbents as stationary phases and direct quantification by instrumental methods, in the technique of HPTLC.

(i) The main difference between HPTLC and conventional TLC is the particle size of the stationary phase. The smaller particle size (2-7 μm) is used in HPTLC as compared to that in TLC (150-250 μm). Also, the pore size is more uniform in HPTLC as compared to that in TLC. Thickness of the stationary phase is 0.2 mm as against 1-2 mm in TLC. This greatly reduces the time of analysis (1 to 5 min per sample) and increases the performance in HPTLC.

(ii) In conventional TLC, the solid support most widely used is silica gel or alumina. Recent developments in HPTLC have expanded the solid supports from silica to many bonded phases. This can provide a surface for reverse phase chromatography. Thus, in addition to silica plates, C_8 or C_{18} plates are also available

Table 9.4: Comparison between HPLC and TLC

Sr. No.	HPLC	TLC
1	Unsuitable when large number of compounds is present in the sample.	Suitable even when more compounds are present in the sample.
2	Use of a large number of solvents is inconvenient and costly.	Large number of solvents can be used at a fairly reasonable cost.
3	Mixture of solute and solvent is eluted out and hence, there is a possibility of interference in the measurement of absorbance of a solute.	Solvent is lost before the detection of a solute and hence, there is no possibility of interference in measurement of absorbance of a solute.
4	Very slow eluting compounds can spoil the column.	No danger of a plate getting spoilt even when the interaction of a solute with the stationary phase is more.
5	Column is costly.	Plate is cheaper compared to a column.

commercially.

(iii) A major drawback of HPTLC is the small sample capacity. To obtain optimum resolution and sensitivity in HPTLC, the band should be no greater than 3-6 mm in width [**Fig. 9.45(a)**]. This can accommodate a sample size of only 6 to 20 ì L. For delivering such a small quantity to a plate, following devices are required to be used.

(a) Hamilton syringe coupled to a micrometer screw, or

(b) A platinum-iridium (Pt – Ir) capillary

These devices pose the problem when a viscous solution is to be transferred to the plate.

In order to separate samples on mg scale, a band width of 190 mm [**Fig. 9.45(b)**] can be spotted, which can accommodate about 500 μL (approximately 5-20 mg) of the sample.

(iv) As in TLC, ascending, descending, circular and horizontal developments of plates are possible in HPTLC also but in addition, a simultaneous flow from opposite directions may also be applied in HPTLC. This is possible because, the sample can be spotted in two rows at the centre of the plate, as shown in **Fig. 9.45(a)**, and the mobile phase is passed in two opposite directions. Thus, this technique essentially doubles the number of samples that can be run at a time as compared to that in TLC. As many as 20 samples can be analyzed at a time per plate by using a technique of HPTLC.

(v) In TLC, semi-quantitative analysis of the compounds is carried out by comparing the intensity of spots in an UV cabinet or an iodine chamber, visually. For quantitative analysis, the stationary phase on the plate is scraped off and the quantity of the compound is determined by recording absorbance in the UV region or by using some other methods. However, this method does not provide accurate quantification. This drawback of TLC is overcome in HPTLC. The biggest advantage of HPTLC is the ease of quantification. In HPTLC, *in situ* measurement of the absorbance or intensity of fluorescence of a solute at the required λ_{max} value is possible. Such instruments, which measure the absorbance when the solute is still on the stationary phase are called *scanning densitometers*. This makes HPTLC more sensitive than TLC. For non-

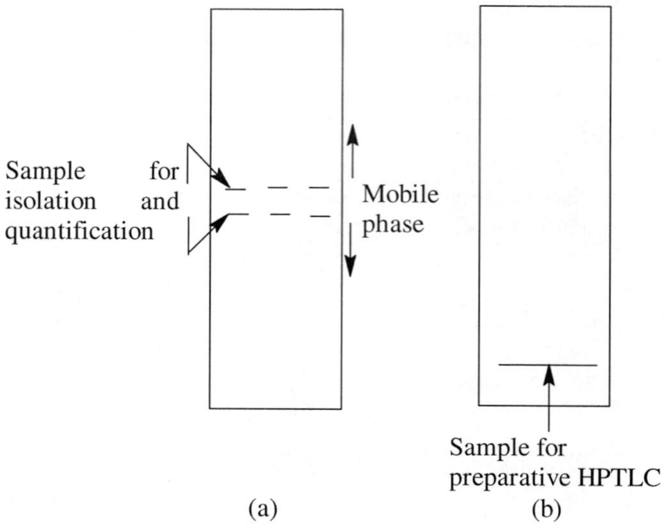

Fig. 9.45: Sample spotting and flow of mobile phase in HPTLC

Table 9.5: Comparison between TLC and HPTLC

Sr. No.	TLC	HPTLC
1	Limited number of surfaces is available commercially as stationary phases.	Along with silica gel and alumina, C_8 and C_{18} plates are also available commonly.
2	Particle size (150-250 μm) and pore size of the stationary phase is bigger and non-uniform.	Particle size (5-10 μm) and pore size of the stationary phase is smaller and more uniform.
3	Thickness of the stationary phase is 1-2 mm. Hence, more time is required for completion of analysis.	Thickness of the stationary phase is 0.2 mm. Hence, analysis is complete in a short time period.
4	Sample capacity is comparatively larger (100 μL).	Sample capacity is smaller (6 to 20 μL).
5	All the plate developmental methods are used except for the simultaneous development in two directions.	Simultaneous development in two directions along with the usual developmental methods makes possible analysis of more compounds at the same time.

absorbing and non-fluorescing compounds, derivatization can be carried out to impart the appropriate characteristics.

The comparison between TLC and HPTLC is given briefly in **Table 9.5**.

4) Stationary phase

Stationary phase used in HPTLC is silica gel or alumina. In addition to silica plates, C_8 or C_{18} plates are also available commercially. The most preferred and the frequently used stationary phase in HPTLC is silica gel. The particle size of the stationary phase is in the range of 2-7 μm. The thickness of the stationary phase is about 0.2 mm. The smaller thickness of the stationary phase allows higher resolution and faster separation of compounds. Nowadays, pre-coated plates are available in the market.

5) Sample application

In HPTLC, the plate is positioned on the movable stage with the help of an aluminium lever. The stage moves automatically to the positions where the samples are to be spotted on the plate. A number of vials are filled with the sample solutions and placed in the vial rack. With the help of a syringe, each sample is spotted in the form of a *band* and not as a *circular spot* as in case of TLC, under the pressure of nitrogen gas. The pressure of about 60-90 psi (4-6 bar) of nitrogen is used. The special *automatic sample applicators* are made use of for this purpose. They provide the following advantages.

(i) The bands are positioned accurately on the plate.
(ii) The accurate sample volumes are delivered.
(iii) Sharp peaks are obtained in the chromatogram.

6) Mobile phase

Like other chromatographic techniques, the mobile phase used in HPTLC is either a single solvent or a mixture of solvents. The common organic solvents like chloroform, methanol, toluene, acetonitrile, etc. can be used as mobile phases. The mobile phase at room temperature is passed through the plate under normal pressure.

7) Quantitative estimation by HPTLC

The developed plates are observed in the UV cabinet, using wavelengths as 254 nm or 366 nm, for identifying the isolated compounds.

For quantitative estimation, a special device called *scanner* is used in HPTLC. It provides following advantages.

(i) The quantitative estimation of different compounds at their λ_{max} values can be carried out, since the scanner provides measurement at the wavelengths in the range of 200-800 nm.

(ii) In the scanner, each sample band is brought in the path of a required wavelength and the interaction of a solute with the wavelength is recorded quantitatively, without the removal of an isolated spot from the stationary phase.

Thus, the scanner makes possible *in situ* and accurate quantification by HPTLC. The quantification of the separated compounds on the plate itself makes HPTLC more accurate and hence, it is very commonly used for quantitative estimation of compounds.

8) Instrumentation in HPTLC

The instrument used for the quantitative estimation of compounds by HPTLC is known as *scanning densitometer*. A scanning densitometer has the following compounds.

(i) A light source
(ii) A collimating lens
(iii) A monochromator
(iv) A converging lens
(v) A detector
(vi) A stepping motor

(i) A light source

A scanning densitometer makes use of a source of radiation required to be focused on the separated compounds. A hydrogen lamp, a mercury vapor lamp or a xenon lamp is used for this purpose. The advantages and disadvantages of these sources are as discussed under UV spectrometry (**Chapter 2, Section 2.4.1**)

(ii) A collimating lens

A beam of radiation coming out from an entrance slit is made parallel, before it enters the monochromator by passing it through a collimating lens.

(iii) A monochromator

A monochromator in the form of either a prism or a grating is commonly used in densitometers. Either a single or a double monochromator is used depending on the type of a densitometer. A mono-wavelength densitometer makes use of a single monochromator, whereas a dual-wavelength densitometer makes use of two monochromators.

(iv) A converging lens to concentrate or focus the beams

A beam of radiation coming out from the monochromator is converged by passing it through a converging lens in order to focus it on the compounds separated on the plate. The beam when gets reflected back, falls on the detector.

(v) A detector

In order to find the concentration of the separated compounds accurately, an effective detector, such as a photomultiplier tube, is employed for the measurement of the intensity of the reflected beam. A signal produced by the detector indicates the concentration of a compound present in that spot.

(vi) A stepping motor

In HPTLC, compounds in the sample are separated at different positions on the plate. In order to bring each spot in the focus of a converged beam of radiation, an additional device called a *stepping motor*, is used in densitometers. A stepping motor moves a plate under the focused light beam in order to scan the plate.

Densitometers are of different types, which are discussed below.

(A) A single beam densitometer
(B) A double beam densitometer
(C) A dual wavelength densitometer

(A) A single beam densitometer

As shown in **Fig. 9.46**, in a single beam densitometer, there is only a single beam containing a narrow range of radiation, coming out from the monochromator. This beam when falls on

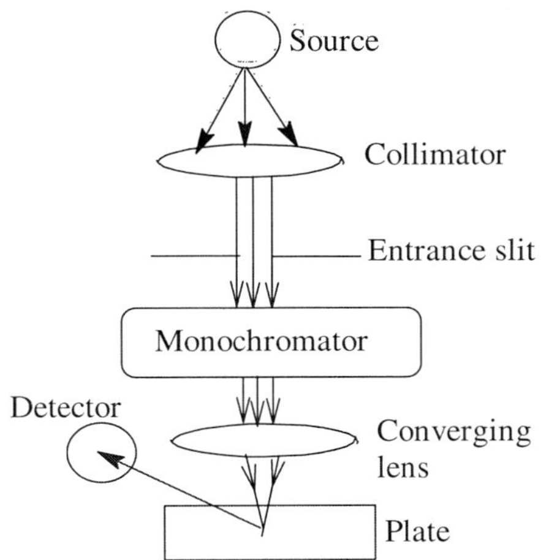

Fig. 9.46: Single beam densitometer

the plate, where sample spots are not present, produces an output corresponding to the blank reading. Then the beam falls on the separated compounds and produces some output. The two signals produced are then processed by the instrument so as to produce a net signal, which corresponds to the concentration of the compound in that spot.

(B) A double beam densitometer

In a double beam densitometer, as shown in **Fig. 9.47**, a single beam coming out from the monochromator falls on the beam splitter, which splits it into two beams. One beam falls on the plate, where there are no spots separated and another beam falls exactly at a point where a separated compound is present. These two beams reflect

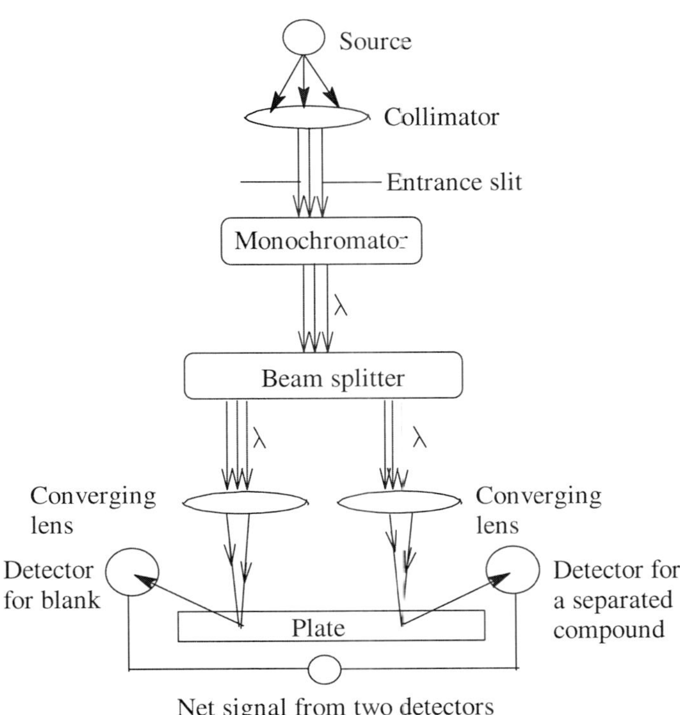

Fig. 9.47: Double beam densitometer

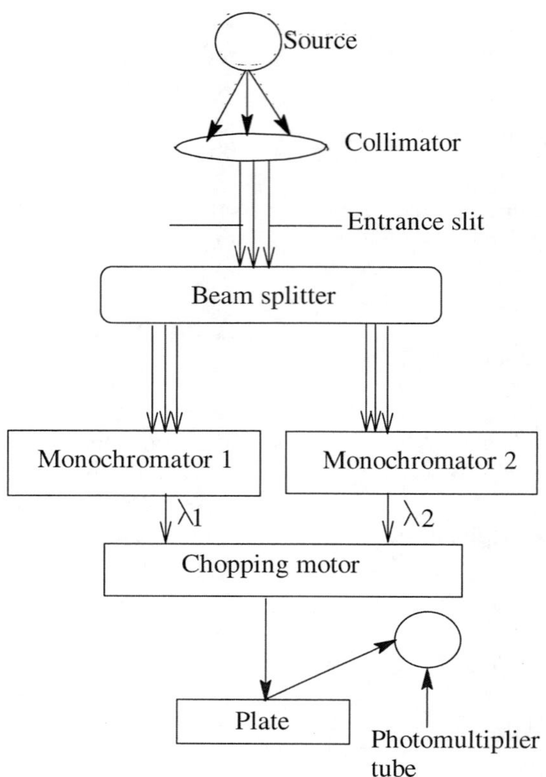

Fig. 9.48: Dual wavelength densitometer

back and fall on the separate detectors in the form of photomultiplier tubes. The output from the two detectors is processed so as to produce a signal corresponding to the concentration of a compound in that spot.

(C) A dual wavelength densitometer

In a dual wavelength densitometer, as shown in **Fig. 9.48**, a single beam coming out from the source falls on the beam splitter, which splits it into two beams. Two beams enter two different monochromators. Thus, two separate beams coming out from two monochromators correspond to two different wavelengths. These two wavelengths fall alternately, on each spot on the plate. Thus, the absorbance of each spot at two different wavelengths is recorded. In order to record the absorbance of a particular spot at one particular wavelength, a chopper is placed between the monochromators and a plate, which allows only one wavelength to fall on the plate at a time. After the interaction of radiation with the compounds on the plate, the reflected beam is collected by a photomultiplier tube, which produces a signal corresponding to the concentration of a compound at that spot.

Thus, densitometry is superior to thin layer chromatography because of clean separation, higher selectivity, *in situ* measurement of the concentration and the greater accuracy in quantification.

COMMON NOTATIONS USED IN LIQUID CHROMATOGRAPHY

1. K = distribution coefficient or partition coefficient
2. C_S = concentration of a solute in the stationary phase
3. C_M = concentration of a solute in the mobile phase
4. N = column efficiency in terms of total number of plates in the column
5. H = column efficiency in terms of height equivalent to one theoretical plate or HETP value
6. L = length of column packing
7. R_S = resolution between two peaks
8. t_R = retention time of the retained compound measured from the injection to peak maximum
9. t_M = retention time of the species that is not retained by the column packing and is taken as the retention time of the mobile phase or air
10. w = width of the peak at the base
11. σ = the peak standard deviation ($4\sigma = w$)
12. k' = capacity factor for a solute
13. V_S = volume of stationary phase
14. V_M = volume of mobile phase
15. α = column selectivity or selectivity factor
16. u = flow rate of the mobile phase

FORMULAE USED IN LIQUID CHROMATOGRAPHY

1) $$K = \frac{C_S}{C_M}$$

2) $$N = \frac{L}{H}$$

3) $$R_S = \frac{t_{R2} - t_{R1}}{\frac{w_2 + w_1}{2}} = \frac{2\,\Delta t}{w_2 + w_1}$$

OR

$$R_S = \frac{2\,\Delta t}{2\,w} = \frac{\Delta t}{w}$$

where, t_{R1} and t_{R2} are retention times of compounds 1 and 2,
w_1 and w_2 are the peak widths for compounds 1 and 2.
If $w_1 = w_2 = w$, then $w_1 + w_2 = 2w$

4) $$N = \left(\frac{t_R}{\sigma}\right)^2 = 16\left(\frac{t_R}{w}\right)^2$$

5) $$t_R = t_M\,(1 + k') = t_M\left(1 + K\frac{V_S}{V_M}\right)$$

6) $$k' = K\frac{V_S}{V_M} = \frac{C_S}{C_M} \times \frac{V_S}{V_M}$$

$$k' = \frac{t_R - t_M}{t_M}$$

7) $$R_S = \frac{\sqrt{N}}{4}\,\frac{(\alpha - 1)}{\alpha}\,\frac{k'_Y}{1 + k'_Y}$$

where, α = Selectivity facor

$$= \frac{(t_R)_Y - t_M}{(t_R)_X - t_M} = \frac{(t_R)_Y}{(t_R)_X}$$

$$= \frac{k'_Y}{k'_X} = \frac{\text{Capacity factor for solute Y}}{\text{Capacity factor for solute X}}$$

$$= \frac{K_Y \dfrac{V_S}{V_M}}{K_X \dfrac{V_S}{V_M}} = \frac{\left(\dfrac{C_S}{C_M}\right)_Y \dfrac{V_S}{V_M}}{\left(\dfrac{C_S}{C_M}\right)_X \dfrac{V_S}{V_M}}$$

Since the ratio of volume of stationary phase to that of mobile phase is same for both the solutes, X and Y,

$$\alpha = \text{Selectivity factor} = \frac{\left(\dfrac{C_S}{C_M}\right)_Y}{\left(\dfrac{C_S}{C_M}\right)_X}$$

$$= \frac{K_Y}{K_X} = \frac{\text{Partition coefficient for Y}}{\text{Partition coefficient for X}}$$

8) $$N = 16\,R_S^2\left(\frac{\alpha}{\alpha - 1}\right)^2\left(\frac{1 + k'_Y}{k'_Y}\right)^2$$

k'_Y = capacity factor for solute Y

9) $$(t_R)_Y = \frac{N.H.(1 + k'_Y)}{u} \text{ OR}$$

$$(t_R)_Y = \frac{16\,R_S^2\,H}{u}\left(\frac{\alpha}{\alpha - 1}\right)^2\frac{(1 + k'_Y)^3}{k'^2_Y}$$

10) $$\log\frac{(K_X)_1}{(K_X)_2} = A_X\left(\varepsilon_2^0 - \varepsilon_1^0\right)$$

where, $(K_X)_1$ and $(K_X)_2$ are the partition coefficients of a solute X in two mobile phases, 1 and 2, respectively.
A_X is the molecular size of the solute X
ε_1° and ε_2° are the eluent strengths of two mobile phases, i.e. solvent 1 and 2, respectively.

CHAPTER 10

GAS CHROMATOGRAPHY

In gas chromatography, gas is the mobile phase and solid or liquid is the stationary phase. Accordingly, the following two techniques are used under gas chromatography.

10.1. Gas solid chromatography

10.2. Gas liquid chromatography

10.1. GAS SOLID CHROMATOGRAPHY (GSC)

10.1.1. Principle

Gas solid chromatography makes use of gas as the mobile phase and solid as the stationary phase. This technique has somewhat limited applications as compared to gas liquid chromatography (GLC). This is because the interaction of solutes with the stationary phase is in the form of their adsorption on it and this adsorption is non-linear. This does not keep the ratio of the concentration of a solute in the stationary phase (C_S) to that in the mobile phase (C_M) constant, i. e. the distribution coefficient of a solute ($K = C_S/C_M$) does not remain constant during the separation. Since, all the chromatographic equations are derived on the assumption that the ratio C_S/C_M remains constant throughout the separation, it is difficult to apply the general principles of chromatography to gas solid chromatography, under this situation. Secondly, the distribution coefficients of solutes are generally much larger than those for GLC. Hence, the solutes in the gaseous form are not eluted out completely from the solid stationary phase. This leads to a semi-permanent retention of solutes on the stationary phase and further causes elution of solutes over a longer time period. Because of this, it is difficult to record narrow peaks for solutes in GSC, instead it results in a problem of tailing or broadening of elution peaks. This tailing brings about remixing of the separated compounds. Hence, this technique is useful for the separation of species such as H_2S, CS_2, nitrogen oxides, CO, CO_2 and rare gases that are not retained on liquid columns.

10.1.2. Stationary Phase

The most common stationary phase in GSC is the molecular sieves or porous polymers.

10.1.2.1. Molecular Sieves

The molecular sieves are the resins like zeolites, which are manufactured carefully so as to control the pore size in them. These pores or holes are of molecular dimensions. The molecules that are smaller than the pores, penetrate into the interior of the sieve particles, where they can be adsorbed. The bigger molecules cannot enter the interstices of the sieve. Thus, for the smaller molecules, a larger surface area is available for the adsorption as compared to that for the larger molecules. Hence, sieves can be used to separate solutes based on their size and adsorption coefficients. The molecules having smaller size, e.g. O_2, N_2, CO, H_2 and methanol, are able to enter the interstices of the molecular sieves but still can be separated from each other because of the differences in their adsorption coefficients. One problem with molecular sieves as the stationary phase is that the polar compounds like CO_2 are permanently adsorbed in the pores of the sieves and thus, block the surface to other species.

10.1.2.2. Porous Polymers

The stationary phase in GSC can be in the form of porous polymeric beads of uniform size. A polymer can be in the form of styrene cross-linked with divinyl benzene. This polymer is available in the market under the trade name of *Porapak*. The pore size of this polymer is controlled by controlling the degree of polymerization. Being hydrophobic, this polymer finds its main use in the separation of gases, which are polar in nature. Thus, the separation of the polar species like H_2S, oxides of nitrogen, H_2O, CO_2, CH_3OH and vinyl chloride is possible with this stationary phase.

10.2. GAS LIQUID CHROMATOGRAPHY (GLC)

Unlike GSC, GLC is very widely used for the separation of gaseous samples. In this technique, gas is used as the mobile phase and the liquid, which is immobilized by supporting on some solid matrix, is used as the stationary phase.

10.2.1. Principle

In GLC, gas which is used as a mobile phase, does not interact much with the solutes to be separated. The major role of the mobile phase is to push the solutes, which are desorbed from the stationary phase, out of the column. Hence, the mobile phase is usually referred to as a *carrier gas*.

An essential condition for the analysis by GLC is that the sample should be in the form of vapor. The vapor of the sample is introduced at the head of the column. The solutes from the mixture interact with the stationary phase by dissolving in it. The solutes having greater solubility in the stationary liquid phase remain in the higher concentration in it, whereas the solutes having lesser solubility in the stationary liquid phase remain in the smaller concentration in it. Thus, the solutes distribute themselves between the phases according to their distribution coefficients. The solutes having lesser interaction with the stationary phase are easily desorbed from it and are eluted out faster. The elution of the desorbed compounds is achieved by forcing an inert carrier gas such as nitrogen or helium through the column. Like in other chromatograms, a chromatogram obtained in GLC, also records the elution curves for the eluted compounds, which are bell-shaped.

All the equations used in liquid chromatography, as listed at the end of the chapter on Liquid Chromatography (**Chapter 9**), are also applicable to gas chromatography and can be used to calculate column efficiency, resolution and elution time. Thus, all the general principles of liquid chromatography are applicable to GLC also with minor modifications that arise from the compressibility of the gaseous mobile phase.

10.2.2. Instrumentation

The basic components of GLC are as follows.

10.2.2.1. Carrier gas supply
10.2.2.2. Sample injection system
10.2.2.3. Columns
10.2.2.4. Thermostat
10.2.2.5. Detectors
10.2.2.6. Recorders

10.2.2.1. Carrier Gas Supply

The carrier gas used in GLC must be chemically inert. Gases like helium, argon, nitrogen and hydrogen are used most of the times. Helium is the most widely used carrier gas. All these gases are supplied commercially in the pressurized cylinders. Along with the gas cylinders, other accessories like pressure regulators (in order to adjust the pressure or flow rate of the carrier gas), pressure gauges (to record the pressure used), flow meters (to record the flow rate of the carrier gas) and the molecular sieves (to remove H_2O or other impurities from the carrier gas) are also provided.

The pressure of the carrier gas at the inlet is usually in the range of 10-50 psi above the room pressure, which provides the flow rates of 25-50 mL/min. Most of the times, it is observed that the flow rate remains more or less constant if the inlet pressure of the carrier gas remains constant The pressure or the flow rate can be measured either at the inlet or at the outlet of the column. The flow rates can be measured at the inlet by using a device called a *rotameter*, but this device is not very accurate. Instead, a simple *soap bubble flow meter*, as shown in **Fig. 10.1**, is employed to measure the flow rate at the end of the column.

Soap bubble flow meter

It consists of a graduated glass column

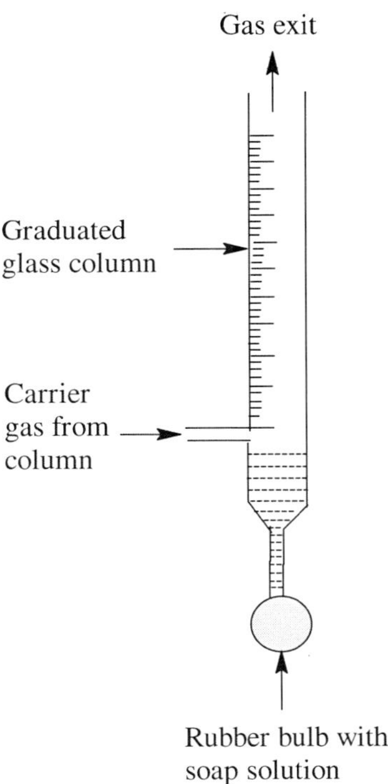

Fig. 10.1: Soap bubble flow meter

having a side tubing, which is connected to an analytical column. At the lower end of the column, a rubber bulb containing an aqueous solution of soap or detergent, is attached. When this rubber bulb is squeezed, a soap film is formed in the path of the carrier gas. When the carrier gas enters the glass column, it pushes the soap film in the column in upward direction. The time required for this soap film to move between two graduations on the glass column is noted. This information is used to calculate the flow rate of the carrier gas.

10.2.2.2. Sample Injection System

In order to get a peak, which is sharp enough and provides the accuracy in the quantification, a sample of the suitable size should be introduced as a "*plug*" of vapor, i. e. it should be introduced at once. The slow injection or the oversized samples bring about spreading of the sample and therefore, are responsible for poor resolution. For injecting the sample into a heated *sample port* located at the head of the column, a *microsyringe* is used. It is injected through a *rubber* or a *silicone diaphragm*. The sample port is usually maintained at about 50 °C above the boiling point of an analyte.

Usually, the sample size ranges from a few tenths to 10 μL. The capillary columns require much smaller sample size. In order to introduce the small amounts of the sample accurately to the column head, an additional device known as a *sample splitter* is employed. In this case, initially, a large volume of the sample is introduced. The sample is split into different streams with the help of a sample splitter and one small stream is allowed to pass through the port. The remaining sample goes as a waste.

10.2.2.3. Columns

1) Types of columns

Two types of columns, viz. *capillary columns* and *packed columns* are employed in GLC and are described below.

(A) Capillary columns

The capillary column is nothing but a capillary tubing of internal diameter of about 0.3 -0.5 mm. The inner walls of the capillary tubing are coated with a very thin film (about 1μm) of the liquid, which acts as the stationary phase. The capillary columns offer negligible resistance to the flow of the mobile phase and hence, the pressure drop across the two ends of the capillary column is negligible. Therefore, the columns as long as 10-100 m or more can be used. These longer length columns consist of several hundred thousand theoretical plates. The ratio of the volume of the stationary phase to the mobile phase (Vs/V_M) for these columns ranges from 100-300. This is the major reason that explains their high efficiency. Since these columns contain limited amount of the stationary phase, they suffer from very low sample loading capacities (< 0.01μL). The loading capacity of the capillary columns can be increased by coating the inner walls of the capillary with a porous material such as graphite, metal oxide or silicate. The porous materials provide increased surface area for the coating of the stationary phase, which automatically increases the loading capacity of the column.

(B) Packed columns

The packed columns are made up of glass or tubes of stainless steel, copper or aluminium, with the internal diameter of the order of 1-8 mm. These columns are filled with solid supports, which adsorb liquid used as the stationary phase for the separation. The packed stationary phase in these columns offers some resistance to the flow of the mobile phase and hence, there is some pressure drop across the two ends of the column. Therefore, these columns are not as long as the capillary columns, but the normal length of the column ranges from 2-20 m. The column is made compact so as to fit it in the limited space inside the thermostat of the chromatograph, by folding it or by coiling it.

The ratio of the volume of the stationary phase to the mobile phase (Vs/V_M) for these columns ranges from 10-20. The number of theoretical plates per foot length of the column is 100-1000. The best packed columns have a total of 20,000 or more theoretical plates. For these columns, though the ratio of the volume of stationary phase to the mobile phase (Vs/V_M) is less than that for the capillary columns, the total amount of the stationary phase is more and hence, their sample loading capacity is higher. However, because of the greater number of theoretical plates in the capillary columns, their efficiency for the separation is higher as compared to the packed columns.

The comparison between the capillary and the packed columns is given in **Table 10.1**.

2) Solid supports for packed columns

The ideal solid support used in packed columns should satisfy the following conditions.

(i) It should have small, spherical and uniform particle size.

(ii) It should have good mechanical strength.

(iii) It should have high specific surface area, at least of the order of 1 m^2/g.

(iv) It should be inert even at elevated temperatures.

(v) It should be readily wetted by the liquid phase, which is to be used as the stationary phase, so as to give an uniform coating.

There is no such perfectly ideal solid support available yet, but the two most common supports are derived from the diatomaceous earth. The commonly used solid supports for the packed columns include *Firebrick* and *Kieselguhr*.

(a) Firebrick, which is sold under the trade names

Table 10.1: Comparison between packed and capillary columns

Sr. No.	Parameter	Capillary columns	Packed columns
1	Internal diameter	0.3 – 0.5 mm	1-8 mm
2	Length	10-100 m	2-20 m
3	V_S/V_M	100-300	10-20
4	No. of theoretical plates	several hundred thousands	Around 20,000
5	Sample loading capacity	Lower	Higher
6	Efficiency of separation	Higher	Comparatively lower

such as *Chromosorb P*, *C 22* and *Sterchamol*, provides greater strength and larger surface area as compared to Kieselguhr, but is more active. This can lead to a semi-permanent retention of the gaseous compounds of the mixture on the stationary phase. Its disadvantage lies in the fact that it cannot be employed with polar compounds.

(b) Kieselguhr, which is sold under the trade names such as *Chromosorb W*, *Celite*, *Embacel* and *Celatom*, provides smaller surface area as compared to Firebrick, and is fragile. As compared to Firebrick, it is less active and does not lead to a semi-permanent retention of the gaseous compounds of the mixture on the stationary phase.

3) Stationary phase used in the column

The stationary phase used in GLC is liquid, which is immobilized on a solid support. Desirable properties of the immobilized liquid phase in GLC are listed below.

(i) Low volatility

The liquid used as the stationary phase should not be volatile, since GLC is carried out at sufficiently high temperature. Ideally, the liquid used as the stationary phase should have boiling point, which is at least 200 °C higher than the maximum operating temperature of the column.

(ii) High thermal stability

The liquid used as the stationary phase should not get destroyed or degraded at the operating temperature of the column.

(iii) Chemical inertness

The liquid used as the stationary phase should neither react with the solid support nor with the compounds to be separated.

(iv) Solvent characteristics

The liquid used as the stationary phase should possess the selectivity factor (α, alpha, Gr.) and the capacity factor (k') for the solutes to be resolved, within a suitable range.

No such ideal liquid, which satisfies all these requirements, is available. As a consequence, GLC makes use of several interchangeable columns, each with a different stationary phase. A variety of liquids can be used as stationary phases in GLC. The stationary phase in GLC determines the retention time of a solute in the column. The solutes having small distribution coefficients do not interact much with the stationary phase and pass through the column so rapidly that no significant separation occurs. On the other hand, when the distribution coefficients are large, the solutes interact strongly with the stationary phase and a long time is required to elute them out of the column. To have a reasonable residence time of solutes in the column, a solute must interact with the stationary phase to a limited extent but definitely not very strongly. For this purpose, the polarities of the two substances should be somewhat alike. For the separation of non-polar compounds like hydrocarbons or ethers, a non-polar stationary phase, *squalane* (a high molecular weight saturated hydrocarbon) can be used as the stationary phase. On the other hand, a more polar stationary phase such as polyethylene glycol would probably be more effective for separating alcohols or amines. Solutes with nearly identical boiling points but different polarities can be separated by GLC. Solutes having similar polarities can also be separated using GLC if they differ in boiling points. The order of elution for such compounds is in the increasing order of boiling points.

4) Column preparation in GLC

The support material of the required particle size range is obtained by using proper sieves. A liquid that is to be used as a stationary phase is poured in it so as to get the slurry of proper consistency. The amount of the liquid to be used as the stationary phase is calculated so as to achieve a thin coating (5-10 μm) on all the solid particles of the support. After evaporation of excess solvent, dry and free flowing particles are obtained. These coated support particles are then filled, with gentle tapping and shaking, into the column so as to provide a uniformly packed column. A special care is taken to avoid channeling, which may otherwise lead to the broadening of the peaks. After the column has been packed, it is bent or coiled into an appropriate shape so that it can be fitted in a compact space of the oven of the gas chromatograph. A properly prepared column may be employed for the separation of compounds from several samples.

10.2.2.4. Thermostat

Gas column chromatography makes use of a sample in the form of vapor. Hence, the column is operated at high temperature. The column temperature is an important parameter in GLC, since the variation in temperature results in the change in the retention time of a compound. Hence, it is absolutely important to control the temperature of the column, strictly to a few tenths of a degree, by employing a thermostat in the oven. The optimum column temperature depends upon the boiling point of the sample to be analyzed and also on the degree of separation required. Usually, a temperature higher than the average boiling point of a sample is employed for the separation. If a sample contains a large number of compounds with a broad range of boiling points, then a facility of temperature programming, provided in the equipment, is utilized. This allows an increase in the temperature of the column in increments, thereby allowing elution of all the compounds of the mixture within a reasonable time period, which ranges from 2-30 min.

10.2.2.5. Detectors

Detector used in gas chromatography should satisfy the following conditions.

(i) It should *respond rapidly*. This is because solute passes over the detector very rapidly (1 sec or less) and therefore, detector should produce response during this short time interval.

(ii)It should be *highly sensitive* so as to produce a large response to lower concentrations of solutes. This is particularly required in gas chromatography, since a solute is eluted out along with a large volume of the carrier gas.

(iii)It should produce response *linear* to the concentration of solutes in the eluate.

(iv)It should respond to a wide variety of compounds.

(v) It should not, as far as possible, destroy the sample.

No single detector satisfies all these conditions. The most commonly used detectors in GLC are described below.

1) Thermal conductivity detector [TCD] or a Katharometer

Principle

Thermal conductivity detector is also called a *Katharometer* and is based upon the changes in the thermal conductivity of the gas stream. Thermal conductivity detector works on the principle of Whetstone's bridge, which consists of four resistances in the circuit. Out of four resistances, the magnitude of three resistances remains constant and the fourth one varies as per the change in the temperature. The change in the temperature of the resistance wire is because of the difference in the capacity of the solute and the carrier gas to absorb heat, i.e. the difference in their thermal conductivities, when they are passed over the heated element. The change in the temperature changes the resistance, which in turn brings about the change in the current in the circuit. This gives the idea of the concentration of a solute in the eluate.

Construction

As shown in **Fig. 10.2**, two coils A and B (corresponding to resistance R_1 and R_4, respectively) are kept at constant temperature, by passing a constant current through them. One coil (A) is placed in the gas stream before the sample injection system and another coil (B) is kept beyond the column. The coils are made up of fine platinum or tungsten wires or alternatively a semi-conducting thermostat is made use of. Two more resistances, R_2 and R_3, are connected with these coils as shown in **Fig. 10.2** and the circuitry is joined so as to amplify and record the signal.

Working

A standing current is passed through two coils A and B by connecting them to a source of constant electric voltage. The passage of a constant current through these coils maintains them at constant temperature. The values of the two resistances, R_1 and R_2, are constant throughout the separation. When the carrier gas is passed over coil A, which is placed before the sample injection system, depending on its thermal conductivity, it removes some heat from the coil. The temperature of this coil A remains constant throughout the separation, since only the carrier gas passes over it. This constant temperature of the coil offers a constant resistance R_1 to the flow of current. The carrier gas also passes over coil B, kept beyond the column. The temperature of this coil B also attains certain value, when only the carrier gas is passing over it and offers resistance R_4 to the flow of current. The current in the circuit is made zero (null point) by adjusting the value of resistance R_3 in the circuit so that **equation (10.1)** is satisfied.

$$\frac{R_1}{R_2} = \frac{R_4}{R_3} \quad ...(10.1)$$

In this way, the thermal conductivity of the carrier gas is cancelled and the effects of variation in the flow rate, pressure and electrical power are minimized.

When the eluate contains a solute, a mixture of a solute and the carrier gas passes over second coil B, whereas only the carrier gas passes over coil A. The thermal conductivity of the carrier gas alone and of a mixture of a solute and the carrier gas in the eluate are different. Hence, when a solute is eluted out in the carrier gas, this mixture removes different amount of heat from coil B as compared to when only the carrier gas passes over it. The temperature of coil B now depends on the thermal conductivity of this mixture and not on the thermal conductivity of the carrier gas alone. The resistance offered by coil B depends on the actual temperature of this coil. The change in the resistance of this coil disturbs the null point in the circuit. The resistance R_3 in the circuit is again adjusted so as to get zero current in the circuit. This is achieved only under the condition expressed by **equation (10.1)**. The change in the resistance R_4 of coil B provides information about the concentration of a solute in the eluate.

The carrier gas used in GLC is either hydrogen (H_2) or helium (He). The thermal conductivities of H_2 and He are roughly 6 to 10 times greater than those of the most the organic compounds. Thus, the presence of even small amount of an organic compound in the carrier gas brings about a relatively large decrease in the thermal conductivity of the eluate. This results in a marked rise in the temperature of the detector. This is not the case when nitrogen (N_2) or carbon-di-oxide (CO_2) is used as the carrier gas, since their conductivities are almost the same as those of

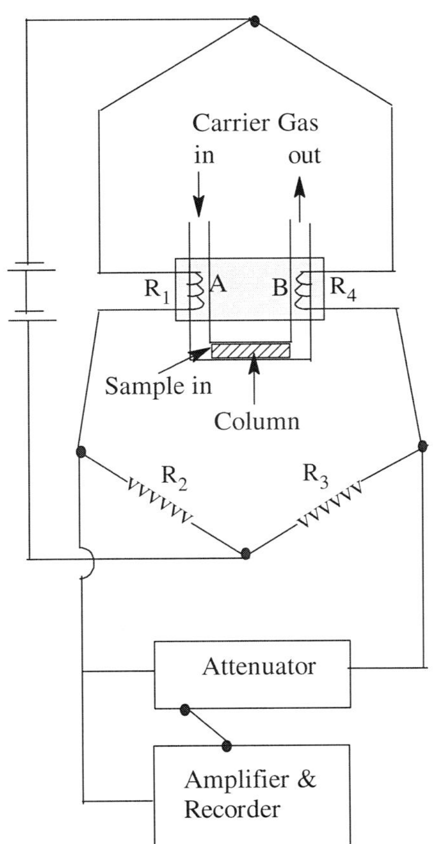

Fig. 10.2: Thermal conductivity detector

the organic compounds. Thus, the presence of a small amount of an organic compound in these carrier gases does not bring about a noticeable change in the thermal conductivity of the eluate. Hence, detection of organic compounds by thermal conductivity detector, in presence of N_2 or CO_2 as a carrier gas, is less sensitive.

Advantages

(i) Thermal conductivity detector is a relatively simple, rugged and an inexpensive detector.
(ii) It can be used for detecting a wide variety of substances and hence, it is a broadly applicable detection system.
(iii) It is non-destructive of the sample.
(iv) It provides accurate results.

Disadvantages

(i) Thermal conductivity detector is a non-selective detector.
(ii) It is not very sensitive as compared to other detectors.
(iii) Detection of organic compounds by thermal conductivity detector, in the presence of N_2 or CO_2 as a carrier gas, is less sensitive.

2) Flame ionization detector (FID)

This detector is described in detail under Liquid Chromatography (**Chapter 9, Section 9.10.2.7**).

3) Electron capture detector (ECD)

Principle

A beam of electrons is generated from an element, which acts as an electron emitter. These electrons generate a standing current in the circuit, which remains constant in absence of an organic compound. If an organic compound, which is capable of capturing electrons, comes in the path of this electron beam, suddenly the number of electrons is decreased and it results in the change in the current in the circuit. This change in the current gives indication about the presence of an organic compound in the eluate and also about its concentration in it.

Construction

As shown in **Fig. 10.3**, an electron capture detector consists of a β-emitter such as nickel (Ni^{63}) or tritium (H^3), adsorbed on platinum or titanium

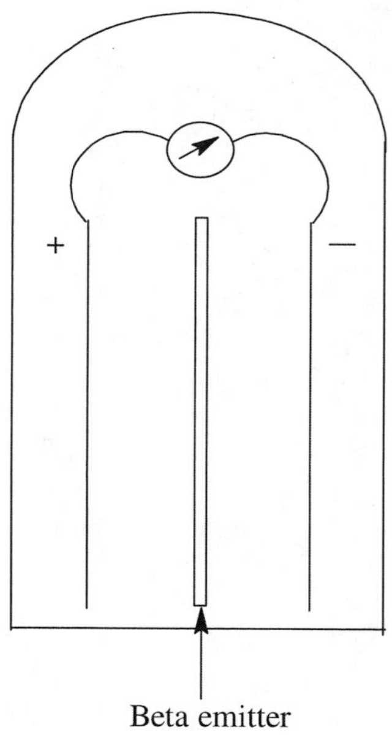

Fig. 10.3: Electron capture detector

foil. Two electrodes, acathode and an anode, are kept on either side of this β-emitter. Two electrodes are connected to an ammeter in order to record the current produced in the circuit.

Working

The effluent from the column is passed over a β-emitter. When a solute is not eluted out from the column, only the carrier gas (which is usually N_2 gas) passes over the β-emitter. A beam of electrons from the β-emitter causes ionization of the carrier gas and results in the production of a shower of electrons. In the absence of any organic solute in the eluate, ionization of the carrier gas produces a constant standing current between a pair of electrodes. When a solute is eluted out from the column, and when this solute is able to capture electrons towards it, the current decreases. The decrease in the current gives idea about the concentration of a solute in the sample.

Advantages

(i) Electron capture detector is selective in its response.
(ii) It is highly sensitive towards the organic compounds possessing electronegative functional groups such as halogens, peroxides, quinines, nitro and so on. It is very commonly used for the detection and determination of chlorinated insecticides. It is insensitive to compounds such as amines, alcohols and hydrocarbons.
(iii) In contrast to flame ionization detector, it does not alter the sample significantly.

Disadvantage

The response from electron capture detector is non-linear unless the potential across the detector is pulsed.

10.2.3. Applications of GLC

1) Gas liquid chromatography is used for the qualitative and the quantitative analysis. Under carefully controlled conditions, an accuracy of 1.3 % is attainable.
2) Gas liquid chromatography is commonly used for the analysis of volatile compounds or the compounds which can be vaporized at the temperature of the sample port of the gas chromatograph.
3) This technique is specifically applied for the separation of complex mixtures, organo-metallic compounds and bio-chemical systems.
4) Gas chromatograms are widely used as criteria of purity for volatile compounds. Contaminants, if present, are revealed by the appearance of the additional peaks. The area under these peaks provides rough estimate of the extent of contamination. The technique is also useful for evaluating the effectiveness of purification processes.
5) It is very commonly used as a powerful fractionating tool in conjunction with superior analytical instruments such as mass, UV, IR and NMR spectrometers.

10.2.3.1. Qualitative Analysis by GLC

Gas liquid chromatography is less useful as a tool for identifying the separated compounds. However, some parameters are made use of in order to confirm the presence of certain compounds in the mixture. The parameters used for qualitative analysis of compounds are described below.

1) Retention time (t_R)

The retention time is a characteristic

parameter of solutes, which can help in their identification. However, it changes considerably with the changes in the temperature of the column and in the flow rate and pressure of the carrier gas. Thus, in the absence of a precise control on the temperature, this parameter may lead to wrong information. Hence, whenever retention time is to be used for the identification of compounds, a chromatogram is to be recorded number of times. The average of at least three retention time measurements is considered to be satisfactory in qualitative analysis. Many a times, the retention time for an unknown sample and a standard is recorded together since retention time for both is found to vary similarly as these operating conditions are varied. This enhances the probability of identifying the standard as well asthe compounds in the sample. The retention time for the standard and an analyte is also recorded by using two or more columns. This almost confirms the identity of a standard and an unknown. Recording a chromatogram number of times becomes tedious as well as expensive and hence, usually, the separated compounds are identified by spectrometric techniques.

2) Relative retention time (α, alpha, Gr.)

Relative retention time is nothing but the selectivity factor for a solute for a definite combination of a stationary phase and a mobile phase and it describes the retention time of a solute in relation with the retention time of a standard. It is expressed mathematically by the **equation (10.2)**.

$$\alpha = \frac{(t_R)_Y - (t_R)_M}{(t_R)_X - (t_R)_M} \quad \ldots(10.2)$$

where, $(t_R)_Y$ and $(t_R)_X$ are the retention time of stanard Y and a solute X, respectively, and $(t_R)_M$ is the retention time of a compound which is not retained by the column. Thus, $(t_R)_M$ is the retention time of the mobile phase. The parameters, $(t_R)_Y$, $(t_R)_X$ and $(t_R)_M$ can be readily obtained from a chromatogram, when an internal standard (Y) is introduced into a sample containing an analyte (X). The only requirement for calculating the relative retention time for a solute is that the peaks for X and Y should not overlap and the two species X and Y should be different chemically.

3) Retention volume (V_R)

Another useful parameter for qualitative analysis is the retention volume. It is defined as the total volume of the carrier gas required to elute out the compound completely from the column. Though the measurement of the retention volume requires the measurement of the retention time as well, the product of the average flow rate (F) of the carrier gas within the column and the retention time (t_R) of a compound, gives the retention volume (V_R), which remains constant irrespective of the changes in the temperature of the column. This is because if the column temperature is increased, the volume of the gas is increased, because of which the flow rate (F) of the carrier gas (expressed as volume of gas collected per unit time) is also increased, but the retention time (t_R) is reduced. Therefore, the product of t_R and F remains constant even if the temperature of the column varies. The expression for the retention volume (V_R) is given by **equation (10.3)**.

$$V_R = t_R\, F \quad \ldots. (10.3)$$

4) Specific retention volume (V_g)

The specific retention volume (V_g) is a better parameter for the qualitative analysis by GC as compared to the previous parameters. This is because it depends only upon the distribution coefficient of a solute (K), the temperature of the column (T_C) and the density (ρ_S) of the stationary phase. This is clear from **equation (10.4)**.

$$V_g = \frac{K}{\rho_S} \times \frac{273}{T_c} \quad \ldots(10.4)$$

Volume of the gas per unit weight of the stationary phase, required to elute the compound completely, is called the *specific retention volume* of that compound. Hence, specific retention volume is defined by **equation (10.5)**.

$$V_g = \frac{V_R - V_M}{w} \times \frac{273}{T_c} \quad \ldots(10.5)$$

where, V_g = specific retention volume,

V_R = retention volume of a solute in the column and $V_R = t_R F$,

t_R = retention time of a solute in the column,

V_M = retention volume of a species not retained by the column (usually, air or carrier gas), and

$V_M = t_M F$,

t_M = column retention time of a species not retained by the column,

T_C = column temperature in Kelvin, and

w = mass of the stationary phase

Both the quantities, V_M and V_R, depend upon the average pressure within the column = a quantitity that lies between the inlet pressure P_i and the outlet pressure P_o.

To obtain the specific retention volume (V_g) of a compound, the average flow rate (F) within the column must be known. The flow rate at the end of the column (F_m) is readily obtained by means of a soap bubble meter and the average flow of the gas within the column (F) can be calculated from F_m as follows by using **equation 10.6**.

$$F = F_m \frac{T_C}{T} \left(\frac{P - P_{H_2O}}{P} \right) \quad \ldots(10.6)$$

where,

T_C = column temperature in degree Kelvin,

T = temperature of the gas at the bubble meter (usually taken as room temperature),

P = pressure at the end of the column (usually taken as normal pressure), and

P_{H_2O} = vapor pressure of H_2O. The presence of moisture develops some pressure inside the column, which is subtracted from the observed pressure to get the actual pressure of the carrier gas inside the column.

5) Retention index (I_x)

It is used as a qualitative parameter mainly for a homologous series. Here, the standard used is normal paraffin. It is based upon a comparison between the position of an analyte peak $(t_R)_x$ and the peaks for two or more normal paraffins, $(t_R)_n$ and $(t_R)_{n+1}$, where 'n' stands for the number of carbon atoms in one normal paraffin and (n +1) stands for the number of carbon atoms in the higher homologue of the normal paraffin containing 'n' number of carbon atoms. By definition, the retention index (I_x) for a normal paraffin is equal to 100 times the number of carbon atoms in that paraffin, regardless of the type of column used or the chromatographic conditions followed. Hence, for n-pentane, the retention index (I_x) is always 500 and that for n-octane, it is 800. Thus, the retention index increases with the increase in the number of carbon atoms in a compound [**Fig. 10.4(a)**]. The retention time and the retention volume also increase with the increase in the number of carbon atoms in a compound. Hence, as shown in **Fig. 10.4(b)**, for a particular homologous series, a plot of the logarithm of the retention time or the retention volume against the number of carbon atoms is linear. Consequently, a plot of logarithm of the corrected retention time, (t_R - t_M), versus the retention index, for a series of normal paraffins, is also a straight line as shown in **Fig. 10.5**.

The retention index (I_X) for an analyte X is defined by **equation 10.7**.

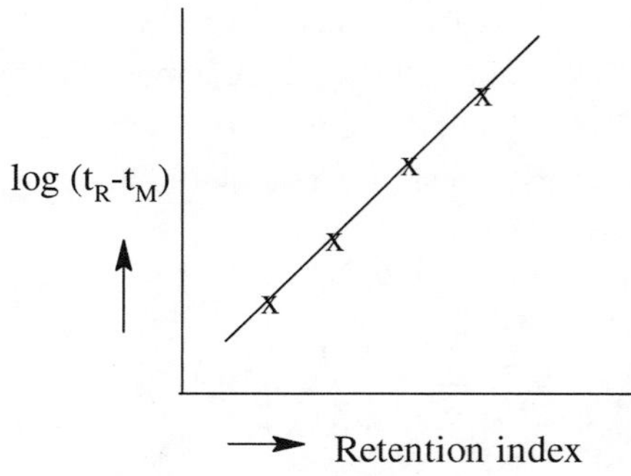

Fig. 10.5: A plot of corrected retention time versus the retention index for a series of normal paraffins

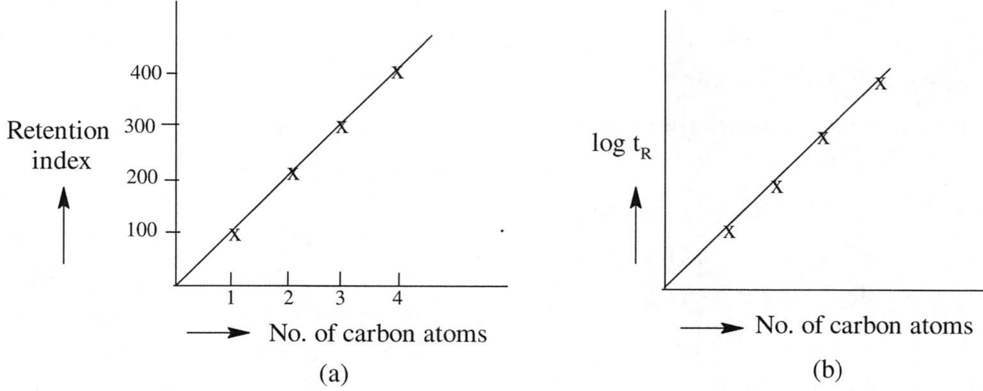

Fig. 10.4: A plot of (a) retention index and (b) the logarithm of retention time against the number of carbon atoms

$$I_X = 100\left[\frac{\log (t'_R)_X - \log (t_R)_M}{\log (t'_R)_{n+1} - \log (t'_R)_n}\right] + 100\,n \quad ...(10.7)$$

where, $(t'_R)_X$ is the corrected retention time for a solute X in the mixture, i. e. $n' = (t_R - t_M)$,

$(t_R)_M$ is the retention time for the species not retained by the column,

$(t'_R)_{n+1}$ is the corrected retention time for the paraffin containing (n + 1) carbon atoms, and

$(t'_R)_n$ is the corrected retention time for the paraffin containing 'n' carbon atoms.

From the chromatogram, the retention time of a solute can be found out. By extrapolating this value of retention time on a standard calibration curve, as shown in **Fig. 10.4(b)**, the number of carbon atoms in that solute can be predicted. The retention time can also be extrapolated on a standard calibration curve, shown in **Fig. 10.5**, to get the retention index for a particular solute. Using this value of retention index, the number of carbon atoms in that solute can be found out. The retention index can also be calculated using **equation (10.7)**, since all the retention time values, $(t'_R)_X$, $(t_R)_M$, $(t'_R)_{n+1}$ and $(t'_R)_n$, are available from the chromatogram and the value of 'n', i. e. the number of carbon atoms in a standard paraffin, is known.

Note: The subscripts 'n' and (n+1) describe the number of carbon atoms in two different paraffins, which are used as standards. They do not indicate the number of carbon atoms in an analyte. The number of carbon atoms in an analyte is obtained from the retention index, I_X, since $I_X = (100 \times n')$, where, n' is the number of carbon atoms in an analyte.

Sometimes, a single gas chromatogram does not provide sufficient information to identify solutes in their mixture. Hence, many a times, the retention index is determined for the solutes by injecting the sample into three columns containing the stationary phases of different polarities. If an identical retention index is obtained for a solute on all the three columns, then the presence of a particular analyte in the sample can be confirmed.

6) Retention time plots

A linear relationship between the log t_R and the number of carbon atoms for the members of a homologous series can be used for qualitative analysis of any homologous series like aldehydes, ketones, alcohols, etc.

Another useful plot, which can be used for different homologous series, is obtained by injecting the sample into two columns with the stationary phases that differ in polarity. The retention time of solutes on two different columns is determined and a plot of the logarithm of the retention time on one column (t_{R1}) versus that on the other (t_{R2}) is prepared. This plot yields a straight line. For different homologous series, lines with different intercepts and different slopes are obtained. This is shown in **Fig. 10.6**.

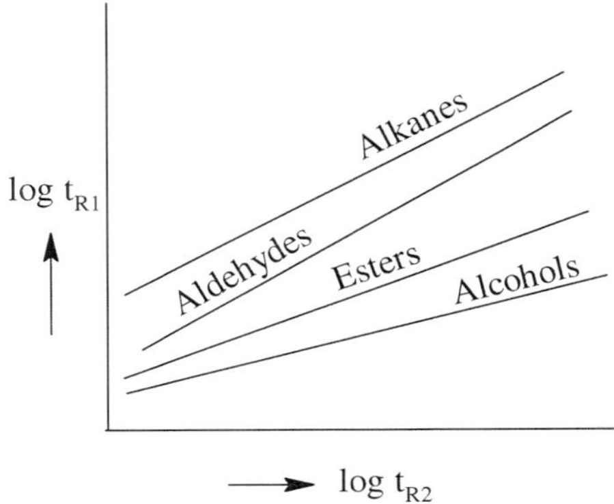

Fig. 10.6: A plot of the logarithm of retention time of a compound on two columns for homologous series

These plots help in the identification of compounds with similar boiling points but having differing polarities. A combination of the retention time of a solute on two different columns decides its position on a line having a particular slope, thereby helping to identify the functional group in it. This technique is quite analogous to two-dimensional paper chromatography.

In spite of all these qualitative parameters, identification with GLC is difficult, since the exact retention time (t_R) and the retention volume (V_R) are not obtained as they require very rigid control on the temperature of the column and also on the pressure as well as the flow rate of the carrier gas. Moreover, most of the detection systems used are non-selective and hence, respond almost in the similar way to all the solutes, which are eluted out from a column. The employment of the selective or the specific detectors in GLC, however, makes possible a good combination of the tremendous separatory power of GLC with the superior analytical qualities of the instruments.

After the separation of the solutes using GLC, they can be identified by using two different approaches.

(i) The first approach is to collect the vapor of the eluted solutes as the separate fractions in a cold trap and then identify them by NMR, IR, mass or other spectrometric techniques. The main drawback of this approach is that a solute is present in a very small quantity in the eluate, which can lead to less intense signals in the detector.

(ii) A second general method is to use a selective detector to monitor the column effluent continuously.

Some of the selective detectors in GLC are described below.

10.2.3.2. Quantitative Analysis

Quantitative analysis in GLC is carried out by exactly the same methods as described under liquid chromatography in **Chapter 9**, **Section 9.7.2** or by using cetain selective detectors as describbed under the **Section 10.2.4** of this chapter.

10.2.4. GLC with Selective Detectors

10.2.4.1. Automatic Titration Detectors

Gas liquid chromatography with automatic titration detector is used either for volatile aromatic and aliphatic fatty acids or for amines. In this method, the effluent from the column is continuously led directly into a cell containing a solution of an acid-base indicator. The absorbance of this solution is monitored continuously, photometrically. When an acidic or an alkaline solute is not present in the eluate, the color of an acid-base indicator remains unchanged and a constant absorbance reading is obtained. As soon as an acidic or an alkaline solute appears in the eluate, the color of an acid-base indicator changes. This results in the change in the absorbance of an acid-base indicator. This change in the absorbance provides information about the quantity of a solute in the eluate. Addition of a suitable titrant to this eluate also provides an idea about the concentration of an acid or a base in the eluate. The wavelength of absorption of a compound helps in identifying the compound. Thus, the qualitative as well as the quantitative information is obtained in this manner. This method is commonly employed in the analysis of various chlorinated compounds contained in the pesticide residues.

10.2.4.2. Coupling of Gas Chromatography to Mass Spectrometry

Nowadays, chromatographic columns are commonly coupled to mass spectrometers. As soon as the solute is eluted out from the column, it is passed into a mass spectrometer. Here, the solute is ionized and undergoes fragmentation, thereby producing a number of ionic species. A signal is obtained for each ionic species, which results in the production of a mass spectrum. This spectrum makes possible the identification and also the quantification of a large number of compounds present in the sample. Hence, it is particularly used for the analysis of compounds from the natural origin and also for the biological systems. For example, it is used for characterization of the odors and flavors of foods and identification of pollutants. It is also used to diagnose certain volatile compounds like alcohol in breath and to find the presence or the absence of certain drugs or drug metabolites in the body fluids.

A major problem in this method is the presence of a large volume of the carrier gas in the eluate, which dilutes the eluted compounds enormously and weakens the signal. This is not, however, a major drawback of this method, since several separators can be employed in order to separate solute from a large volume of the carrier gas before the eluate is passed to the mass spectrometer. This is discussed in detail in **Chapter 5, Section 5.8.**

Coupling of mass spectrometer with efficient separatory devices such as chromatographs, provides an important tool for the separation and identification of compounds from a complex mixture. Such techniques are referred to as the *hyphenated techniques*.

10.2.4.3. Coupling of Gas Chromatography to IR Spectrometry

In this case, the effluent from the gas chromatograph is passed first through a separator to remove most of the carrier gas and then through a Fourier transform IR spectrometer. This provides an IR spectrum of an eluted solute, which helps in its identification. The spectra for solutes can be stored in a computer or can be printed out to derive the required information, whenever needed.

FORMULAE USED IN GAS CHROMATOGRAPHY

1. $V_R = t_R F$

V_R = total volume of the carrier gas required to elute out the compound completely

t_R = retention time of a solute in the column

F = average flow rate of the carrier gas within the column

2. $$V_g = \frac{K}{\rho_S} \times \frac{273}{T_c}$$

V_g = specific retention volume of a solute

K = distribution coefficient of a solute

ρ_S = density of the stationary phase

T_C = temperature of the column

3. $$V_g = \frac{V_R - V_M}{W} \times \frac{273}{T_c}$$

V_M = retention volume of a species not retained by the column (usually, air or carrier gas) = t_M F

w = mass of the stationary phase

4. $$F = F_m \frac{T_C}{T}\left(\frac{P - P_{H_2O}}{P}\right)$$

F = average flow rate of the gas within the column

F_m = flow rate of the gas at the end of the column

P = pressure of the gas at the end of the column usually taken as the normal pressure

P_{H2O} = vapor pressure of H_2O

T = temperature of the gas at the bubble meter (usually taken as room temperature)

5. $$I_X = 100\left[\frac{\log(t'_R)_X - \log(t_R)_M}{\log(t'_R)_{n+1} - \log(t'_R)_n}\right] + 100\,n$$

I_X = retention index for an analyte X

$(t'_R)_X$ = the corrected retention time for a solute X in the mixture, i. e. $t'_R = (t_R - t_M)$

$(t_R)_M$ = the retention time for the species not retained by the column

$(t'_R)_{n+1}$ = the corrected retention time for a paraffin containing (n + 1) carbon atoms

$(t'_R)_n$ = the corrected retention time for the paraffin containing ‘n’ carbon atoms.

CHAPTER 11

POLAROGRAPHY AND AMPEROMETRY

ELECTROCHEMICAL METHODS

In electrochemical methods, the extent of a chemical reaction is measured based on the variation in some electrical parameter. One or more electrically related parameters such as charge, voltage or current, are measured and then correlated with the concentration of a compound in a sample. Different techniques included under electrochemical methods are -

1) Polarography
2) Potentiometry
3) Conductimetry
4) Electrogravimetry
5) Coulometry

11.1. INTRODUCTION TO POLAROGRAPHY

Polarography is an electrochemical method of analysis, which involves controlled electrolysis of the sample to be analyzed. In polarography, the substance to be analyzed undergoes electrolysis under the influence of an externally applied potential difference (PD), as a result of which, electrolysis current is generated in the electrolytic cell. This current is measured and plotted against the PD applied across the electrodes so as to get a current vs. voltage (c-v) curve. Only a minute fraction of the analyte is electrolyzed at the surface of the microelectrode in polarography. During electrolysis, cations of an electrolyte undergo reduction at cathode. In order to achieve controlled electrolysis in polarography, the external PD is properly controlled. Thus, the electrolysis current is very small (usually < 50 μA) and the extent of reduction due to electrolysis is negligible so that the same solution may be repeatedly used for analysis, without significant change in its c-v curve.

An electrical apparatus used for supplying voltage for electrolysis and measuring the current produced due to electrolysis of an electrolyte is known as a *polarograph*. It consists of a potentiometer, an electrolytic cell or a polarographic cell (PC) and a galvanometer (G), as shown in **Fig. 11.1**. Detailed description of a polarograph is given under **Section 11.3**.

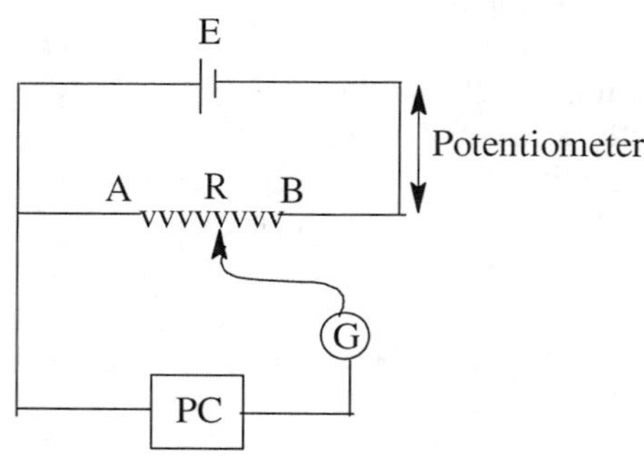

Fig. 11.1: A polarograph

Difference between voltammetry and potentiometry

In **voltammetry**, a definite PD is applied across the electrodes of the cell or a definite current is allowed to pass through an electrochemical cell, which causes electrolysis of an electrolyte. The extent of electrolysis may vary from complete electrolysis in *electrogravimetry* and in *coulometry* to a limited or controlled electrolysis in *polarography* and *amperometry*.

In case of **potentiometry**, one records the PD or the electramotive force across the electrodes in an electrochemical cell when no current passes through the cell. Thus, potentiometry is voltammetry at zero current.

In polarography, the PD across the electrodes of a polarographic cell is increased slowly and the current resulting from the electrolysis is measured. A graph of current (c) along Y-axis vs. voltage (v) along X-axis is plotted. This current-voltage (c-v) curve is called a *polarogram*. The c-v curve has a characteristic 'S' shape, as shown in **Fig. 11.2**, and is used for qualitative as well as quantitative analysis of electro-reducible and electro-oxidizable species.

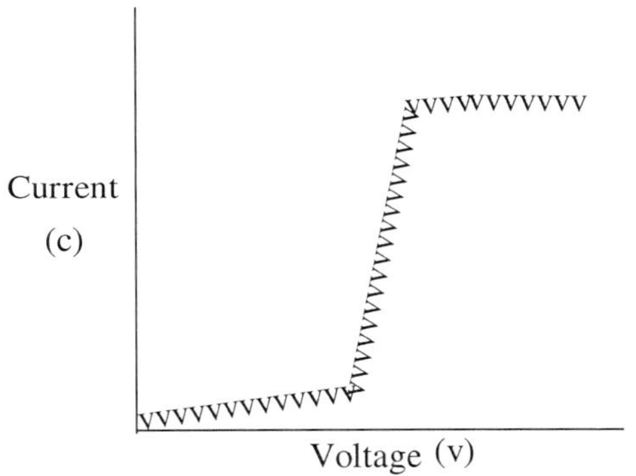

Fig. 11.2: S-shaped polarogram

Reactions occurring in a polarographic cell are as follows.

(a) Dissociation of an electrolyte

If an electrolyte is lead chloride ($PbCl_2$), it dissociates in an aqueous solution as follows.

$$PbCl_2 \rightleftharpoons Pb^{+2} + Cl^-$$

(b) At Cathode

Reduction of cations takes place at cathode.

$$Pb^{+2} + 2e \longrightarrow Pb$$

(c) At Anode

Oxidation of anions takes place at anode.

$$2\,Cl^- \longrightarrow Cl_2 + 2\,e$$

11.2. APPLICATIONS OF POLAROGRAPHY

1) The polarographic technique is useful for the estimation of those ions which get reduced to a stable lower oxidation state, especially to the zero valent state and then amalgamate with mercury, e. g. Bi^{+3}, Cd^{+2}, Pb^{+2}, etc.
2) Oxygen gas is electro-reducible and hence, it can be analyzed by polarography. The estimation of oxygen from water is carried out to find the extent of river pollution. The microbes or creatures consume dissolved oxygen in river water. Hence, the content of oxygen is reduced considerably in the presence of higher degree of contamination of water.
3) Polarography can be directly applied to analyze compounds from the biological fluids such as plasma, urine, bile etc. and hence, drugs and metabolites can be analyzed from these body fluids, accurately.
4) Polarography is commonly used to analyze inorganic salts, but it can also be used for analyzing certain organic compounds. When it is used for analyzing organic compounds, the method is termed as *organic polarography*.
5) The compounds which are not active polarographically, i.e. those which are not electro-reducible or electro-oxidizable, can also be analyzed indirectly by polarography. In such a case, polarographically inactive compounds are derivatized chemically so as to introduce a functional group in them, which is either reducible or oxidizable. For example, organic hydrocarbons are nitrated. Nitro group can be easily reduced to an amino group and hence, after nitration, these hydrocarbons can be analyzed by polarography. Certain hormones and steroids are nitrosated. Nitroso group can also be reduced very easily and hence, the nitrosated compounds can be analyzed polarographically. Bromo derivatives are also easily reducible. Hence, polarographically inactive compounds can be brominated in order to make them polarographically active.

11.3. INSTRUMENTAL SET UP FOR POLAROGRAPHY

As shown in **Fig. 11.1**, a polarograph

consists of the following three components.

11.3.1.A *potentiometer* for providing a known PD across the electrodes in the polarographic cell

11.3.2.An *electrolytic* or a *polarographic cell*

11.3.3.A *galvanometer* or an *ammeter* for measuring electrolysis current

11.3.1. A potentiometer

A potentiometer consists of an electrolytic cell (E) and a resistance R, connected in series. The required PD is set across the electrodes in the polarographic cell by adjusting the position of a jockey or a movable pointer, connected to a galvanometer, on a resistance wire (R) between the points A and B (**Fig.11.1**). The PD between points A and B across the resistance wire (R) is equal to the electromotive force (e. m. f., E) of a galvanic cell. Point A is at positive potential, since it is connected to the positive electrode of a galvanic cell and point B is at negative potential, since it is connected to the negative electrode of a galvanic cell. Thus, potential drops down from the positive to the negative value as one moves from point A to point B. If the length of the resistance wire is 10 units, then a potential drop per unit length of resistance wire is E/10. The position of the jockey on the resistance wire decides the potential of the negative electrode of an electrolytic cell. Thus, the change in the position of the jockey on the resistance wire provides the varying PD across the electrodes of an electrolytic cell (Potential at point A is always fixed and is equal to the potential of the positive electrode of a galvanic cell). Hence, the change in PD across electrodes reflects the change in the potential of the negative electrode.

11.3.2. Polarographic Cell or an Electrolytic Cell

A polarographic cell is H shaped as shown in **Fig. 11.3**. One arm of H shaped cell contains the solution of a sample to be analyzed (analyte) and another arm contains saturated KCl solution or KCl solution of known strength. Dropping Mercury Electrode (DME) is used as a cathode and is

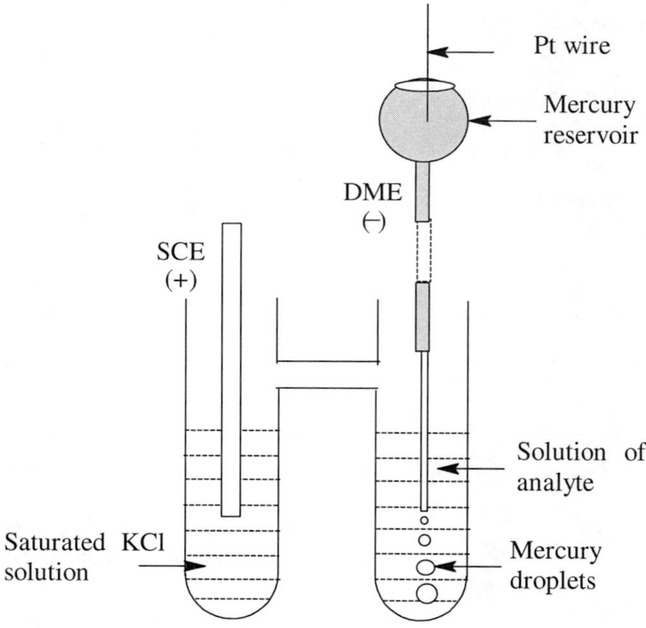

Fig. 11.3: H shaped polarographic cell

dipped in the solution of an analyte. Saturated Calomel Electrode (SCE) is used as an anode and is dipped in a saturated solution of KCl.

11.3.2.1. Dropping Mercury Electrode (DME)

Construction

Normally, electrodes are used in the form of solid rods or solid plates. Dropping mercury electrode (DME) exists in the form of small droplets of mercury formed at the tip of a capillary, as shown in **Fig. 11.4**. It consists of a short length of glass capillary tubing having internal diameter in the range of 0.03 to 0.05 mm. The size of a capillary decides the size of droplets formed at its tip. Capillary tubing is attached to a short but large bore glass tubing, which is connected to a mercury reservoir via a piece of a rubber tubing. Height of mercury column above the tip of the capillary tubing is maintained by changing the level of mercury reservoir bulb. Constant height of the mercury column above the tip of the capillary tubing is essential in order to maintain the flow rate of mercury or to determine the number of droplets of mercury formed per unit time. Each droplet goes through a definite sequence at the tip of the capillary. Initially, a small droplet is formed at the tip of the capillary, then the droplet slowly grows in size, attains a critical mass and then detaches from the capillary. Negative potential is applied to mercury droplets by introducing a platinum wire in Hg reservoir. Platinum wire is maintained at negative potential by connecting it to an anode of a *galvanic cell*, which acts as a source of electrons to it. Difference between the *galvanic* and the *voltaic cell* or an *electrolytic cell* (a polarographic cell) is explained under the **Section 11.4.6** of this chapter.

Working

Because of the availability of electrons at DME, the positive ions of an analyte are attracted towards it during electrolysis. Once the cations of the analyte are in the vicinity of DME, at a particular potential at DME, cations are reduced. If $PbCl_2$ is an analyte, Pb^{+2} ions are reduced to Pb atoms as shown in the following reaction.

$$Pb^{+2} + 2e \longrightarrow Pb$$

Thus, DME is used as a cathode in the polarographic cell.

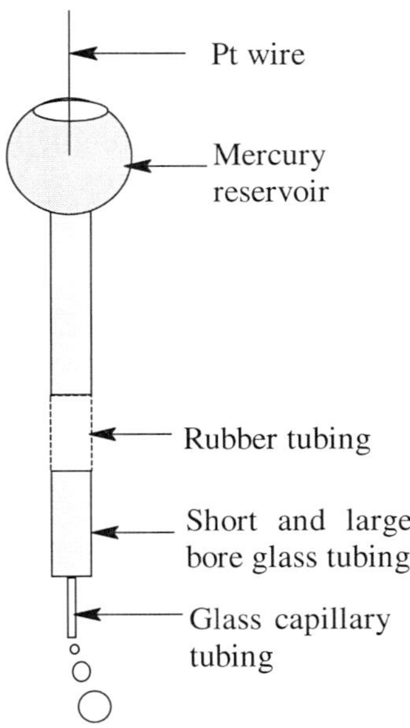

Fig. 11.4: Dropping mercury electrode

Advantages of DME

1) In case of a solid electrode in the form of a rod or a plate, the electrode reaction takes place at the surface of an electrode. The products of the reduction reaction accumulate on the surface of an electrode. This deposition of products does not make available the electrons on the electrode for the reduction of other cations near electrode. Thus, accumulation of the electrode reaction products adversely affects the potential at the surface of a solid electrode.

   Dropping mercury electrode is not a solid electrode. The negatively charged droplets of mercury are continuously formed at the tip of the capillary. Hence, even if the products are accumulated on one drop, the next drop, which is formed freshly at the tip of the capillary, is made available for the reduction of other cations in the vicinity of a mercury droplet. Thus, because of the renewal of the surface of the drop, always a fresh surface is available for the reduction reaction. Therefore, accumulation of the electrode reaction products does not adversely affect the potential at the surface of mercury droplets. For example, if $PbCl_2$ is to be analyzed polarographically, it first dissociates into Pb^{+2} ions and Cl^- ions. The Pb^{+2} ions get reduced to Pb atoms, which further form an amalgam (Pb.Hg) with a mercury droplet. This product ultimately collects at the bottom of an electrolytic cell when a mercury droplet detaches from the capillary. New droplet formed at the tip of the capillary, provides the fresh surface for the reduction of few more Pb^{+2} ions.

2) Though DME is not a solid electrode, surface area of each mercury droplet can be easily calculated by using a formula for the surface area of a sphere. As long as the capillary of the same dimension is used throughout the polarographic studies, there is no change in the dimensions of mercury droplets. Thus, the reproducible surface area of the drop can be readily calculated at any time during the drop life.

3) Mercury droplet forms amalgam (solid solution) with many metals, which is formed at its surface after reduction of ionic species. Because of this, species get reduced at lower potentials.

4) Dropping mercury electrode can be used up to -1.6 V in acidic medium and up to -2.6 V in basic solution or in non-aqueous solution, when used in combination with saturated calomel electrode. With other solid microelectrodes, it is not possible to achieve reduction at such a low voltage. Voltage required for the reduction of H^+ ions (available from aqueous solution) at DME is higher as compared to that required for the reduction of most of the cations or electro-reducible species The reduction of H^+ ions leads to the evolution of hydrogen gas. This involves the risk of explosion at the electrode.

$$2\,H^+ + 2e \longrightarrow H_2$$

If most of the species get reduced at DME at a potential which is lower than that required to reduce H^+ ions, then automatically the risk of explosion due to the formation of hydrogen gas is avoided. Thus, *high overvoltage of hydrogen** at DME makes possible the safe electro-reduction of many species at negative potentials, which are unattainable on solid microelectrodes.

5) A minute current flows through DME, since it is a microelectrode. This brings about controlled electrolysis in polarography. Since electrolysis

*** Hydrogen overvoltage**

Hydrogen is reduced at DME according to the following equations -

$$H + H^+ \rightarrow H_2^+ \quad \text{and} \quad H_2^+ + e \rightarrow H_2$$

Thus, molecular hydrogen is formed by the combination of a hydrogen atom, formed by electrolysis, with H^+ ion. The theoretical potential E at which H^+ ions are reduced at DME at 25 °C is given by the equation -

$$E = E_{Ho} + 0.0592 \log [H^+]$$

where, E_{Ho} is the standard potential of the normal hydrogen electrode and $[H^+]$ is the concentration of hydrogen ions. In practice, a potential higher than E is required before hydrogen is evolved at the electrode. The difference between these two potentials is known as *hydrogen overvoltage*. Its magnitude depends on the type of electrode, concentration of hydrogen ions $[H^+]$, temperature, etc. In polarography, it also depends on the presence of other ions in solution. The high hydrogen overvoltage of DME extends its voltage range to about -2.0 V with respect to SCE, if the pH and the supporting electrolyte are selected carefully.

current is very small (usually < 50 μA), the extent of reduction of an analyte is negligible and hence, several polarograms can be run on the same solution without appreciable change.

6) Diffusion current (i_d, as shown in **Fig. 11.8**) reaches a steady value rapidly and is reproducible, when DME is used as cathode.

Disadvantages of DME

1) Mercury is oxidized at an applied potential of about + 0.4 V (vs. SCE) and hence, it has a very limited potential range as an anode. Thus, high positive potentials cannot be maintained at DME.
2) In DME, mercury droplets are used as cathode. The surface area of these droplets (i.e. of an electrode) is constantly changing because drops form, grow in size, attain a constant weight, and then detach from the capillary. The change in the surface area of these droplets gives rise to current oscillations. Hence, the S-shaped c-v curve is not smooth, but consists of wavy lines, as shown in **Fig. 11.2**.
3) The potential applied to DME, affects the interfacial tension between the mercury droplet and an analyte solution. This affects the size of mercury droplets. While recording a polarogram, the potential at DME is gradually changed. This leads to the changes in the size of droplets and hence, in its surface area. Since surface area is required for the calculation of concentration of a solute, this changing surface area leads to a change in the calculated value of the concentration of an analyte. The size of droplets is also influenced by chemical agents, which can affect this interfacial tension between the mercury droplet and an analyte solution.

11.3.2.2. Calomel Electrode

Construction

As shown in **Fig. 11.5**, this electrode consists of pure mercury in contact with a mixture of mercury and calomel (Hg_2Cl_2) and a solution of potassium chloride.

Working

The reaction which determines the potential of this electrode is given below.

$$Hg_2Cl_2\ (s) + 2e \longrightarrow 2\ Hg + 2\ Cl^-$$

Commonly, 0.1N, 1N or saturated solution of KCl is used for the polarographic studies. When the saturated solution is used in the preparation of calomel electrode, the electrode is called as *saturated calomel electrode* (SCE). The potential of calomel electrode depends both on the temperature and the concentration of KCl solution. (The potentials of the calomel electrode vs. the normal hydrogen electrode in saturated, 1N and 0.1N KCl solutions are + 250, + 286 and + 338 mV, respectively, at 20°C and + 246, + 285 and + 338 mV at 25°C, respectively).

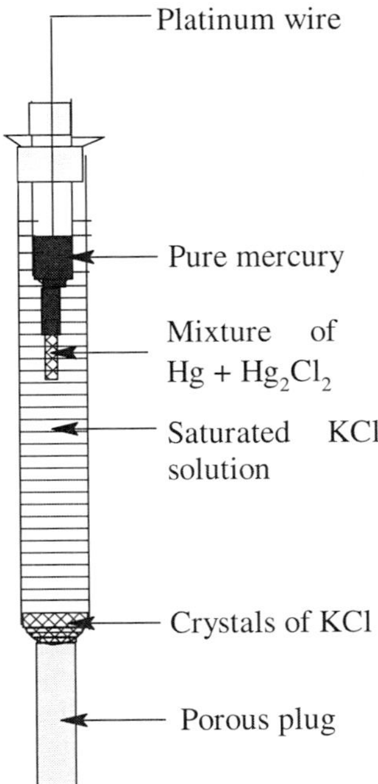

Fig. 11.5: Calomel electrode

Saturated calomel electrode acts as an anode. The anion of an analyte undergoes oxidation with the deposition of electrons on it. In case of $PbCl_2$ as an analyte, the Cl^- ions get oxidized at SCE as shown below.

$$2Cl^- \longrightarrow Cl_2 + 2e$$

Advantages

(i) Saturated calomel electrode is easy to prepare.
(ii) It provides consistent potential.

Hence, it is the most widely used reference electrode.

Disadvantage

Saturated calomel electrode suffers from a drawback of having a high temperature coefficient for voltage and is of the order of -0.76 mV/°C, i.e. the potential of SCE changes by 0.76 mV with the change in the temperature by 1 °C. This change in potential leads to the errors in the analysis and hence, is of significance in accurate analysis.

Thus, in polarography, two electrodes used are DME and SCE. When cathode other than DME (such as solid platinum electrode) is used, the method is known as *voltammetry* and the resulting c-v curve is referred to as a *voltammogram*.

11.3.2.3. Comparison between DME and SCE

1) Dropping mercury electrode is used as a *cathode*, where reduction of an analyte takes place and saturated calomel electrode is used as an *anode*, where oxidation occurs.
2) Cathode is in the form of droplets and is termed as a *microelectrode*. In SCE, platinum wire or rod is used for electric contact and hence, it is a *macroelectrode*.
3) When external e.m.f. is applied across the electrolysis cell, the electrons are supplied to the cathode, which spread over a smaller surface area of a droplet. Because of high electron density (number of electrons per unit surface area), a mercury droplet gets polarized. Hence, DME is termed as a *polarizable* electrode. In a circuit, the same number of electrons flow through anode also but because of the larger surface area of anode, the electron density is much lower as compared to that in DME. Therefore, it does not get polarized. Hence, SCE is termed as a *non-polarizable* electrode.
4) Since the electron density at DME changes with the change in the PD across the electrodes of a polarographic cell, the potential of cathode (DME) goes on changing as the PD across the electrodes is changed. However, the potential of anode remains almost constant even if the PD across the cell is changed, because of its non-polarizable character or because electron density on it remains almost constant at all the potential values. Since the potential of SCE remains almost constant, it is termed as a *reference electrode*, whereas DME is termed as an *indicator electrode*.

The comparison between DME and SCE is tabulated in **Table 11.1**.

Table 11.1: Comparison between DME and SCE

Sr. No.	DME	SCE
1	Acts as a cathode.	Acts as an anode.
2	It is a microelectrode.	It is a macroelectrode.
3	It is a polarizable electrode.	It is a non-polarizable electrode.
4	It acts as an indicator electrode	It acts as a reference electrode

Thus, in polarography, when PD across wo electrodes is changed, the potential of SCE remains unaltered, whereas the potential of DME changes. The actual applied potential across the electrodes is equal to the potential of the large surfaced SCE less the potential of the polarized electrode, DME. When the potential of SCE remains constant, the PD across the electrodes is equal to the potential of DME (E_{appl}). This external potential (E_{appl}) is applied by means of a potentiometer.

11.3.3. A Galvanometer or an Ammeter for Measuring Electrolysis Current

When external potential is applied to the electrodes in the polarographic cell, the electrolysis of an analyte occurs. The current produced due to electrolysis is measured using either a fast responding galvanometer or a damped galvanometer. A fast responding galvanometer records the maximum current produced during electrolysis, whereas a damped galvanometer records the average current produced during electrolysis.

11.4. BASIC CONCEPTS OF ELECTROCHEMISTRY

In order to understand polarographic technique, it is recommended that a reader should go through few basic concepts of electrochemistry.

11.4.1. Anode

Any electrode, at which oxidation reaction occurs, is termed as an *anode*. Hence, the term *anodic oxidation* is commonly used in electrochemistry.

11.4.2. Cathode

Any electrode, at which reduction reaction occurs, is termed as a *cathode*. Hence, the term *cathodic reduction* is common in electrochemistry.

11.4.3. Electric Current in Solution

The movement of the positively charged ions towards the negative electrode and the movement of the negatively charged ions towards the positive electrode constitute an *electric current* in solution.

11.4.4. Potential

The magnitude of the charge on an object is termed as its *potential.*

11.4.5. Voltage

Voltage is nothing but the potential difference between two objects.

11.4.6. Difference between the Galvanic and an Electrolytic Cell (Voltaic Cell)

A *galvanic cell* acts as a source of electricity to an electrolytic cell. The galvanic cell *converts chemical energy to electrical energy.*

An *electrolytic cell* or a *voltaic cell* makes use of an electrical energy provided by a galvanic cell and *converts this electrical energy to chemical energy* so as to bring about either oxidation or reduction of an electrolyte at the electrodes.

11.4.6.1. A Galvanic Cell

Daniel cell is an example of a galvanic cell. As shown in **Fig. 11.6**, it consists of two electrodes. Zinc electrode is dipped in the solution of zinc sulphate, whereas copper electrode is dipped in the solution of copper sulphate. Each electrode, along with the solution in which it is dipped, is termed as a '*half cell*'. Thus, a Daniel cell consists of two half cells.

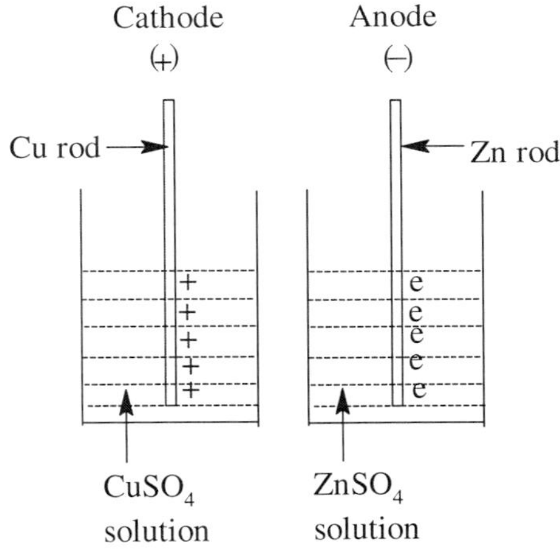

Fig. 11.6: Daniel cell or a galvanic cell

Electrode Reactions in the galvanic cell

(a) In one half cell, zinc passes into solution and gets oxidized to Zn^{+2} ions.

$$Zn \longrightarrow Zn^{+2} + 2e \ \ldots \text{(Anodic oxidation)}$$

Since zero-valent zinc is oxidized to a divalent zinc ion, this reaction is an *oxidation* reaction. Hence, zinc electrode is termed as an *anode* (Anodic oxidation). The electrons, which are liberated during this oxidation reaction, are deposited on zinc electrode and hence, this electrode gains negative charge. Though it is negatively charged, it is still referred to as an anode, since the oxidation reaction occurs at this electrode.

(b) In another half cell, cupric ions are reduced to atomic copper, which are deposited on the surface of an electrode.

$$Cu^{+2} + 2e \longrightarrow Cu \ \ldots \text{(Cathodic reduction)}$$

Since divalent cupric ions are reduced to a zero valent copper, this reaction is a *reduction* reaction. Hence, copper electrode is termed as a *cathode*. During reduction, electrons are consumed by Cu^{+2} ions and these electrons are obtained from the

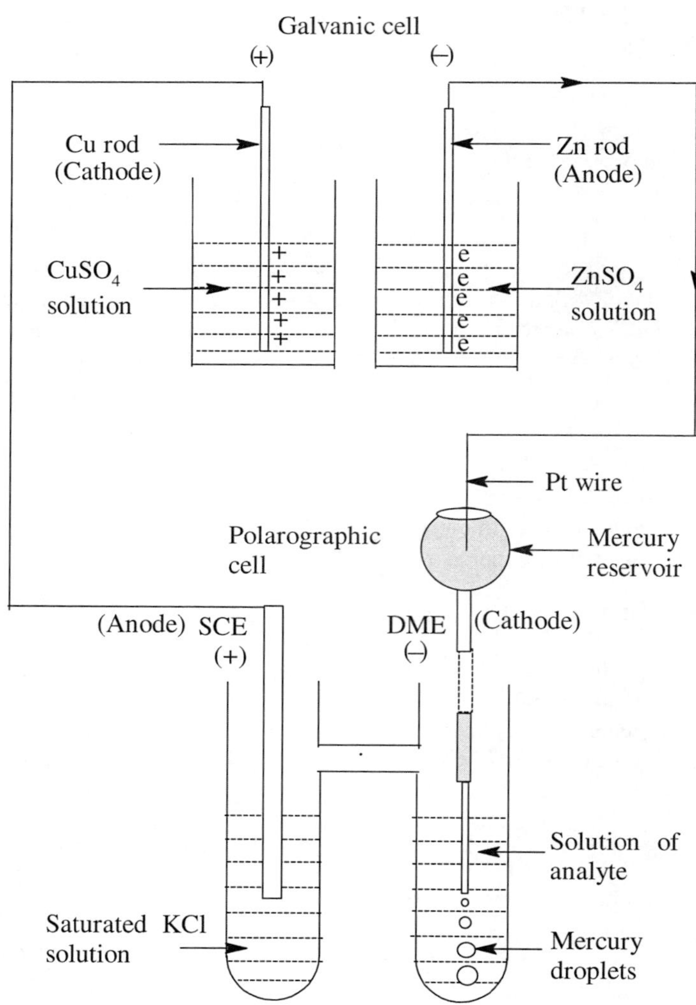

Fig. 11.7: Supply of electrons to DME from a galvanic cell

copper rod itself. Thus, copper rod attains positive potential. Though it is positively charged, it is still referred to as a cathode, since the reduction reaction occurs at this electrode.

11.4.6.2. Electrolytic Cell or a Voltaic Cell (Polarographic Cell)

A polarographic cell is an example of an electrolytic cell or a voltaic cell. In an electrolytic cell, cathode (dropping mercury electrode in case of polarography) is connected to zinc electrode of the galvanic cell, with the help of a metallic wire. The electrons accumulated on zinc rod are thus, supplied to the cathode. Hence, the cathode of an electrolytic cell is at negative potential. This is shown in **Fig. 11.7**. The electrons supplied to the cathode are used up for the reduction of the cations of an analyte. Thus, in a galvanic cell, cathode is positively charged, whereas in an electrolytic or a polarographic cell, cathode is negatively charged.

11.5. COMPONENTS OF A POLAROGRAM (c-v Curve)

The solution of an analyte is prepared, usually, in water. In order to remove an electro-reducible impurity of dissolved oxygen from an analyte solution, nitrogen gas is bubbled through it for several minutes. Otherwise, dissolved oxygen would interfere with the c-v curve of an analyte. A gradually increasing voltage is applied to the electrodes and the corresponding current is measured. A polarogram for an analyte is then obtained by plotting current on Y-axis and voltage (E_{appl}) across the electrodes or the potential of DME on X-axis. A separate polarogram is also run on a blank solution devoid of an analyte. This provides the correct value of the residual current (i_r) in the circuit, required for an accurate determination of concentration of an analyte. A typical S-shaped polarogram is shown in **Fig. 11.8**.

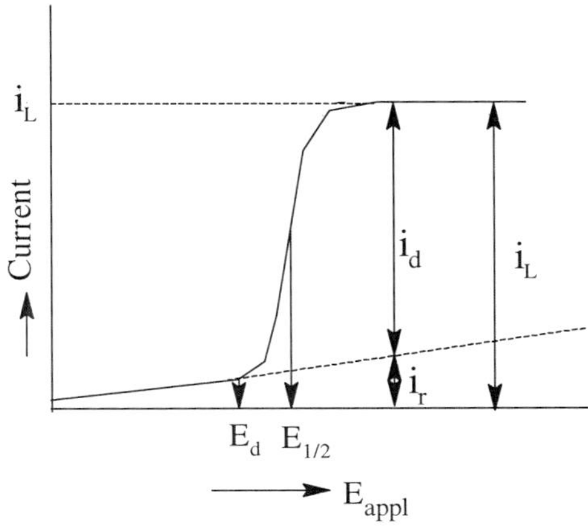

Fig. 11.8: S-shaped c-v curve in polarography

Meaning of the abbreviations used in **Fig. 11.8** is explained below.

i_r = residual current

i_d = diffusion current, which is proportional to the concentration of electro-reducible ions present in the sample. Thus, it is a quantitative parameter in polarography.

i_L = limiting current, which is the maximum current obtained during polarography.

Recording of a polarogram is continued till limiting current is obtained.

E_d = decomposition potential of the species, which depends both on the species getting reduced and also on the electrode at which a species is getting reduced.

At decomposition potential, an electrolyte starts getting reduced near electrode.

$E_{1/2}$ = half wave potential, which produces a current midway along the steeply rising portion of the S-shaped curve. It is a characteristic of the species being analyzed and hence, is a parameter used for qualitative analysis. The most important point is that it is independent of the electrodes used.

As PD across electrodes is changed, a typical S-shaped c-v curve is obtained due to changes in the flow of current through the cell. The flow of current depends on many factors, which are described below.

11.6. FACTORS INFLUENCING FLOW OF CURRENT DURING CONTROLLED ELECTROLYSIS

In electrolysis, when an external e.m.f. is applied to the electrolytic cell, the electrons are supplied to the cathode. At a particular potential of a microelectrode (DME), it gets *polarized* and transfers the electrons to the electro-reducible substance at the electrode surface. The reduction of an electro-reducible species occurs at cathode, where electrons are supplied by the cathode to an electrolyte. Oxidation of an electro-oxidizable species occurs at anode, where electrons are received from an electrolyte. The consumption of electrons from cathode and the yield of electrons at anode are responsible for the production of current in the circuit.

Electrolysis of any species involves at least three factors which control the flow of current. In order to find the current produced in the circuit, based on the concentration of an electrolyte in the cell, the cations of an electrolyte from the bulk of a solution should first reach cathode or DME (**Mass Transfer**). Once near cathode, an electrode should provide the required number of electrons for the reduction of these cations (**Electron Transport**). After the electrode reaction, the products formed at the electrode should be removed so that the next species that approaches the electrode, experiences the same potential at the electrode (**Removal of product from electrode**). All these steps are discussed in detail below.

11.6.1. Mass Transfer

11.6.1.1. Migration
11.6.1.2. Convection
11.6.1.3. Diffusion

11.6.2. Electron Transfer

11.6.2.1. Reversible electrode reactions
11.6.2.2. Irreversible electrode reactions

11.6.3. Removal of the product

Control on all the above mentioned factors assists in obtaining accurate value of current required for quantitative estimation of analytes.

11.6.1. Mass Transfer

Three basic mechanisms are involved in the mass transfer of an analyte from the bulk of the solution to the polarized electrode surface, where it can be reduced. These mechanisms are migration, convection and diffusion.

11.6.1.1. Migration

In a polarographic cell, an electrolyte exists in the dissociated form. Hence, the positively charged cations and the negatively charged anions are present in solution. The electropositive species of an electrolyte are attracted towards the negatively charged and polarized DME, while the electronegative species of an electrolyte are attracted towards the positively charged SCE. This mass transfer of ions from bulk to the electrodes is not based on the concentration gradient, but is based on the potential gradient produced in the solution. Hence, this means of transport does not provide information about the concentration of an analyte in the cell, and therefore, *mass transfer by migration is not preferred in polarography.*

However, the attraction between the charged ions of an electrolyte and the charged electrodes cannot be avoided, but it can be minimized by the addition of a large excess of an inert substance called the *supporting electrolyte* (SE) to the solution of an analyte. For example, if the supporting electrolyte used is 0.1 M KCl solution, it is completely ionized in the solution and exists in the form of K^+ ions and Cl^- ions. The K^+ ions migrate towards cathode and the Cl^- ions migrate towards anode. Compared to the amount of the supporting electrolyte, the amount of an analyte ($PbCl_2$ in **Fig. 11.9**) is less. Hence, the cations of an analyte do not get attracted towards a cathode, DME. Since, K^+ ions are not reduced at the selected applied potential to the cathode, they simply form a layer of charged particles around the microelectrode and avoid the attraction of cations of an electrolyte by the electrode. This is shown in **Fig. 11.9** for $PbCl_2$ as an analyte. Thus, mass transfer by migration is avoided by using a large excess of an inert electrolyte.

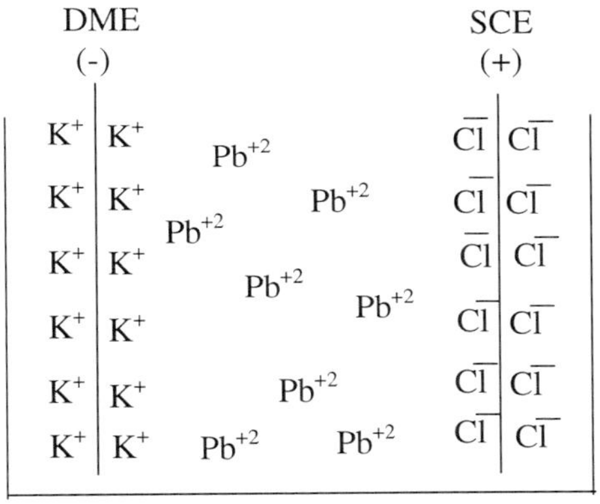

DME (-) SCE (+)

K^+ | K^+ Pb^{+2} Cl^- | Cl^-

K^+ | K^+ Pb^{+2} Pb^{+2} Cl^- | Cl^-

K^+ | K^+ Pb^{+2} Pb^{+2} Cl^- | Cl^-

K^+ | K^+ Cl^- | Cl^-

K^+ | K^+ Pb^{+2} Cl^- | Cl^-

K^+ | K^+ Pb^{+2} Pb^{+2} Cl^- | Cl^-

Fig. 11.9: Role of supporting electrolyte in polarography

11.6.1.2. Convection

This means of transport operates when the solution is agitated. The agitation may be caused by the difference in the density or temperature in various parts of an electrolytic cell or it may be produced by some form of mechanical stirring. For example, when mercury droplets detach from the capillary tubing and fall down in an electrolyte solution, they cause agitation. Because of agitation, a layer of K^+ ions around DME is disturbed. This allows more of electro-active substance (i.e. Pb^{+2} ions) to reach the electrode surface and leads to an increase in the current flow, which is not a real measure of the actual concentration of an electrolyte in the cell.

11.6.1.3. Diffusion

Diffusion brings about mass transfer of an electro-active species based on the concentration gradient. Below the decomposition potential (potential required to start the reduction of cations at DME), the concentration of an electrolyte in bulk [C_b] and near electrode [C_e] is sufficient. Hence, the concentration gradient (C_b - C_e) is not sufficiently large. The concentration gradient is the driving force which drives cations from bulk towards an electrode, where they get reduced and contribute to the current in the circuit.

When the potential corresponding to the decomposition potential of an analyte is applied to DME, slowly, ions near DME start getting reduced and hence, the concentration of the reducible species (e.g. Pb^{+2} ions) at the electrode surface [C_e] is rapidly reduced. The concentration of an electrolyte in the bulk [C_b], however, does not change much, even when some of the cations are reduced near cathode, because the concentration or the number of ions of an electrolyte in the bulk is much higher than the number of ions that get reduced near DME. Since [C_b] is almost constant and [C_e] is reduced, the difference between [C_b] and [C_e], i.e. the concentration gradient (C_b - C_e), is increased. Since the driving force which is responsible for bringing ions from bulk to the electrode increases, more and more cations are transferred from bulk to the electrode. This leads to an increase in the mass transfer. When the concentration gradient remains constant, i.e. when C_e = zero and (C_b - C_e) = (C_b - 0) = C_b, a constant current, called as a *limiting current*, is obtained in the circuit. This change in current in different portions of c-v curve is explained in detail, later in this chapter. The limiting current provides information about the concentration of an analyte in the sample. The limiting current is lower in an unstirred system as compared to that in the stirred system. Stirring of the solution brings more of electro-reducible species near the electrode and increases the limiting current. A constant limiting current value can only be achieved in an unstirred solution (as in case of polarography) or in solutions stirred at a constant rate (as in case of voltammetry). The magnitude of the limiting current is also related to the factors such as diffusion coefficient of an analyte in a particular medium and the surface area (A) of the microelectrode.

11.6.2. Electron Transfer

Once the electro-reducible species is brought near DME, it is reduced only if proper potential is applied to DME. The potential at which the reduction of an electro-reducible species starts at the electrode is termed as its *decomposition potential* (E_d). The potential of an electrode indicates the availability of electrons from it. At lower potentials (beyond E_d), DME makes available few electrons to an electro-active species near it and hence, only few cations are reduced at DME, thereby producing a small current in the circuit. At higher potentials, DME makes available a larger number of electrons to the cations near it and hence, more cations are reduced at DME, thereby producing higher current in the circuit.

The electron transfer process occurs on the electrode surface between the electrode and the electro-active species like Pb^{+2} ions. If this species is in equilibrium with other species, like $PbCl_2$ (as shown in the dissociation reaction below), then the equilibrium must shift towards right side to produce more of the active species (Pb^{+2} ions), so that it is reduced at the electrode during electron transfer process, thereby producing current in the circuit.

$$PbCl_2 \rightleftharpoons Pb^{+2} + 2\,Cl^- \text{... (Dissociation)}$$

This equilibrium shift to produce more of the electro-active species occurs either at the electrode surface or in the bulk of the solution. The electron transfer process is *reversible* or *irreversible*. It is *reversible* only while the product (Pb atoms obtained by the reduction of Pb^{+2} ions by the gain of electrons from the electrode) is at the electrode surface. This is because when the product (Pb) is at the electrode, it can donate two electrons gained by it during its reduction, back to the electrode and get converted to Pb^{+2} ions. Under this condition, the two electron transfer rates (the rate of accepting electrons from an electrode and the rate of donating electrons to the electrode) differ only in their directions. The reversible electrode reaction occurs when the forward and the reverse electron transfer rates are much greater than the mass transfer rates.

$$Pb^{+2} + 2\,e \rightleftharpoons Pb \text{ ... (Reduction)}$$

The electrode process is *irreversible* when the mass transfer rate is much faster than the electron transfer rate. When many electro-active species are present near electrode, the reversible reaction so as to convert product back to an electro-active species does not get preference over the normal electrode reaction.

11.6.3. Removal of the Product

Accumulation of the product at the electrode surface does not allow an electro-active species to feel the actual potential applied to the electrode, since the accumulated product acts as a barrier between the electrode and an electro-active species, as shown in **Fig. 11.10**. The product

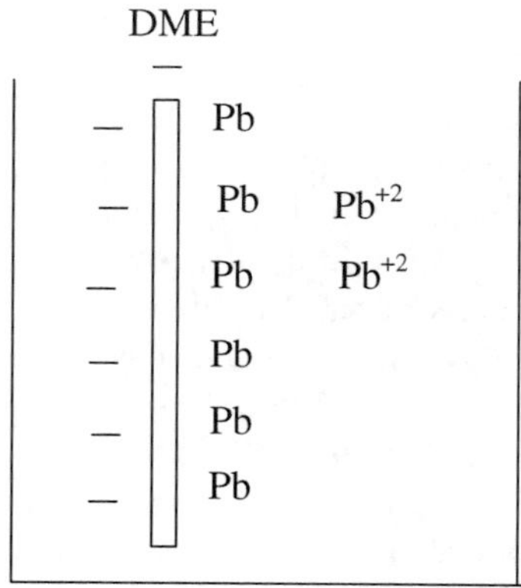

Fig. 11.10: Barrier of an accumulated product between electrode and an analyte

accumulation affects the electron transfer process as well as the mass transfer process, both of which are important in deciding the magnitude of the limiting current and hence, of the actual concentration of an analyte. In case of DME, accumulation of the product at the electrode surface does not come into picture, since the electrode is in the form of droplets and always a fresh surface is available for the electrode reaction.

11.7. NATURE OF c-v CURVE

Explanation of variation in the current in the current-voltage curve in polarography can be explained with the help of **Fig. 11.11**. A typical polarogram consists of three parts.

11.7.1. Part AB, corresponding to the *residual current*, i_r

11.7.2. Part BC, corresponding to the *diffusion current*, i_d

11.7.3. Part CD, corresponding to the *limiting current*, i_L

Point B corresponds to the *decomposition potential* (E_d) of an analyte.

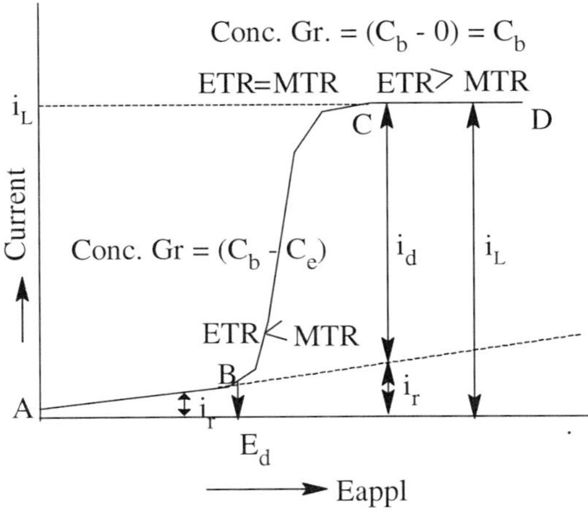

Fig. 11.11: Different parts in c-v curve of a polarogram

11.7.1. Part AB

When an external potential, less than the decomposition potential (E_d) of an analyte, is applied to DME, a small electrolysis current is produced, provided some soluble electro-reducible substances or impurities are present in the electrolytic cell, which get reduced at potential less than the decomposition potential (E_d) of an electrolyte. The current flowing across the solution-electrode interface is called the *faradic current* (i_f). Below the decomposition potential, this faradic current is due to the reduction of trace impurities in an analyte. For example, water used for preparing solution of an analyte contains traces of O_2. It is very difficult to remove last traces of O_2 from water even after bubbling N_2 gas through the solution. Similarly, ordinary distilled water often contains traces of copper. An impurity of Hg^{+2} ions can also be present in solution if the solutions are deoxygenated in presence of pool anode, with the formation of H_2O_2. Since all these impurities are present in traces, the faradic current is very minute. The major contribution to the residual current is from the *condenser current* (i_c), which is produced due to the formation of Helmholtz double layer. The formation of Helmholtz double layer or a condenser or a capacitor at the mercury droplet-solution interface, is shown in **Fig. 11.12**.

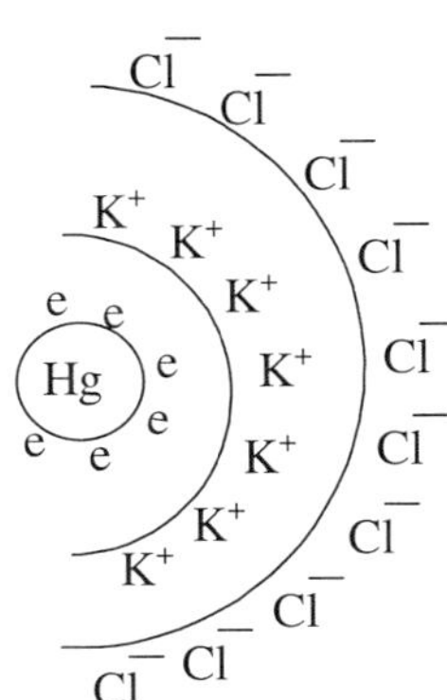

Fig. 11.12: Formation of Helmholtz double layer

The positively charged K^+ ions of the supporting electrolyte (KCl) form a layer around the negatively charged Hg droplets, which in turn are surrounded by a layer of the negatively charged Cl^- ions. The formation of this double layer produces a condenser current. Thus, a residual current, which is produced below decomposition potential, is the sum of the faradic current (i_f) and the condenser current (i_c).

$$i_r = i_f + i_c \quad ... (11.1)$$

Since the impurities are present in smaller concentration, the magnitude of the faradic current is smaller and since, the supporting electrolyte is present in greater amount, the magnitude of the condenser current is greater.

11.7.2. Part BC

If $PbCl_2$ is the analyte in polarography, initially it is dissociated into Pb^{+2} ions and Cl^- ions. The reduction of Pb^{+2} ions starts at point B, which is the decomposition potential of Pb^{+2} ions. As the potential at DME is increased, more Pb^{+2} ions are reduced at DME. The number of Pb^{+2} ions that are reduced near DME depends on the electron transfer rate (ETR). At lower potentials, ETR is low. Hence, all the Pb^{+2} ions, which are present near DME, are not reduced. When few Pb^{+2} ions are reduced, the concentration of Pb^{+2} ions near DME (C_e) is depleted and the concentration gradient (C_b - C_e), increases. As the concentration gradient increases, the driving force, which is responsible for bringing more Pb^{+2} ions near DME, also increases. This increases the rate of mass transfer (MTR) of Pb^{+2} ions from bulk to DME, and hence, more of Pb^{+2} ions are brought near DME. When the increasing negative potential is applied to DME, more and more electrons are provided to it. This increases the rate of electron transfer (ETR). With the increase in ETR, more of Pb^{+2} ions are reduced at DME, which further reduces the concentration of Pb^{+2} ions near DME. Reducing the concentration of Pb^{+2} ions near DME, further increases the concentration gradient. Thus, in part BC, both ETR and MTR go on increasing. Since more and more Pb^{+2} ions are reduced at DME, a continuously increasing current is obtained in this part. At point B (**Fig. 11.11**), ETR is low and MTR is moderate, because C_e has some value greater than zero. Over the portion, BC, both ETR and MTR continue to rise, but ETR is always less than MTR.

11.7.3. Part CD

At point C, the magnitudes of both ETR and MTR become exactly equal. The electron transfer rate is so high that whatever number of Pb^{+2} ions is brought near DME, all are reduced. Beyond point C, ETR is always more than MTR. Because of this, the concentration of Pb^{+2} ions near DME (C_e) becomes zero. Hence, (C_b - Ce) = (C_b - 0) = C_b, where, C_b is the concentration of an analyte in bulk. It is also equal to the original concentration of an analyte, since the extent of electrolysis is very low in polarography. Therefore, in this portion, the

1. Limiting Current (i_L): It is the total current read in an ammeter. It includes residual current (i_r), diffusion current (i_d) and sometimes, migration current (i_m) of a reducible substance, if this is not adequately suppressed.

$$i_L = i_r + i_d + i_m$$

In presence of excess supporting electrolyte, $i_m = 0$.

2. Residual current (i_r): It is the current obtained below decomposition potential and is the sum of the faradic current (i_f) and the condenser current (i_c).

$$i_r = i_f + i_c$$

3. Migration Current (i_m): Undesirable contribution to the cathodic current is referred to as the migration current. The migration current is mainly produced due to the mass transfer from bulk to DME because of potential gradient, i.e. due to attraction of cations of an electrolyte by DME. This current is undesirable in polarography. It is eliminated by the addition of a large excess of an inert electrolyte like potassium chloride, which conducts nearly the total current across the electrolysis cell but does not interfere with the electrode reaction of interest.

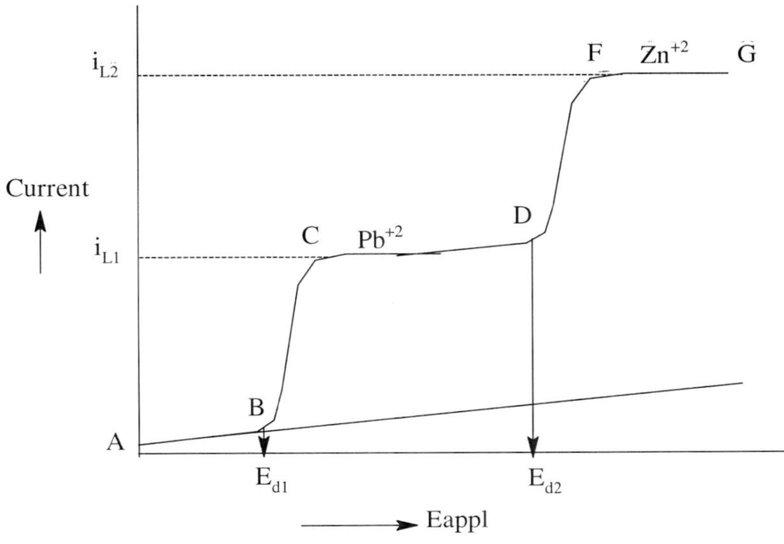

Fig. 11.13: Polarogram for a mixture of Pb^{+2} ions and Zn^{+2} ions

concentration gradient remains constant, which is equal to C_b. Since the concentration gradient remains constant, always a constant number of Pb^{+2} ions are brought from bulk to DME. Reduction of a constant number of Pb^{+2} ions at any potential of DME in this portion produces a constant current. Hence, a plateau is produced. This constant value of current is called as a *limiting current* (i_L). When this current is obtained, recording of the polarogram is stopped. The limiting current is the sum of the residual current (i_r) and the diffusion current (i_d).

$$i_L = i_r + i_d$$

If a solution of an analyte contains two different ions, as the voltage is raised, after the limiting current for one ion has been reached, the potential eventually rises to a value at which cations of another metal are reduced. Consequently, the current voltage curve begins to rise again after the horizontal stretch. Thus, determination of different ions is possible if the reduction potentials of ions to be detected vary by more than 0.2V. For example, if the solution contains, Pb^{+2} ions and Zn^{+2} ions in the mixture, then a polarogram with two S-shaped curves is obtained as shown in **Fig. 11.13**.

The first wave on the polarogram is for the reduction of Pb^{+2} ions.

$$Pb^{+2} + 2e \rightarrow Pb \rightarrow \underset{\text{Amalgam}}{Pb(Hg)}$$

The second wave is for the reduction of Zn^{+2} ions present in the solution.

$$Zn^{+2} + 2e \rightarrow Zn \rightarrow \underset{\text{Amalgam}}{Zn(Hg)}$$

Many a times, the adjustment of pH of the solution is required so that the reduction potentials of two or more cations do not coincide. Sometimes, in order to remove interference of one cation in the analysis of another cation, a substance forming complex with a particular ion is also added.

In order to confirm that proper conditions are maintained during polarographic analysis, the diffusion currents for the sample and the standard solutions are measured under identical conditions and the concentration of the sample is calculated from the ratio of the diffusion currents for the sample ($i_{unknown}$) to the standard ($i_{standard}$). Concentration of the unknown sample is calculated from the following formula.

$$\frac{C_{unknown}}{C_{Standard}} = \frac{i_{unknown}}{i_{standard}} \quad \cdots (11.2)$$

where, $C_{unknown}$ is the concentration of sample and $C_{standard}$ is the concentration of a standard.

11.8. SIMPLE MANUAL POLAROGRAPH

Construction

The simplest instrument commonly used for recording polarograms is known as a *simple manual polarograph*. The circuitry of a simple manual polarograph is as shown in **Fig. 11.14**. It consists of a *potentiometer* made up of a *battery* (B) and a *resistance* (R_1). The position (P) of the pointer or a *jockey* (J_1), on the resistance wire (R_1) supplies the required negative potential to DME of the polarographic cell (C). Saturated calomel electrode is connected to another jockey (J_2), which can move on the shunt (R_2), so that the magnitude of current in an ammeter can be adjusted. The instrument is switched on and off by means of a switch (S). With the help of a jockey (J_1), voltage (V) between DME and SCE can be varied.

Working

To plot a polarogram, the value of resistance (R_2) is kept maximum, so that the sensitivity of the instrument is minimum. Under this position, large current cannot pass through an ammeter. Thus, the high resistance (R_2), protects an ammeter. If this resistance is kept to the minimum, a large current can pass through the circuit, which can destroy an ammeter. Hence, resistance (R_2) is also called as a *shunt*. The instrument is then switched on by means of a switch (S).

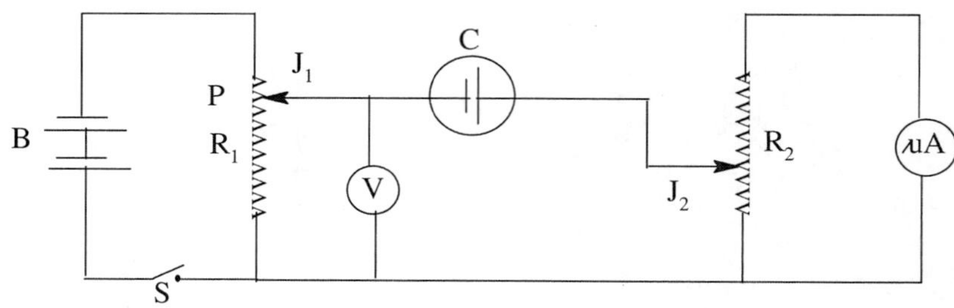

Fig. 11.14: A simple manual polarograph

By adjusting the position of a jockey on (R_1) of a potentiometer, a suitable potential (around 0.1 V) is applied, which is indicated by a voltmeter V. The magnitude of current in an ammeter is recorded. If this current is too low, which cannot be measured accurately, then the resistance (R_2) is reduced and the sensitivity is increased. Reduction in resistance of a shunt allows more current to pass through it so that higher accuracy is obtained in the measurement. Once the position of J_2 on R_2 is adjusted, it is kept fixed for the subsequent readings. The negative potential of DME is then increased with the help of a jockey J_1 and the magnitude of the current produced is recorded. This process is repeated until a sufficient number of readings, which can provide S-shaped curve, are recorded or till a constant current (limiting current) is obtained in the circuit. A polarogram is then plotted for the negative potentials applied to DME and the currents produced in the circuit.

Disadvantage

One obvious disadvantage of a simple manual

polarograph is that it makes use of an uncalibrated potentiometer and hence, it cannot be used for very accurate measurements, unless a standardizing circuit is incorporated.

11.9. ILKOVIC EQUATION

In order to confirm that the current obtained is diffusion controlled and is not governed by any other factors, a theoretical equation is derived for it. The theoretical expression for diffusion current is known as *Ilkovic equation*. This equation takes into account the factors which affect diffusion of an analyte in the electrolytic cell. It is expressed as follows.

$$i_d = k.\, n\, D^{1/2}\, c.\, m^{2/3}.\, t^{1/6} \quad \ldots(11.3)$$

where, k = a constant = 607 or 706. Its value is obtained from a combination of numerical constants, which include geometry of the mercury drop, Faraday number (F) in coulombs, density of mercury, etc. When average diffusion current is measured by using a damped galvanometer, $i_d = (i_d)_{avg}$ and k = 607. When the maximum diffusion current is measured by using a fast responding galvanometer, $i_d = (i_d)_{max}$ and k = 706. The relation between $(i_d)_{avg}$ and $(i_d)_{max}$ is as given in **equation 11.4**.

$$(i_d)_{max} = \frac{7}{6}(i_d)_{avg} \quad \ldots(11.4)$$

The explanation for $(i_d)_{avg}$ and $(i_d)_{max}$ is given under the **Section 11.9.1.1 (2)**.

In **equation 11.3**, n = number of electrons involved in electrode reaction. For example, n = 2 for the reduction of Pb^{+2} ions, since it consumes two electrons from the electrode.

D = diffusion coefficient of the reducible or the oxidizable substance. Its value depends on the temperature of an electrolytic solution.

c = concentration of a reducible or an oxidizable substance (mol/L),

m = flow rate of Hg from the capillary of DME (mg/sec),

t = average life time of mercury droplets at the tip of the capillary (sec). It is also referred to as drop time. It is usually measured when the potential corresponding to the half wave potential ($E_{1/2}$) is applied to DME.

Values of both, the flow rate of Hg and the drop time, depend on the factors like internal diameter of the capillary, height of the Hg reservoir, i.e. pressure of Hg at the tip of the capillary, the potential applied to DME, the temperature of an analyte and the composition of the solution.

Rearranging Ilkovic **equation (11.3)**, **equation (11.5)** is obtained.

$$k.\, n\, D^{1/2} = \frac{i_d}{c.\, m^{2/3}.\, t^{1/6}} \quad \cdots(11.5)$$

All the terms on the left hand side of **equation (11.5)** are constant and the product, $knD^{1/2}$, is called *diffusion current constant*. All the parameters in this term are independent of electrodes and instrument used. The product on the right hand side, $m^{2/3}\, t^{1/6}$, is called *capillary characteristics*. The terms, 'm' and 't', remain constant when all the experimental conditions, like height of mercury in mercury column, temperature, etc. are properly maintained. Thus, in **equation (11.5)**, all the terms, except diffusion current (i_d) and concentration (c), are constant. Hence, **equation (11.5)** can be written as follows.

$$\left(k.\, n\, D^{1/2}\right)\left(m^{2/3}.\, t^{1/6}\right) = \frac{i_d}{c} = \text{constant}$$

$$\text{Since, } \frac{i_d}{c} = \text{constant}, \; i_d \propto c$$

i.e. diffusion current $\propto$ concentration

Hence, an accurate measurement of diffusion current provides concentration of an analyte.

Putting proper values of all the parameters in **equation (11.3)**, theoretical value of diffusion current $(i_d)_{calc}$ can be obtained. Diffusion current measured from the polarogram $(i_d)_{exp}$ is compared with the theoretical value of diffusion current $(i_d)_{calc}$. If these two match exactly, then it confirms that electrolysis is diffusion controlled. If these two do not match, then the electrolysis current is governed, along with the concentration gradient, by the other factor also.

11.9.1. The Factors Influencing Diffusion Current

For the comparison of the experimental $(i_d)_{exp}$ and the theoretical $(i_d)_{calc}$ values of diffusion current, it is absolutely essential to measure the experimentally obtained diffusion current on a polarogram, accurately and it is also essential to calculate the theoretical diffusion current accurately. Following factors should be controlled to get a correct match between $(i_d)_{exp}$ and $(i_d)_{calc}$.

11.9.1.1. Determination of Diffusion Current (i_d)

1) Determination of the experimental value of diffusion current $(i_d)_{exp}$

For comparing theoretical and practical values of diffusion current, it is essential to measure diffusion current on a polarogram, accurately. If it is measured at different values of potentials at DME, the magnitude of the residual current varies. This can produce error in the measured values of diffusion current. Hence, diffusion current is always measured at a potential, where the interfacial tension (explained under the **Section 11.9.1.3**) at the mercury droplet-analyte solution interface remains constant. Exact values of the limiting current (i_L) and the residual current (i_r) are thus, measured at the same potential. The difference between the two gives $(i_d)_{exp}$. It is also essential to run a separate polarogram on the blank solution (containing no analyte) in order to get the exact value of the residual current.

2) Determination of the theoretical value of diffusion current $(i_d)_{calc}$

In order to calculate the theoretical value of diffusion current $(i_d)_{calc}$ accurately, it is essential to know the value of constant 'k' to be used (607 or 706) in the Ilkovic **equation (11.3)**, i.e. it is essential to know whether an ammeter is recording an *average current* or the *maximum current*. A *slow ammeter* or a *damped ammeter* records the average current and makes use of k = 607 for the calculation of diffusion current. A *fast responding ammeter* records the maximum current produced in the circuit and makes use of k = 706 for the calculation of diffusion current.

In case of DME, the size of a droplet varies at the tip of the capillary. A small droplet, formed in the beginning, slowly grows in size, becomes large and then detaches from the tip of the capillary. At a particular applied potential to DME, a definite number of electrons is provided to a mercury droplet. As mercury droplet grows in size, the electron density (charge per unit area) on it decreases. Thus, during the formation of a droplet, because of the change in its volume or surface area, the current produced also varies. When a droplet is smaller in size, the electron density on it is higher and correspondingly, current produced is higher. On the other hand, when a droplet grows in size, electron density on it decreases and correspondingly, current produced is also reduced. The change in the electron density with the change in the size of a droplet is shown in **Fig. 11.15**.

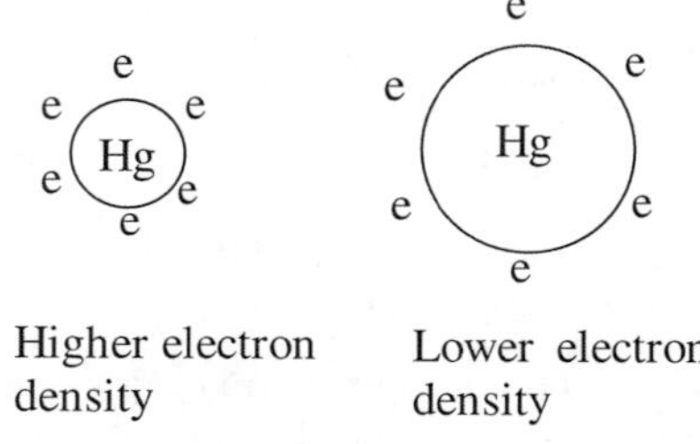

Fig. 11.15: Change in electron density with change in size of a mercury droplet

A fast responding ammeter is able to respond fast to the changes in the electron density on a mercury droplet and hence, to the changes in the current in the circuit. Thus, it can measure the maximum and the minimum values of current in the circuit. On the other hand, a damped galvanometer or a slow responding ammeter can neither respond to the maximum value (point B in **Fig.11.16)** nor to the minimum value (point C in **Fig. 11.16**) of current in the circuit. Let us consider a slow responding ammeter, shown in **Fig. 11.16**. At point A, it shows an average value of current. An ammeter pointer moves anticlockwise, when current is reduced and moves clockwise, when current is increased. When the droplet is small, more current is produced in the circuit and pointer in an ammeter tries to move towards B, but it cannot reach point B because it responds slowly as compared to the rate at which the current is changed. As a droplet grows bigger and bigger, current in the circuit is reduced and the pointer in an ammeter tries to move towards C, but it cannot reach point C also because it is a slow responding ammeter. Thus, a damped ammeter is not able to respond fast to the changes in the current in the circuit and thus, provides an average value of current.

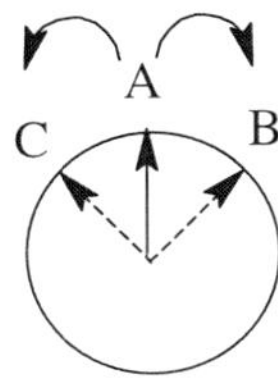

Fig. 11.16: Response in a damped ammeter

Thus, in order to calculate an accurate value of the theoretical current $(i_d)_{calc}$, it is essential to know the type of a galvanometer used so that the correct value of constant `k' can be selected. This helps in providing a correct match between the theoretical and the experimental diffusion currents.

11.9.1.2. Height of Mercury Column (h)

In Ilkovic equation, the values of two parameters, viz., flow rate of mercury (m) and life time (t) of a mercury droplet at the tip of the capillary, are dependent on two factors - dimensions of capillary of DME and the height of mercury column above the tip of the capillary. An increase in the height of a mercury column (h) does not increase the size of a mercury droplet, because size is exclusively determined by the internal diameter of the capillary of DME, but it definitely increases the pressure at the tip of the capillary and hence, automatically, there is an increase in the flow rate of mercury. Since flow rate increases, the number of drops formed per unit time also increases. This reduces the life time of each droplet at the tip of the capillary. Thus, 'm' varies linearly whereas 't' varies inversely with the height of mercury column. The relations between the flow rate and the height of a mercury column and between the life time of a droplet and the height of a mercury column are given by the **equations (11.6)** and **(11.7)**, respectively.

$$m \propto h_{corr}$$

$$\therefore m = k\, h_{corr} \quad \ldots (11.6)$$

$$\text{and } t \propto \frac{1}{h_{corr}}$$

$$\therefore t = k' \frac{1}{h_{corr}} \quad \ldots (11.7)$$

where, k and k' are constants and h_{corr} is the height of a mercury column in centimeters, above the tip of the capillary of DME, corrected for back pressure (h_{back}) due to the interfacial tension between a mercury droplet and an analyte solution. Its value can be calculated by using **equation (11.8)**.

$$h_{corr} = h - h_{back} \quad \ldots (11.8)$$

where, h is the height of mercury observed in the mercury column.

For aqueous solutions, the back pressure is given by **equation (11.9)**.

$$h_{back} = \frac{3.1}{m^{1/3}\, t^{1/3}} \quad \ldots (11.9)$$

If **equations (11.6)** and **(11.7)** are substituted in Ilkovic **equation (11.3)**, and provided all other factors which could affect diffusion current remain constant, then it can be shown that diffusion current (i_d) varies with the square root of h_{corr}.

$$\text{i.e. } i_d \propto \sqrt{h_{corr}} \quad \cdots(11.10)$$

Equation (11.10) provides a means of ascertaining whether current is actually diffusion controlled.

11.9.1.3. The Applied Potential (E_{appl})

The life time (t) of a mercury droplet at the tip of the capillary is affected by the applied potential at DME. Actually, the value of 't' is affected by the interfacial tension between the mercury droplet and an analyte solution, which in turn is affected by the potential applied to DME. The variation in the interfacial tension between the mercury droplet and an analyte solution with the potential applied to DME is shown graphically in **Fig. 11.17**.

As shown in **Fig. 11.17**, as the negative applied potential (E_{appl}) is increased, an interfacial tension between a mercury droplet and the analyte solution interface passes through a maximum at approximately - 0.52 V against SCE and then decreases rapidly. Interfacial tension between a mercury droplet and an aqueous solution is found to remain constant in the range AB. In this range, therefore, the drop life also remains constant. Hence, it is measured when the applied potential is in this range. In practice, since the product $m^{2/3}\,t^{1/6}$ is influenced by the 6th root of 't', it is considered almost constant as it varies less than 0.5 % over the applied potential range of 0-1 V (negative potential). However, at more negative potentials, interfacial tension is reduced. If interfacial tension is less, h_{back} is less and h_{corr} is more [**equation (11.8)**]. Therefore, value of 't' is less [**equation (11.7)**]. Hence, the product, $m^{2/3}\,t^{1/6}$, shows a more rapid decline in its value, which must be taken into account. Values of the drop life (t) and the diffusion current (i_d) should be measured at the same potential, when the experimental value of diffusion current i_d is to be compared with its calculated value .

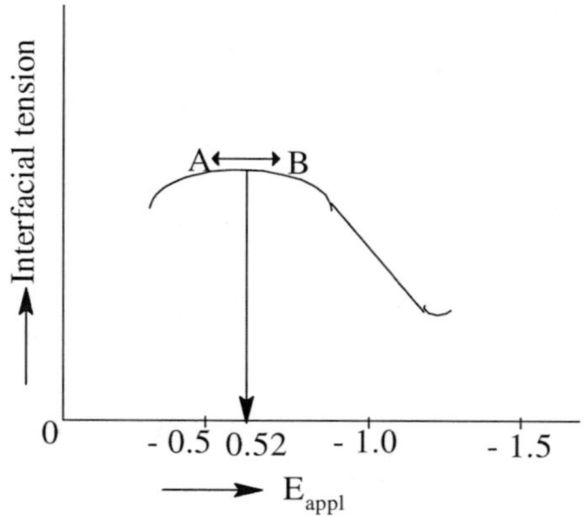

Fig. 11.17: Relation between interfacial tension and potential applied to DME

11.9.1.4. Effect of Temperature

Change in temperature brings about the changes in viscosity of an electrolyte, which can in turn bring about the changes in the mobility of ions. This leads to the change in the diffusion coefficient (D) in an Ilkovic **equation (11.3)**. Thus, though the temperature term does not appear in Ilkovic equation, the change in temperature affects every term in it, except the number of electrons (n) involved in an electrode reaction. Change in temperature by 1– 2 °C changes diffusion current by 1 -2 %. Hence, the temperature control, to the extent of ± 0.25 to ± 0.50 °C, for the working temperature of 25 °C, is required to maintain an error within 1 %.

11.9.1.5. Viscosity of Solution

Change in the viscosity of a solution changes the mobility of ions and hence, the value of diffusion coefficient (D). This leads to the change in the magnitude of diffusion current. One of the reasons for the change in viscosity of an electrolyte is the use of a very large excess, i.e.

more than 10 % of the supporting electrolyte. Another reason for the change in the viscosity is the complex formation of an analyte with the supporting electrolyte or with some other component of the solution used for analysis.

11.10. AMPEROMETRY

11.10.1. Principle

Amperometry is based on the principle of polarography. Polarography is carried out by recording current produced in the circuit when potential at DME is varied. In polarography, current is plotted against voltage and S-shaped curve is obtained. In the c-v curve of any analyte, limiting current is independent of the voltage applied to DME. The only factor affecting the limiting current is the concentration of an analyte. The higher the concentration of an analyte, the greater is the magnitude of diffusion current and vice versa. Thus, diffusion current is directly proportional to the concentration of an analyte. This is shown diagrammatically in **Fig. 11.18**.

As against polarography, in amperometry, a constant potential is applied to DME. Any potential between X and Y (**Fig. 11.18**) can be selected, where magnitude of current would vary only if there is a change in the concentration of an analyte. At a fixed potential of DME, if the concentration of an analyte is slowly reduced during a chemical reaction, by the addition of a titrant, the limiting current goes on decreasing.

For amperometric analysis, it is essential to know the nature of a polarogram of an analyte and a titrant. In amperometry, current is plotted against the volume of a titrant to obtain a titration curve. Different kinds of titration curves are obtained, which are discussed below. Titration curves are used to find the end point or the equivalence point of titrations. The end point is the point of intersection of two lines giving the change of current before and after the equivalence point.

11.10.2. Method and Titration Curves

It is very essential to know the current-voltage curve of the titrant and also of an analyte in the supporting electrolyte in which the titration is to be carried out. Amperometric titration is carried out at a constant voltage. The voltage applied at DME, during titration is such that the total diffusion current of the titrant or of an analyte to be titrated or of both is obtained. Depending on the

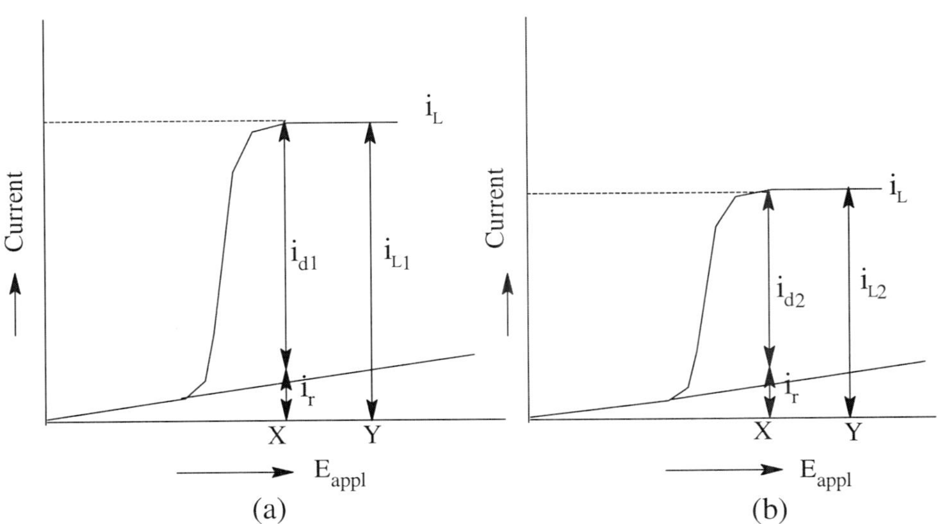

Fig. 11.18: Diffusion current at (a) higher and (b) lower concentrations

voltage applied to DME, following types of curves, which are most commonly encountered in amperometric titrations, are obtained.

11.10.2.1. Curve 1

In **Fig. 11.19(a)**, polarograms of solute to be analyzed (S) and that of the titrant (T) are shown. If amperometry is carried out using a potential between X and Y, where only the solute to be titrated gives full diffusion current, a titration curve as shown in **Fig. 11.19(b)** is obtained. Initially, when no titrant is added, the current in the circuit is equal to the limiting current corresponding to the concentration of a solute. As the titrant is added to a solute, a chemical reaction between the solute and a titrant occurs and the concentration of a solute starts decreasing. With the decrease in the concentration of a solute, diffusion current also decreases. This decrease in the current with the addition of a titrant is shown in **Fig. 11.19(b)**. When all the solute is reacted with the titrant, diffusion current becomes zero. With the addition of an excess titrant to an electrolytic cell, the current still remains zero because a titrant does not contribute to the diffusion current when the potential between X and Y is applied to DME. Hence, once the solute is totally consumed during the titration, current remains constant (zero) for any additional volume of the titrant. Thus, a titration curve as shown in **Fig. 11.19(b)** is obtained.

The slight rounding off in the vicinity of the equivalence point is due to the solubility of the precipitate in the solution or due to dilution of the solution with the addition of a titrant. In spite of the curvature, a sharp end point for the titration can be obtained by putting a tangent on the curve and by extrapolating the linear part backward. The point of intersection of the two, provides correct information about the equivalence point for the titration.

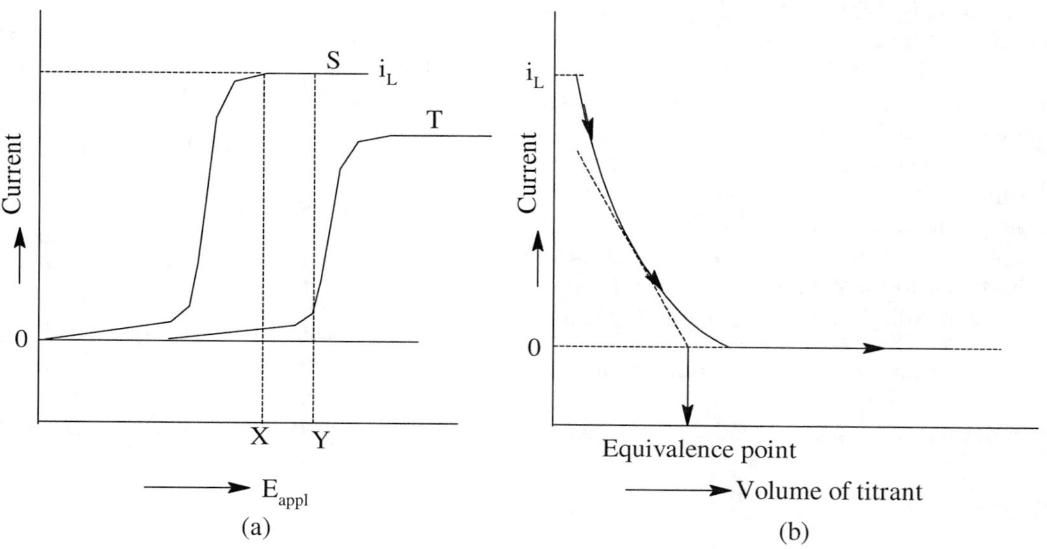

Fig. 11.19: (a) Polarograms for the solute and a titrant (b) titration curve 1

An example of this kind of amperometry is the titration of lead ions (Pb^{+2}) with oxalate ions (sodium oxalate) or sulphate ions (sodium sulphate), wherein lead ions are precipitated as lead oxalate or lead sulphate.

11.10.2.2. Curve 2

In **Fig. 11.20(a)**, polarograms of solute to

be analyzed (S) and that of the titrant (T) are shown. In this case, the solute gives no diffusion current at the voltage between X and Y, but the titrant does produce it. Initially, before the titration is begun, only the solute, which does not produce any diffusion current between X and Y, is present in the cell. Hence, initially, current is zero, as shown in **Fig. 11.20(b)**. With the addition of the titrant, a solute reacts with it and hence, its concentration decreases. This decrease in concentration of a solute does not alter magnitude of current in the circuit, since solute is not contributing to the diffusion current at the voltage between X and Y. Hence, in the titration curve [**Fig. 11.20(b)**], current continues to remain zero even with the addition of a titrant. When all the solute is completely reacted, addition of further aliquots of a titrant in the cell slowly increases the current in the circuit, because

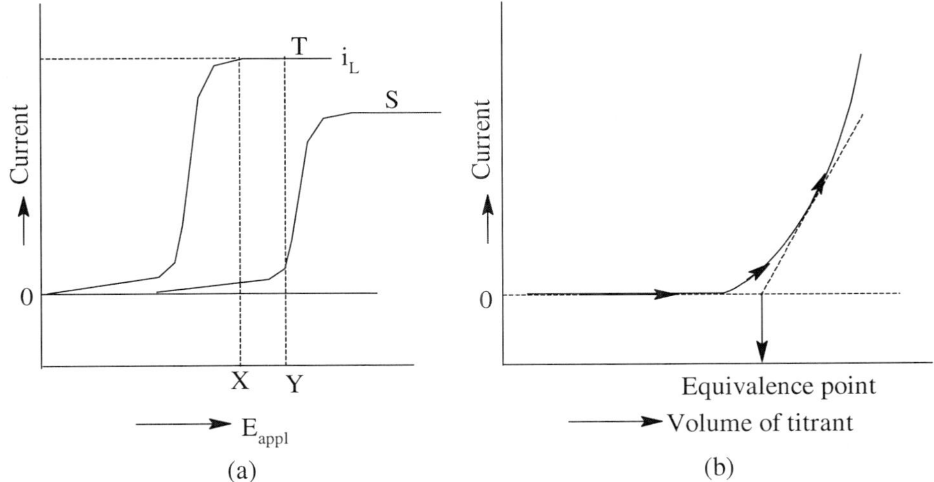

Fig. 11.20: (a) Polarograms for the solute and a titrant (b) titration curve2

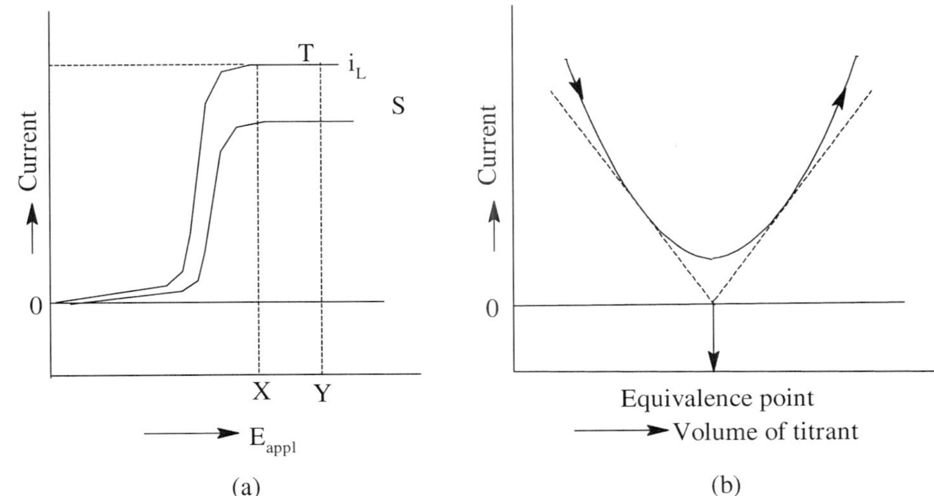

Fig. 11.21: (a) Polarograms for the solute and a titrant (b) titration curve 3

titrant produces diffusion current at the voltage between X and Y. With the increasing volume of the titrant, the magnitude of diffusion current also increases and hence, a plot as shown in **Fig. 11.20(b)** is obtained. The correct equivalence point is obtained by extrapolating two parts of the plot so as to get a point of intersection.

An example of this kind of amperometry is the titration of sulphate ions (SO_4^{-2}) with barium ions (barium nitrate) or lead ions (lead nitrate or lead acetate), wherein the sulphate ions are precipitated as barium sulphate or lead sulphate.

11.10.2.3. Curve 3

In **Fig. 11.21(a)**, polarograms of solute to be analyzed (S) and that of the titrant (T) are shown. Here, solute as well as titrant produce diffusion current at the voltage between X and Y. Initially, before the titration is begun, only the solute is there in the cell. Hence, the limiting current corresponding to its concentration is produced in the circuit. As the titrant is added to the cell, solute starts reacting with it and its concentration goes on decreasing. Since, the solute contributes to the diffusion current, with the decrease in its concentration, current in the circuit decreases. When all the solute reacts with the titrant, current reaches to zero. With the addition of more titrant, the current starts rising, since titrant also contributes to diffusion current. The correct equivalence point is obtained by putting tangents on both the sides of the curve so as to get a point of intersection.

An example of this kind of amperometry is the titration of lead ions (Pb^{+2}) with dichromate ions (potassium dichromate).

11.10.2.4. Curve 4

In **Fig. 11.22(a)**, polarograms of solute to be analyzed (S) and that of the titrant (T) are shown. At any voltage, between X and Y, a solute is not reduced but is oxidized and a titrant is reduced. Thus, both the solute and the titrant produce diffusion currents but the solute produces an

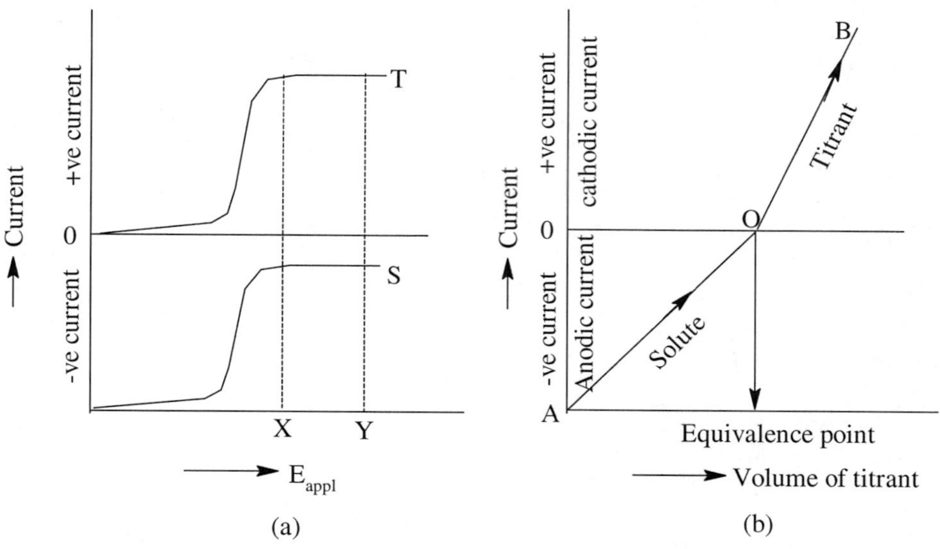

Fig. 11.22: (a) Polarograms for the solute and a titrant (b) titration curve 4

anodic diffusion current and the titrant produces a *cathodic diffusion current*. These two currents are recorded in the opposite directions in an ammeter, as shown in **Fig. 11.23**. Before titration, the solute is present in the cell in full concentration. When any potential between X and Y is applied, the solute produces an anodic diffusion current, i.e. it gets oxidized at DME. When the titrant is added, slowly a solute starts reacting with it and its

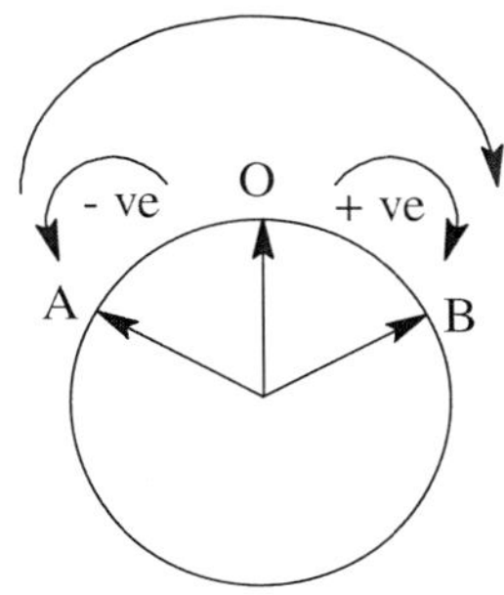

Fig. 11.23: Anodic (negative) and cathodic (positive) current in amperometry

concentration starts decreasing. As the concentration of a solute decreases, the anodic current, which is indicated as the negative current, decreases and hence, a pointer in an ammeter starts moving from position A to position O [**Fig. 11.22(b)** and **11.23**)]. Thus, when solute is reacting with the titrant, the anodic current or the negative current goes on decreasing. When all the solute reacts completely with the titrant, the anodic current becomes zero. With the addition of more titrant, current in the circuit starts increasing, since at the same potential, titrant produces cathodic diffusion current, which is shown in the positive direction in **Figures 11.22** and **11.23**. The change in current from anodic to cathodic is indicated by the change in the position of a pointer in an ammeter from A to O and from O to B. The end point of the titration is indicated by a zero current in the circuit. The slopes of two lines, AO and OB [**Fig. 11.22(b)**], depend on the rate of change of current in these regions.

The example of this particular titration is the titration of iodide ions (I^-) with mercuric ions (Hg^{+2}) or of chloride ions (Cl^-) with silver ions (Ag^+) and also, the titration of titanic ions (Ti^{+3}) in an acidified tartrate medium with ferric ions (Fe^{+3}).

In order to understand reactions that occur in this type of amperometric titration, consider a reaction between an electro-oxidizable analyte potassium iodide (KI) with mercuric nitrate [$Hg(NO_3)_2$]. The negative or the anodic diffusion current in **Fig. 11.22(b)** is produced due to oxidation of I^- ions. Though there is no change in the oxidation state of iodine, the reaction taking place is oxidation, since two electrons are released in the reaction. The positive or the cathodic diffusion current in **Fig. 11.22(a)** is produced due to reduction of mercuric ions (Hg^{+2}) to mercury atoms. These oxidation-reduction reactions (electrode reactions) are shown below.

Reduction of titrant:

$$Hg^{+2} + 2e \longrightarrow Hg$$

Oxidation of an analyte:

$$2I^- + 2Hg \longrightarrow Hg_2I_2 + 2e$$

Amperometric titrations can sometimes be used to carry out analysis when neither an analyte nor the titrant yields a polarographic wave. Under this situation, a polarographic indicator, i.e. one which can produce diffusion current at the applied potential, may be used in the titration. For example, in the analysis of aluminium salts using fluoride ions as a titrant, if an indicator containing ferric ions is used, then it is possible to carry out amperometric titration. Both aluminium and fluoride ions are polarographically inactive. The titrant (fluoride ions) can form complexes with aluminium as well as with iron, but the complex of aluminium is more stable as compared to that of iron. During the titration, diffusion current falls gradually and then very rapidly near the end point, which corresponds to a zero current.

11.10.3. Advantages of Amperometric Titrations

(i) Very dilute solutions may be titrated accurately (± 0.3 %) and rapidly.

(ii) Results of amperometric titrations are

independent of the capillary characteristics and temperature, provided that there is no change during a titration.

(iii)Substances which are not oxidizable or not reducible, i.e. the substances which are polarographically inactive, may also be titrated if the titrant gives diffusion current or if the titrant is active polarographically.

(iv)Precipitation titrations cannot be used effectively for solutes possessing appreciable solubility in the reaction mixture. Such solutes can be analyzed using amperometric titrations.

(v)Amperometry is also useful under the conditions where potentiometric and conductimetric titrations cannot be carried out.

(vi)In case of highly colored solutions, use of chemical indicators does not provide distinct end point. Under this situation, amperometry is found to be extremely useful.

11.10.4. Drawback of Amperometric Titrations

Apart from the normal sources of errors in volumetric determinations, impurities which give diffusion current, may have to be removed by preliminary chemical separation or the conditions (e.g. selection of potential at DME) are so chosen that these impurities do not contribute to the current.

CHAPTER 12

POTENTIOMETRY

12.1. INTRODUCTION

Potentiometry is an electrochemical method of analysis, in which the electromotive force (e.m.f.) developed across the electrodes, due to chemical reactions occurring in an electrochemical cell, is measured. In potentiometry, either the potential (E) of an electrode is measured or the changes in the e.m.f. or the potential difference (PD) across the electrodes of the cell, with the increase in the volume of a titrant, are measured. This can be used to determine the concentration of a wide range of solutes.

The instrumental set-up used in potentiometry is shown in **Fig. 12.1**. It includes an *electrochemical cell* consisting of a *reference electrode* and an *indicator electrode*. The electrodes are dipped in an analyte solution whose concentration is to be determined. The potential of a reference electrode (E_{Ref}) is independent of the nature and composition of a solution into which it is placed. The potential of an indicator electrode (E_{Ind}) varies with the nature of the solution in which it is dipped and it provides the information about the concentration of a species involved in an electron exchange.

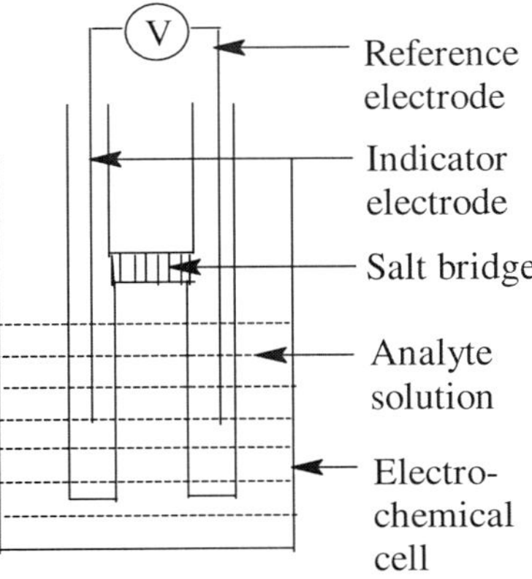

Fig. 12.1: Instrumental set-up for potentiometry

When two electrodes are connected to a voltmeter, the PD or the change in the PD across the electrodes with the progress of a chemical reaction can be measured. The e.m.f. of the cell is expressed by **equation (12.1)**.

$$E_{Cell} = E_{Ref} + E_{Ind} + E_{Jun} \quad \dots (12.1)$$

where, E_{Ref} is the potential of a reference electrode,

E_{Ind} is the potential of an indicator electrode, and

E_{Jun} is the liquid junction potential

The liquid junction potential is easily eliminated by the use of an appropriate salt bridge. As soon as an electrode is dipped in a particular solution, it assumes a potential close to its standard electrode potential (SEP). In a pair of electrodes, one electrode becomes positive with respect to another electrode. A spontaneous chemical reaction occurs with the passage of electrons through the external circuit from the more negative electrode (cathode) to the more positive electrode (anode). The reduction of a species occurs at cathode and the oxidation occurs at anode. Each electrode responds to a particular species, i.e. either to a cation or to an anion. Many ion-selective electrodes or gas sensitive or enzyme sensitive electrodes can be used in combination with the reference electrode. Such electrodes find application in the analysis of biogenic compounds.

12.2. APPLICATIONS

1) Potentiometry is used for the quantitative estimation, i.e. to find the concentration of a solute, from the voltage developed across the

electrodes as a result of a chemical reaction in the cell.

2) It is also used to find the pH of a solution.

12.3. THEORY OF POTENTIOMETRY

The relationship between the concentration of a species at a particular electrode and the voltage generated in an electrochemical cell is represented by *Nernst equation*, which is very widely used in all the electrochemical techniques. Since the potential of a reference electrode remains constant, the change in the PD between the electrodes of an electrochemical cell indicates the change in the potential of an indicator electrode at which the chemical reaction of interest occurs.

Nernst equation for cations (cationic electrode)

For any cation, M^{+z}, the reduction reaction can be written as follows.

$$M^{+z} + z\,e \longrightarrow M$$

The potential of an electrode, where cations are reduced to the neutral elements, is given by **equation (12.2)**.

$$E = E^0_{M^{+z},\ M} + \frac{RT}{zF} \ln a_{M^{+z}} \quad \cdots (12.2)$$

For any anion, X^{-z}, the oxidation reaction can be written as follows.

$$X^{-z} \longrightarrow X + z\,e$$

The potential of an electrode, where anions are oxidized to the neutral elements, is given by **equation (12.3)**.

$$E = E^0_{X^{-z},\ X} - \frac{RT}{zF} \ln a_{X^{-z}} \quad \cdots (12.3)$$

The potential of an electrode involved in the oxidation as well as reduction reactions is given by **equation (12.4)**.

$$E = E^0_{Ox,\,Red} + \frac{RT}{zF} \ln \frac{a_{Ox}}{a_{Red}} \quad \cdots (12.4)$$

In **equations (12.2)**, **(12.3)** and **(12.4)**,

E^o is the standard electrode potential (SEP) or the reduction potential of the half cell involved. It is defined as the potential of an electrode when all the species involved in the Nernst equation are at unit activity.

The term 'a' represents the thermodynamic activity of the ion to which the electrode is sensitive.

R is the Gas constant,

T is the absolute temperature (°K),

F is the Faraday constant, and

z is the number of electrons involved in the electrode reaction.

The SEPs of different electrodes are determined using the *standard hydrogen gas electrode* as a reference electrode at 25 °C or 298 °K. The SEP for the hydrogen gas electrode is arbitrarily taken as zero. For this reference electrode, H^+ ion activity is considered to be unity and a hydrogen fugacity (thermodynamic pressure) is considered to be 1 atmosphere. The SEPs of many electrodes are listed together in a series, commonly referred to as the *electrochemical series*.

12.4. ELECTRODES USED IN POTENTIOMETRY

12.4.1. Reference Electrodes

12.4.1.1. Calomel Electrode

Calomel electrode is described in detail in **Chapter 11**, **Section 11.3.2.2** with reference to **Fig. 11.5**.

12.4.1.2. Mercury (I) Sulphate Electrode

This electrode is prepared exactly in the same way as that of the calomel electrode. The only difference is that instead of a mixture of potassium chloride and calomel (mercurous chloride, Hg_2Cl_2), it makes use of 0.05 M sulphuric acid saturated with mercurous sulphate (Hg_2SO_4). It provides a potential of 682 mV as against the hydrogen electrode. The potential of this electrode is determined by the following half reaction.

$$Hg_2SO_4\ (s) + 2\ e \longrightarrow 2\ Hg\ (s) + SO_4^{-2}$$

12.4.1.3. Silver–Silver Chloride Electrode

Construction

The silver-silver chloride electrode consists of a silver wire having a thin layer of silver chloride on its surface. A thin coat of silver chloride is obtained by electrolytic deposition of silver chloride on silver wire, when silver wire is dipped in a solution of potassium chloride.

$$KCl \longrightarrow K^+ + Cl^-$$
$$2\ Cl^- \longrightarrow Cl_2 + 2\ e$$
$$\underset{\text{(from wire)}}{2Ag} + Cl_2 \longrightarrow AgCl$$

The potential of this electrode is determined by the following half reaction.

$$AgCl\ (s) + e \longrightarrow Ag\ (s) + Cl^-$$

Advantages

1) Silver-silver chloride electrode is very convenient to use.
2) It can provide different potentials in the presence of different concentrations of potassium chloride solution, e.g. in the presence of a saturated solution, 1M and 0.1M solutions, it provides potentials of +200, +235.5 and +288 mV, respectively, at 25 °C.

Disadvantages

1) It is an expensive electrode.
2) Its fabrication is not easy.

12.5. SALT BRIDGES

When two solutions of different compositions come in contact with each other, the transfer of ions across their boundary leads to the development of PD between them. This PD is known as *diffusion potential* or *liquid junction potential*. Development of the liquid junction potential can be completely nullified with the use of a salt bridge. A salt bridge consists of a saturated solution of salts like potassium chloride (KCl), potassium nitrate (KNO_3) or ammonium nitrate (NH_4NO_3). The salt solutions are usually solidified by adding a small quantity of agar in them. When such a salt bridge is present between two half cells, i.e. between the solution in the reference electrode compartment and the solution in the indicator electrode compartment, as shown in **Fig. 12.1**, the possible contamination of two solutions can be prevented. Thus, the salt bridge reduces or eliminates the liquid junction potential almost to zero and therefore, the term, E_{Jun}, in **equation (12.1)** becomes insignificant.

12.6. INDICATOR ELECTRODES

12.6.1. Hydrogen Electrode

Construction

The hydrogen electrode consists of a thin wire or a foil of platinum, coated with a porous material. An electrolytic coating of platinum black on the platinum wire provides enough porosity for the adsorption of hydrogen gas on it. As long as the surface of platinum metal remains in contact with hydrogen gas, the electrode acts as an electrode of *metallic hydrogen*. Potential at the platinum surface depends on the H^+ ion concentration of the solution and on the partial pressure of H_2 used to saturate the solution with gas.

Advantages

1) The potential of the hydrogen electrode is arbitrarily assigned to be zero and hence, it is a very widely used reference electrode in the electrochemical series.
2) As an indicator electrode, it is widely used for the determination of pH.
3) It is very easy to fabricate.
4) It provides consistent potential.

12.6.2. Glass Electrode

Construction

As shown in **Fig. 12.2**, a glass electrode consists of three parts as described below.

(i) Thick walled glass tubing, providing very high electrical resistance, is attached at its bottom to a glass bulb.

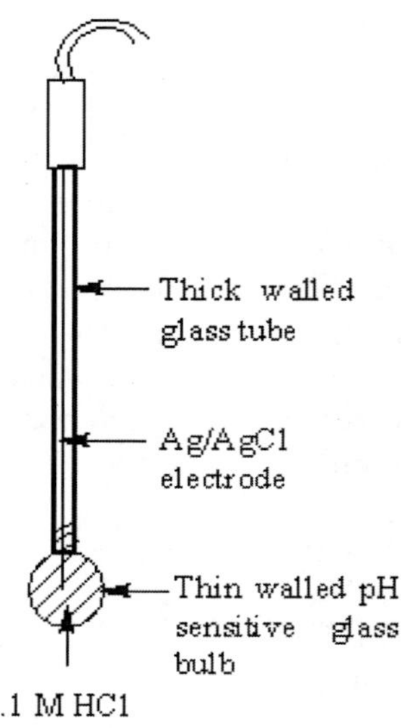

Fig. 12.2: Glass electrode

(ii) A *glass bulb*, which is the real sensing element of the electrode, is mainly used to respond to the changes in H^+ ion concentration. It is made up of a thin wall or a membrane from oxides of sodium, calcium and silicon. The specific composition of these oxides provides the pH responsive glass. The glass bulb is filled with 0.1M hydrochloric acid.

(iii) A silver wire, coated with silver chloride, is dipped in 0.1M hydrochloric acid inside the bulb so as to make an electrical contact. It also acts as a reference electrode. The potential of this reference electrode is not affected by the changes in the pH of a solution.

Applications

1) Glass electrode is commonly used to find the pH of solutions.
2) It is also used as an indicator electrode for titrations involving neutralization.

Equation (12.5) is used to find the pH of a sample solution.

$$E = k + 0.0592\,(pH_1 - pH_2) \quad \dots (12.5)$$

where, E is the potential of the glass electrode when dipped in a test solution, pH_2 is the pH of the test solution and pH_1 is the pH of the solution inside the bulb. Most of the times, the bulb is filled with 0.1M HCl. Knowing the value of pH_1 for 0.1 M HCl and then substituting its value in **equation (12.5)**, **equation (12.6)** is obtained.

$$pH_1 = -\log_{10}[H^+]$$

$$pH_1 = \log_{10}\frac{1}{[H^+]}$$

$$\therefore pH_1 = \log_{10}\frac{1}{[0.1]}$$

$$\therefore pH_1 = \log_{10}\frac{1}{[10^{-1}]}$$

$$\therefore pH_1 = \log_{10}[10]$$

$$\therefore pH_1 = 1$$

Since, $E = k + 0.0592\,(pH_1 - pH_2)$

$$E = k + 0.0592\,(1 - pH_2)$$

$$\therefore E = k + 0.0592 - 0.0592\,pH_2$$

In this equation, k is a constant and hence, (k + 0.0592) is another constant (K).

$$\therefore E = K - 0.0592\,pH_2 \quad \dots (12.6)$$

The constant K is known as *asymmetry potential*,

the value of which depends on the factors such as thickness of the glass bulb, strains in the glass and the composition of the solution inside the bulb.

Advantages

The advantages of the glass electrode are as follows.

1) The response of the glass electrode for the slight change in the pH of the test solution is very fast.
2) The response from the glass electrode is unaffected by the presence of the electro-oxidizable or electro-reducible substances in the test solution. Similarly, dissolved gases, highly colored liquids, or the presence of moderate concentrations of salts, except for the sodium salts, do not affect the response of the glass electrode.
3) In case of a glass membrane, made up of lithium and silica, the measurements over a wider range of pH are possible.
4) A combination of the glass electrode and the reference electrode in one single unit has increased the ease of handling the system.

Disadvantages

The disadvantages of the glass electrode are as follows.

1) Glass electrode is fragile and hence, needs careful handling.
2) Scratches on the glass bulb alter the response from the glass electrode.
3) Glass electrode cannot be used for dehydrating agents and colloidal substances, since they do not provide accuracy in the measurements.
4) Glass electrode provides a very high internal resistance and hence, is not useful in simple potentiometers.

Rejuvenation of glass electrode

With the increased usage of glass electrode, its efficiency goes down. The decreased efficiency leads to the following problems.

1) With the change in the pH of the test solution, this electrode does not provide fast response. The slow response from an electrode can lead to wrong information.
2) In case of the lowered efficiency of the glass electrode, it shows undue sensitivity, i.e. the slight physical movement of the electrode leads to a sudden increase or sudden decrease in the pH values.
3) In case of the lowered efficiency, the response from the electrode against a pair of buffers cannot be calibrated. Normally, the pH meters are calibrated by first dipping the glass electrode in a buffer of pH 4. If the instrument does not produce a digital display of pH 4, the knob is adjusted so as to adjust the pH value in the instrument to 4. Then the electrode is washed with water, wiped with a tissue paper and dipped in another buffer of pH 9. At this stage, if the instrument produces a digital display of pH 9, then the glass electrode is considered to be efficient. On the contrary, if a display of pH 9 is not obtained in the instrument at this stage, then the glass electrode is assumed to be reduced in its efficiency.
4) Under the reduced electrode efficiency, electrode cannot be standardized in the range of meter's asymmetry potential control [i.e. the value of K in **equation (12.6)** does not remain constant].

In case of the lowered efficiency of the glass electrode, it can be rejuvenated and reused. The electrode usually becomes useless after its rejuvenation twice or thrice. The glass electrode can be rejuvenated by using the following steps.

1) In order to remove the residual sodium ions from the surface of a glass membrane, the glass electrode is just dipped once in 0.1 M HCl. If this treatment does not provide a responsive surface, the next treatment is undertaken.
2) The glass electrode is dipped alternately in the acidic and alkaline solutions.
3) If the second method also fails, then the glass electrode is dipped in 20 % ammonium fluoride (NH_4F) solution for 3 minutes or in 10 % hydrofluoric acid (HF) for 15 seconds. After this treatment, the electrode is washed thoroughly with water. Then it is again dipped in 5 M HCl to remove the traces of fluorides and ultimately washed with distilled water.

After rejuvenation, glass electrode should be stored in the acidified distilled water so as to maintain its efficiency.

12.6.3. Redox Electrodes

A redox electrode is a metallic electrode, made up of an inert metal like gold, platinum or palladium. It is the indicator electrode that responds to an oxidation/reduction system. The commonly used metallic indicators respond either to particular cations or anions. There are certain *cationic electrodes,* which respond to different types of cations [e.g. a *mercury indicator electrode* for determination of calcium (Ca^{+2}) ions or *copper indicator electrode* for determination of cupric (Cu^{+2}) ions]. Similarly, there are certain *anionic electrodes* which respond to different types of anions [e.g. *silver indicator electrode* for determination of halide (Cl^{-1}, Br^{-1} or I^{-1}) ions]. In the cationic or anionic electrodes, only one chemical species is associated with the electrode. A redox electrode is in contact with the readily soluble oxidized and the reduced forms of an analyte. For example, the potential of a platinum electrode in a solution containing cerous (Ce^{+3}) ions and ceric ions (Ce^{+4}) is given by **equation (12.7)**.

$$E_{Ind} = E^{o} - 0.0592 \log \frac{a_{Ce^{+3}}}{a_{Ce^{+4}}} \quad \cdots (12.7)$$

12.6.4. Ion Selective Electrodes

Like glass electrode, ion selective electrode is a membrane electrode. In case of metallic electrodes, the potential is due to the oxidation/reduction reaction at an electrode surface. However, in membrane electrodes, the potential at the electrode is somewhat similar to the liquid junction potential, which is developed across a membrane that separates reference and analyte solutions from each other. Glass electrode is selective to the concentration of H^+ ions. The other membrane electrodes are selective either to the concentration of cations (like Ca^{+2} ions) or anions (like NO^-_3 ions). Glass electrode allows calculation of pH of an analyte solution, whereas calcium or nitrate ion selective electrodes allow calculation of pCa or pNO_3 of analyte solutions, which indicate concentration of Ca^{+2} ions or NO^-_3 ions, respectively, in solution. The membrane electrodes show ion selectivity by ion exchange mechanism or by crystallization or complexation.

Construction

Ion selective electrode consists of an inner and an outer container. Inner container contains a reference solution and an outer container contains an analyte solution. A thin and a porous membrane, which can conduct electricity, separates two solutions. A potential is developed across this membrane. An ion exchanger is introduced in the outer container. An ion of interest is sometimes incorporated in solution in an organic solvent. Hence, the ion selective electrode is also termed as *liquid ion exchange electrode*. Most of the times, the ion exchanger is present in a solid inert matrix

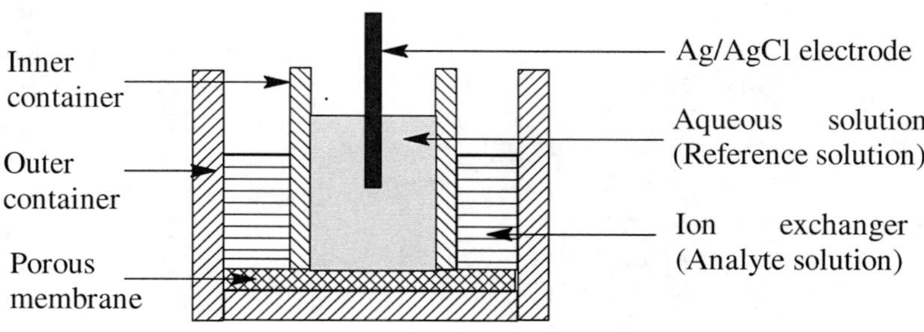

Fig. 12.3: Liquid ion exchange electrode

such as PVC, polythene or silicone rubber. A typical liquid ion exchange electrode is shown in **Fig. 12.3**. Ion selective electrode is used in combination with a reference electrode. Silver-silver chloride reference electrode is introduced in the inner container.

Advantages

1) Ion exchange electrodes are highly versatile and hence, allow selective analysis of ions from their mixture.
2) They are very easy to handle.

Disadvantage

1) Most of the ion-selective electrodes are not selective, in real sense, exclusively for one particular ion, but are able to interact to some degree with many other ions possessing the same charge or having similar chemical nature.

12.7. POTENTIOMETRIC TITRATIONS

12.7.1. Principle

In potentiometric titrations, a substance to be analyzed is titrated using a suitable titrant. With the addition of a titrant to an analyte solution, the potential of an indicator electrode, i.e. the change in the PD between the reference and the indicator electrodes is measured. The titration curve is then obtained by plotting either the potential (E) of the indicator electrode or the change in the PD per unit volume of the titrant ($\Delta E/\Delta V$) against the volume of the titrant. Instead of potential, pH of an analyte solution and instead of ($\Delta E/\Delta V$), the term ($\Delta pH/\Delta V$) can also be used to plot a graph. The equivalence point in the titration curve shown in **Fig. 12.4(a)** is indicated by a marked inflection in the titration curve. The equivalence point in the titration curve shown in **Fig. 12.4(b)** is determined by recording the burette reading, which produces the maximum change in the PD or pH per unit volume of the titrant.

12.7.2. Apparatus

Construction

The apparatus required for the potentiometric titration is shown in **Fig. 12.5**. It consists of the following components.

1) A potentiometer or a pH meter (Not shown in figure).
2) A container containing an analyte solution with a reference electrode and an indicator electrode
3) Magnetic or a mechanical stirrer
5) Burette

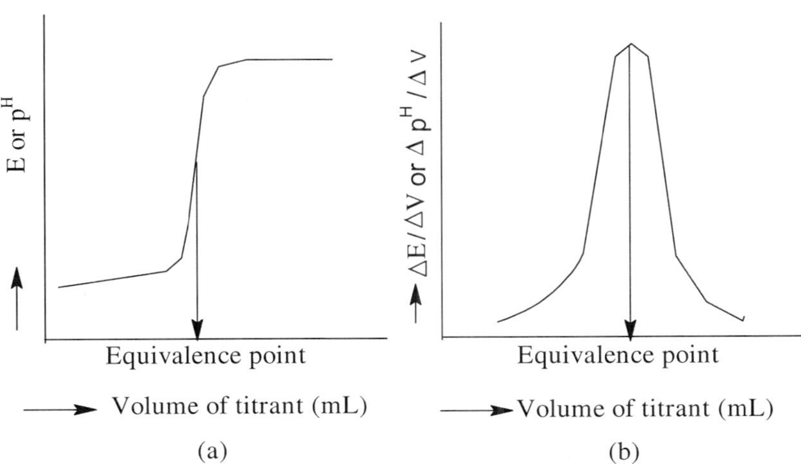

Fig. 12.4: (a) Normal and (b) first derivative titration curves in potentiometric titrations

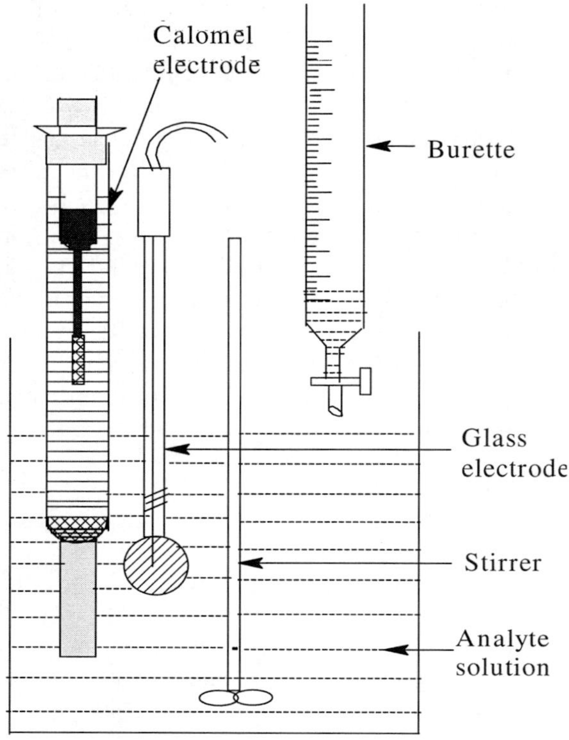

Fig. 12.5: Apparatus for potentiometric titration

Working

1. Usually, any reference electrode, whose potential remains constant throughout the titration, may be used in potentiometry. The choice of an indicator electrode is based on the system to be analyzed. In case of acid-base titrations, glass electrode is used as an indicator electrode, whereas for redox titrations, platinum electrode is used as an indicator electrode.
2. The electrodes are immersed in the solution to be titrated.
3. The electrodes are connected to two ends of wires, which are in turn connected to the voltmeter or to the pH meter to record the PD developed between the electrodes or to record the change in the pH of a solution during titration.
4. A titrant is then slowly added to an analyte and the solution is stirred continuously.
5. The PD values or the pH values for different aliquots of the titrant are recorded for plotting a graph as shown in **Fig. 12.4(a)**. The change in the PD or the change in the pH values, for unit volume of the titrant, is calculated from these readings for plotting a graph as shown in **Fig. 12.4(b)**.
6. The two curves, as shown in **Figures 12.4(a)** and **(b)**, are plotted to obtain the end point graphically.
7. The equivalence point from these two graphs is determined as explained before.
8. If the change in the PD or pH of a solution with respect to the volume of a titrant is slow, then the slope of the curve, shown in **Fig. 12.4(a)**, is very gradual and it becomes difficult to find the equivalence point from such a curve. Under this condition, a differential curve, as shown in **Fig. 12.4(b)**, is obtained by plotting the change in the PD per unit volume of the titrant ($\Delta E/\Delta V$) or the change in the pH per unit volume of the titrant ($\Delta pH/\Delta V$) against the volume of the titrant. This curve helps in determining the equivalence point accurately.

12.7.3. TYPES OF POTENTIOMETRIC TITRATIONS

Potentiometric titrations fall in the following three categories.

12.7.3.1. Acid–base titrations
12.7.3.2. Redox titrations
12.7.3.3. Precipitation titrations

12.7.3.1. Acid–Base Titrations

In acid-base titrations, instead of potential (E) of an indicator electrode or the PD across the electrodes, the pH or the change in the pH of an analyte solution per unit volume of a titrant ($\Delta pH/\Delta V$) is measured. For acid-base titrations, glass electrode is used as an indicator electrode. The potential of a glass electrode at the equivalence point is given by **equation (12.6)**.

$$E = K - 0.0592\ pH_2 \quad \ldots (12.6)$$

potentiometry for acid-base titrations can be

carried out for the following applications.

1) To find normality or molarity of an acidic or a basic solution.
2) To analyze a mixture of a weak acid and a strong acid or a mixture of a weak base and a strong base.

In case of a single acid, the pH of an analyte or the change in the pH of an analyte is recorded and plotted against the volume of a titrant. The equivalence point is obtained graphically, as shown in **Figures 12.4(a)** and **(b)**.

In case of a mixture of a weak acid (e.g. acetic acid) and a strong acid (e.g. hydrochloric acid), if the dissociation constants of both the acids are sufficiently different, then the graphs as shown in **Figures 12.6(a)** and **(b)** are obtained. The first inflection in the titration curve occurs when the stronger acid is neutralized and the second inflection occurs when the neutralization is complete. Thus, normality of both the acids can be calculated from the equivalence points.

The imaginary values, for the titration of an acid with an alkali, are given in **Table 12.1**, to make clear how two graphs [**12.6 (a)** and **(b)**] are plotted so as to get the equivalence point. If 10 ml of 0.1 M solution of HCl is titrated with 0.1 M NaOH, then the equivalence point should be obtained when 10 ml of NaOH is added to the acid. In potentiometry, it is essential to record readings, even after the equivalence point is reached. This helps in getting an accurate equivalence point.

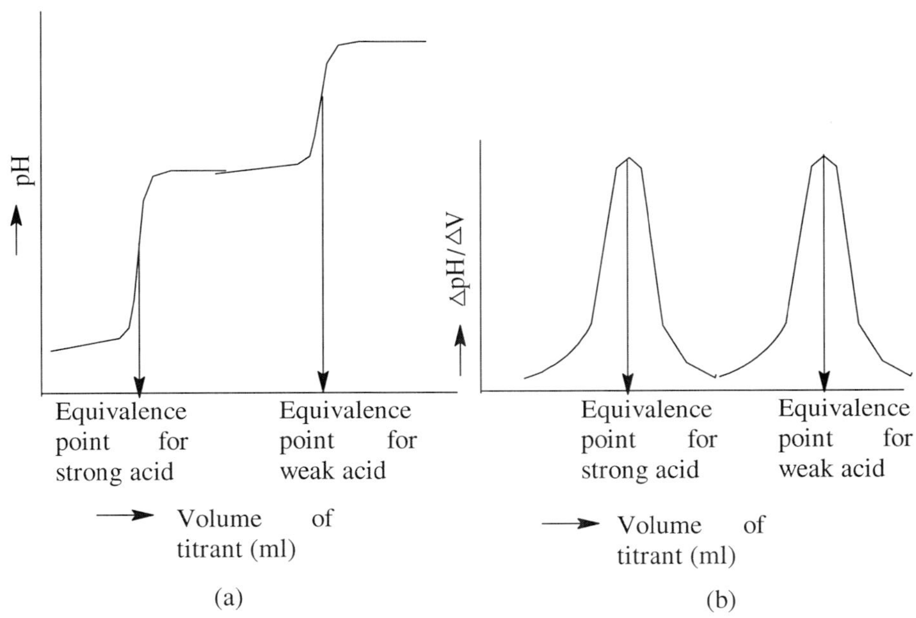

Fig. 12.6: Titration curves for potentiometric titration of a weak acid and a strong acid

From the data given in **Table 12.1**, it is clear that when 10 ml of NaOH is added to HCl, ΔpH/ÄV value is highest. Hence, that is the equivalence point for that titration.

12.7.3.2. Redox Titrations

For redox titrations, platinum electrode is used as an indicator electrode. The potential at the equivalence point is given by **equation (12.8)**.

Table 12.1: Imaginary values for the titration of an acid with an alkali

Redg. No.	pH	Volume of titrant added (V ml)	ΔpH	ΔV (ml)	ΔpH/ΔV
1	1.0	0.0			
2	1.1	5.0	0.1	5.0	0.02
3	1.2	7.0	0.1	2.0	0.05
4	1.4	8.0	0.2	1.0	0.2
5	1.7	9.0	0.3	1.0	0.3
6	2.2	9.5	0.5	0.5	1.0
7	2.7	9.7	0.5	0.2	2.5
8	3.3	9.8	0.6	0.1	6.0
9	4.3	9.9	1.0	0.1	10.0
10	7.0	10.0	2.7	0.1	27
11	7.4	10.1	0.4	0.1	4.0
12	7.8	10.3	0.4	0.2	2.0
13	8.3	10.5	0.5	0.2	2.5
14	9.1	11.0	0.8	0.5	1.6
15	10.0	12.0	0.9	1.0	0.9

Thus, the potential of an indicator electrode depends on the ratio of the concentrations of the oxidized to the reduced forms of an ion. The reference electrode can be any electrode, which provides the constant potential throughout the titration. An example of the redox titration is the

$$E = E^0_{Ox, Red} + \frac{RT}{zF} \ln \frac{a_{Ox}}{a_{Red}} \cdots \quad (12.8)$$

analysis of ferrous ions using permanganate solution. The following reaction takes place during the redox titration.

$$Fe^{+2} \longrightarrow Fe^{+3}$$

A graph of the potential (E) or the change in the potential per unit volume of the titrant (ΔE/ΔV) against the volume of the titrant is plotted in this case. The titration curves similar to those shown in **Figures 12.4(a)** and **(b)** are obtained. The equivalence point in this type of titration is obtained as shown in the titration curves.

12.7.3.3. Precipitation Titrations

In precipitation titrations, silver electrode is used as an indicator electrode. The reference electrode used is silver-silver chloride electrode. The potential of an indicator electrode is given by **equation (12.2)** for cationic electrodes.

$$E = E^0_{M^{+z}, M} + \frac{RT}{zF} \ln a_{M^{+z}} \cdots (12.2)$$

An example of precipitation titration is analysis of potassium chloride solution using silver nitrate solution in presence of nitric acid. The following reaction takes place during the titration.

$$AgNO_3 + KCl \rightarrow AgCl \downarrow + KNO_3$$

Before titration, the concentration of chloride ions is high. With the addition of silver nitrate solution, silver chloride gets precipitated out, since the solubility product of AgCl is exceeded, i.e. the product of the concentration of silver ions [Ag^+] and chloride ions [Cl^-] exceeds the solubility product (K_S) for AgCl.

$$[Ag^+]\ [Cl^-] > K_S \text{ i.e. } 1.56 \times 10^{-10}$$

As more and more of Cl^- ions from KCl are removed from the solution, at one point, the product of the concentrations of silver ions [Ag^+] and chloride ions [Cl^-] becomes exactly equal to the solubility product of AgCl. At this moment, the precipitation of AgCl stops. The addition of more of $AgNO_3$ then increases the concentration of Ag^+ ions in the solution. The change in the concentration of ions leads to the change in the potential of silver electrode, which provides the information about the equivalence point for the titration.

12.7.4. Advantages of Potentiometric Titrations

1) Potentiometric titrations do not depend on the visual observations and the color change of an indicator. Hence, they are used when highly colored solutions are to be analyzed.
2) They find use when suitable indicators are not available for titrations, e.g. they can be used for very dilute solutions, which do not give clear end point for the titrations involving indicator.
3) They provide high accuracy.

12.7.5. Disadvantages of Potentiometric Titrations

1) A large number of readings are required to be recorded.
2) Plotting of the graph is essential.
3) It needs electrodes, some of which are costly.
4) Maintenance of electrodes is absolutely essential.

CHAPTER 13

CONDUCTIMETRY

Conductimetry is an electrochemical method of analysis, in which the progress of a chemical reaction is studied with the help of changes in conductance of a solution.

13.1. THEORY OF CONDUCTIMETRY

The method of conductimetry is based on Ohm's law, which states that the potential difference (PD, V volts), developed between the electrodes is the product of current (i amperes) flowing through the cell and resistance (R ohms, Ω - Capital omega, Gr.) offered by the solution to the flow of current. Ohm's law can be expressed mathematically as follows.

$$V = iR$$

In general, resistance of any element is directly proportional to its length (l) and inversely proportional to its area (a). Thus, resistance can be expressed in terms of these parameters by **equation (13.1)**.

$$R \propto l$$

$$R \propto \frac{1}{a}$$

$$\therefore R \propto \frac{l}{a}$$

$$\text{or } R = \rho \left(\frac{l}{a}\right) \cdots (13.1)$$

where, ρ (rho, Gr.) is a constant of proportionality and is termed as *specific resistance* or *resistivity*. The term (l/a), is referred to as a *cell constant*.

Conductance (G) of a solution is the reciprocal of its resistance (R) and is expressed in siemen (s, Ω^{-1} or mho). Mathematically, it is expressed as follows.

$$G = \frac{1}{R} = \frac{1}{\rho} \frac{1}{\left(\frac{l}{a}\right)}$$

$$\therefore G = \kappa \frac{1}{\left(\frac{l}{a}\right)}$$

$$\therefore G = \frac{\kappa}{\left(\frac{l}{a}\right)} \cdots (13.2)$$

where, κ (kappa, Gr.) is a constant of proportionality and is termed as *specific conductance* or *conductivity*.

13.2. DEFINITIONS OF SOME COMMON TERMS

Definitions of some of the common terms used in conductimetry are as follows.

13.2.1. Metallic Conductance

Metals conduct an electric current due to the flow of electrons in them. This type of conductance is called as *metallic conductance*.

13.2.2. Electrolytic Conductance

Electrolytes like acids, bases and salts, conduct electricity due to the flow of ions present in them or formed during electrolysis. This type of conductance is called an *electrolytic conductance*.

13.2.3. Equivalent Conductance

Conductance of an electrolyte solution depends on the degree of dilution. While studying the variation in conductance of electrolytes, it is essential to take into account the degree of dilution. This is especially important when the comparison of conductance of two electrolyte solutions, containing identical amount of solutes, is to be made. This may be achieved by expressing conductance in terms of *equivalent conductance*. Equivalent conductance, expressed by using a symbol, capital lambda (Λ, Gr.), is obtained by multiplying the specific conductance (κ) of a solution by the volume in milliliters (V_e) of a solution containing 1 gram equivalent of a solute. Mathematically, equivalent conductance can be expressed by **equation (13.3)**.

$$\Lambda = \kappa \times V_e \ \ldots (13.3)$$

If 'c' gram equivalents are present in 1 liter or 1000 mL of a solution, then the volume containing 1 gram equivalent of a solute (V_e mL) can be expressed as –

$$V_e = \frac{1000}{c}$$

$$\therefore \Lambda = \frac{1000\ \kappa}{c} \cdots (13.4)$$

With dilution, the concentration 'c' of an electrolyte solution goes on changing. Calculation by using **equation (13.4)** takes into account the change in equivalent conductance with dilution.

Since the normality of solution is defined as the number of equivalents present in 1 liter of a solution, the normality of a solution containing 'c' equivalents per liter is 'c'. Substituting the concentration term (c) in **equation (13.4)**, by the normality (N) of the solution, **equation (13.5)** is obtained.

$$\Lambda = \frac{1000\ \kappa}{N} \cdots (13.5)$$

For example, the equivalent conductance of 0.01 N KCl solution, which has a specific conductance of 0.001413 mho/cm, may be calculated in the following two ways by using **equations (13.3)** and **(13.5)**.

A 0.01 N solution contains 0.01 equivalents of KCl in 1000 mL of its solution. Therefore, volume containing 1 equivalent of KCl (V_e) would be 100,000 mL. Substituting this value of V_e in **equation (13.3)**, the following equivalent conductance is obtained.

$$\Lambda = \kappa \times V_e$$

Using **equation 13.5** also, the same value of equivalent conductance is obtained as shown below.

$$\Lambda = \frac{1000\ \kappa}{c}$$

$$\therefore \Lambda = \frac{1000 \times 0.001413}{0.01} = 141.3\ \text{mho. cm2 /eq.}$$

13.2.4. Molar Conductance

Molar conductance, represented by a symbol ($\overline{\Lambda}$ read as lambda bar), is obtained by multiplying the specific conductance (κ) of a solution by the volume in milliliters (V_m) of a solution containing 1 mole of a solute. Mathematically, molar conductance can be expressed by the following equation.

$$\overline{\Lambda} = \kappa \times V_m \ \ldots (13.6)$$

If 'c' moles are present in 1 liter or 1000 mL of a solution, then the volume containing 1 mole of a solute (V_m mL) can be expressed as –

$$V_m = \frac{1000}{c}$$

$$\therefore \bar{\wedge} = \frac{1000\ \kappa}{c} \cdots (13.7)$$

Since molarity of a solution is defined as the number of moles present in 1 liter of a solution, the molarity of a solution containing 'c' moles per liter is 'c'. Substituting the concentration term (c) in **equation (13.7)** by the molarity 'M' of the solution, **equation (13.8)** is obtained.

$$\bar{\wedge} = \frac{1000\ \kappa}{M} \cdots (13.8)$$

Both the equivalent conductance and the molar conductance are inversely proportional to the concentration of a solute in the solution. The higher the concentration, the lower is the conductance. Thus, conductance increases with dilution, since ions can move freely in it without any ionic interaction. Hence, the maximum value of conductivity, indicated by the symbol, Λ^o, is reached at infinite dilution.

13.3. INSTRUMENTATION

Since conductance is merely the reciprocal of the resistance of a solution, it is determined by measuring electrical resistance, commonly with a *Wheatstone bridge apparatus*.

Construction

The instrument used for determining conductance of a solution consists of a conductivity cell made up of glass or quartz. The cell contains two inert electrodes made up of platinum or gold, coated with a porous substance like platinum black to absorb gases. Wheatstone bridge is constructed by introducing the conductivity cell and a standard resistance (R_S) in the circuit along with a resistance wire, over which a jockey can move so as to get the *null point*. An oscillator, to generate an alternating current of a frequency of about 1000 cps, is used in the circuit. An alternating current reverses the electrolysis and does not allow electrolysis of an electrolyte under study. A null point is obtained by sliding a jockey on the resistance wire. Ammeter (A) records the current in the circuit. Wheatstone bridge, used for the measurement of conductance, is shown in **Fig. 13.1**.

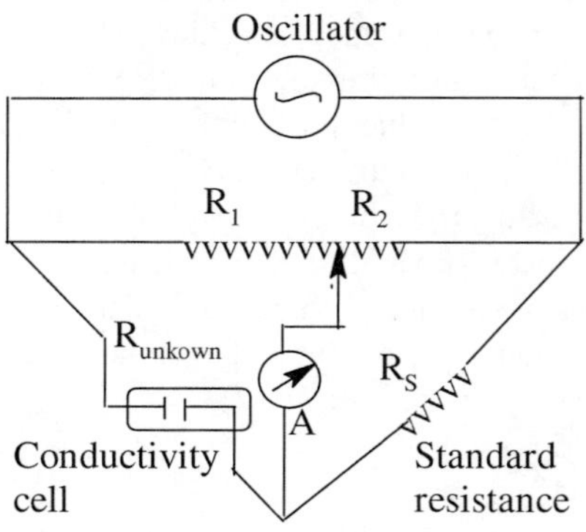

Fig. 13.1: Wheatstone bridge for the measurement of conductance

Working

1) Determination of conductance of a solution

In order to determine conductance of a solution, the electrodes of proper size are selected and the distance between the electrodes is adjusted so as to get a measurable quantity of current in the circuit. Electrolytic resistance, like metallic resistance, varies directly with the length of the conducting medium and inversely with its cross sectional area. Since, resistance is directly proportional to the factor (l/a), the higher resistance is offered by the solution when the distance between the two electrodes (l, the length of the solution which offers resistance to the flow of current through it) is large and the area (a) of electrodes is small. Since the resistance is high, conductance of this solution is small and hence, very small current flows through the circuit. Such a small current can involve error in its measurement. In order to avoid this, either the distance between the two electrodes (l) can be reduced or the area (a) of electrodes can be increased. Similarly, when the resistance of a solution is too low, conductance is very high and hence, the current flowing through the circuit is also very high. This high current can destroy the instrument. In order to reduce the current flowing through the circuit, resistance of the solution is to be increased, either by increasing the distance (l) between the electrodes in a conductivity cell or by decreasing the area (a) of electrodes. Thus, the size of the electrodes and the distance between them may be varied to increase the accuracy and the precision of the measurement.

The solution whose conductance is to be determined is placed in a conductivity cell. A standard or a known resistance (R_S) is included in the circuit. An alternating current is passed across the electrodes. A jockey is moved on the resistance wire, the position of which determines the values of R_1 and R_2 so that no current passes through the circuit (null point). The resistance ($R_{Unknown}$) of the solution to the flow of current is then calculated by the **equation (13.9)**, used commonly in Wheatstone bridge method.

$$\frac{R_1}{R_{Unknown}} = \frac{R_2}{R_S} \cdots (13.9)$$

Conductance of the solution in a conductivity cell is then calculated by taking the reciprocal of $R_{Unknown}$, the units of which are reciprocal ohms (also called as mhos).

$$\therefore G = \frac{1}{R_{Unknown}}$$

The magnitude of the conductivity or conductance (G) of a solution varies with the dimensions of the electrodes and also with the distance between the electrodes. Hence, the value of conductance for the same solution is different in different conductivity cells. In order to avoid this cell to cell variation, instead of determining conductance of a solution, its specific conductance (κ) is determined. Specific conductance of a solution is the conductance in a cell having electrodes of 1 sq. cm cross-sectional area, which are 1cm apart from each other. Since the area of electrodes and the distance between them is fixed, the value of specific conductance does not vary from cell to cell.

2) Determination of specific conductance of a solution

Conductance and the specific conductance are related to each other by **equation (13.2)**.

$$G = \frac{\kappa}{\left(\frac{l}{a}\right)} \cdots (13.2)$$

In order to find the value of specific conductance (κ), other terms in **equation (13.2)** should be known. Conductance (G) of a solution can be determined as described above. The term (l/a) can be calculated, if the dimensions of the electrodes and the distance between them is known. While fabricating the conductivity cells, the electrodes are not placed at a distance of 1 cm from each other. Similarly, electrodes of exactly 1 sq. cm cross-sectional area are also not used. The term (l/a) is known as a *cell constant*, the magnitude of which varies from cell to cell. If the value of a cell constant is known, the specific conductance of a solution can be calculated. The cell constant is determined experimentally as follows.

3) Determination of the cell constant (l/a)

In order to determine the magnitude of the cell constant for any cell, the terms G and κ in **equation (13.2)** should be known. Hence, a conductivity cell is filled with a standard solution of known specific conductance (κ). A solution of 0.1 M or 0.01 M pure potassium chloride (KCl) is used as a standard for this purpose. For calibration of a conductivity cell, repeatedly recrystallized potassium chloride should be used. Similarly, high purity conductivity water (resistivity > 2 x 10^5 Ωm) should be used. Conductance (G) of this solution is then measured using Wheatstone bridge method. From the values of G and κ, the cell constant (*l*/a), for any cell can be calculated using **equation (13.2)**. Thus, even if the distance between the electrodes (*l*) and the dimensions of the electrodes (a) are not known, their ratio (*l*/a), i.e. a cell constant, can be calculated experimentally.

Once the cell constant is known for different cells, the measurement of conductance (G) of a particular solution in different cells provides a constant value of specific conductance (κ) of a solution. Thus, the conductance (G) varies from cell to cell, but the specific conductance of a solution is independent of the cells used.

13.4. CONDUCTIMETRIC TITRATIONS

In conductimetric titrations, either an absolute conductance (G) or the change in conductance (ΔG) of a solution, on addition of a titrant, is usually recorded. In case of the measurement of an absolute conductance of a solution, the calibration of the conductivity cell to find the cell constant (*l*/a) is required to be carried out as described above.

13.4.1. Ionic Conductivities

Each ion makes a definite contribution to the total conductance of a solution and this contribution is independent of other ions present in the solution. This becomes clear when molar conductivities of pairs of salts having an ion in common, such as KCl – NaCl or KNO_3 - $NaNO_3$, are compared. The replacement of one ion by another, i.e. K^+ ion by Na^+ ion, always leads to a constant difference in conductance. For a solution containing '$n_{(+)}$' number of cations and '$n_{(-)}$' number of anions, let $\Lambda^o_{(+)}$ and $\Lambda^o_{(-)}$ be the molar ionic conductivities at infinite dilution. For such a salt, maximum molar conductivity of a solution (Λ^o) can be expressed as the sum of the maximum molar ionic conductivities of cations and anions. Mathematically, it can be expressed as follows.

$$\Lambda^o = n_{(+)} \Lambda^o_{(+)} + n_{(-)} \Lambda^o_{(-)} \quad \dots (13.10)$$

The molar ionic conductivity of most of the ions increases with the temperature because the increase in the temperature increases mobility of ions. Hence, the conductimetric titrations are carried out at constant temperature.

13.4.2. Applications of Conductimetric Titrations

In conductimetric titrations, when a titrant is added to a sample to be analyzed, the conductivity of the solution changes depending on the relative mobility of the ions added or removed from the solution. The change in conductance, before and after the equivalence point is recorded with the addition of regular aliquots of the titrant to the solution of an analyte. A graph of actual conductance (G) or the change in conductance (ΔG) on Y-axis and the volume of titrant on X-axis is plotted. A point of intersection of two straight lines provides the equivalence point for that titration (**Fig. 13.3**).

During the titration, only the chemical reaction between the titrant and an analyte should bring about the changes in conductance of a solution. However, addition of a titrant dilutes an analyte solution and brings about changes in conductance of a solution. In order to avoid the effect of dilution on conductance, the change in the volume throughout the course of a titration should be kept small by employing a titrant which is at least 100 times more concentrated than the solution being titrated. In case of dilute solutions, a correction for the dilution effect may be applied by multiplying each conductance reading by the ratio of the total volume (V) to the initial volume (v) of the solution in the conductivity cell.

In the region of the equivalence point, a slight curvature is obtained instead of two absolutely straight lines, because of the hydrolysis, dissociation or solubility of the reaction product.

13.4.3. Types of Conductimetric Titrations

Conductimetric titrations find wide applications in the following areas.

13.4.3.1. Neutralization titrations
13.4.3.2. Precipitation titrations
13.4.3.3. Complexometric titrations

13.4.3.1. Neutralization Titrations

A neutralization reaction is a reaction between an acid and a base so as to produce salt and water. The titration curves in these titrations consist of an initial decrease followed by a rise in conductance. This can be explained with the ionic conductivities for different ions in solution. The molar ionic conductivity of four ions is tabulated in **Table 13.1**. An example of neutralization titration is the titration of sodium hydroxide with hydrochloric acid [**Fig. 13.2(a)**], the reaction for which is shown below.

$$2\,NaOH + HCl \rightarrow NaCl + H_2O$$

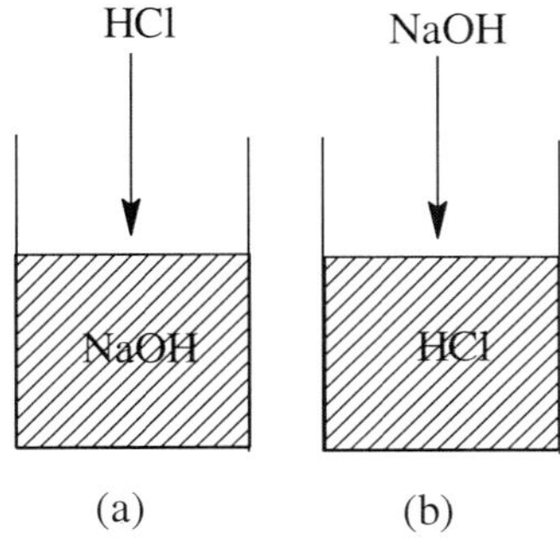

Fig. 13.2: Titration between an acid and a base

In this titration, initially, the concentration of OH^- ions in the solution to be titrated is more. When hydrochloric acid is added to a solution of NaOH, concentration of OH^- ions decreases. With the reduction of OH^- ions, the concentration of chloride ions increases because of the formation of a salt, NaCl, during neutralization reaction. Thus, decrease in conductance is due to the replacement of the hydroxyl ions with a molar ionic conductivity of 199, by the chloride ions with a molar conductivity of 76. At the equivalence point, all NaOH is completely reacted. Hence, there are no more OH^- ions in the reaction mixture. Beyond the equivalence point, if more of titrant (HCl) is added to the reaction mixture, then the increase in the conductivity is due to the increase in the concentration of H^+ ions of very high molar conductivity (350).

As shown in **Fig. 13.2(b)**, when HCl is titrated against NaOH, the initial decrease in conductivity is because of the decrease in the concentration of H^+ ions of very high molar conductivity (350), which are replaced by Na^+ ions with low conductivity (50). Beyond the equivalence point, the rise in the conductivity is due to the excess of high ionic conductivity of OH^- ions (199) in the reaction mixture. The equivalence point is obtained graphically by the intersection of two lines. In case of stronger solutions of NaOH and HCl, meeting of two absolutely straight lines, as shown in **Fig. 13.3(a)**, provides a sharp, accurate and definite end point.

Table 13.1: Molar ionic conductivities of ions

Ionic species	Molar ionic conductivity
H^+	350
Na^+	50
OH^-	199
Cl^-	76

In case of a titration of a weak acid with a strong base or a weak base with a strong acid, initially, a small conductance is produced, as shown in **Fig. 13.3(b)**. As the titration progresses, conductance increases, since the concentration of the salt increases. Near the equivalence point, a distinct curvature or *rounding off* is observed due to pronounced hydrolysis of the salt produced during titration. Beyond the equivalence point, the increase in conductance is because of the increase in the concentration of a high conductivity ion from the titrant. Extension of two lines, before and after the curvature, is required to get the correct end point in this case.

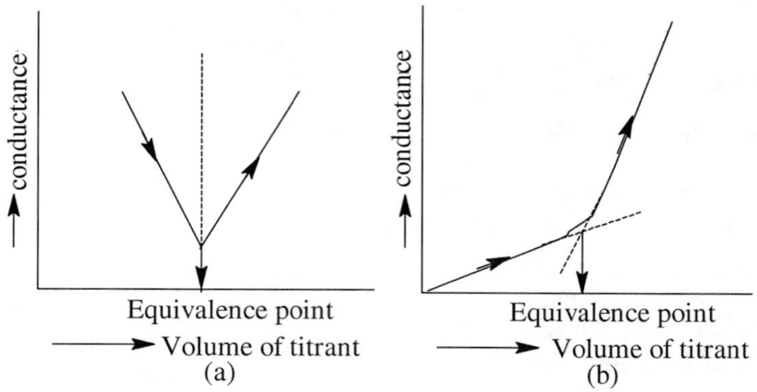

Fig. 13.3: Titration curves for conductimetric titration of (a) a strong acid with a strong base and (b) a weak acid with a strong base

Weak acids like phenols, which produce colored salts, can be titrated conveniently by conductimetry. Similarly, weak bases like alkaloids, amines and certain dyes, which pose difficulties when titrated by aqueous or non-aqueous acid-base titrations using indicators (since the color change is not distinct at the end point due to initial color of the substance to be titrated), can also be titrated by conductimetry. The conductimetric titrations find special application in the analysis of such compounds.

13.4.3.2. Precipitation Titrations

The conductimetric titrations are also used to study precipitation reactions when a suitable indicator cannot be used in the conventional precipitation titrations. The equivalence point for these titrations is determined by finding out the point of intersection of two lines obtained in the titration curve. An accurate end point is obtained when the precipitate is formed rapidly and when it is sparingly soluble. Similarly, proper selection of a titrant is also absolutely essential. One more requirement for accuracy in such titrations is that the precipitate (such as AgCl) should not adsorb any of the chemicals involved in the experiment.

13.4.3.3. Complexometric Titrations

The conductimetric titrations are also found to be applicable to the reactions involving complex formation. The equivalence point for these titrations is found exactly by the same method as described for the previous two types. The approximate molar ionic conductivity of ions in water at infinite dilution at 25 °C is given in **Table 13.2**.

Thus, conductimetric titrations provide a simple alternative for analyzing substances, which otherwise are difficult to analyze by other titrimetric procedures.

Table 13.2: Approximate molar ionic conductivity of ions in water at infinite dilution at 25 °C

Cation	$10^4 \Lambda^o_+ / \Omega^{-1}$ $m^2 mol^{-1}$	Anion	$10^4 \Lambda^o_- / \Omega^{-1}$ $m^2 mol^{-1}$
H^+	350	OH^{-1}	199
Li^+	39	Cl^{-1}	76
Na^+	50	Br^{-1}	78
K^+	74	I^{-1}	77
NH_4^+	74	NO_3^{-1}	71
Ag^+	62	HCO_3^{-1}	45

CHAPTER 14

ELECTROPHORESIS

14.1. INTRODUCTION

The technique of electrophoresis is mainly used for the separation of charged species from each other. It finds major applications in the field of biochemistry or molecular biology. The separation of charged particles by electrophoresis is based on the principle of difference in the mobility or the rates of migration in an electric field. The compounds can have a charge for many reasons, some of which are given below.

1) Certain compounds, when dispersed in water, adsorb hydroxyl ions on their surface and acquire a negative charge. Some compounds are also able to adsorb, preferentially, certain ions present in solution. These compounds then carry the charge depending on the charge present on the adsorbed ions.
2) Certain polar compounds like amines, phenols, carboxylic acids, etc. can ionize in solution and acquire charge on their surface.
3) Sometimes, solids acquire charge because of the difference in the dielectric constant between the dispersed particles and the dispersion medium.

14.2. THE ELECTRIC DOUBLE LAYER

Most of the compounds, when dispersed in a dispersion medium, adsorb either cations or anions from the solution and acquire positive or negative charge on their surface. The ions which are directly adsorbed by the compounds and give charge to their surface are referred to as *potential determining ions*. These ions, in turn, attract the oppositely charged ions towards them and form a *secondary layer*. The ions having a charge opposite to the potential determining ions are known as *counter-ions* or *gegenions*. These counter ions are in turn surrounded by the oppositely charged ions. The potential determining ions and the counter ions together form a double layer of charge, as shown in **Fig. 14.1**. The first layer is tightly bound and a second

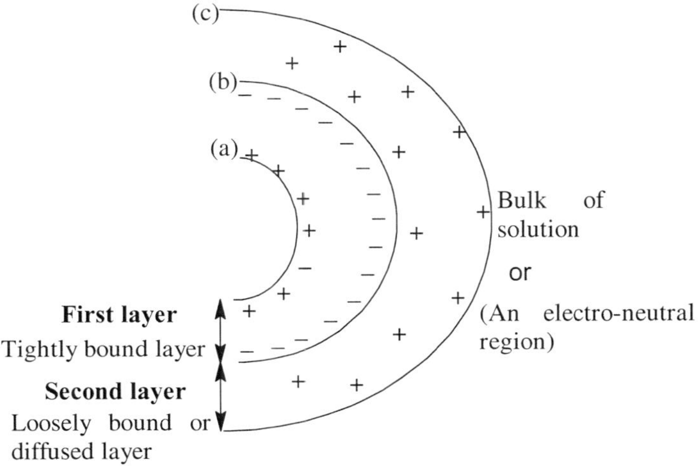

Fig. 14.1: Formation of a Helmholtz double layer

layer is loosely bound or is diffused. Hence, the double layer is called as *diffused double layer*. Since this phenomenon was first put forth by the scientist, Helmholtz, the double layer is also called as *Helmholtz double layer*.

14.3. NERNST POTENTIAL AND ZETA POTENTIAL

The potential at the solid surface (a) **(Fig. 14.1)**, due to the potential determining ions, is called *Nernst potential* (E). It depends on the degree of charge present on that surface. It is defined as the difference in the potential at the solid surface (a) and the electro-neutral region of the solution, i.e. bulk of the solution.

The potential at the surface (b), due to the counter-ions or gegenions, is called *zeta potential*. It is defined as the difference in the potential at the surface of the tightly bound layer (b) and the electro-neutral region of the solution. Zeta potential governs the degree of repulsion between the adjacent, similarly charged dispersed particles. Hence, it finds special application in determining the stability of suspensions or any system containing dispersed particles. If zeta potential is below a certain value, the force of repulsion between the adjacent particles is reduced and attractive forces exceed the repulsive forces. Hence, the suspended particles come together and settle down. This results in *flocculation*. The reduction in the zeta potential is observed with the increasing concentration of *electrolytes* like sodium chloride or potassium chloride in the system. When the concentration of electrolytes is increased, due to the increased screening effect, the counter ions of the solute of interest are less attracted by the first layer. As a result, the thickness of the double layer shrinks, i.e. the second layer becomes more diffused and the potential falls off more rapidly with distance. When the zeta potential on a particle is more, the repulsion between the two neighboring particles is also more. At a particular value of zeta potential, the particles remain apart from each other and remain suspended in the dispersion medium. Thus, proper adjustment of the zeta potential is necessary to avoid sedimentation of particles and to formulate stable suspensions. Apart from the stability of suspensions, the stability of colloids and micelles, which determines solubilizing capacity of surfactants, also depends on the magnitude of the zeta potential. Hence, measurement of the zeta potential is important in the field of pharmacy. The methodology for determination of the zeta potential is discussed later in this chapter under the **Section 14.4.1.1**.

14.4. ELECTROKINETIC PHENOMENA

There are four electrokinetic phenomena which are based on the movement of a charged surface with respect to an adjacent liquid phase. They are described below.

14.4.1. Electrophoresis
14.4.2. Electro-osmosis
14.4.3. Sedimentation potential
14.4.4. Streaming potential

14.4.1. Electrophoresis

In this technique, charged particles move through a stationary or an immobilized liquid, under the influence of an applied potential difference (PD).

14.4.2. Electro-osmosis

In this technique, solids are immobilized by converting them into a plug and liquid moves through this plug of solids under the influence of an applied PD.

14.4.3. Sedimentation Potential

It is just the reverse of electrophoresis. The sedimentation potential is the PD developed when the charged particles are in motion or when the charged particles undergo sedimentation.

14.4.4. Streaming Potential

It is the reverse of electro-osmosis. It is the PD developed when the liquid is forced to flow through a plug or bed of particles.

14.4.1. Electrophoresis

When electrophoresis is carried out by using capillary columns, the technique is called as *capillary electrophoresis* or *capillary zone electrophoresis*.

14.4.1.1. Determination of Zeta Potential

Technique of electrophoresis can be well explained based on the determination of zeta potential for a system.

Instrumentation

In order to measure zeta potential on particles in a suspension or a colloid, an electrophoretic cell containing two platinum electrodes is made use of. A suspension or a colloid under study is filled in an electrophoretic cell and a definite PD is applied across the electrodes. The instrumental set-up is shown in **Fig. 14.2**.

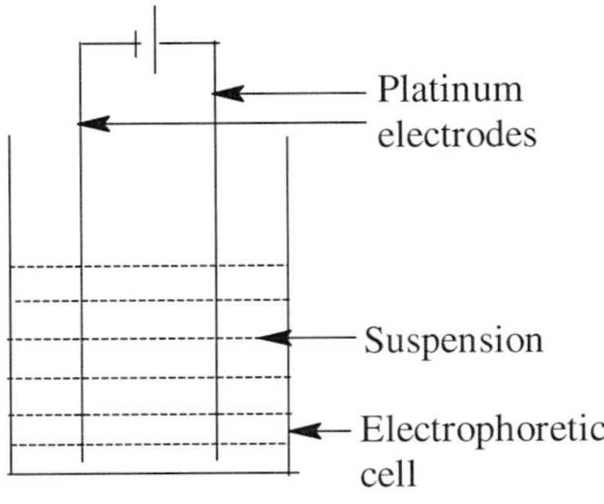

Fig. 14.2: An electrophoretic cell

Working

When an appropriate PD (E) is applied to platinum electrodes, separated by a distance (d), a potential gradient, E/d volts/cm, is produced. Under its influence, the particles of the suspension or an emulsion, move towards the electrode (electrophoresis) having charge opposite to the charge present on their surface. The movement of the particles of the suspension or an emulsion in the electrophoretic cell is observed under the microscope or an ultra-microscope. From the movement of the particle, its rate of migration can be calculated. This in turn, is a function of the charge on the particle. As the shear plane or a loosely bound layer of the particles is located at the periphery of the tightly bound layer **(Fig. 14.1)**, the rate-determining potential is the zeta potential. The size and shape of a particle do not affect its zeta potential.

From the direction of the movement of the particle, the charge on its surface can be determined. By using *Smoluchowski equation* **(equation 14.1)**, the sign and the magnitude of the zeta potential may be determined.

$$\zeta = \left(\frac{4\pi\eta}{D}\right)\left(\frac{v}{E/d}\right) = \left(\frac{4\pi\eta}{D}\right) u \cdots (14.1)$$

where, ζ (Zeta, Gr.) = zeta potential of the sample,

η (Eta, Gr.)= viscosity of the medium in poise (dynes.sec/cm^2),

D= dielectric constant of a medium,

v = velocity of migration of a particle in cm/sec or microns/sec,

E = potential across two electrodes of an electrophoretic cell,

d = distance between two electrodes in an electrophoretic cell,

E/d= potential gradient in volts/cm, and

$u = \text{electrophoretic mobility} = \left(\frac{v}{E/d}\right)$. It is defined as the velocity (v) of a particle when the potential gradient of 1 volt/cm is applied across the electrodes.

Applications of electrophoresis

1) By adjusting the magnitude of zeta potential, the stability of suspensions and emulsions can be increased.
2) Like the particles in the suspensions and emulsions, other species such as bacteria, erythrocytes, isolated cells from the plant origin and the particles of many other contaminants, can also be seen under microscope. Hence, electrophoresis is also used for the identification and the quantitative estimation of samples containing these species.

When the particles cannot be observed individually using a microscope or an ultra-microscope, other electrophoresis methods are employed, which are discussed below.

14.4.1.2. Moving Boundary Electrophoresis

Moving boundary electrophoresis makes use of an electrophoretic cell, as shown in **Fig. 14.2**. In this method, the movement of one particular particle is not measured, but when many particles move together, a clear boundary between the dispersed particles and the pure dispersion medium is seen under the influence of an electric field. Thus, the movement of this boundary is studied. In case of a colorless dispersed phase, the boundary is located by the refractive index gradient. When two or more species are present in the sample and if their mobility is different, then each species forms a separate and a distinct boundary, moving with a characteristic velocity. This allows identification of more than one species at a time.

Applications

1) Measurement of the electrophoretic mobility of each species helps in their identification.
2) The relative amounts of different species in their mixture can also be estimated.

14.4.1.3. Zone Electrophoresis

Instrumental set-up

The instrumental set-up for zone electrophoresis is extremely simple. A strip of a fitter paper or a gel is saturated with a conducting buffer solution. The cellulose acetate membrane, agar, starch or polyacrylamide gels, cut into strips, can also be used. Two platinum wires are embedded into the strip of the filter paper or a gel, as shown in **Fig. 14.3**. During the separation, the strip should not be allowed to dry. When current is passed through the strip, it produces heat, which can cause evaporation of water from the strip. This can be minimized by immersing the strip in a cooling liquid or sandwiching the strip between impervious solid sheets.

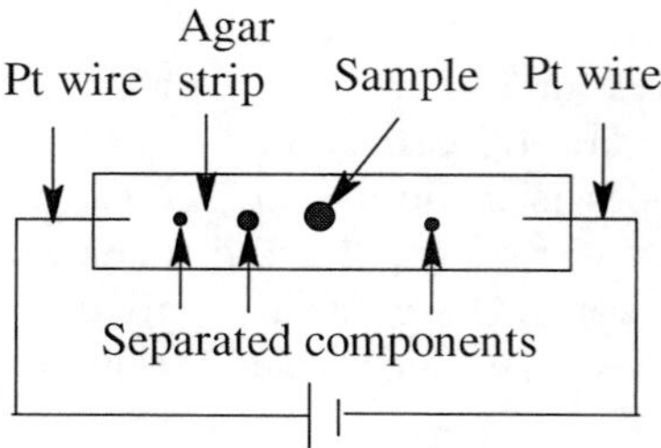

Fig. 14.3: Instrumental set-up for zone electrophoresis

Working

The sample to be analyzed is introduced on the strip in the form of a circular spot or a narrow band. A PD is applied across two ends of the strip via an electrical contact through platinum wires. The components of the sample move in particular directions, depending on the charge present on them. Different species are separated in the form of zones or bands on the filter paper, based on their electrophoretic mobility. Once the separation is complete, the strip is removed and dried. The position of the spots or bands corresponding to the individual components is detected by a color reaction or the radioactivity counting.

Advantages

1) Zone electrophoresis requires much smaller sample than that required for moving boundary electrophoresis.
2) The instrument required is very simple and cheap.

3) Since the sample is present on an inert and the porous strip, there is no convection during the separation.
4) Several samples can be analyzed simultaneously.

Uses

Because of the requirement of a smaller sample size, zone electrophoresis is used widely to study the proteins in the body fluids such as blood serum, lymph, cerebrospinal fluid, saliva, gastric juices, pancreatic juices and bile.

14.4.1.4. Immuno-electrophoresis

Immuno-electrophoresis is commonly used for the identification of different proteins from their mixture or from the body fluids. It is also used for the identification of antigens in the body, responsible for causing a disease. Thus, immuno-electrophoresis is used as a powerful diagnostic tool in the field of pathology.

The instrumental set-up used for this technique is exactly same as that shown in **Fig. 14.3**. The proteins in the body fluids, including antigens, are first separated by zone electrophoresis. Immuno-diffusion combined with electrophoresis is called immuno-electrophoresis. After the separation, different proteins appear on the strip, in the form of bands or spots. If the spots are not visible, a specific reagent like a ninhydrin reagent, which produces pink colored complexes with proteins, is used to locate different proteins on the strip. The separated protein bands are cut into pieces and are kept in an antibody solution. On standing, a particular antigen reacts with an antibody and forms the precipitate. If this precipitate is not visible, some stains can be made use of.

The standard electrophoretic pattern of different body fluids is available in the literature. If an electrophoretic pattern of a body fluid is found to vary, the presence of some antibodies in it, corresponding to a certain infection, can be predicted. Thus, the presence of a particular antigen in the body fluid can be detected. This helps in the diagnosis of a disease.

14.4.1.5. Isoelectric Focusing

Proteins are chains of polypeptides, which are chains of up to 300 amino acids. They have a carboxylic group as an acidic moiety and an amino group as a basic moiety. An amino group in proteins is protonated in the acidic medium. The carboxylic group is ionized to a carboxylate anion in the neutral and alkaline media. Thus, in the acidic as well as in the basic medium, these compounds remain in the ionized forms. Hence, proteins are amphoteric in nature. Dissociation of proteins in the acidic and an alkaline medium is shown in **Fig. 14.4**. However, at one particular pH, the carboxylic group and an amino group, both remain unionized. The pH at which proteins remain unionized is referred to as an *isoelectric pH*. At this pH, proteins are precipitated quantitatively. An isoelectric pH is a characteristic of a particular protein.

$$H_2N - (CH_2)_n - COOH \xrightarrow{\text{Acidic pH}} \overset{+}{H_3N} - (CH_2)_n - COOH$$

And

$$H_2N - (CH_2)_n - COOH \xrightarrow{\text{Basic pH}} H_2N - (CH_2)_n - COO^-$$

Fig. 14.4: Ionization of amino acids in acidic and basic media

Isoelectric focusing is a method for the separation of proteins by electrophoresis based on their isoelectric pH values. At isoelectric pH, proteins do not carry any charge on them and hence, do not migrate in an electric field.

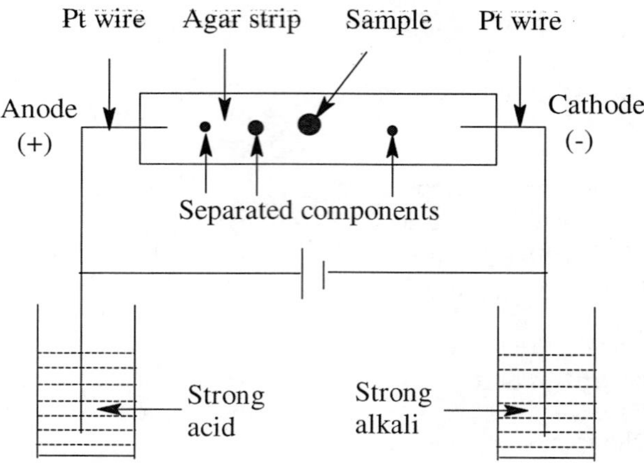

Fig. 14.5: Instrumental set-up for isoelectric focusing

An instrumental set-up for an isoelectric focusing method is similar to that used for zone electrophoresis and is shown in **Fig. 14.5**. In order to carry out separation of proteins by immuno-electrophoresis, across a strip of filter paper or an agar, a pH gradient is imposed by dipping anode in a strong acid and cathode in a strong alkali. A sample containing a mixture of proteins is spotted at the centre of the strip. In an aqueous medium, all the proteins are initially present in the ionized form. When a PD is applied across two ends of the strip, the proteins start moving towards two electrodes, depending on the charge present on their surface. As they move across the strip, they experience the pH gradient. When a protein reaches the spot on the strip, where the pH corresponds to its isoelectric pH, the charge on its surface becomes zero. Thus, at this spot, protein precipitates out and stops migrating. The protein with the highest isoelectric pH is located nearest to the cathode, which is immersed in a strong base. The protein with the lowest isoelectric pH is located nearest to the anode, immersed in a strong acid. The other proteins settle at the intermediate positions, where the pH values are intermediate and equal to their isoelectric pH.

Thus, different techniques in electrophoresis provide a simple method for the separation and identification of complex compounds.

CHAPTER 15

LIGHT SCATTERING SPECTROMETRY

In the light scattering technique, there are two methods.

1) Turbidimetry
2) Nephelometry

Both these methods are used to measure the concentration of the dispersed particles in various samples, i.e. when the sample is turbid. Emulsions, suspensions and colloidal solutions are the common examples of dispersion, wherein one phase is dispersed into the other. Thus, in dispersions, a dispersed phase is present in a dispersing medium. The light scattering technique is commonly employed in determining the properties of macro-molecules like polymers and proteins.

15.1. PRINCIPLE

When a beam of radiation is passed through a sample of a colloidal solution, a part of the radiation is absorbed, a part of it gets reflected, a part of it gets transmitted and the remaining gets scattered. The colloidal particles have at least one dimension in the range of 10 to 100 A° on the lower side and a few microns (μ) or micrometers (μm) on the upper side (1 μ or 1 μm = 10^4 A°).

The scattering of light is observed only under the following conditions.

1) When the size of the particles of the dispersed phase is significantly smaller than the wavelength of the incident radiation, the scattering of radiation is observed commonly. The scattering by molecules or aggregates of molecules in such a case is referred to as *Rayleigh scattering*.
2) Scattering of radiation is also observed when the refractive index of the dispersing medium is different from that of the dispersed particles.

The intensity of the scattered radiation increases with the particle size. With particles of the colloidal dimensions, scattering becomes so intense that it can be observed by the naked eyes also. Thus, a beam of light passing through a colloidal suspension gets scattered and produces a *pencil of light* or a *cone of light*, as shown in **Fig. 15.1**. This effect was first observed by Tyndall and hence, is known as *Tyndall effect*. The colloidal particles having the particle size between 10 -100 A° (i.e.1-10 nm) bring about scattering of UV (2000-4000 A°) and visible (4000 – 8000 A°) radiation. This effect indicates the presence of suspended particles in the sample.

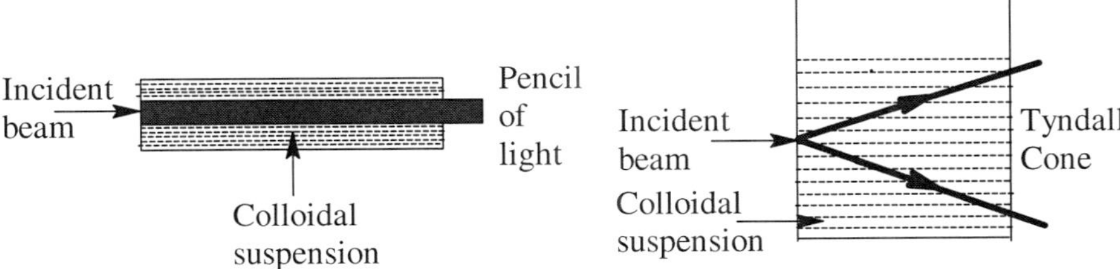

Fig. 15.1: Tyndall effect

1 Angstrom unit, 1 A° = 10^{-8} cm = 10^{-10} m
1 Nanometer, 1 nm = 10^{-9} m
1 μ or 1 μm = 10^4 A° = 10^{-6} m
1 μ = 10^3 mμ = 10^{-6} m
1 mμ = 10^{-9} m
1 nm = 1 mμ

15.2. DIFFERENCE BETWEEN TURBIDIMETRY AND NEPHELOMETRY

The intensity of the scattered light can be measured in two directions –

1) When the turbidity is high, the intensity of the scattered light is also high. In such a case, the turbidity is measured in the direction of the incident radiation, i.e. at 0° angle and the method is called as *turbidimetry*.
2) When the turbidity is low, the intensity of the scattered light is also low. In such a case, in order to measure the intensity of the scattered light accurately, turbidity is measured at any angle between 75 and 135°, usually at 90° angle, to the incident beam. This is because along 0° angle, the loss in the intensity is much higher than that along 90° angle. The higher the intensity of the scattered light, the higher is the accuracy of the measurement. (Thus, when the suspension is dilute and when the intensity of the scattered light is less, in order to increase the accuracy in the measurement of the intensity of the scattered light, an angle of 90° is selected, where, the loss in the intensity is minimum). When the turbidity is measured at any angle between 75 and 135° to the incident radiation, the method is called as *nephelometry*. The difference in the turbidimetry and nephelometry is indicated diagrammatically in **Fig. 15.2**.

Turbidity (τ) of any dispersion is defined by an **equation (15.1)**.

$$\tau = \frac{1}{l} \ln \frac{I_o}{I_t} \cdots (15.1)$$

where, I_o and I_t are the intensities of the incident and the transmitted beams and '*l*' is the path length through which light passes in the dispersion.

15.3. INSTRUMENTATION

Visual and photoelectric colorimeters may be used as turbidimeters or nephelometers. The components of a turbidimeter and a nephelometer are very much similar to the UV-visible spectrometer, and are described below.

1) A source

Either a monochromatic source like a mercury lamp or a polychromatic source like a tungsten lamp is very commonly used in

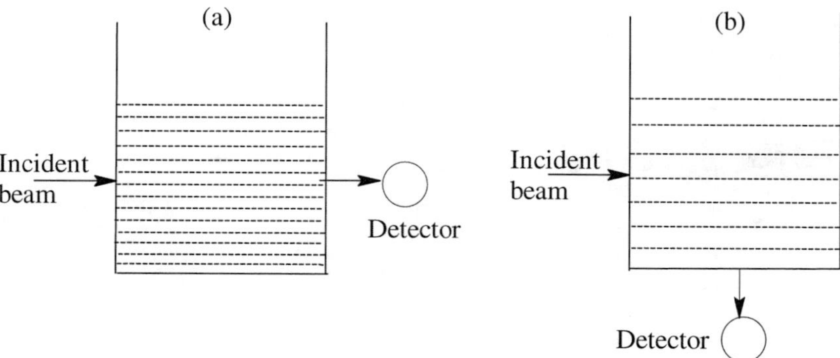

Fig. 15.2: Measurement of intensity of scattered radiation in (a) turbidimetry and (b) nephelometry

turbidimetry and nephelometry.

2) A monochromator

Commonly, the filters are used as monochromators in turbidimetry and nephelometry. The scattered radiation usually falls in the UV-visible range. A filter of the same color as that of the color of the dispersion is used, but a blue filter usually results in the greater sensitivity.

3) A sample holder

A sample holder is made up of quartz, which is transparent to UV-visible radiation.

4) A Detector

A detector used in most of the cases is usually a photocell.

5) A recorder

The intensity of the scattered beam can be recorded so as to get a graph of intensity vs. concentration.

The light transmitted by a turbid solution does not generally obey Beer-Lambert law precisely. Hence, in case of turbidimetry, a

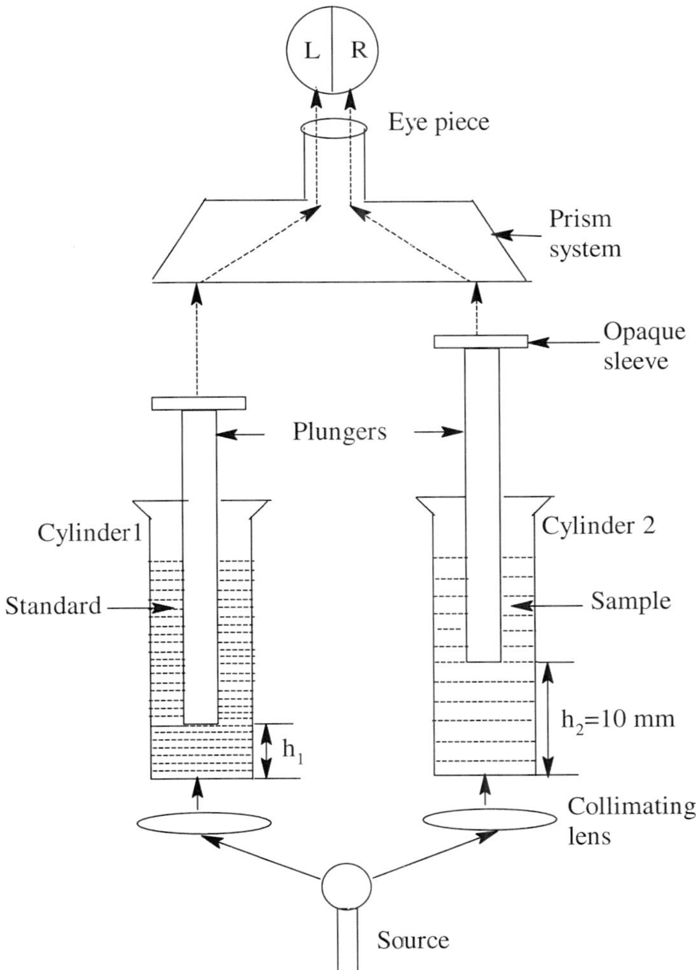

Fig. 15.3: Duboscq turbidimeter

calibration curve must be constructed using several standard dispersions.

15.3.1. Duboscq Colorimeter

Construction

Duboscq colorimeter or a turbidimeter is a piston type or a plunger type of a colorimeter. As shown in **Fig. 15.3**, it consists of two identical and calibrated *quartz cylinders*. In case of a *Duboscq turbidimeter*, quartz cylinders possess a polished bottom for the passage of light through them. In case of a *Duboscq nephelometer*, since the intensity of the scattered light is to be measured at right angles to the incident beam, the quartz cylinders possess a polished surface or a window on the lower side of one of the vertical sides of the cylinders, but they are opaque at the bottom. Light is passed from these side windows into quartz cylinders. This is shown in **Fig. 15.4**. Inside the cylinders, the quartz *pistons* or *plungers* are fitted with the help of *opaque sleeves*. Plungers can move up and down but do not slide down freely. Thus, they can be moved and kept fixed at a definite height inside the cylinder. Light passing through both the cylinders is allowed to enter the eye piece through a prism system, where two halves, left (L) and right (R), of the *field of view*, get illuminated.

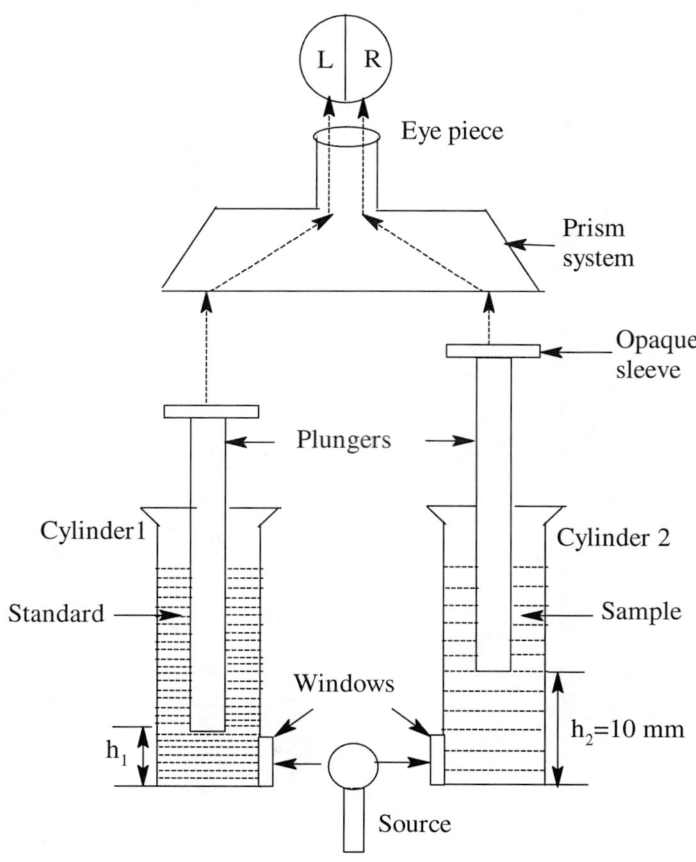

Fig. 15.4: Duboscq nephelometer

Working

A defined volume of the standard solution, containing more turbidity than that of the sample, is taken in *cylinder 1*. Equal volume of the sample is introduced in *cylinder 2*. Initially, the plungers just touch the bottom of the cylinders. The height of the plunger in the sample is set at 10 mm from the bottom of the cylinder.

The radiation from the source falls on the dispersions in two cylinders. A part of the light is absorbed and a part of it is scattered. The two beams of light are then brought to a common axis by a prism system. On looking through the eyepiece, a wide circular field is visible. The light from one cylinder illuminates one half of the field and the light from the second cylinder illuminates another half of the field. The illumination in two halves matches when the intensity of the scattered light from the two cylinders becomes exactly the same. This happens when the light in both the cylinders interacts with the same number of particles. The height of the plunger in the standard dispersion is adjusted until the intensities of the scattered beams received in two fields of the eye piece are matched exactly. Care should be taken so that the plungers always remain below the surface of the liquid in cylinders. For a more turbid dispersion in cylinder 1, the plunger height (h_1), required to be raised above the bottom of the cylinder, so as to get equal illumination in two halves, is lesser as compared to the height of the plunger (h_2 = 10 mm) set in cylinder 2. This is because cylinder 1 contains denser (higher concentration) dispersion as compared to that in cylinder 2. Hence, the same number of particles, responsible for scattering the light from 10 mm height (h_2) in cylinder 2, is available in a smaller height (h_1) in cylinder1.

In order to get the accurate value of the turbidity of a sample solution, i.e. to find concentration of sample accurately by using Duboscq colorimeter, it is essential to record the readings at least 6 times. The exact concentration of an unknown sample is then determined by calculating the average of all these readings.

The amount of light scattered by the particles depends on the number of particles coming in the path of radiation from the base of the cylinder to the base of the plunger. The more the particles below the base of the plunger, the more is the scattering and the higher is the intensity of the scattered beam coming out from the top of the plunger. Thus, the concentration (c) of the solution is inversely proportional to the depth (h) of the solution below the plunger. This depth is normally read directly from the calibrations on the quartz cylinder.

Thus, $$c \propto \frac{1}{h}$$

$$\text{or } c.h = \text{constant}$$

When the intensity of illuminations in two halves of an eye piece matches with each other, the product of the concentration and height of the plunger from the bottom of the cylinder, is exactly same for both the cylinders. This can be expressed mathematically by **equation (15.2)**.

$$c_1 h_1 = c_2 h_2 \quad \dots (15.2)$$

where, c_1 = concentration of a standard,

c_2 = concentration of a sample,

h_1 = height of the plunger from the bottom of cylinder 1, and

h_2 = height of the plunger from the bottom of cylinder 2 = 10 mm

For cylinder 2, containing a sample, h_2 = 10 mm. Hence, **equation (15.2)** takes the form as follows.

$$c_1 h_1 = c_2 \times 10 \quad \dots (15.3)$$

The concentration (c_1) of the standard solution is known. The height (h_1) of the plunger from the bottom of cylinder 1 for the standard is measured. Hence, the concentration (c_2) of the sample can be calculated by using **equation (15.4)**.

$$c_2 = \frac{c_1\, h_1}{10} \cdots (15.4)$$

If the percent concentration of the sample is to be determined, then both the sides of **equation (15.4)** are multiplied by 100 to get **equation (15.5)**.

$$100\, c_2 = 100\left(\frac{c_1\, h_1}{10}\right) \cdots (15.5)$$

$$\text{or} \quad \%\, c_2 = 10 \times (c_1\, h_1) \ldots (15.6)$$

Advantages

1) Plotting of a calibration curve is not required.
2) The apparatus used is very simple and cheap.

Drawbacks

1) Determination of the turbidity using a Duboscq turbidimeter is based on the visual matching of illumination in two halves of an eye piece. Therefore, it is difficult to detect the small differences in the illumination in two halves. Hence, the accuracy in the measurements is less.
2) Personal variation may occur in the measurements.
3) An average of 5 to 6 readings is required for the accurate determination of the concentration of the sample. Since eyes get fatigued while matching intensity in two halves, recording more readings, makes an already tedious process, the more tedious.

15.3.2. Eel's Nephelometer

Construction

As shown in **Fig. 15.5**, an Eel's nephelometer makes use of mercury or a tungsten lamp. A monochromator used is a filter. Quartz tube is used as a sample holder. In order to reflect the scattered light to the detector, which is usually a photocell, a reflector is provided. A photocell is kept at the bottom of the sample tube. A reflector is mounted above the photocell itself. The photocell is connected to a galvanometer. The whole assembly is enclosed in a chamber. The top of the sample holder, which is outside the chamber, is covered with a metallic lid. When the instrument is in use, the metal cap fits over the sample holder. If the cap is removed by mistake, while working with the instrument, a micro switch inside the instrument is operated to disconnect the photocell from the galvanometer. This arrangement is provided to prevent the damage to the photocell and galvanometer, by the large current resulting from the sudden entry of an external light.

Working

The light is allowed to pass vertically through a window onto the filter. A blue filter or a filter having the same color as that of the sample is selected as a monochromator. The radiation coming out of the filter passes into the sample holder. The light is scattered by the multiple reflections by the particles of the turbid suspension. Such a scattered light is collected by the reflector and directed towards the photocell. The photocell generates current depending on the intensity of the scattered light. The current so generated is recorded by a sensitive galvanometer. It gives idea about the concentration of a substance in the sample.

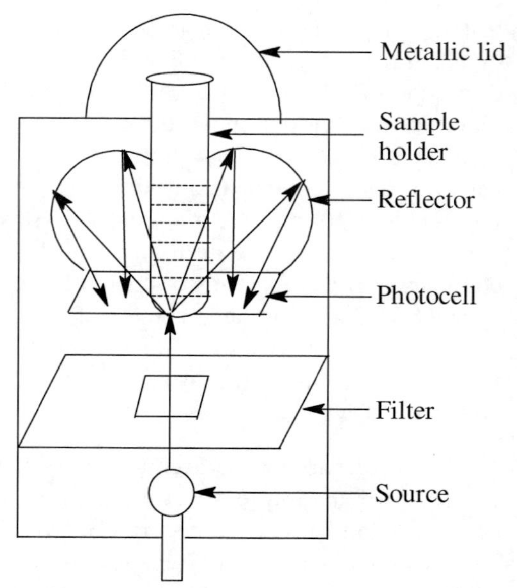

Fig. 15.5: An Eel's nephelometer

A standard suspension of known concentration is prepared. Various dilutions are prepared from this stock suspension so as to get 5-6 suspensions of known concentration. The intensity of the scattered light is then recorded for all these standard suspensions in the decreasing order of the turbidity. A calibration curve is prepared by plotting the intensity of the scattered light from the suspensions against their concentrations. Intensity (I_s) of the scattered beam is ultimately recorded for a sample by replacing the standard suspension from the sample tube with the sample suspension. The concentration (c_s) of the sample is determined by extrapolating the intensity of the scattered light on the concentration axis, as shown in **Fig. 15.6**.

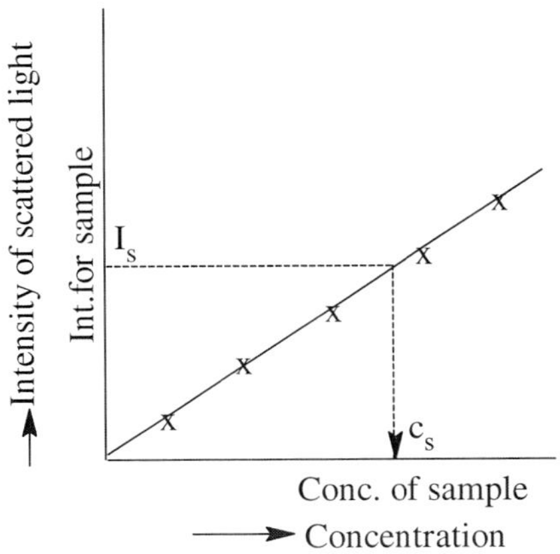

Fig. 15.6: Calibration curve in nephelometry

Advantages

1) The measurement of the intensity of the scattered radiation is not done visually in Eel's nephelometry. Hence, it does not involve man to man variation.
2) Eel's nehelometer provides higher accuracy compared to Duboscq nephelometer.
3) It does not cause a problem of fatigue to the eyes of an operator.

Disadvantages

1) It requires plotting of the calibration curve.
2) The fabrication of Eel's nephelometer is not as simple as Duboscq nephelometer.

Thus, both the methods have their own advantages and disadvantages. In Duboscq colorimeter, plotting of the calibration curve is not required, but the intensity of the scattered light is measured 5-6 times to get higher accuracy. In Eel's nephelometer, a plotting of the calibration curve is required, using 5-6 dilutions, but readings are more accurate.

15.4. APPLICATIONS OF TURBIDIMETRY

1) Turbidimetry is used to determine the concentration of the dispersed particles in suspensions.
2) It is also used to determine the number of microorganisms in the nutrient medium during antimicrobial testing. In such a case, a definite turbidity is obtained by mixing a fixed amount of barium chloride and sulphuric acid so as to get a fixed quantity of the precipitate of barium sulphate. The turbidity or opalescence of the microbial suspension is then matched with the turbidity of barium sulphate. This ensures the use of a definite number of microorganisms during antimicrobial testing. The precipitate of barium sulphate is obtained according to the following chemical reaction.

$$BaCl_2 + H_2SO_4 \rightarrow BaSO_4 \downarrow + 2\ HCl$$

3) The light scattering techniques are used for the determination of the molecular weight of macromolecules such as polymers or proteins.

Thus, the light scattering techniques provide a very simple means for the quantitative estimation of the dispersed media.

CHAPTER 16

SEPARATION TECHNIQUES

Many a times, substances of interest are not available in the pure form. They are often mixed with other substances, which may act as impurities. The presence of impurities can make selective and accurate analysis of compounds difficult. In order to avoid this, an analyte is separated from the interfering impurities using various separation techniques. Similarly, these techniques are used in the field of pharmacy to separate active principles, i.e. drugs from the formulations like tinctures, extracts, pills, tablets, suspensions, ointments, etc. The separation techniques can also be used to isolate vitamins, enzymes, hormones, alkaloids, etc. from their natural sources in order to analyze them without any interference.

Some of the methods for the separation of compounds from each other include methods such as chromatography, crystallization, filtration, distillation, sublimation and extraction. This chapter deals with the separation methods using extraction.

16.1. EXTRACTION METHODS

Extraction methods can be classified as follows.

16.1.1. Solid–liquid extraction
16.1.2. Liquid–liquid extraction
16.1.3. Counter-current extraction

16.1.1. Solid˘Liquid Extraction

A solid is extracted by using a suitable solvent in three different ways.

1) Maceration
2) Percolation
3)Continuous extraction by using Soxhlet apparatus

1) Maceration

In this method of extraction, a sample to be extracted is kept in an enclosed container. A suitable solvent such as water, methanol, ethanol, etc. is then added to it. It is left alone at room temperature for 2-3 days for complete extraction. The mixture may be stirred intermittently to enhance the rate of extraction. After complete extraction, the mixture is filtered through the muslin cloth and the residue (marc) on the muslin cloth is pressed to obtain the maximum volume of the extract. A clear extract is then obtained by filtration and is treated further as per the requirements.

Advantage

Maceration is a *cold extraction method*, wherein the sample is not exposed to heat. Hence, it is especially useful for extracting heat labile substances.

Drawback

Maceration may not extract the sample completely in some cases because of cold conditions.

2) Percolation

In case of percolation, a sample to be extracted is placed in a percolator, as shown in **Fig. 16.1**. A percolator is a cone shaped vessel having cock at the bottom. A sample to be extracted is placed in the percolator. A solvent used for the extraction is added from the top of the percolator, while keeping the cock open. When solvent is about to leave the percolator, the cock is closed. The additional amount of the solvent is added so as to get its level above the sample to be extracted. The percolator is then covered from the top and the sample is allowed to macerate for 24 hours. At the end of that period, the cock is opened and the percolate (extract) of the sample is allowed to fall slowly from the bottom. The mass in the percolator is then pressed and the percolate is collected. Sufficient volume of the solvent is then added so as to get the required volume. The percolate is then filtered to get the clear extract.

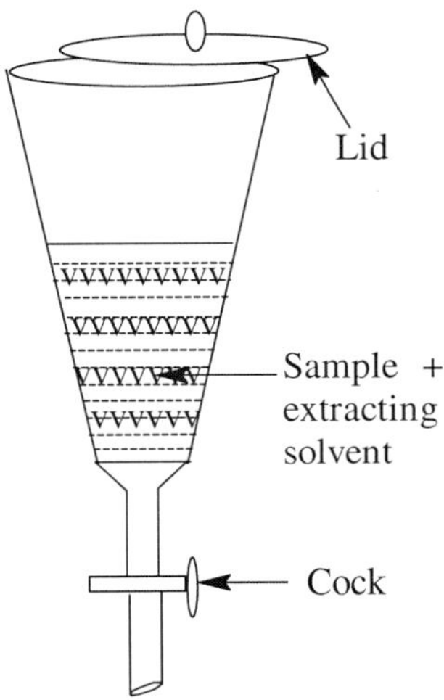

Fig. 16.1: Extraction by percolation

Advantages

(i) One advantage of this method is that the sample and the solvent can be added from time to time into the percolator. This helps in the maximum extraction of a large quantity of the sample in a minimum time period.

(ii) Heat labile substances can be extracted.

Percolation method is commonly used for the preparation of tinctures.

3) Continuous extraction by using Soxhlet apparatus

The Soxhlet apparatus, as shown in **Fig. 16.2**, consists of three parts.

(i) A round bottom flask with solvent

(ii) A thimble containing sample to be extracted

(iii) Condenser

The sample to be extracted is kept inside the thimble. The top end of the thimble is attached to a condenser. The bottom of the thimble is fitted into a round bottom flask, containing an extracting solvent. The flask is heated so as to generate vapor of the extracting solvent, which passes through the side arm of the flask into the condenser. The condensed extracting solvent falls on the sample in the thimble and extracts the active material. The extract then returns back to the round bottom flask containing an extracting solvent through a siphon, as shown in **Fig. 16.2**.

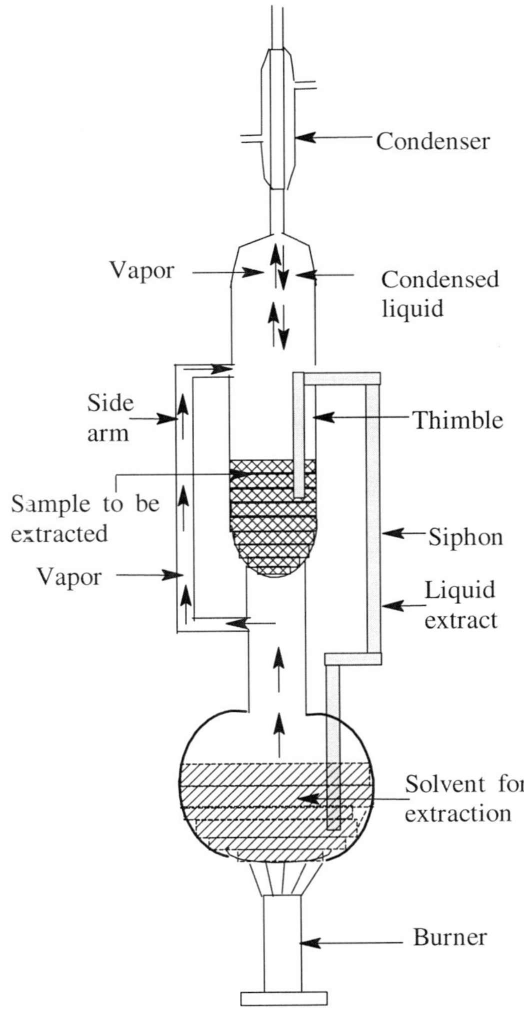

Fig. 16.2: Continuous extraction using Soxhlet apparatus

Advantage

Since the extract falls back into the round bottom flask, same solvent is used over and over again during continuous extraction. This makes possible the continuous extraction of the material using small volumes of a solvent.

Drawback

The extracted material is collected in the round bottom flask containing a solvent which is continuously heated. Hence, the heat labile substances cannot be extracted by this method.

Continuous extraction is used when the substance to be extracted has low solubility in the extracting solvent.

16.1.2. Liquid˘Liquid Extraction

16.1.2.1. Principle

This is also one of the separation techniques, wherein a solute present in one liquid is extracted into another immiscible liquid. The principle behind this separation technique is based on the *Nernst Law*, which states that "the ratio of the activities (i.e. concentrations) of a solute in two immiscible liquids at equilibrium is always constant". The ratio of concentrations of a solute in two immiscible solvents is called the '*distribution coefficient*' or '*partition coefficient*' (K).

$$K = C_u / C_l$$

where, C_u = concentration of a solute in the solvent forming an upper layer (a lighter liquid),

and C_l = concentration of a solute in the solvent forming a lower layer (a heavier liquid).

Partition coefficient can be found out by using separating funnels or by using a *shake flask method.* In this method, a liquid containing a solute to be extracted is mixed with another liquid in an enclosed flask. The flask is shaken continuously by keeping it over a mechanical shaker. Sufficient time is allowed to reach the equilibrium between the phases, and the concentration of a solute in each phase is determined.

16.1.2.2. Difference between Distribution Coefficient (Partition Coefficient) and Distribution Ratio

Distribution coefficient and distribution ratio of a solute differ from each other. Distribution coefficient or partition coefficient is the ratio of concentrations of only undissociated or unionized solute in two immiscible solvents, whereas distribution ratio is the ratio of the concentrations of undissociated as well as dissociated forms of a substance in two different solvents. This can be explained with the help of dissociation of benzoic acid as shown in **Fig. 16.3**. When benzoic acid is added to water, a part of it gets dissociated into benzoate anions and protons. When another immiscible liquid like ether is added to it, it extracts only the undissociated benzoic acid, whereas water retains both, the dissociated as well as undissociated acid.

$$C_6H_5COOH \rightleftharpoons C_6H_5COOH + C_6H_5COO^- + H^+$$

Undissociated acid — Dissociated acid (Benzoate anion)

Fig. 16.3: Dissociation of benzoic acid

Distribution coefficient (K) for benzoic acid in ether and water is expressed by **equation (16.1).**

$$K = \frac{[C_6H_5COOH]_{ether}}{[C_6H_5COOH]_{water}} \quad \ldots (16.1)$$

Distribution ratio (K_D) is expressed by **equation (16.2).**

$$K_D = \frac{[C_6H_5COOH]_{ether}}{[C_6H_5COOH]_{water} + [C_6H_5COO^-]_{water}} \quad \ldots (16.2)$$

Thus, if a substance dissociates in solution, the values of K and K_D would differ. Similarly, for solutes which associate or get polymerized in solution, the values of K and K_D would differ. When the partitioning of benzoic acid in benzene and water is studied, distribution coefficient and the distribution ratio are calculated by **equations (16.3)** and **(16.4)**.

When benzoic acid is extracted in benzene, it undergoes association and exists as a dimer **(Fig.16.4)**. In water, part of benzoic acid gets dissociated into benzoate anion ($C_6H_5COO^-$) and protons.

$$\therefore K = \frac{[\text{Dimer}]_{\text{benzene}}}{[\text{Benzoic acid}]^2_{\text{water}}} \quad \cdots (16.3)$$

and

$$K_D = \frac{[\text{Dimer}]_{\text{benzene}}}{[C_6H_5COOH]_{\text{water}} + [C_6H_5COO^-]_{\text{water}}} \quad \cdots (16.4)$$

Application of liquid-liquid extraction can be understood from an example of selective separation of aniline (a basic liquid) from nitrobenzene (a neutral liquid), when they are present together. Both being liquids and miscible with each other, cannot be separated unless aniline is converted to a water soluble hydrochloride salt. The separation of two liquids from their mixture is thus carried out by dissolving them in a non-aqueous solvent like benzene or ether and extracting a basic compound (aniline) in an aqueous solution containing dilute hydrochloric acid. Aniline gets converted to aniline hydrochloride and enters into an aqueous layer, thereby leaving nitrobenzene in the non-aqueous layer. The process of extraction is repeated till complete separation is achieved.

The separation of two compounds from each other can be achieved by liquid-liquid extraction, but if there are more than two or three constituents in a mixture, their clear separation from each other is difficult unless distribution coefficients of all the constituents are distinctly different.

The magnitude of partition coefficient decides the efficiency as well as the ease of separation of compounds from their mixture. Hence, it is absolutely essential to determine the partition coefficients of solutes. In order to get a reproducible value of distribution coefficient or partition coefficient, certain conditions are required to be maintained. The change in certain factors can change the partition coefficient of solutes, which may either facilitate or hamper their extraction from one phase to the other.

16.1.2.3. Factors Affecting Magnitude of Partition Coefficient

The factors which affect the partition coefficient of a solute are described below.

1) Solvent used for extraction

(i) Two solvents involved in extraction should have different density and polarity so that they are immiscible with each other.

(ii) Solvents should have low toxicity and low inflammability.

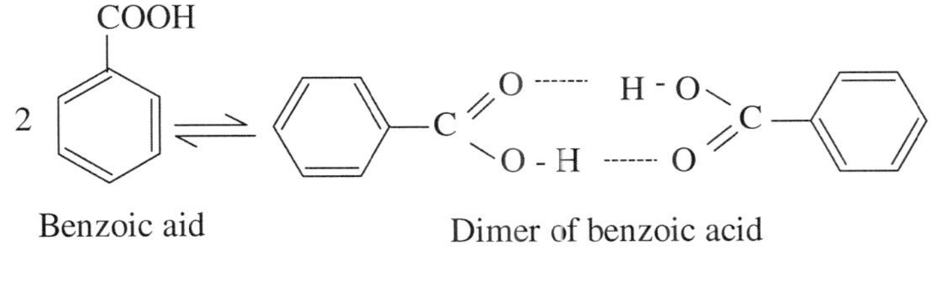

Fig. 16.4: Dimer of benzoic acid

(iii) Solvents should be cheap, easily available and should be easily recovered after extraction.
(iv) It should be selective for a solute.
(v) Commonly used solvents are chloroform, ether, carbon tetra chloride, benzene, petroleum ether, ethylene dichloride and so on.
(vi) Volume of solvent used for extraction also decides the partition coefficient of a solute. If volume of a solvent is increased, its extraction power is also increased.

2) pH of the solution

The pH of a solution decides solubility of a substance in a particular solvent. For example, extraction of alkaloids from plants requires adjustment of pH of a solution. Alcoholic extracts or ether extracts dissolve alkaloids along with other plant constituents such as tannins, starch, chlorophyll, etc. To separate alkaloids from such plant constituents, the extract is made acidic. Acid forms salts with alkaloids, which are basic in nature because of the presence of nitrogen in them. These salts being polar, dissolve in polar solvents easily. Thus, if dilute hydrochloric or sulphuric acid is added to an ether extract of plants containing alkaloids, acidic aqueous layer selectively extracts alkaloids, leaving behind the unwanted plant constituents (tannins, starch, chlorophyll, etc.) in ether layer. The aqueous acidic layer is separated from the ether layer. The extracted salts of the alkaloids are precipitated out from the aqueous solution by converting them back to the original bases by the addition of an alkali. These precipitated bases are then extracted in ether to have further separation of alkaloids from water soluble impurities. Thus, extraction of a substance from one liquid to the other or its partition coefficient would depend on the pH of the extracting solvent.

3) Salting-out effect

The salting-out effect is generally used to decrease the solubility of a water soluble component or to increase the solubility of a compound in the non–aqueous phase. The reduction of solubility by increasing the ionic strength of a solution is known as *salting-out effect*. For example, benzoic acid or ephedrine has sufficient solubility in water. To extract them completely from aqueous extracts and to increase their concentration in an organic phase, a salt having very high solubility in water, e.g. NaCl, is added to an aqueous phase. Sodium chloride dissolves in water and displaces a substance which has lower solubility than it, and forces it to enter into an organic phase.

16.1.2.4. Methods of Liquid-Liquid Extraction

Liquid–liquid extraction by using two immiscible liquids can be carried out by using two techniques.

1) Batch extraction
2) Continuous extraction

1) Batch extraction

The *batch extraction* is carried out by using a set of separating funnels. A solution from which a substance is to be extracted and an immiscible extracting solvent are introduced in a separating funnel. Two phases are mixed thoroughly in order to extract the substance from one phase to the other. If the extracting solvent is heavier, it would form a lower layer in the separating funnel. This heavier layer, containing the extracted material, is removed and stored in a separate container. For more effective and complete separation, more of fresh extracting solvent is added to the lighter layer which is retained in the separating funnel and the extraction is continued. This procedure is repeated till the extraction is almost complete. If the extracting solvent is lighter, it would form an upper layer in the separating funnel. In such a case, the lower layer is removed and transferred to another separating funnel, containing fresh extracting solvent. The extraction is completed by repeating the procedure twice or thrice. Extraction by this method is carried out when the partition coefficient of a solute is high. Method is simple and quick and hence, is widely used for the extraction on a small scale. For extraction on a large scale, a continuous extraction process is applicable.

2) Continuous extraction

The continuous extraction method is carried out when the partition coefficient of solutes is low. An immiscible extracting liquid is kept flowing continuously through the solution from which a solute is to be extracted. Although there is not enough time for the equilibrium to reach, a solute is extracted continuously in this extraction method.

This method requires a special kind of extractor, depending on whether the solvent used for extraction is lighter or heavier than the sample solution.

(i) Extracting solvent lighter than the sample solution

Apparatus used for this type of extraction is shown in **Fig. 16.5**. It is similar to that of the Soxhlet apparatus but instead of one solvent, two solvents are used in this case.

The extracting solvent (e.g. a non-aqueous solvent), which is lighter than the sample solution (e.g. an aqueous solution), is placed in a container (A). It is connected to a thimble (B) holding the

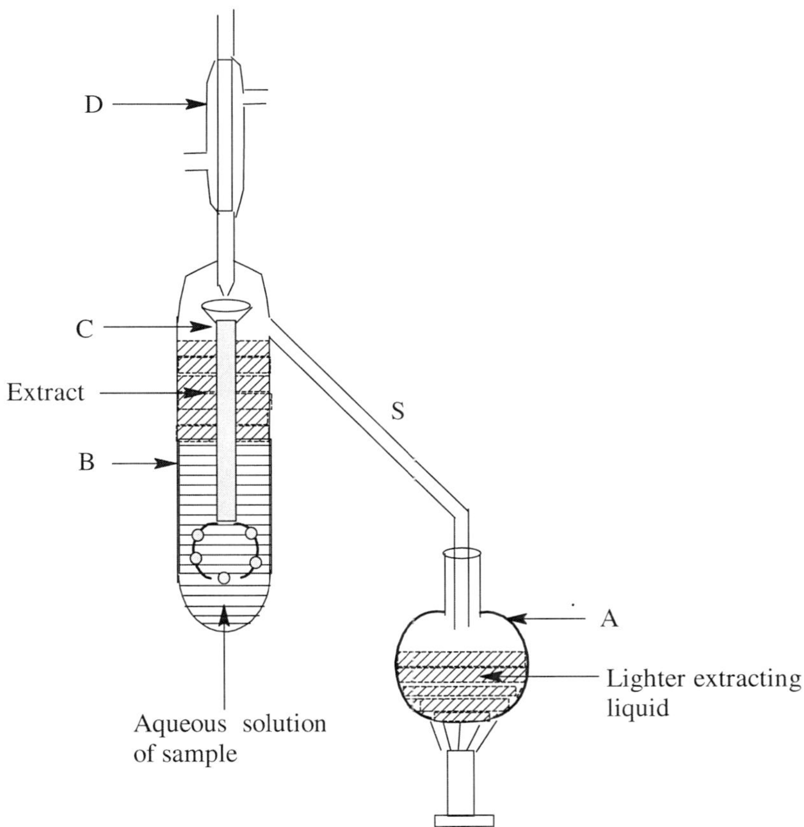

Fig. 16.5: Extraction using extracting solvent lighter than the sample solution

sample solution to half its capacity. A glass tube (C), having a funnel shaped opening at one end and a glass bulb with holes at another end, is placed inside the thimble. This body is then connected to a condenser (D), which is attached at the upper end of the thimble. The extracting solvent in the container (A) is heated. Vapor of the extracting solvent passes through the thimble into the condenser and falls as droplets into the funnel type glass tube (C). The droplets of the extracting liquid enter the glass tube and then escape through the holes in the glass bulb. The extracting solvent being lighter than the solution to be extracted, passes through the sample solution. In this process, it extracts the solute and gets accumulated on the top of the sample solution. When sufficient quantity of the extracting liquid gets collected in the thimble, it overflows back to the flask (A) from the side arm (S). The process is continued till the extraction is complete.

(ii) Extracting solvent heavier than the sample solution

The apparatus used for this type of

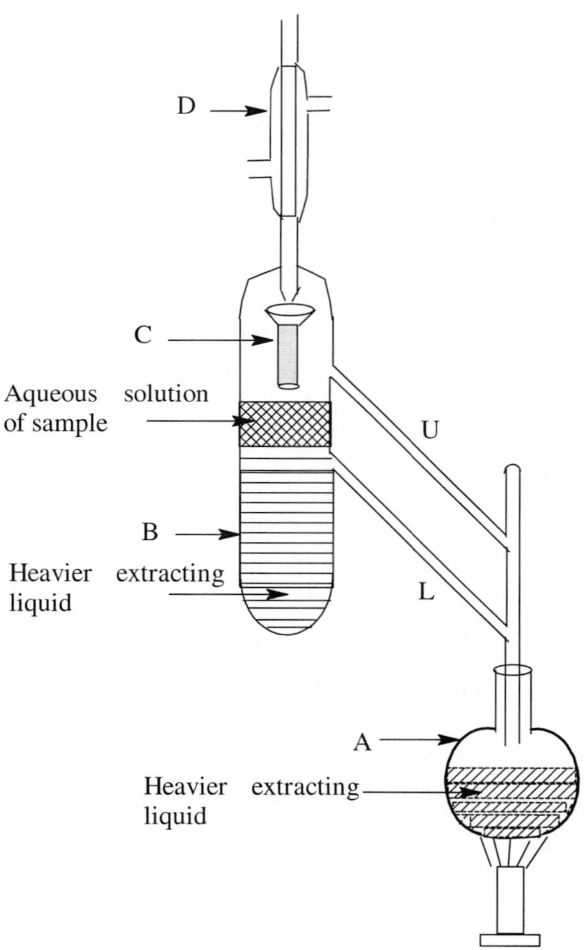

Fig. 16.6: Extraction using extracting solvent heavier than the sample solution

extraction is shown in **Fig. 16.6**. The extracting solvent is placed in a round bottom flask (A) and is heated. The sample solution to be extracted is present at the centre of the thimble (B). The vapor of the solvent passes from the upper side tube (U) of the flask into the thimble and then to the condenser (D) attached at the top of the thimble. On cooling, the droplets of the heavier extracting solvent drop down in the glass tube (C) and pass through the sample solution. In this process, it extracts the solute and gets accumulated at the bottom of the thimble, from where it overflows into the flask (A) through the lower side tube (L). The rate of heating of the extracting solvent in the flask (A) is adjusted so as to maintain the level of the sample solution between two side tubes (U) and (L) of the flask, so that the sample solution does not overflow at any time during the extraction process. This is continued till the complete extraction is achieved. This method of extraction is used when the material to be extracted has low partition coefficient for a pair of solvents.

16.1.3. Counter˘Current Extraction

If a sample contains two or more substances having distribution coefficients close to each other, then simple liquid-liquid extraction using separating funnels is not effective. Even after using a large number of separating funnels, complete extraction cannot be achieved under this condition. In order to achieve complete extraction of compounds from such a mixture, the extraction procedure is modified and made more effective.

In this modified method, two immiscible solvents are used to carry out a series of extractions in multiple tubes and one phase is allowed to pass to the next tube in the series, independently.

16.1.3.1. Principle of Counter-Current Extraction

At any time, the fraction of solute entering the upper phase (f_u) is given by **equation (16.5)**.

$$f_u = \frac{\text{Amount of solute in upper phase}}{\text{Total amount of solute}} \quad \cdots (16.5)$$

Similarly, the fraction of solute in the lower phase (f_l) is given by **equation (16.6)**.

$$f_l = \frac{\text{Amount of solute in lower phase}}{\text{Total amount of solute}} \quad \cdots (16.6)$$

$$f_u + f_l = 1 \ldots (16.7)$$

The amount of solute in the upper phase = C_uV_u,

The amount of solute in the lower phase = C_lV_l,

C_u = concentration of a solute in the upper layer,

C_l = concentration of a solute in the lower layer,

V_u = volume of the solvent forming the upper layer, and

V_l = volume of the solvent forming the lower layer

Substituting the values of amount of a solute in the upper and the lower layers in **equations (16.5)** and **(16.6)** respectively, **equations (16.8)** and **(16.9)** are obtained.

$$\therefore f_u = \frac{C_uV_u}{C_uV_u + C_lV_l} \quad \cdots (16.8)$$

$$\text{and} \quad f_l = \frac{C_lV_l}{C_uV_u + C_lV_l} \quad \cdots (16.9)$$

Dividing each term in **equations (16.8)** and **(16.9)** by C_lV_l, **equations (16.10) and (16.11)**, respectively, are obtained.

$$\therefore f_u = \frac{\frac{C_uV_u}{C_lV_l}}{\frac{C_uV_u}{C_lV_l} + \frac{C_lV_l}{C_lV_l}} \quad \cdots (16.10)$$

$$\text{and} \quad f_l = \frac{\frac{C_lV_l}{C_lV_l}}{\frac{C_uV_u}{C_lV_l} + \frac{C_lV_l}{C_lV_l}} \quad \cdots (16.11)$$

In **equations (16.10)** and (**16.11**),

$$\frac{C_u}{C_l} = K = \text{Partition coefficient}$$

Let $\frac{V_u}{V_l}$ be equal to R.

$$\therefore f_u = \frac{KR}{KR+1} \cdots (16.12)$$

and $$f_l = \frac{1}{KR+1} \cdots (16.13)$$

If the solvent forming an upper layer is an extracting solvent (non-aqueous) and the solvent forming the lower layer (an aqueous layer) contains a solute to be extracted, then for an effective separation, values of K and R, i.e. the partition coefficient of a solute and the ratio of the volume of an upper layer to the volume of the lower layer, should be more.

16.1.3.2. Instrumentation

In order to achieve multiple extraction simultaneously, a special apparatus is used. Craig apparatus performs multiple extraction of each phase, semi- automatically.

Construction

In Craig apparatus, a series of special type of separating tubes are connected in such a way that the outlet of one tube is the inlet of the next tube. As shown in **Fig. 16.7**, **Tube 1** is positioned in a slanting manner, whereas **Tube 2** is positioned vertically. The combination of these two tubes forms one unit. Craig apparatus consists of a number of such units. Each unit can be rotated about a pivot (P), separately.

Working

The slanted tube in each unit (**Tube 1**, **Tube 3** and so on) contains the heavier liquid (lower phase) and the vertical tube in each unit (**Tube 2**, **Tube 4** and so on) contains the lighter liquid (upper phase), which is the extracting liquid. The slanted tube in **Unit 1** contains heavier liquid along with the sample, from which the components are to be extracted.

When **Unit 1** is tilted *clockwise* by an angle of 45°, the lighter liquid from **Tube 2** enters **Tube 1**. **Unit 1** is rocked back and forth around the pivot (P) so as to allow the extraction of the sample from the heavier liquid into the lighter liquid. Shaking is continued till lighter liquid gets saturated with the sample. The two phases are then allowed to settle in **Tube 1**. Once the equilibrium is reached between the two phases, an assembly is rotated through 45°, *anticlockwise*. The lighter liquid in **Tube 1** now enters **Tube 2**. Some components, which have larger distribution coefficient, are extracted faster in the lighter liquid.

Unit 1 is then rotated *clockwise* through 90°. The lighter liquid, saturated with the components having high partition coefficient, is thus, transferred from **Tube 2** of **Unit 1** into **Tube 3** of **Unit 2**. **Tube 3** contains heavier liquid. **Unit 2** is rotated *clockwise* through 45° to mix more of lighter liquid into **Tube 3**. **Unit 2** is then rocked back and forth around pivot (P). The components extracted in the lighter liquid in **Unit 1** again get partitioned between the fresh heavier liquid in **Tube 3** and the fresh lighter liquid from **Tube 4**. This allows further separation of components in two liquids. The compounds having higher affinity for the lighter liquid, get concentrated in the lighter liquid present in vertical tubes of all the units, whereas compounds having high affinity for the heavier liquid get concentrated in the heavier liquid present in the slanted tubes of all units. The process is repeated till the separation of all the compounds in the mixture is achieved.

Consider that the sample in **Unit 1** contains two components X and Y. If the partition coefficient of X (K_X) is more than the partition coefficient of Y (K_Y), then X has more affinity for the upper phase, i.e. for a lighter liquid. Since the partition coefficient of Y (K_Y) is less than that of X (K_X), it has more affinity for the lower phase, i.e. for the heavier liquid. When $K_X > K_Y$, in the first few units (**Unit 1** and **Unit 2**), the component X gets saturated in all the vertical tubes, whereas the

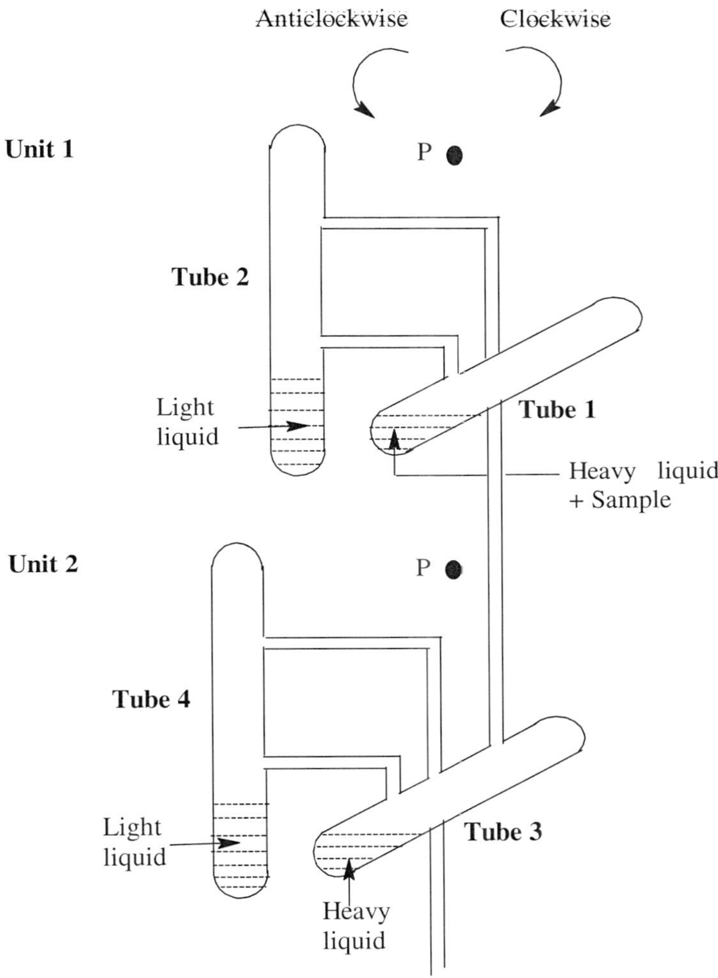

Fig. 16.7: Extraction using Craig apparatus

component Y gets saturated in all the slanted tubes. Thus, the last vertical tube contains pure X, whereas the last slanted tube contains pure Y.

The amount of compound present in each tube in each round of extraction can be calculated as follows.

Let us assume that –

1. There is only one compound to be extracted from the heavier liquid into the lighter liquid.
2. Quantity of this compound in a heavier liquid is 100 mg.
3. The partition coefficient of this compound is 1 (K =1), when equal volumes of the heavier and the lighter liquids are used.

Table 16.1 gives the amount of compound present in each tube in the first round of extraction using ten units. The heavier liquid containing 100 mg of the compound in **Tube 1**, when extracted by the lighter liquid in **Tube 2**, gets partitioned between two liquids. The lighter liquid containing 50 mg of the compound, when transferred to **Tube 3**, gets partitioned between the heavier and the lighter liquid. This process is continued in a number of units.

After the first round of extraction, **Tube 1** contains 50 mg of the compound in the heavier liquid. In the second round, this compound is further extracted. The compound gets partitioned between the heavier and the lighter liquid in the subsequent tubes, as shown in **Table 16.2**. This process is continued in a number of units. **Table 16.2** gives the amount of compound present in each tube in the second round of extraction using ten units.

Table 16.1: Amount of compound present in each tube in the first round of extraction

Unit No.	Tube No.	Amount of comd. (mg)
(100 mg of compound is present in Tube 1 before extraction procedure)		
1	1	50
	2	50
2	3	25
	4	25
3	5	12.5
	6	12.5
4	7	6.25
	8	6.25
5	9	3.125
	10	3.125
6	11	1.562
	12	1.562
7	13	0.781
	14	0.781
8	15	0.391
	16	0.391
9	17	0.195
	18	0.195
10	19	0.097
	20	0.097

Table 16.2: Amount of compound present in each tube in the second round of extraction

Unit No.	Tube No.	Amount of comd. (mg)
Second round of extraction (50 mg of compound is present in Tube 1 before second round of extraction) Fresh lighter liquid added to Tube 2		
1	1	25
	2	25
2	3	12.5
	4	12.5
3	5	6.25
	6	6.25
4	7	3.125
	8	3.125
5	9	1.562
	10	1.562
6	11	0.781
	12	0.781
7	13	0.391
	14	0.391
8	15	0.195
	16	0.195
9	17	0.097
	18	0.097
10	19	0.0487
	20	0.0487

At the beginning of the third round of extraction, **Tube 1** contains 25 mg of the compound in the heavier liquid, which gets partitioned between the heavier and the lighter liquid. The number of rounds of extraction are repeated till all the compound is extracted from the heavier liquid.

16.1.3.3. Applications of Counter-Current Extraction in Pharmaceutical Sciences

1. The counter-current extraction is used for the effective separation of compounds from each other, when the number of components to be separated is more and components possess partition coefficients closer to each other.
2. The separation is especially of importance when the presence of one compound affects the stability of another product in the mixture.
3. Crude plant extracts can be purified.
4. Samples extracted from the biological fluids can be characterized for the presence of drugs and their metabolites, after separating the components using counter-current extraction.

Thus, counter-current extraction provides an efficient method for the extraction of compounds with low partition coefficient.

CHAPTER 17

PROBLEMS ON SPECTROMETRY

PROBLEMS BASED ON BEER'S LAW

Example-1: $A_{1cm}^{1\%}$ for procaine hydrochloride at 290 nm is 680. An injection of procaine and adrenaline, when diluted by a factor of 2000, gave an absorbance of 0.68 when measured in 1 cm cell at 290 nm. Calculate the concentration of procaine hydrochloride in the injection.

Given:

$$A_{1\ cm}^{1\ \%} = 680$$

$$A = 0.68$$

Dilution factor = 2000

$$b = 1\ cm$$

Solution:

$$A = A_{1cm}^{1\%} .b .c$$

$$\therefore 0.68 = 680 \times 1 \times c$$

$$\therefore c = \frac{0.68}{680}$$

$$= 0.001\ g / 100\ mL$$

$$= 1\ mg / 100\ mL$$

This is the concentration of procaine hydrochloride when the injection is diluted 2000 times.
Therefore, concentration of procaine hydrochloride in its original injection is -
0.001 x 2000 = 2 g / 100 mL

= 2 % w/v

Example-2: The absorbance of a standard solution of caffeine at a concentration of 1 mg /100 mL, measured at 272 nm was 0.51 and a sample of caffeine showed an absorbance of 0.450 at 272 nm. Calculate the concentration of caffeine in the sample and its molar absorptivity. (Mol. wt. of caffeine = 212 and b = 1 cm)

Given:

$c_{std} = 1 \text{ mg} / 100 \text{ mL}$

$A_{std} = 0.51$

$A_{sample} = 0.450$

Mol. wt. of caffeine = 212

b = 1 cm

Solution:

$$A_{std} = \varepsilon.\ b.\ c_{std} \ldots (1)$$

$$A_{sample} = \varepsilon.\ b.\ c_{sample} \ldots (2)$$

$$\therefore \frac{A_{std}}{A_{sample}} = \frac{c_{std}}{c_{sample}} \ldots (3)$$

Conc. of standard = c_{std} = 1 mg / 100 mL

= 10 mg / 1000 mL

= 0.010 g /1000 mL

Mol. wt. of caffeine = 212 g

212 g of caffeine ≡ 1 mole of caffeine

0.010 g ≡ 0.000047 moles of caffeine

= 4.7×10^{-5} moles

$c_{std} = 4.7 \times 10^{-5}$ mol / L

Substituting values in **equation (3)**, we get -

$$\frac{0.51}{0.45} = \frac{4.7 \times 10^{-5}}{c_{sample}}$$

$$\therefore c_{sample} = 4.147 \times 10^{-5} \text{ mol / L}$$

To find molar absorptivity, consider either **equation (1)** or **equation (2)**.

Equation (1):

$A_{std} = \varepsilon \times b \times c_{std}$

$$0.51 = \varepsilon \times 1 \times 4.7 \times 10^{-5}$$

$$\varepsilon = \frac{0.51}{4.7 \times 10^{-5}}$$

$$= \frac{0.51 \times 10^{5}}{4.7}$$

$$= 0.1085 \times 10^{5}$$

$$= 10850 \text{ cm}^{-1} \text{ mol}^{-1}\text{L}$$

Equation (2):

$$A_{sample} = \boldsymbol{\varepsilon} \text{ b. c}_{.sample}$$

$$0.45 = \boldsymbol{\varepsilon} \times 1 \times 4.147 \times 10^{-5}$$

$$\varepsilon = \frac{0.45}{4.147 \times 10^{-5}}$$

$$= \frac{0.45 \times 10^{5}}{4.147}$$

$$= 0.10851 \times 10^{5}$$

$$= 10851 \text{ cm}^{-1} \text{ mol}^{-1} \text{ L}$$

Example-3: $A_{1cm}^{1\%}$ of a drug at its wavelength of maximum absorption is 700. One mL of an injection containing the drug, when diluted to 1 liter for analysis, gave an absorbance of 0.68 at the wavelength of maximum absorption, when measured in 1 cm cell. Calculate the amount of drug in the injection.

Given:

$$A_{1\text{ cm}}^{1\,\%} = 700$$

$$A = 0.68$$

$$b = 1 \text{ cm}$$

Dilution factor = 1000

Solution:

$$A = A_{1cm}^{1\%} \times b \times c$$

$$0.68 = 700 \times 1 \times c$$

$$\therefore c = \frac{0.68}{700}$$

$$\therefore c = 0.00097 \text{ g / 100 mL}$$

$$c = 0.97 \times 10^{-3} \text{ g /100 mL}$$

This is the concentration of the drug when the injection is diluted 1000 times. Therefore, the concentration of the drug in the original injection is -

$$c = 0.97 \times 10^{-3} \times 10^{3} \text{ g /100 mL}$$

$$= 0.97 \text{ g / 100 mL}$$

$$= 0.97 \%$$

Example-4: A cardiac drug of molecular weight 207 has a molar absorptivity of 703 at 262 nm. When a tablet of the drug is dissolved in water and the solution diluted to 2.5 liters, the resulting solution gave an absorbance of 0.52 at 262 nm in 1 cm cell. Calculate the amount of drug in the tablet.

Given:

Mol. wt. = 207

$\varepsilon = 703$

A= 0.52

b = 1 cm

Dilution factor = 2.5 L or 2500 mL

Solution:

$$A = \varepsilon \times b \times c$$

$$0.52 = 703 \times 1 \times c$$

$$\therefore c = \frac{0.52}{703}$$

$$= 0.00074 \text{ mol / L}$$

$$= 0.74 \times 10^{-3} \text{ mol / L}$$

This is the concentration of the drug when original solution is diluted to 2.5 liters.

Therefore, concentration of the drug in the original solution or amount of drug in a tablet is =

$$c = 0.74 \times 10^{-3} \times 2.5 \text{ mol / tablet}$$

$$= 0.00185 \text{ mol / tablet}$$

$$= 0.185 \times 10^{-2} \text{ mol / tablet}$$

$$1 \text{ mole of a drug} \equiv 207 \text{ g}$$

$$0.185 \times 10^{-2} \text{ moles} \equiv 0.185 \times 10^{-2} \times 207 \text{ g}$$

$\therefore$ 0.3829 g of drug is present in one tablet

Example-5: In the determination of acetone in blood, 6 mg /100 mL standard solution, when measured in 1 cm cell, showed an absorbance of 0.182. Calculate its molar absorptivity. What is the acetone concentration of a blood sample if the absorbance of the blood sample in 1 cm cell was found to be 0.423?

Given:

$$c_{std} = 6 \text{ mg /100 mL}$$

$$b = 1 \text{ cm}$$

$$A_{std} = 0.182$$

$$A_{sample} = 0.423$$

Solution:

(i) To find ε

For a standard acetone solution

$$A_{std} = \varepsilon \times b \times c_{std}$$

$$0.182 = \varepsilon \times 1 \times c_{std}$$

$$c_{std} = 6 \text{ mg /100 mL}$$

$$= 60 \text{ mg / 1000 mL}$$

$$= 0.060 \text{ g / 1000 mL}$$

Mol. wt. of acetone CH_3COCH_3 (C_3H_6O) = 36 + 6 +16= 58

58 g of acetone = 1 mole of acetone

$$0.060 \text{ g of acetone} \equiv 0.001 \text{ mol / L} = c_{std}$$

$$\therefore A_{std} = \varepsilon \times b \times c_{std}$$

$$0.182 = \varepsilon \times 1 \times 0.001$$

$$\varepsilon = \frac{0.182}{0.001}$$

$$\therefore \ \varepsilon = 0.182 \times 10^3 = 182 \ cm^{-1} \ mol^{-1} \ L$$

(ii) To find c_{sample}

$$A_{sample} = \varepsilon \times b \times c_{sample}$$

$$0.423 = 182 \times 1 \times c_{sample}$$

$$\therefore c_{Sample} = \frac{0.423}{182} \ mol/L$$

$$= 0.0023 \ mol / L$$

1 Mole of acetone = 58 g

0.0023 moles of acetone = 0.116 g / L

= 11.6 mg / 100 mL

Example-6: $A_{1cm}^{1\%}$ of a drug with molecular weight 375 is found to be 250. What will be its molar absorbance? What should be the concentration of the drug that will show an absorbance of 0.472 in 1 cm cell?

Given:

$$A_{1cm}^{1\%} = 250$$

Mol. wt. = 375

A = 0.472 and b = 1 cm

Solution:

(i) To find Molar absorbance (ε):

$A_{1cm}^{1\%}$ of a drug is 250. That means a solution of 1 % concentration, i.e.1 g / 100 mL concentration, would show absorbance of 250 in 1 cm cell. Hence -

$$A = A_{1cm}^{1\%} \times b \times c = 250$$

To find å, the concentration in mol / L should be found out.

Since, 1 g of a drug is present in 100 mL, 10 g of a drug should be present in 1000 mL of its solution.

375 g of drug ≡ 1mole of a drug

10 g of drug ≡ 0.0266 moles

$$\therefore c = 0.0266 \ mol / L$$

$$A = \varepsilon \times b \times c$$

$$\therefore 250 = \varepsilon \times 1 \times 0.0266$$

$$\therefore \varepsilon = \frac{250}{0.0266}$$

$$\therefore \varepsilon = 9398 \text{ cm}^{-1} \text{ mol}^{-1} \text{ L}$$

(ii) To find concentration

$$A = \varepsilon \text{ x } b \text{ x } c$$

$$\therefore 0.472 = 9398 \text{ x } 1 \text{ x } c$$

$$\therefore c = \frac{0.472}{9398} \text{ mol / L}$$

$$\therefore c = 5.02 \text{ x } 10^{-5} \text{ mol / L of a drug}$$

Example-7: Calculate the absorptivity of a compound with molecular weight of 144, if 1 x 10^{-5} g / mL solution exhibits an absorbance of 0.400 when optical path is unity.

Given:

Mol. wt. = 144

A = 0.400

c = 1 x 10^{-5} g / mL

Solution :

To find molar absorptivity (ε):

$$c = 1 \text{ x } 10^{-5} \text{ g / mL}$$

$$\text{or } 10^{-5} \text{ x } 10^{3} \text{ g / L} = 10^{-2} \text{ g / L}$$

$$144 \text{ g of a drug} = 1 \text{ mole}$$

$$10^{-2} \text{ g} = 10^{-2} / 144 \text{ moles}$$

$$= 0.0000694 \text{ moles}$$

$$\therefore c = 0.694 \text{ x } 10^{-4} \text{ mol / L}$$

$$A = \varepsilon \text{ x } b \text{ x } c$$

$$\therefore 0.400 = \varepsilon \text{ x } 1 \text{ x } 0.694 \text{ x } 10^{-4}$$

$$\varepsilon = \frac{0.400}{0.694 \text{ x } 10^{-4}}$$

$$\therefore \varepsilon = 0.5763 \text{ x } 10^{4} = 5763 \text{ cm}^{-1} \text{ mol}^{-1} \text{ L}$$

Example-8: Convert absorbance of 0.523 to percent transmittance and convert 75 % transmittance to absorbance.

Solution:

$$\text{Absorbance} = -\log_{10} T$$

$$\therefore \text{Absorbance} = \log_{10}\left(\frac{1}{T}\right)$$

$$A = \log_{10}\left(\frac{100}{T \times 100}\right)$$

$$A = \log_{10}\left(\frac{100}{\% T}\right)$$

$$A = \log_{10}(100) - \log_{10}(\% T)$$

(i) Conversion of absorbance to transmittance

$$A = \log_{10}(100) - \log_{10}(\% T)$$

$$\therefore 0.523 = \log_{10}(100) - \log_{10}(\% T)$$

$$\therefore \log_{10}(\% T) = 2.000 - 0.523$$

$$= 1.477$$

$$\therefore \% T = \text{Antilog}(1.477)$$

$$= 29.99$$

(ii) Conversion of % transmittance to absorbance

$$A = \log_{10}(100) - \log_{10}(\% T)$$

$$A = \log_{10}(100) - \log_{10}(75)$$

$$\therefore A = 2.000 - 1.875$$

$$\therefore A = 0.1249$$

Examples for practice

Example-1: A solution of a drug, when diluted by a factor of 2500, gave an absorbance of 0.45 when measured in 1 cm cell at 320 nm. $A_{1cm}^{1\%}$ for the drug at 320 nm is 450. Calculate the concentration of the drug in the solution.

Answer: 2.5 % w/v

Example-2: A standard drug with molecular weight 157 was dissolved in a solvent so as to produce the concentration of 4 mg /100 mL. The solution showed an absorbance of 0.65, when measured in 1 cm cell at 254 nm. A sample of the same drug showed an absorbance of 0.52 at 254 nm. Calculate the concentration of the drug in the sample and its molar absorptivity.

Answer: $c_{sample} = 2.037 \times 10^{-4}$ mol /L

$\varepsilon = 2552\ cm^{-1}\ mol^{-1}L$

Example-3: Convert absorbance of 0.45 to percent transmittance and convert 65 % transmittance to absorbance.

Answer: % T = 35.48 and A = 0.187

PROBLEMS BASED ON FIESER AND WOODWARD RULES

Fieser and Woodward have formulated an empirical method to predict the absorption characteristics of organic compounds. In this method, the base value of absorption is set for certain skeletons of molecules from different classes. Similarly, certain values are also assigned to the absorption by various functional groups, such as alkyl groups, double bonds and other substituents. Calculation of absorption maxima of compounds from different classes is illustrated below.

Some of the observations in case of compounds containing ethylenic chromophore are as follows.

1) An isolated ethylenic chromophore shows intense absorption due to π to π transition.
2) The alkyl substitution or an attachment of a hetero-atom (nitrogen or a sulphur atom), bearing a non bonding electron pair, to the ethylenic linkage, shifts the absorption peak towards a longer wavelength or brings about a *bathochromic shift*.
3) The absorption characteristics of cycloalkenes are equivalent to that of acyclic compounds. Thus, absorption characteristics of cyclohexene are equivalent to that of hexene. The absorption of cycloalkenes is independent of their ring size.
4) In acyclic conjugated dienes, 1, 3–butadiene is considered to be a parent compound, whose base value for absorption maximum is taken as 217nm.

$$H_2{}^1C = {}^2CH - {}^3CH = {}^4CH_2$$

1, 3–Butadiene

5) If a compound exists in the form of cis and trans isomers, the trans isomer absorbs at a longer wavelength and with greater intensity. The cis form absorbs at a shorter wavelength and with lesser intensity.

The common terms used while calculating the wavelength of maximum absorption (λ_{max}) of compounds are given below.

1) Homoannular and heteroannular systems

Cyclic dienes can be either *homoannular* or *heteroannular* in nature. Both the systems contain two double bonds, which are necessarily conjugated. In a homoannular system, two double bonds are in the same ring, whereas in a heteroannular system, two double bonds are in two separate rings, which are fused to each other.

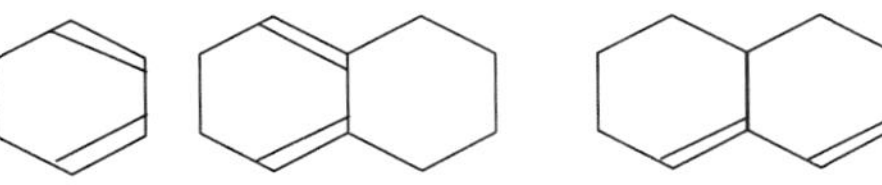

Homoannular systems | Heteroannular system

Base value = 253 | **Base value = 214**

The base value for a homoannular system is 253 nm, whereas for a heteroannular system, it is 214 nm.

2) Ring residue

The term *ring residue* refers to the part of the ring present as a substituent on the atoms in a ring in a particular system. In the following structure, the sides of the rings, shown by thick lines at C_1 and C_3 are the ring residues for 1,3-butadiene system, whereas the thick lines at C_4 indicate the substituents.

3) An exocyclic double bond

An *exocyclic* double bond is a double bond which is present outside the ring but is directly attached to it. The examples of compounds possessing an exocyclic double bond are given below. An exocyclic double bond can be a part of another ring as shown in compound (b). Double bond in ring A in structure (b) is exocyclic to ring B. Double bond in structure (c) is exocyclic to both the rings.

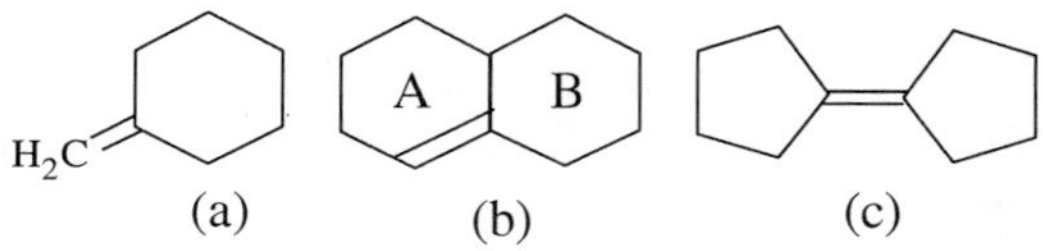

(a) (b) (c)

I- RULES FOR PREDICTING ABSORPTION MAXIMA IN COMPOUNDS CONTAINING 1,3–BUTADIENE SYSTEM

The rules for predicting the bathochromic shift in 1, 3-butadienes are based mainly on the work carried out by Fieser and Woodward. These rules are summarized below.

1.	Base value for1, 3–butadiene system	217
	Increments for -	
(i)	Each alkyl group or ring residue	+ 5
(ii)	One exocyclic double bond	+ 5
(iii)	Double bond exocyclic to two rings = (5 x 2)	+ 10
(iv)	Homoannular unit	+ 39

Calculation of λ_{max} value for compounds possessing 1,3-butadiene system

1) Example-1: Find λ_{max} for compound 1

Compound 1

The structure of **compound 1** fits in the system of 1,3-butadiene. It has one exocyclic double bond at C_3. Similarly, two thick lines on C_4 represent two substituents in this system. Two thick lines at C_1 and C_3 represent two ring residues. Hence, its λ_{max} value can be calculated as follows.

> **Note:** A bond between C_2 and C_3 is not considered as a residue, since it is a part of 1,3-butadiene skeleton. Thick lines at positions 1 and 3 are considered as ring residues since they do not form a part of skeleton of 1, 3–butadiene system.

1.	Base value for1, 3–butadiene system	217
2.	One exocyclic double bond	+ 5
3.	Two substituents at C_4 = (2 x 5)	+ 10
4.	One ring residue each at C_1 and C_3 = (2 x 5)	+ 10
	Hence, the predicted λ_{max} for **compound 1** is	**242**

2) Example 2: Find λ_{max} for compound 2

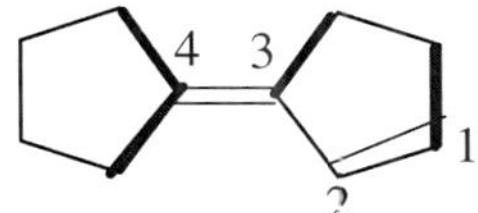

Compound 2

The structure of **compound 2** fits in the system of 1,3-butadiene. It has one double bond between C_3 and C_4, which is exocyclic to both the rings. Two thick lines on C_4 and one thick line, each on C_1 and C_3, represent four ring residues. Hence, its λ_{max} value can be calculated as follows.

1.	Base value for1, 3–butadiene system	217
2.	One double bond exocyclic to two rings = (2 x 5)	+ 10
3.	Two ring residues at C_4 = (2 x 5)	+ 10
4.	One ring residue each at C_1 and C_3 = (2 x 5)	+ 10
	Hence, the predicted λ_{max} for **compound 2** is	**247**

3) Example 3: Find λ_{max} for compound 3

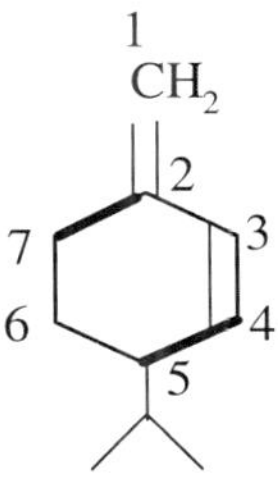

Compound 3

The structure of **compound 3** fits in the system of 1,3-butadiene. It has one double bond at C_2, which is exocyclic to the ring. One thick line, each at C_2 and C_4, represents two ring residues. Hence, its λ_{max} value can be calculated as follows.

1.	Base value for1, 3–butadiene system	217
2.	One exocyclic double bond at C_2	+ 5
3.	One ring residue each at C_2 and C_4 = (2 x 5)	+ 10
	Hence, the predicted λ_{max} for **compound 3** is	**232**
	The observed λ_{max} for **compound 3** is	**231**

4) Example-4: Find λ_{max} for compound 4

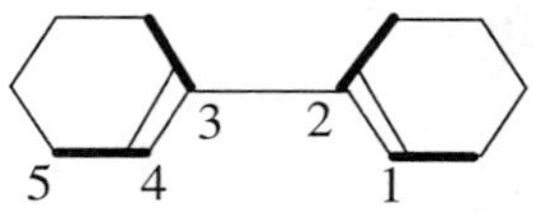

3 2

5 4 1

Compound 4

The structure of **compound 4** fits in the system of 1,3-butadiene. It has no exocyclic double bond. Four thick lines at C_1, C_2, C_3 and C_4, represent four ring residues. Hence, its λ_{max} value can be calculated as follows.

1.	Base value for1, 3–butadiene system	217
2.	One ring residue each at C_1, C_2, C_3 and C_4 = (4 x 5)	+ 20
3.	Hence, the predicted λ_{max} for **compound 4** is	**237**
	The observed λ_{max} for **compound 4** is	**236**

II - RULES FOR PREDICTING ABSORPTION MAXIMA IN COMPOUNDS CONTAINING HOMOANNULAR AND HETEROANNULAR SYSTEMS

The prediction for the position of absorption by homoannular and heteroannular systems is based mainly on the work by Fieser. These rules are as given below.

1.	Base value for heteroannular diene system	214
2.	Base value for homoannular diene system	253
	Increments for -	
(i)	Each alkyl group or ring residue	+ 5
(ii)	One exocyclic double bond	+ 5
(iii)	Double bond exocyclic to two rings (5 x 2)	+ 10
(iv)	Double bond extending conjugation	+ 30
(v)	Polar groups	
	a) O – Alkyl	+ 6
	b) S – Alkyl	+ 30
	c) N – $(Alkyl)_2$	+ 60
	d) Cl or Br	+ 5
	e) OAc	+ 0

Calculation of λ_{max} value for compounds containing homoannular and heteroannular systems

5) Example-5: Find λ_{max} for compound 5

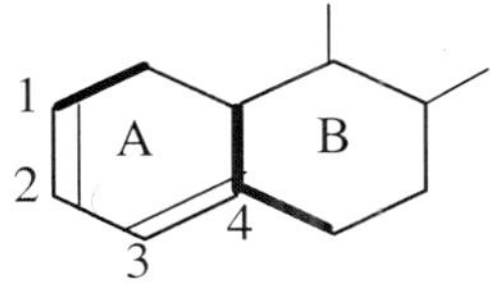

Compound 5

In **compound 5**, both the double bonds are in the same ring (A) and hence, it is an example of a homoannular system. Out of the two double bonds, a double bond between C_3 and C_4 is outside the ring B and is directly attached to it. Hence, this double bond is an exocyclic double bond. Two thick lines at C_4 and one thick line at C_1 represent three ring residues. Hence, its λ_{max} value can be calculated as follows.

1.	Base value for homoannular system	253
2.	Three ring residues at C_1 and C_4= (3 x 5)	+ 15
3	One exocyclic double bond	+ 5
	Hence, the predicted λ_{max} for **compound 5** is	**273**
	The observed λ_{max} for **compound 5** is	**275**

6) Example-6: Find λ_{max} for compound 6

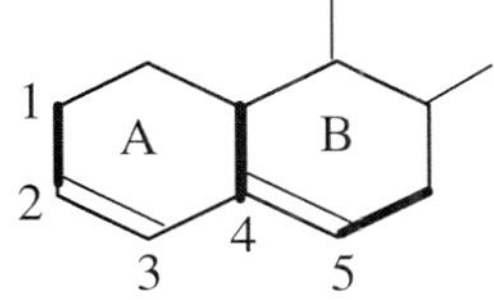

Compound 6

In **compound 6**, two conjugated double bonds are in two separate rings, which are fused with each other and hence, it is an example of a heteroannular system. Out of the two double bonds, a double bond between C_4 and C_5 is outside the ring A and is directly attached to it. Hence, this double bond is an exocyclic double bond. Three thick lines on C_2, C_4, and C_5 represent three ring residues. Hence, its λ_{max} value can be calculated as follows.

1.	Base value for heteroannular system	214
2.	Three ring residues at C_2, C_4 and C_5 = (3 x 5)	+ 15
3.	One exocyclic double bond	+ 5
	Hence, the predicted λ_{max} for **compound 6** is	**234**
	The observed λ_{max} for **compound 6** is	**235**

7) Example-7: Find λ_{max} for compound 7

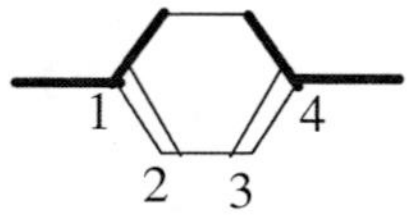

1 4
2 3

Compound 7

In **compound 7**, two double bonds are present at C_1 and C_3. Similarly, both the double bonds are present in the same ring. Hence, it is an example of a 1,3-butadiene system as well as a homoannular ring system. In both the cases, two thick lines at C_1 and C_4, which are part of the ring structure, represent two ring residues. Two thick lines at C_1 and C_4, which are outside the ring, and not the part of the ring structure, represent two substituents. Hence, its λ_{max} value can be calculated as follows.

A - Calculation of λ_{max} based on 1, 3-butadiene system

1.	Base value for 1, 3-butadiene system	217
2.	Two ring residues at C_1 and C_4 = (2 x 5)	+ 10
3.	Two substituents at C_1 and C_4 = (2 x 5)	+ 10
4.	Presence of a homoannular unit	+ 39
	Hence, the predicted λ_{max} for **compound 7** is	**276**
	The observed λ_{max} for **compound 7** is	**265**

B - Calculation of λ_{max} based on a homoannular system

1.	Base value for homoannular system	253
2.	Two ring residues at C_1 and C_4 = (2 x 5)	+ 10
3.	Two substituents at C_1 and C_4 = (2 x 5)	+ 10
	Hence, the predicted λ_{max} for **compound 7** is	**273**
	The observed λ_{max} for **compound 7** is	**265**

8) Example-8: Find λ_{max} for compound 8

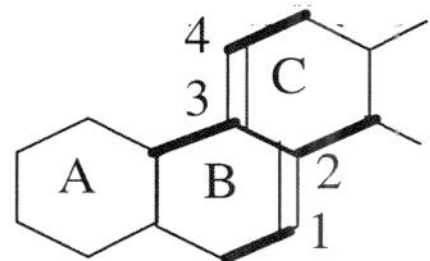

Compound 8

In **compound 8**, two conjugated double bonds are in two separate rings B and C, which are fused with each other and hence, it is an example of a heteroannular system. Out of the two double bonds, a double bond between C_1 and C_2 is outside the ring C and is directly attached to it. Hence, this double bond is an exocyclic double bond. Similarly, a double bond between C_3 and C_4 is outside the ring B and is directly attached to it. Hence, this double bond is also an exocyclic double bond. Four thick lines on C_1, C_2, C_3 and C_4 represent four ring residues. Hence, its λ_{max} value can be calculated as follows.

1.	Base value for heteroannular system	214
2.	Four ring residues at C_2, C_3, C_4 and C_5 = (4 x 5)	+ 20
3	Two exocyclic double bonds = (2 x 5)	+ 10
	Hence, the predicted λ_{max} for **compound 8** is	**244**
	The observed λ_{max} for **compound 8** is	**245**

9) Example-9: Find λ_{max} for compound 9

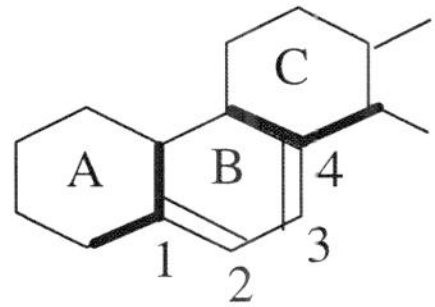

Compound 9

In **compound 9**, two conjugated double bonds are in the same ring B. Hence, it is an example of a homoannular system. Out of the two double bonds, a double bond between C_1 and C_2 is outside the ring A and is directly attached to it. Hence, this double bond is an exocyclic double bond. Similarly, a double bond between C_3 and C_4 is outside the ring C and is directly attached to it. Hence, this double bond is also an exocyclic double bond. Two thick lines, each on C_1 and C_4, represent four ring residues. Hence, its λ_{max} value can be calculated as follows.

1.	Base value for homoannular system	253
2.	Four ring residues at C_1 and C_4 = (4 x 5)	+ 20
3.	Two exocyclic double bonds = (2 x 5)	+ 10
	Hence, the predicted λ_{max} for **compound 9** is	**283**
	The observed λ_{max} for **compound 9** is	**282**

III-RULES FOR PREDICTING ABSORPTION MAXIMA IN COMPOUNDS CONTAINING EXTENDED CONJUGATION

1) For each double bond in conjugation with a homoannular and a heteroannular system, an addition of 30 nm is to be done to the base value.
2) Ring residues or substituents on all the carbon atoms involved in conjugation are to be considered.
3) For each ring residue or a substituent, an addition of 5 nm is to be done.
4) For each homoannular system, addition of 39 nm is to be done to the base value.

Calculation of λ_{max} value for compounds containing homoannular and heteroannular systems with extended conjugation (i.e. more than two double bonds in conjugation)

10) Example-10: Find λ_{max} for compound 10

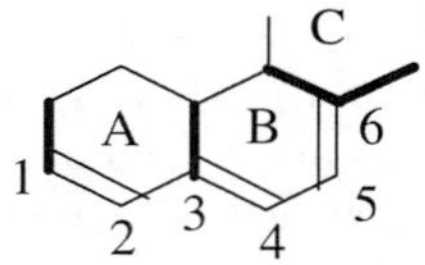

Compound 10

In **compound 10**, two conjugated double bonds between C_3 and C_4 and between C_5 and C_6 are in the same ring B. Hence, it is an example of a homoannular system. Also, two conjugated double bonds between C_1 and C_2 and C_3 and C_4 are present in two different rings A and B. Hence, it is an example of a heteroannular system as well. The value of wavelength of maximum absorption (λ_{max}) for this compound can therefore be calculated based on both the homoannular as well as heteroannular systems. The compound has three double bonds in conjugation and hence, a double bond between C_1 and C_2 is considered as an extended double bond for a homoannular system and a double bond between C_5 and C_6 is considered as an extended double bond for a heteroannular system. A double bond between C_3 and C_4 is outside the ring A and is directly attached to it. Hence, it is an exocyclic double bond. Four thick lines on C_1, C_3 and C_6 represent four ring residues. Hence, its λ_{max} value can be calculated as follows.

A- Calculation of λ_{max} for compound 10 based on homoannular system

1.	Base value for homoannular system	253
2.	Four ring residues at C_1, C_3 and C_6 = (4 x 5)	+ 20
3.	One exocyclic double bond	+ 5
4.	One extended double bond	+ 30
	Hence, the predicted λ_{max} for **compound 10** is	**308**

B- Calculation of λ_{max} for compound 10 based on heteroannular system

1.	Base value for heteroannular system	214
2.	Four ring residues at C_1, C_3 and C_6 =(4 x 5)	+ 20
3.	One exocyclic double bond	+ 5
4.	One extended double bond	+ 30
5.	Homoannular system	+39
	Hence, the predicted λ_{max} for **compound 10** is	**308**

IV - RULES FOR PREDICTING ABSORPTION MAXIMA IN α, β— UNSATURATED KETONES

RULES FOR ENONE AND DIENONE ABSORPTION

$$\underset{\beta}{-C}=\underset{\alpha}{C}-C=O$$

Enone

$$\underset{\delta}{-C}=\underset{\gamma}{C}-\underset{\beta}{C}=\underset{\alpha}{C}-C=O$$

Dienone

Base values for different α, β–unsaturated systems		
1.	Acyclic α, β–unsaturated ketones	215
2.	Six member cyclic α, β–unsaturated ketones	215
3.	Five member cyclic α, β–unsaturated ketones	202
4.	α, β–Unsaturated aldehydes	210
5.	α, β–Unsaturated carboxylic acids and esters	195
	Increments to be added	
(i)	Double bond extending conjugation	+ 30
(ii)	Alkyl group, Ring residue	
	a) - α	+ 10
	b) - β	+ 12
	c) - γ and higher	+ 18
(iii)	Polar Groupings	
(A)	- OH	
	a) - α	+ 35
	b) - β	+ 30
	c) - δ	+ 50
(B)	- OAC	
	a) α, β and δ	+ 6
(C)	- OMe	
	a) - α	+ 35
	b) - β	+ 30
	c) - γ	+ 17
	d) - δ	+ 31
(D)	- S-Alk	
	a) - β	+ 85
(E)	- Cl	
	a) - α	+ 15
	b) - β	+ 12
(F)	- Br	
	a) - α	+ 25
	b) - β	+ 30
(G)	- $N.R_2$	
	a) - β	+ 95
(iv)	Exocyclic double bond	+ 5
(v)	Homoannular system	+ 39

Calculation of λ_{max} value for compounds having α, β—unsaturated system

11) Example-11: Find λ_{max} for compound 11

Compound 11

1.	Base value for α, β–unsaturated ketone	215
2.	One α ring residue	+ 10
3.	One β ring residue	+ 12
	Hence, the predicted λ_{max} for **compound 11** is	**237**
	Observed λ_{max} for **compound 11** is	**232**

12) Example-12: Find λ_{max} for compound 12

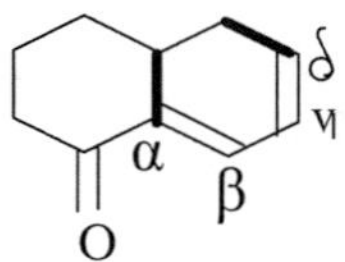

Compound 12

1.	Base value for α, β–unsaturated ketone	215
2.	One α ring residue	+ 10
3.	One δ ring residue	+ 18
4.	One exocyclic double bond (α, β)	+ 5
5.	One extended double bond	+ 30
6.	Homoannular unit	+ 39
	Hence, the predicted λ_{max} for **compound 12** is	**317**

13) Example-13: Find λ_{max} for compound 13

Compound 13

Note: This is **not** an example of extended conjugation, since conjugation should extend in the same direction in order to add up 30 units corresponding to an additional double bond. This is an example of *cross-conjugation*, which has little effect on the λ_{max} of a compound.

1.	Base value for α, β–unsaturated ketone	215
2.	Two β ring residues = (2 x 12)	+ 24
3.	Exocyclic double bond between C_4 and C_5	+ 5
	Hence, the predicted λ_{max} for **compound 13** is	**244**
	Observed λ_{max} for **compound 13** is	**245**

Instead of a double bond between C_4 and C_5, if a double bond between C_1 and C_2 is considered as α, β unsaturation, then there is only one β ring residue (i.e. at C_1) and hence, for this system, the λ_{max} is 215 + 12 = 227. Thus, a better match between the observed and calculated λ_{max} is obtained by considering a highly substituted unit.

14) Example-14: Find λ_{max} for compound 14

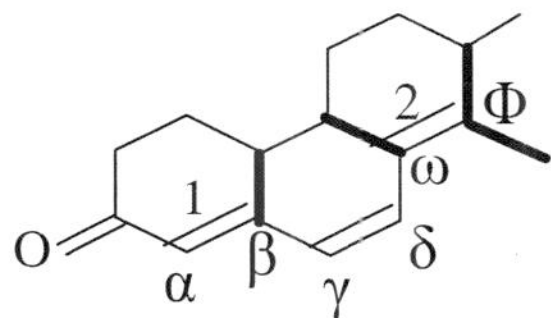

Compound 14

A - Calculation based on Dienone system

1.	Base value for dienone	245
2.	One β– substituent	+ 12
3.	One ω and two Φ substituents = (3 x 18)	+ 54
4.	Two exocyclic double bonds, 1 and 2 = (2 x 5)	+ 10
5.	One extended double bond	+30
	Hence, the predicted λ_{max} for **compound 14** is	**351**

B - Calculation based on Enone system

1.	Base value for enone	215
2.	One β– substituent	+ 12
3.	One ω and two Φ substituents = (3 x 18)	+ 54
4.	Two exocyclic double bonds, 1 and 2 = (2 x 5)	+ 10
5.	Two extended double bonds = (2 x 30)	+ 60
	Hence, the predicted λ_{max} for **compound 14** is	**351**

15) Example-15: Find λ_{max} for compound 15

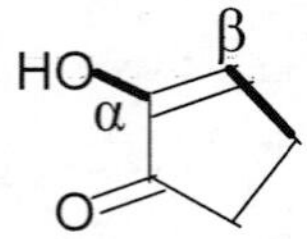

Compound 15

1.	Base value for 5-membered cyclic alpha, beta unsaturated ketone	202
2.	One β– substituent	+ 12
3.	One α-hydroxy substituent	+ 35
	Hence, the predicted λ_{max} for **compound 15** is	**249**
	Observed λ_{max} for **compound 15** is	**247**

Examples for practice

Base values for different compounds

Sr. No.	Compound	Base value
1	1, 3–Butadiene	217
2	Heteroannular system	214
3	Homoannular system	253
4	Acyclic α, β–unsaturated ketone	215
5	6-membered cyclic α, β–unsaturated ketone	215
6	5-membered cyclic α, β–unsaturated ketone	202
7	α, β–unsaturated aldehydes	210
8	α, β–unsaturated carboxylic acids and esters	195

Find λ_{max} values for the following compounds.

1) (Answer: λ_{max} = 313)

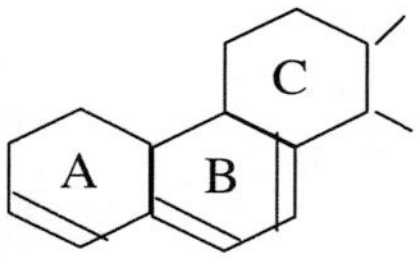

2) (Answer: λ_{max} = 348)

3) (Answer: λ_{max} = 259)

4) (Answer: λ_{max} = 254)

5) (Answer: λ_{max} = 280)

6) (Answer: λ_{max} = 317)

7) (Answer: λ_{max} =262)

PROBLEMS ON INFRARED SPECTROMETRY

Tips for solving problems on IR spectrometry

For solving problems on IR spectrometry, it is essential to know the approximate range of frequencies or wave numbers for certain stretching and bending vibrations corresponding to different functional groups in a molecule. Various *correlation charts*, which correlate wave numbers with these vibrations, are available in the literature.

It should be noted that the structures of compounds cannot be confirmed only from the information of IR spectral data. Information on the NMR and the mass spectra of compounds helps to confirm their proper structures. The IR spectral data helps in predicting the presence or absence of certain functional groups in a molecule.

Wave number ($\bar{\nu}$) is the reciprocal of wavelength (λ) and the frequency (ν) is the ratio of the velocity of light (c) to wavelength (λ).

$$\bar{\nu} = \frac{1}{\lambda} \text{ and}$$

$$\nu = \frac{c}{\lambda}$$

where, c is constant and is equal to 3 x10^{10} cm/sec. Hence, sometimes, wave numbers are often called as frequencies, which is not correct practically.

Table 17.1 gives approximate range of frequencies for different vibrations. From the combination of wave numbers at which the peaks are obtained, the presence of certain functional groups in the molecule can be confirmed.

Table 17.1: Approximate range of wave numbers for certain stretching and bending vibrations corresponding to different functional groups

Sr. No.	Functional group	Type of vibration	Wave number (cm^{-1})	Compounds
1	Hydroxy (-OH)	O - H str*	3650 - 3500	Alcohols, acids, phenols
2	Thiol (-SH) .	S - H str	2600	Mercapto group
3	NH_2 group **(Two peaks in stretching region)**	(i) N - H str Symmetric & Asymmetric str (ii) N - H ben⁺	3500 - 3450 & 3450 -3320 1680 - 1620	Primary amines, Amino acids, Primaryamides
4	N-H group **(Only one peak in stretching region)**	(i) N - H str (ii) N - H ben⁺	3450 - 3320 1680 - 1620	Secondary amines, Secondary amides

5	C – H	(i) C – H str (ii) C – H ben	3000 - 2850 1000 -650	Hydrocarbons, aliphatic compounds & all compounds containing C & H
6	≡ C - H (Acetylenic C-H bond)	C – H str	3300	Alkynes
7	C ≡ N	C ≡ N str	2300 - 2200	Nitriles or cyano compounds
8	C ≡ C	C ≡ C str	2250 - 2100	Alkynes
9	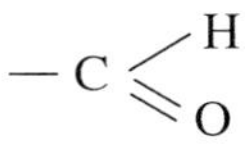 $-C\langle^{H}_{O}$	(i) C – H str (ii) C = O str	2700 1650	Aldehydes
10	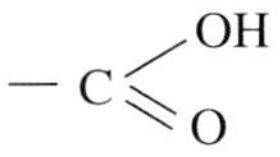 $-C\langle^{OH}_{O}$	(i) O–H str (broad band) (ii) C = O str (iii) O –H ben (iv) Carboxylate anion str 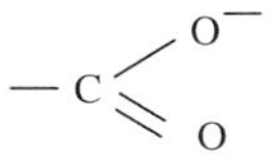 $-C\langle^{O^-}_{O}$	3550 1700 1450 -1400 1300-1200	Carboxylic acids
11	S -H	S – H str	2400	Thiols
12	C = O	(i) C = O str	1820 – 1780 1800 – 1760 1800 – 1740 1740 - 1660 1660 - 1640	Acid anhydrides Acid chlorides Esters Carboxylic acids Aldehydes, Ketones & amides
13	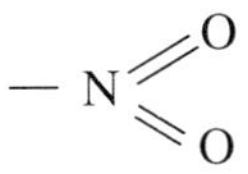 $-N\langle^{O}_{O}$ (**Produces two peaks**)	(i) O=N=O str Symmetrical and Asymmetrical str	1500 & 1300	Nitro compounds

14	$=S(=O)=O$ (Produces two peaks)	(i) O=S=O str Symmetrical and Asymmetrical str	1300 & 1100	Sulfones, sulfonamides
15	C = C **(Two to Four bands in aromatic compounds)**	C = C str	1600, 1550, 1500 & 1450	Aromatic compounds
16	C = C	C = C str	1640 - 1580	Olefins
17	Finger print region		1450 - 980	Used for confirmation of identity of two compounds

str* = Stretching, ben⁺ = Bending

Solved problems on IR spectrometry

1) Example-1:

A compound having molecular formula C_4H_7N produces following peaks in its IR spectrum. Assign the frequencies to the appropriate vibrations and deduce the probable structure. (Cm^{-1}): 2234 and 2947

Solution:

Cm^{-1}	Functional group	Inference
2234	$C\equiv N$ or $C\equiv C$ str	Since nitrogen is present in the structure, nitrile group may be present
2947	C – H str	

Since there are no peaks in the region of 1600 – 1400, this compound is not aromatic in nature. Hence, the probable structure for an aliphatic compound, which fits into the given molecular formula and the IR data, can be as follows.

$$CH_3 — CH_2 — CH_2 — C \equiv N$$

2) Example-2:

A compound having molecular formula C_4H_6 produces following peaks in its IR spectrum. Assign the frequencies to appropriate vibrations and deduce the probable structure. (Cm^{-1}): 3312 and 2867

Solution:

Cm^{-1}	Functional group	Inference
3312	$\equiv C - H$ str	Alkyne may be present
2867	C – H str	

Since there are no peaks in the region of 1600 – 1400, the compound is not aromatic in nature. Hence, the probable structure for an aliphatic compound, which fits into the given molecular formula and the IR data, can be as follows.

$$H - C \equiv C - CH_2 - CH_3$$

Note: 1) The formula C_nH_{2n+2} corresponds to a saturated compound.

2) The formula C_nH_{2n} corresponds to an unsaturated compound, alkene (Presence of a double bond).

3) The formula $C_nH_{(2n-2)}$ corresponds to an unsaturated compound, alkyne (Presence of a triple bond).

3) Example-3:

A compound having molecular formula C_8H_9ON produces following peaks in its IR spectrum. Assign the frequencies to appropriate vibrations and deduce the probable structure.

(Cm^{-1}): 3395, 3010, 1655, 1632, 1587, 1467and1420

Solution:

Cm^{-1}	Functional group	Inference
3395	N - H str	Secondary amine or secondary amide may be present
3010	C – H str	
1655	C = O str or N –H ben	Aldehyde, ketone or an amide may be present. Secondary amine or secondary amide may be present
1632	C = O str or N –H ben	Aldehyde, ketone or an amide may be present. Secondary amine or secondary amide may be present
1587, 1467 and1420	C = C str	Aromatic compound

From the above information, a structure which fits in the given molecular formula may be either (I) or (II).

$NHCOCH_3$ (benzene ring) (I) OR $CONHCH_3$ (benzene ring) (II)

Though the following structures (III), (IV) and (V) fit into the same molecular formula, the given spectral data doesn't match with their structures. Since two peaks (around 3450 – 3320 cm^{-1}) are not obtained corresponding to the primary amino group (-NH_2) in the IR spectrum, the primary amino or primary amido group is not present in the structure. Therefore, structures (III) and (IV) are ruled out. Similarly, structure (V) is an aldehyde. The characteristic peak for C-H stretching in aldehyde (around 2700 cm^{-1}) is not recorded in the IR spectrum. Hence, the compound should be a secondary amide.

$CONH_2$ / CH_3 (o-, m- or p-) (III)

$COCH_3$ / NH_2 (o-, m- or p-) (IV)

CHO / $NHCH_3$ (o-, m- or p-) (V)

4) Example-4:

A compound having molecular formula $C_7H_7O_2N$ produces following peaks in its IR spectrum. Assign the frequencies to appropriate vibrations and deduce the probable structure.

(Cm^{-1}): 3520 (b=broad), 3462, 3395, 2980, 1705, 1640, 1602, 1587, 1435 and1208

Solution:

Cm^{-1}	Functional group	Inference
3520 (b)	O –H str	Alcohols or acids or phenols may be present
3462 and 3395	N - H str	Primary amine or primary amide may be present
2980	C – H str	
1705	C = O str	Esters or acids may be present
1640	N –H ben	Primary amine or primary amide may be present
1602, 1587, 1435	C = C str	Aromatic compound
1208	Carboxylate anion stretching	Carboxylic group may be present

Hence, the probable structure of the compound may be as follows.

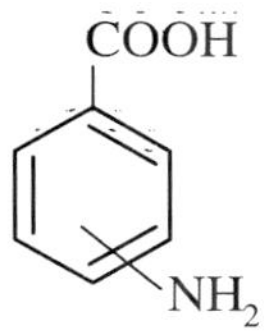

COOH

NH$_2$

(o-, m- or p-)

5) Example-5:

A compound having molecular formula $C_7H_5O_3N$ produces following peaks in its IR spectrum. Assign the frequencies to appropriate vibrations and deduce its possible structure.

(Cm^{-1}): 2980, 2712, 1650, 1609, 1555, 1410 and 1335

Solution:

Cm^{-1}	Functional group	Inference
2980	C – H str	
2712	C – H str	Aldehyde may be present
1650	C = O str	Aldehyde or ketone or amide may be present
1609 and 1410	C = C str	Aromatic compound
1555 and 1335	N = O str (symmetric and asymmetric str)	Nitro group may be present

Hence, the probable structure of the compound may be as follows.

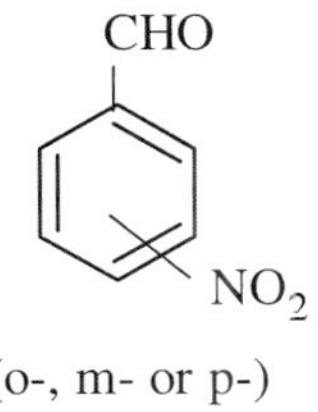

CHO

NO$_2$

(o-, m- or p-)

6) Example-6:

Assign the approximate range of frequencies to the vibrations corresponding to the functional groups in the following structure.

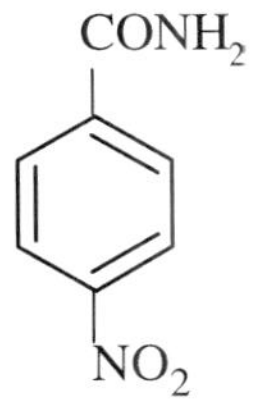

CONH$_2$

NO$_2$

Solution:

Functional group	Cm^{-1}
N– H str	3450 and 3350
C = O str (amide)	1660 - 1640
C – H str	3000
N = O str	1500 and 1300
C = C str (Ar)	1600, 1550, 1500 and 1450

7) Example-7: Differentiate between the following pairs of compounds from their IR spectra.

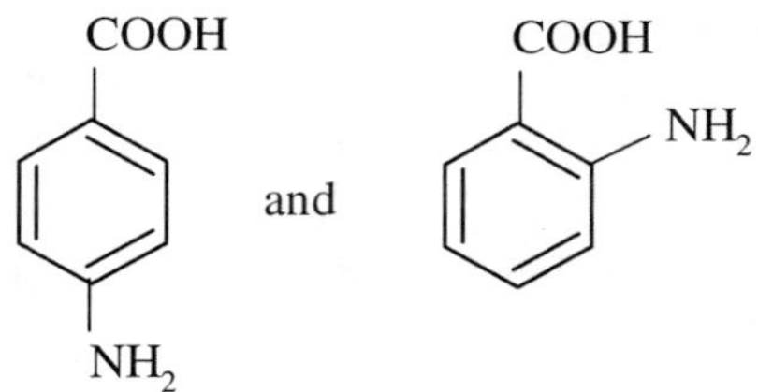

p-Aminobenzoic acid o-Aminobenzoic acid

Solution:

As shown below, o-aminobenzoic acid involves *intra-molecular* hydrogen bonding, and hence, it is not affected by dilution of solution. Bands for N –H stretching and for O –H stretching are shifted towards lower wave numbers in the presence of hydrogen bonding, since hydrogen bonding reduces the vibrational frequency of a bond. In case of p-aminobenzoic acid, *intermolecular* hydrogen bonding is involved. Hence, the peaks for N –H stretching and for O – H stretching are recorded at lower wave numbers as compared to the peaks obtained when there is no hydrogen bonding. As solution is diluted, intermolecular hydrogen bonding is reduced in case of p- aminobenzoic acid. Hence, the position of peaks for O –H and N –H stretching shifts towards left or towards higher wave numbers. Thus, the o- and p- isomers can be distinguished by recording their IR spectra at different dilutions.

o- Aminobenzoic acid
Intra-molecular hydrogen bonding

p- Aminobenzoic acid
Intermolecular hydrogen bonding

Fig. 17.4: Hydrogen bonding in aminoacids

Problems for practice:

Example-1:

Assign the approximate range of frequencies to the vibrations corresponding to the functional groups in the following structures in their IR spectra.

Note: For answers to this question, refer to **Table 17.1**

1)

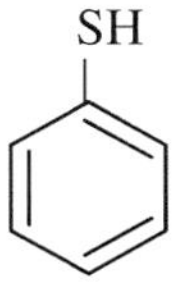

SH

2)

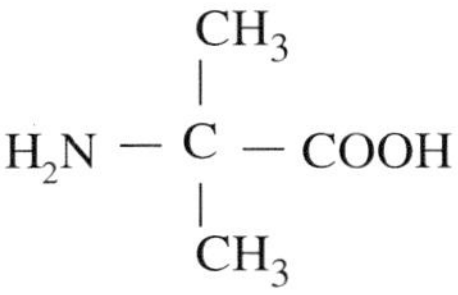

CH_3

$H_2N - C - COOH$

CH_3

3)

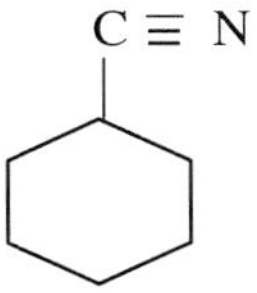

$C \equiv N$

4)

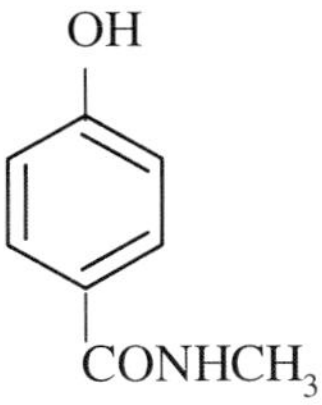

OH

$CONHCH_3$

Example-2:

Differentiate between the following pairs of compounds based on their IR spectra.

(a)

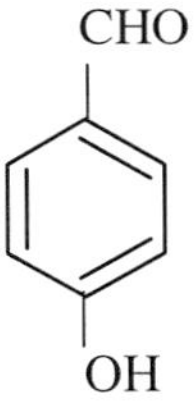

CHO

OH

and

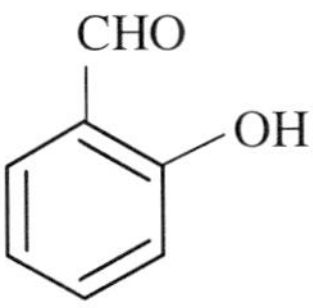

CHO

OH

(b) $COCH_3$ / C_6H_4 / OH (para) and $COCH_3$ / C_6H_4 / OH (ortho)

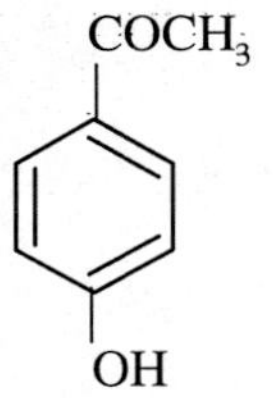

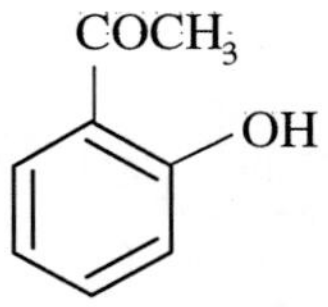

(c) COOH / C_6H_4 / OH (para) and COOH / C_6H_4 / OH (ortho)

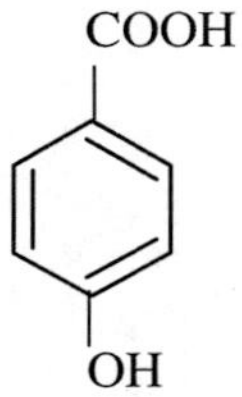

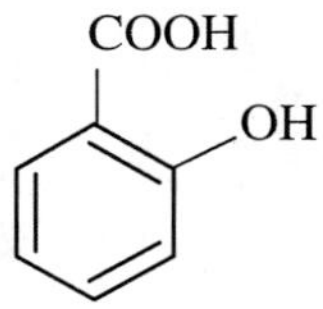

(d) CHO / C_6H_4 / SH (para) and CHO / C_6H_4 / SH (ortho)

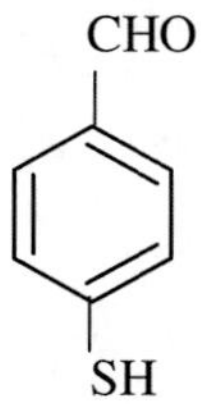

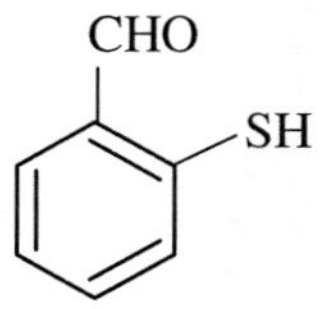

PROBLEMS ON ^{1}H-NMR SPECTROMETRY

For solving problems on NMR spectrometry, the following chemical shift values (approximate values in δ ppm) can be made use of.

Table 17.2: Approximate chemical shift values for different protons

		Type of proton	**Chemical shift of proton in δ ppm**	**Average δ ppm**	
I	1.	$CH_3 - C_{Saturated}$	0.7 -1.3	0.9	Difference of 0.4 & 0.8 in 1 & 2 & 1 & 3, respectively.
	2.	$CH_2 - C_{Saturated}$	1.25 – 1.35	1.3	
	3.	$CH - C_{Saturated}$	1.6 – 1.9	1.7	
II	4.	$CH_3 - C$		0.9	
	5.	$CH_3 - N$		2.5	
	6.	$CH_3 - O$	3.3 – 4.0	3.3	Difference of 0.4 & 0.6 in 6 & 7 & 6 & 8, respectively.
	7.	$CH_2 - O$		3.7	
	8.	$CH - O$		3.9	
III	9.	$CH_3 - Cl$		3.7	
	10.	$CH_3 - Br$		3.5	
	11.	$CH_3 - I$		3.3	
IV	12.	$CH_3 - Br$		2.6	
	13.	$CH_2 Br_2$		4.9	
	14.	$CH Br_3$		6.8	

V	15.	$CH_3 - C = C$	1.6 – 1.9	1.6
	16.	$CH_3 - C = O$	1.9 – 2.6	2.0
	17.	$CH_3 -$ Ph	2.1 – 2.5	2.4
	18.	$CH_3 - O -$ Ph		3.8
	19.	$CH_3 - O - C(=O) - R$		3.8

VI	20.	H - C - C (with bonds above and below C)		1.7
	21.	H – C = C	4.6 -6.4	5.5
	22.	H – C = O		9.7
	23.	$H - C \equiv C$		3.0
	24.	H -Ph		7.3

VII	25.	Aromatic protons in benzene ring	6.0 – 9.5	
VIII		Peak for CH_3 in following structures		
	26.	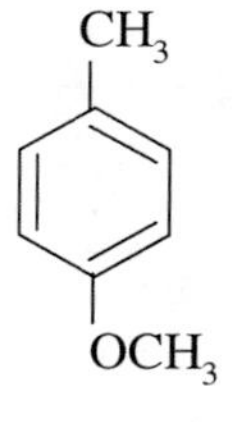 CH_3 – benzene ring – OCH_3 (para)		2.25
	27.	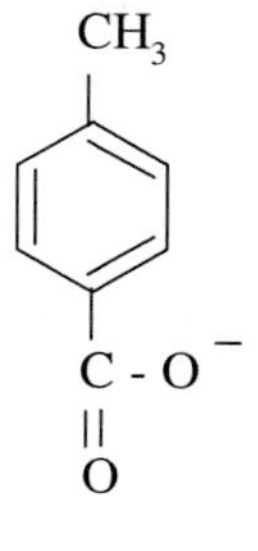 CH_3 – benzene ring – $C(=O)-O^-$ (para)	2.34 – 2.35	2.3

28.	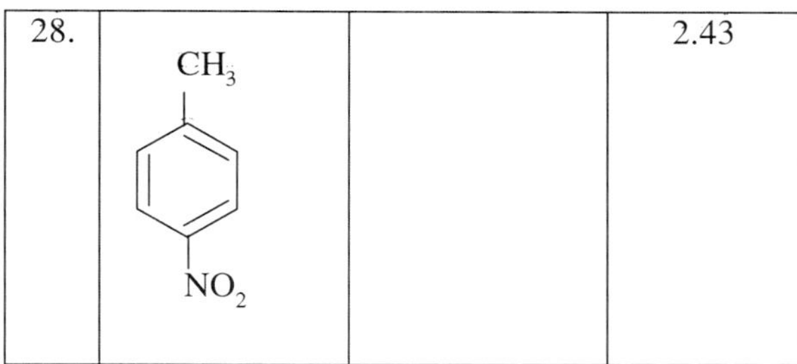		2.43

Tips for solving problems on NMR spectrometry

1. Fluorine atom and phosphorous atom

Fluorine atom and phosphorous atom, like a proton, have I = 1/2 and therefore, they couple with the neighboring protons. Rules for coupling are same in both the cases.

2. Protons on the nitrogen atom

Protons on the nitrogen atom are easily exchangeable.

(a) If the exchange is rapid, NH peak is a sharp singlet and the adjacent C-H protons are not split by the N-H proton. This is observed in case of aliphatic amines.

(b) If the rate of exchange of protons is intermediate, NH peak is a broad singlet. In this case also, the adjacent protons are not split by the NH proton.

(c) When the exchange is very slow, NH peak is broad. In this case, coupling of the NH proton with the adjacent protons is observed. Spin quantum number of nitrogen is 1 (Refer to **Table 4.1** under NMR spectrometry). Hence, proton attached to nitrogen atom experiences (2I + 1) =3 spin states of nitrogen nucleus. This is observed in case of pyrroles, indoles, primary and secondary amides and carbamates.

3. Protons on the oxygen atom

Proton on the oxygen atom is easily exchangeable. Hence, OH peak is a sharp singlet and the adjacent C-H protons are not split by O-H proton. Spin quantum number of oxygen is zero (Refer to **Table 4.1** under NMR spectrometry). Hence, proton attached to oxygen atom experiences (2I + 1) =1 spin state of oxygen nucleus. It can also take part in the intermolecular and intramolecular hydrogen bonding. Thus, because of the exchangeability, O-H proton usually appears as a singlet and it does not couple with the adjacent C-H proton.

Because of hydrogen bonding, the chemical shift of the hydroxyl proton depends on the factors like concentration, temperature and solvent. Hydrogen bonding decreases the electron density around proton and moves proton absorption to lower field, i.e. the peak is shifted downfield. Intermolecular hydrogen bonding is decreased by dilution with a non-polar solvent and with increased temperature. The weakening of hydrogen bonding causes upfield shift of protons. Intra-molecular hydrogen bonding is less affected by their environment.

The rate of exchange of O-H proton in alcohols is decreased by adding anhydrous sodium carbonate, alumina, or molecular sieves. Use of purified deuterated DMSO or acetone also lowers rate of exchange. Under these conditions, the multiplicity of O-H protons and the C-H protons adjacent to O-H protons, can be seen.

Phenolic O-H protons usually produce a sharp singlet because of rapid exchange and hence, do not couple with adjacent protons.

4. Sulfhydryl protons

Sulfhydryl protons (S-H) usually exchange at low rate so that at room temperature, they are coupled to protons on the adjacent carbon atoms. However, the exchange is rapid enough with hydroxyl, carboxylic, enolic protons or with deuterium.

5. Anisotropic Effect

While assigning the chemical shift values to different protons, the following two factors, which influence chemical shift of protons, must be considered.

I- Electron density around a proton, and

II- Anisotropic effect

The first factor is already discussed in detail in chapter 4. The second factor is an anisotropic effect. The term *isotropy* means symmetry. The property of being isotropic means having the same value of a physical property (absorbance, refractive index, density, etc.) when measured in different directions. The term *anisotropy* is exactly opposite to isotropy. The property of being anisotropic means having different values of a physical property when measured in different directions.

Anisotropic effect in NMR spectrometry (different magnitude of magnetic field in different directions) is observed in the following systems.

(i) System containing double bond (alkene)

(ii) System containing triple bond (alkyne)

(iii) System containing benzene ring or aromatic protons

(i) System containing double bond (alkenes)

In **Fig. 17.1**, a molecule of ethylene having one double bond, is placed in the external magnetic field of strength B_o in such a way that a double bond is at right angles to the applied field. Under the influence of an external magnetic field, the ð electrons circulate about the bond so as to produce the induced magnetic field. This induced magnetic field *reinforces* the applied field at the protons. Hence, the protons absorb at lower field and are *deshielded* due to anisotropy. Therefore, the alkenic protons, which are attached to sp^2 hybridized carbon atom, are more deshielded compared to the protons attached to sp^3 hybridized carbon atom and are recorded downfield in the range of 4.5-7.5 ä The more shielded protons in sp^3 hybridized system are recorded upfield in the range of 0.8- 1.5 ä

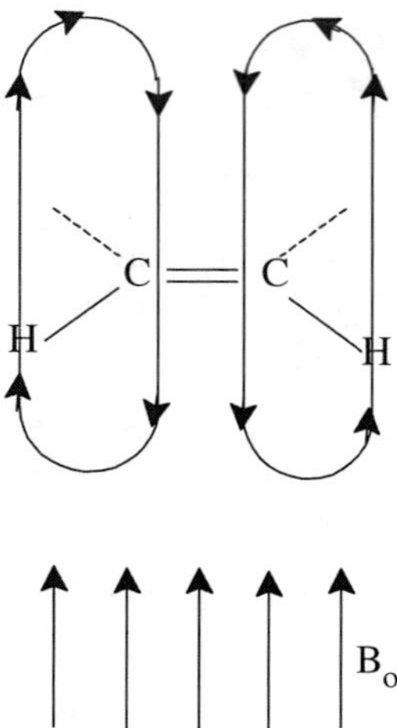

Fig. 17.1: Anisotropic effect in ethylene

(ii) System containing triple bond (alkyne)

In **Fig. 17.2**, a molecule of acetylene having one triple bond, is placed in the external magnetic field of strength B_o in such a way that a triple bond is parallel to the applied field. Under the influence of an external magnetic field, the π electrons circulate about the bond so as to produce the induced magnetic field. At the protons, this induced magnetic field is in the direction opposite to the direction of the applied magnetic field, as shown in **Fig. 17.2**. Hence, the protons absorb at higher field and are *shielded* due to anisotropy. Therefore, the alkynic protons, which are attached to sp hybridized carbon atom, resonate upfield of alkenic protons. Thus, the protons of acetylene resonate at 2.6 δ.

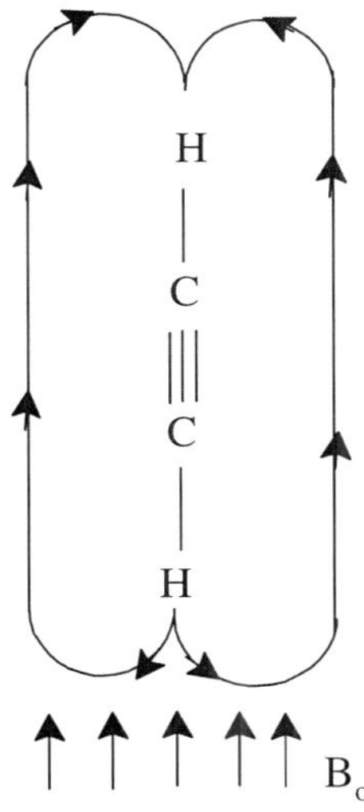

Fig. 17.2: Anisotropic effect in actylene

(iii) System containing benzene ring or aromatic protons

Figure 17.3 shows direction of the induced magnetic field in benzene ring, when placed in the external magnetic field. The π electrons circulate in such a way that the peripheral protons, which are in the plane of the ring, experience the *reinforcement* of the induced magnetic field with the external magnetic field. Hence, these

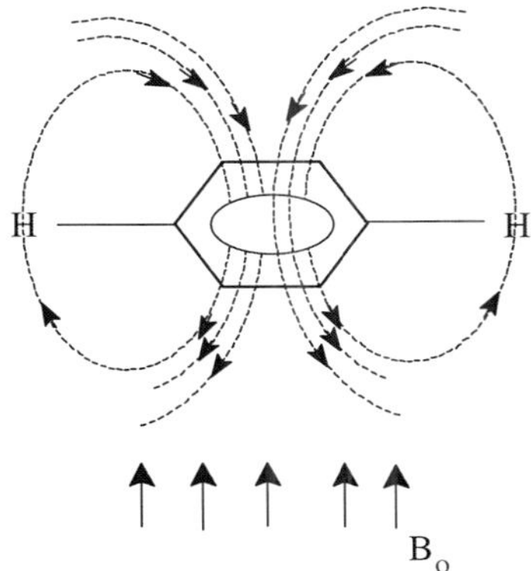

Fig. 17.3: Anisotropic effect in benzene

protons are *deshielded* and resonate at low field with $\delta = 6\text{-}8$. The protons above and below the plane of an aromatic ring are shielded and are recorded upfield.

1) Example-1: Show diagrammatically, the splitting pattern for H_X and H_A protons in the following molecule. (J_{AX} =7 Hz).

$$H_A - \overset{H_A}{\underset{H_A}{C}} - \overset{H_X}{\underset{H_X}{C}} - O - R$$

Solution:

(i) Splitting pattern for H_X: (Production of a quartet for H_X)

In the above molecule, two H_X protons are chemically equivalent. They do not couple with each other. They couple with three neighboring H_A protons. Hence, the multiplicity of two H_X protons is (3 + 1) = 4, i.e. two H_X protons produce a *quartet* in the NMR spectrum. The formation of a quartet is shown below.

As shown in **Fig. 17.4**, in the absence of any coupling, both the H_X protons produce a single peak (*singlet*) in the spectrum, as indicated by a single line in the diagram below. Coupling with the first H_A proton splits the peak for H_X into two, thereby producing a *doublet*, in which the intensity of both the peaks is same (1:1). Coupling with the second H_A proton splits both the peaks of a doublet into two each, thereby producing four peaks, two of which coincide. Thus, it results in a *triplet*, in which the intensity of three peaks is in the ratio of (1: 2: 1). Coupling with the third H_A proton splits all the three peaks of a triplet into two each, thereby producing six peaks, but again, because of overlapping of the peaks, instead of six peaks, only four peaks (*quartet*) are seen in the NMR spectrum, in which the intensity of the peaks is in the ratio of (1: 3: 3:1).

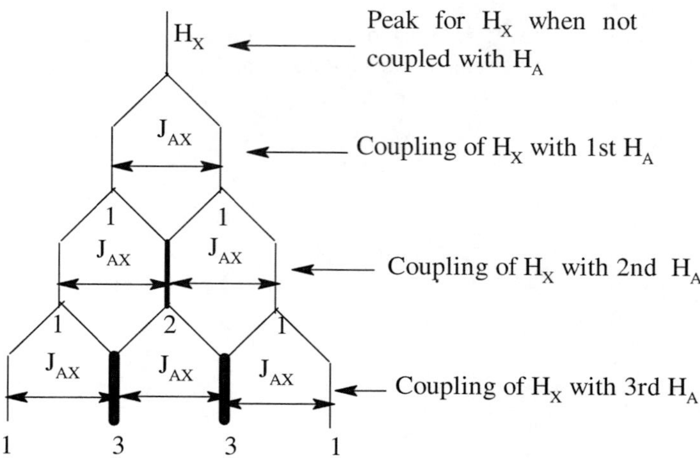

Fig. 17.4: A quartet for H_X protons

(ii) Splitting pattern for H_A: (Production of a triplet for H_A)

In the above molecule, three H_A protons are chemically equivalent. They do not couple with each other. They couple with the two neighboring H_X protons. Hence, the multiplicity of three H_A protons is $(2 + 1) = 3$, i.e. three H_A protons produce *triplet* in the NMR spectrum. The formation of a triplet is explained diagrammatically in **Fig. 17.5**.

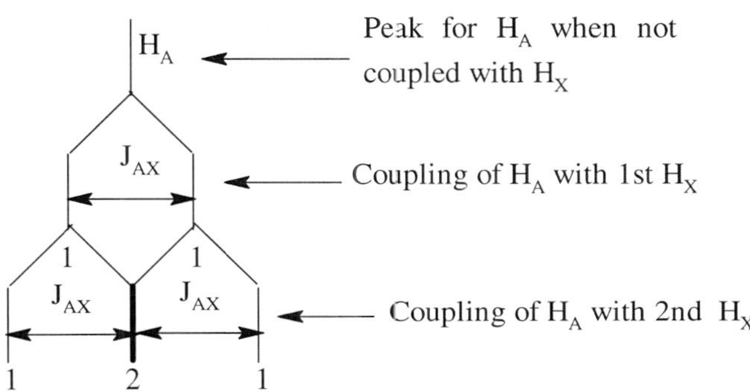

Fig. 17.5: A triplet for H_A protons

2) Example-2: Show diagrammatically, the stepwise splitting pattern for H_A, H_M and H_X protons in the following molecule. (J_{AM} =10 Hz and J_{MX} =5 Hz).

H_A H_M H_X
— C — C — C —

Solution:

(i) Splitting pattern for H_X: (Production of a doublet for H_X)

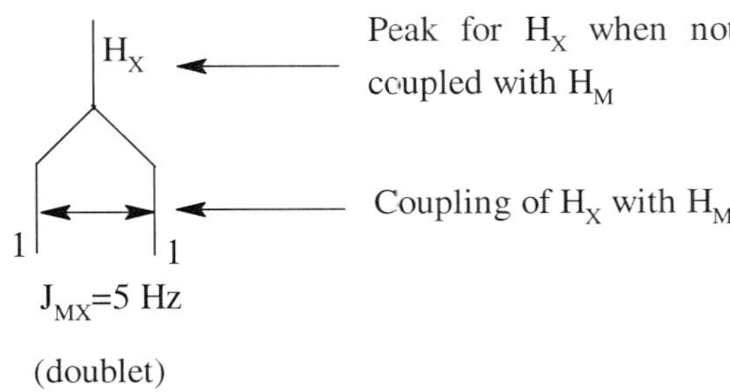

(ii) Splitting pattern for H_A: (Production of a doublet for H_A)

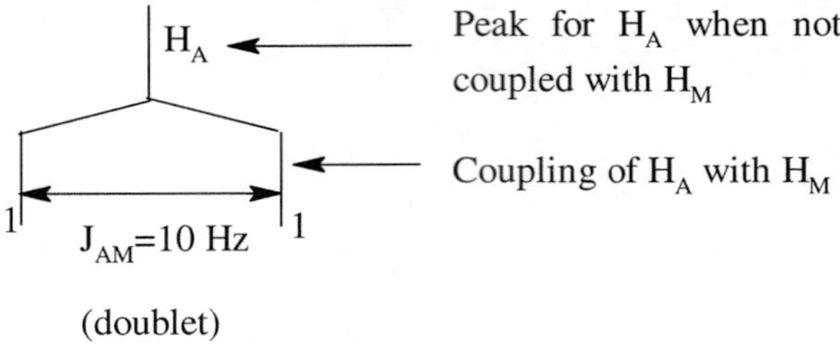

(iii) Splitting pattern for H_M: (Production of a doublet of a doublet for H_M)

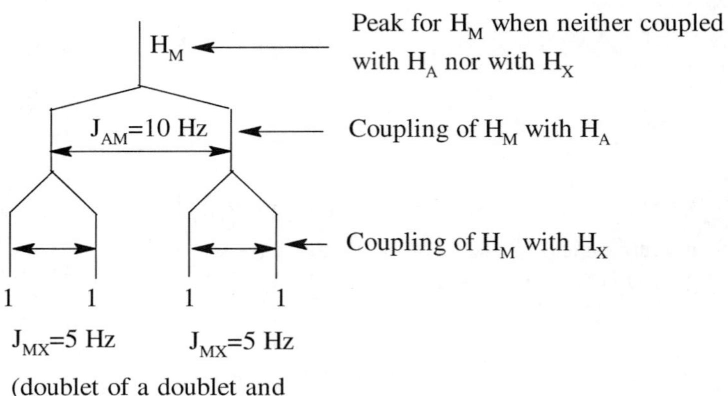

OR

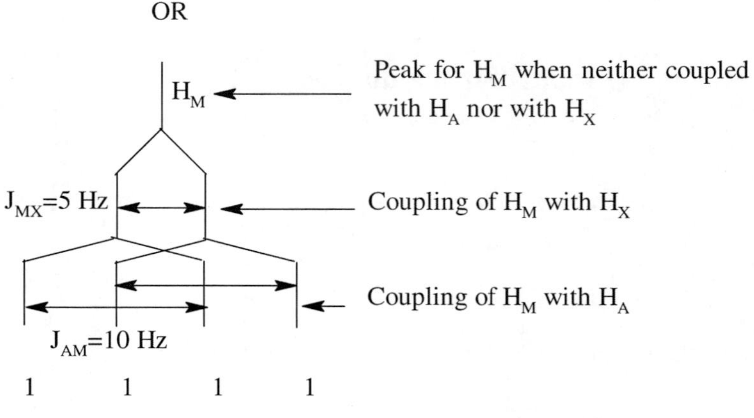

3) Example-3: Assign the chemical shift values (in δ ppm) and the multiplicity to the protons in the following molecule.

$$\overset{A}{H_3C} - O - \overset{B}{CH_2} - \overset{D}{CH_3}$$

Solution:

(i) Protons A: CH_3, **δ** ≈ 3.3 (s, 3H)

Since there are no protons adjacent to these protons, this CH_3 group is recorded as a singlet (s). In the bracket, 3H indicates the integration corresponding to 3 protons in a singlet in the spectrum for these protons.

(ii) Protons B: CH_2, **δ** ≈ 3.7 (q, 2H)

Since there are three protons adjacent to these protons, this CH_2 group is recorded as a quartet (q) (3 + 1) = 4. In the bracket, 2H indicates the presence of 2 protons in a quartet in the spectrum for these protons.

(iii) Protons D: CH_3, **δ** ≈ 1.1 (t, 3H)

Since there are two protons adjacent to these protons, this CH_3 group is recorded as a triplet (t) (2 + 1)= 3. In the bracket, 3H indicates the presence of 3 protons in a quartet in the spectrum for these protons.

Since spins of protons B and protons D influence each other, the coupling constant (J) for these protons should be same and it is in the range of 5 – 8 Hz.

4) Example-4: Assign the chemical shift values (in δ ppm) and the multiplicity to the protons in the following molecule.

E: H_2C — B: CH_2
| |
D: H_2C — O — A: CH_2

Here, protons A and D are chemically equivalent. Hence, they appear at the same chemical shift value in the spectrum. Similarly, protons B and E are chemically equivalent. Hence, they also appear at the same chemical shift value in the spectrum, but the chemical shift for protons A and D is different from the chemical shift for protons B and E. Since protons A and D are near oxygen atom, they are less shielded and absorb at lower magnetic field, or their peak is downfield as compared to the peak for protons B and E.

(i) For protons A and D: δ ≈ 3.7 (t, 4H)

Since, both the protons A and D have two protons each on the adjacent carbon atom (protons B and E, respectively), they appear as a triplet (2+1) = 3. Since this triplet is for 4 protons, the integration of this triplet corresponds to 4 protons. Protons A interact with protons B. and protons D interact with protons E. Therefore, the J value (J_{AB} and J_{DE}) for these protons should be same and it is in the range of 5 – 8 Hz.

(ii) For protons B and E: δ ≈ 1.5 (t, 4H)

Protons B and E are chemically equivalent. Hence, they do not interact or couple with each other. They couple only with protons A and D, respectively. Hence, they also appear as triplet (2+1) corresponding to 4 protons. These protons are away from the electronegative oxygen atom. Hence, they are more shielded. Therefore, they absorb at higher magnetic field and appear upfield to the protons A and D.

5) Example-5: Assign the chemical shift values (in δ ppm) and the multiplicity to the protons in the following molecule.

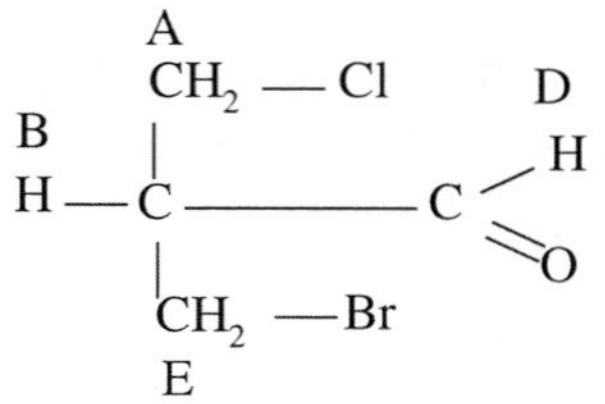

A
CH_2 — Cl D
B H
H — C ———— C = O
CH_2 — Br
E

(i) Protons A and E

In chloromethyl group, CH_2 is attached to the more electronegative chlorine atom and in bromomethyl group, CH_2 is attached to the less electronegative bromine atom. Hence, protons A appear downfield to protons E. Since both the protons A and E have one neighboring proton B, both the methylene protons A and E appear as a doublet corresponding to two protons. Protons A and E interact with proton B. Therefore, their J values (J_{AB} and J_{EB}) are same.

For protons A, $\delta \approx 4.7$ (d, 2H)

For protons E, $\delta \approx 4.5$ (d, 2H)

(ii) Proton B

Proton B is surrounded by 2 protons on either side (protons A and E). It also has one aldehydic proton (proton D) on the adjacent carbon atom. Hence, the number of expected peaks for proton B is 18, as shown below and thus, it results in a multiplet (m) in the spectrum.

$$(2 + 1)\ (2 + 1)\ (1 + 1) = 18$$

For selecting ä value for proton B, compare it with δ value for $CH_3 - C = O$, which is 2. Add 0.8 to it for replacing CH_3 with CH, i.e. $HC - C = O$. This would be more downfield.

Hence, for proton B, $\delta \approx 2.8$ (m, 1H)

(iii) Proton D

Proton D is an aldehydic proton. Because of the presence of an electronegative oxygen atom, the electrons are dragged away from D. Also, because of the presence of a double bond, delocalization of electrons is easy. Hence, the electron density around aldehydic proton is reduced considerably and hence, it is less shielded. Thus, it absorbs at low field and appears much downfield in the spectrum. Because of the neighboring proton B, the aldehydic proton appears as (1+1) = 2, i.e. as a doublet.

Therefore, for proton D, $\delta \approx 9.7$ (d, 1H)

6) Example-6: Assign the chemical shift values (in δ ppm) and the multiplicity to the protons in the following molecule.

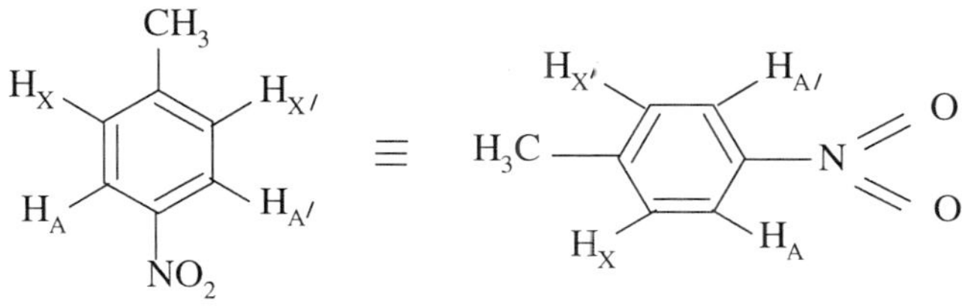

Note: In para substituted aromatic compounds, *meta* and *para* couplings occur. In this case, only *ortho* coupling is considered.

The system containing two different substituents *para* to each other is an example of AA'XX′ system. The spectra of AA'XX′ are always found when a molecule contains two pairs of protons such that the protons within each pair can be imagined to exchange positions by rotation about an axis of symmetry or by reflection at a plane of symmetry.

In the above structure, phenyl ring is attached to a nitro group which is electron withdrawing. This electron withdrawing group withdraws electrons away from methyl protons as well as away from the benzene ring. Hence, all the protons are deshielded or less shielded as compared to when a nitro group is not present on the ring.

(a) Methyl protons

For protons in the methyl group attached to a phenyl ring bearing a nitro group, $\delta \approx 2.4$ (Refer to **Table 17.2**). Because of an electron withdrawing group attached to the benzene ring, δ value for methyl protons is more downfield. Since there is no proton on the adjacent carbon atom, it produces a singlet corresponding to 3 protons. Therefore, for a methyl group, $\delta \approx 2.4$ (s, 3H)

(b) Protons H_A and H_A'

Protons H_A and H_A' are chemically equivalent but magnetically non-equivalent. Hence, each proton gets recorded as a doublet of 1 proton integration. Proton H_A couples with proton H_X and proton H_A' couples with proton H_X'. Most of the times, because of very small difference in the chemical shift of protons H_A and H_A', and because of almost the same values of J_{AX} and $J_{A'X'}$, protons H_A and H_A', get recorded as a doublet corresponding to 2 protons at the same chemical shift value. These two protons are nearer to the electron withdrawing group as compared to the protons H_X and H_X'. Hence, protons H_A and H_A' are more downfield.

(For para substituted compounds, J_{AX} and $J_{A'X'}$ are same, approximately equal to 7-10 Hz).

Therefore, for protons H_A and $H_{A'}$, $\delta \approx 8.1$ (d, 2H)

(c) Protons H_X and $H_{X'}$

Protons H_X and $H_{X'}$ are chemically equivalent but magnetically non-equivalent. Hence, each proton gets recorded as a doublet of 1 proton integration. Proton H_X couples with proton H_A and proton $H_{X'}$ couples with proton $H_{A'}$. Ordinarily, because of very small difference in the chemical shift of protons H_X and $H_{X'}$ and because of almost the same values of J_{AX} and $J_{A'X'}$, protons H_X and $H_{X'}$, get recorded as a doublet corresponding to 2 protons at the same chemical shift value. These two protons are away from the electron withdrawing nitro group, but they are nearer to the electron releasing methyl group. Hence, they produce a peak which is upfield to the peak for the protons H_A and $H_{A'}$.

Therefore, for protons H_X and $H_{X'}$, $\delta \approx 7.2$ (d, 2H)

7) Example-7: Assign the chemical shift values (in δ ppm) and the multiplicity to the protons in the following molecule.

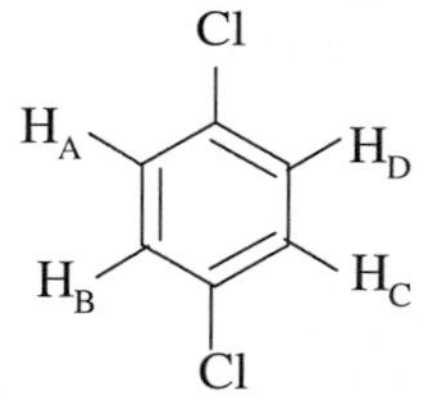

This molecule has symmetrical structure. Because of the plane of symmetry, all the four protons, H_A, H_B, H_C and H_D, are chemically equivalent. Hence, all the four protons get recorded at the same place, as a singlet corresponding to 4 protons. Chlorine is electron withdrawing. Hence, the protons are less shielded. Similarly, all the protons are aromatic protons.

Therefore, for protons H_A, H_B, H_C and H_D, $\delta \approx 7.3$ (s, 4H)

8) Example-8: Assign the chemical shift values (in δ ppm) and the multiplicity to the protons in the following molecule.

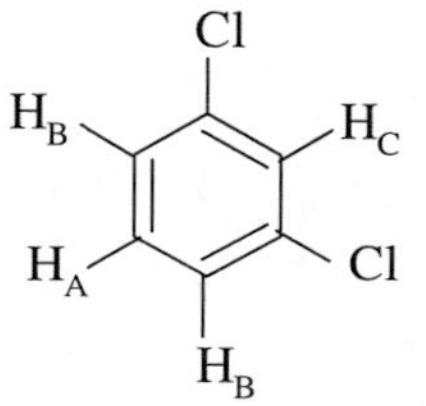

In this case, the coupling of only the *ortho* protons is considered.

(a) Proton H_C

Proton H_C being closer to two chlorine atoms, experiences more dragging of electrons and hence, its peak is produced most downfield compared to the other protons of the ring. Since, there is no other neighboring proton, H_C appears as a singlet.

Therefore, for proton H_C, $\delta \approx 7.35$ (s, 1H)

(b) Protons H_B

Two H_B protons are chemically and magnetically equivalent. These two protons are adjacent to one chlorine atom on one side and one proton on the other side. Hence, their peak is downfield to H_A but upfield to H_C. Because of one adjacent proton H_A, they produce a doublet at the same place.

Therefore, for two H_B protons, $\delta \approx 7.30$ (d, 2H)

(c) Proton H_A

Proton H_A has two neighboring H_B protons, but both being chemically equivalent, produce (2 + 1) = 3 peaks, i.e. a triplet. The intensity of peaks in a triplet is in the ratio of 1:2:1, as shown in **Fig. 17.6(a)**.

Thus, for proton H_A, $\delta \approx$ 7.25 (t, 1H)

Note: In the above structure, if one chlorine atom is replaced by a bromine atom, two H_B protons would be chemically non-equivalent.

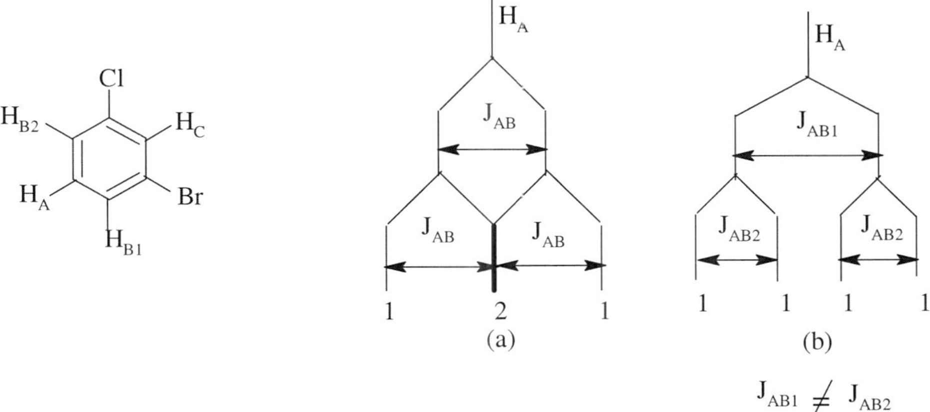

Fig. 17.6: Splitting of a peak for H_A (a) by two chemically equivalent H_B protons and (b) by chemically non-equivalent protons H_{B1} and H_{B2}

For such a structure, protons H_{B1} and H_{B2} are recorded as two doublets at different chemical shift values. Similarly, proton H_A would get recorded as (1 + 1) (1 + 1) = 4 peaks (doublet of a doublet), i.e. in this case, proton H_{B1} couples with proton H_A and splits the peak for H_A into two, as shown in **Fig. 17.6(b)**. Similarly, proton H_{B2} couples with proton H_A and splits two peaks for H_A into two more peaks, as shown in **Fig. 17.6(b)**. Since, the J values for these two couplings are different, the peak for H_A appears as a doublet of a doublet.

9) Example-9: A compound with molecular formula $C_8H_8O_3$ produces following peaks in its PMR spectrum. Assign the most probable structure to the molecule.

^{1}H-NMR:

(δ ppm)	Multiplicity
3.9	(s, 3H)
6.88	(d, 1H)
6.98	(d, 1H)
7.45	(d, 1H)
7.83	(d, 1H)
10.80	(s, 1H) Exchanges with D_2O

Solution:

1) Total number of protons = 8 (Sum of protons given in brackets in the above table).
2) Four protons are present in the aromatic range (δ = 6-8). Therefore, a disubstituted benzene ring may be present.
3) Proton at δ = 10.80 is D_2O exchangeable. Therefore, phenolic or acidic -OH group may be present.
4) Since all the aromatic protons appear as doublets corresponding to one proton each, the two –C-H units must be adjacent to each other, i.e. a compound must be para substituted.
5) Three protons at δ = 3.9, may be from a CH_3 group, attached to an electronegative oxygen atom.
6) Thus, with the units, C_6H_4-, -OCH_3 and one –OH group, 7 C atoms, 8 H atoms and 2 O atoms are accounted for. Still, one C atom and one O atom remain to be accounted for. This can be considered as a keto group.
7) All the four protons, H_A, H_B, H_C and H_D, are chemically non-equivalent and hence, they are recorded as four doublets at different positions.
8) Hence, the possible structure of a compound can be as follows.

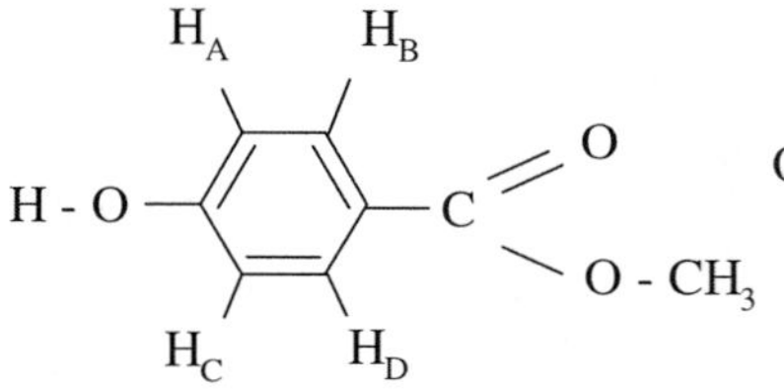

H_A H_B H - O — (benzene ring) — C(=O) — O - CH_3 H_C H_D

OR

H_A H_B H_3 CO — (benzene ring) — C(=O) — O - H H_C H_D

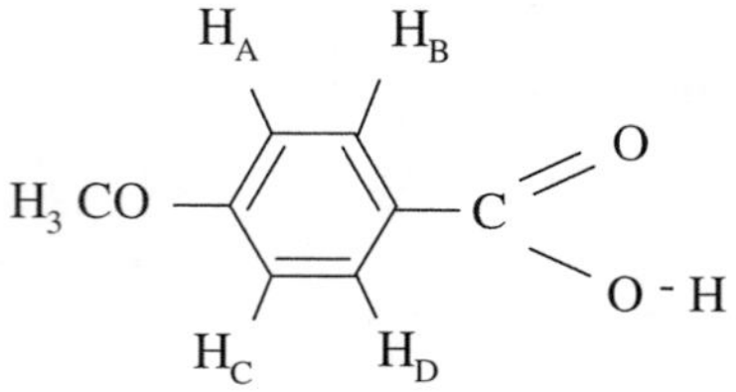

10) Example-10: A compound with molecular formula $C_9H_{11}O_2N$ produces following peaks in its PMR spectrum. Assign the most probable structure to the molecule.

^{1}H-NMR:

(δ ppm)	Multiplicity
2.8	(t, 2H)
3.1	(t, 2H)
4.8	(s, 2H)
7.8	(m, 4H)
10.10	(s, 1H)

Solution:

1) Total number of protons = 11.
2) The peaks at δ = 2.8 and 3.1, each producing a triplet of two protons each, indicate the presence of $-CH_2-CH_2-$ unit.
3) Protons at δ = 4.8 indicate the presence of hydroxy or amino protons. Since the integration corresponds to two protons, it should be because of primary amino protons ($-NH_2$).
4) Four protons at δ = 7.8 are in the aromatic range. Since the integration corresponds to 4 protons, a disubstituted benzene ring may be present.
5) Proton at δ = 10.10 indicates that it can be a hydroxy proton from carboxylic acid or phenol or it can be an aldehydic proton.
6) Since only one proton appears beyond δ = 10 and since two O atoms are present in the molecule, the presence of –COOH group cannot be ruled out. Thus, with the units - C_6H_4, - $CH_2 - CH_2$, $-NH_2$ and one COOH group, all the 9 C atoms, 11 H atoms and 2 O atoms are accounted for.
7) Hence, the possible structures of a compound can be as follows.

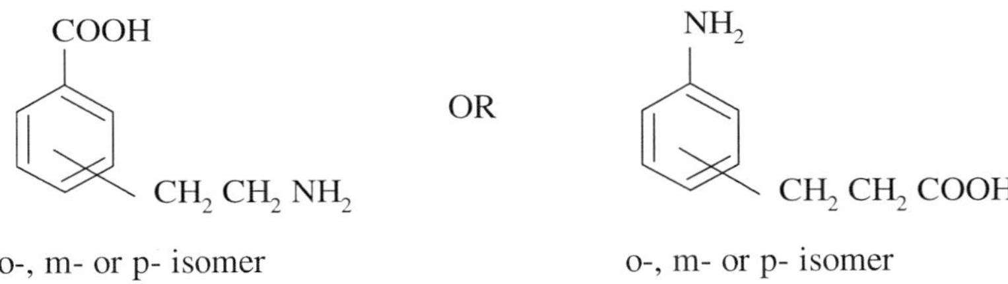

Problems for practice:

Note: Answers to these problems are at the end of this exercise.

Deduce all the possible structures of compounds from the following data.

1) Molecular formula: C_8H_9NO

(δ ppm)	Multiplicity
1.2	(s, 3H)
5.2	(s, 1H)
6.8	(m, 5H)

2) Molecular formula: $C_9H_{10}O$

(δ ppm)	Multiplicity
0.9	(t, 3H)
1.5	(q, 2H)
7.2	(m. 4H)
10.8	(s, 1H)

3) Molecular formula: $C_7H_{14}O_3$

(δ ppm)	Multiplicity
0.9	(t, 60 mm)
2.1	(q, 40 mm)
2.5	(s, 40 mm)

Hint: Figures in mm in the bracket indicate integration of the peaks. The ratio of these figures gives the ratio in which protons are recorded under each peak. For e.g., ratio of 60:40:40 indicates that protons are present in the ratio of 6:4:4 or 3:2:2, i.e. the total number of protons in the molecule can be either 7 (3:2:2) or 14 (6:4:4) or its multiple. Since the molecular formula is given, total number of protons is 14. Hence, the protons under the 1st peak are 6 and under 2nd and 3rd peaks are 4 each.

4) Molecular formula: $C_7H_7NO_2$

(δ ppm)	Multiplicity
4.3	(s, 20 mm)
5.4	(s, 10 mm)
7.2	(m, 40 mm)

5) Molecular formula: $C_5H_6N_2O$

(δ ppm)	Multiplicity
2.1	(d, 10 mm)
2.5	(s, 10 mm)
3.2	(t, 5 mm)
4.7	(s, 5 mm)

6) Molecular formula: $C_7H_6N_2O_3$

(δ ppm)	Multiplicity
4.2	(s, 0.8 mm)
7.8	(m, 1.6 mm)

7) Molecular formula: C_6H_{12}

(δ ppm)	Multiplicity
2.2	(s, 60 mm)

8) Molecular formula: $C_4H_5\ NO_2$

(δ ppm)	Multiplicity
2.7	(t, 10 mm)
2.9	(t, 10 mm)
11.2	(s, 5 mm)

9) A compound has molecular weight = 100 and it exhibits the following spectral characteristics. Deduce its structure.

^{1}H-NMR (ä ppm): 1.3 (d, 48 mm), 4.0 (m, 16 mm), 2.1 (d, 33 mm)

Answers to Problems 1 to 9:

1)

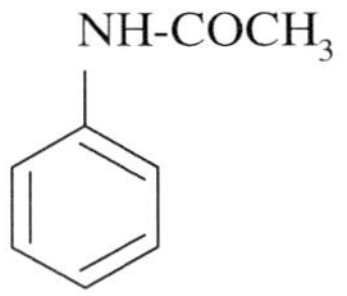

$NH\text{-}COCH_3$ (attached to a benzene ring)

2)

CHO and $CH_2\ CH_3$ (on a benzene ring)

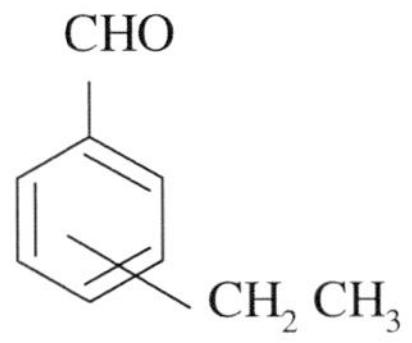

o-, m- or p- isomer

3)

$$H_3C - CH_2 - O - CH_2 - \overset{\overset{\displaystyle O}{||}}{C} - CH_2 - O - CH_2 - CH_3$$

4)

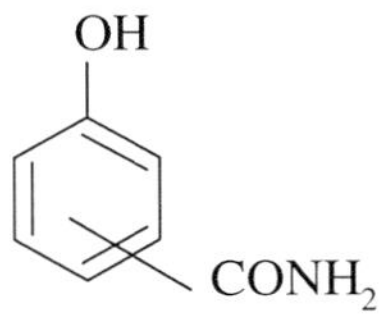

OH and $CONH_2$ (on a benzene ring)

5)

$$CH_2 = CH - \overset{\overset{\displaystyle O}{\|}}{C} - NH - CH_2 - C \equiv N$$

6) 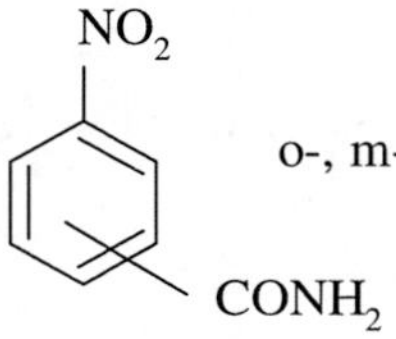 o-, m- or p- isomer

NO_2 — benzene ring — $CONH_2$

7)

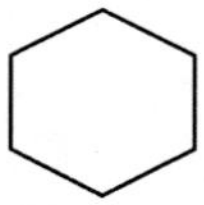

8)

$$N \equiv C - CH_2 - CH_2 - \overset{\overset{\displaystyle O}{\|}}{C} - OH$$

9)

H_3C — CH = CH — CH_3; CH_2 — O — CH_2

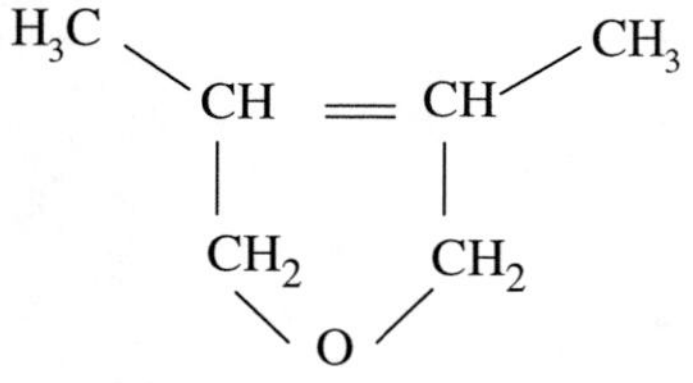

PROBLEMS ON MASS SPECTROMETRY

Table 17.3 lists the loss in weight from the species if certain radicals are lost during fragmentation process.

Table 17.3: Loss of mass for the species lost as radicals

Sr. No.	Loss of mass (units)	Possible species lost as radicals
1	14	CH_2
2	15	CH_3, NH
3	16	NH_2
4	17	OH
5	18	H_2O
6	28	C=O, CH_2=CH_2, N_2
7	29	CH_3-CH_2, CHO
8	31	OCH_3
9	43	CH_3-CH_2-CH_2
10	45	COOH
11	57	CH_3-CH_2-CH_2- CH_2

1) Example-1: Explain the appearance of the peaks corresponding to m/e = 142 (M^+) and m/e = 113 in the following compound.

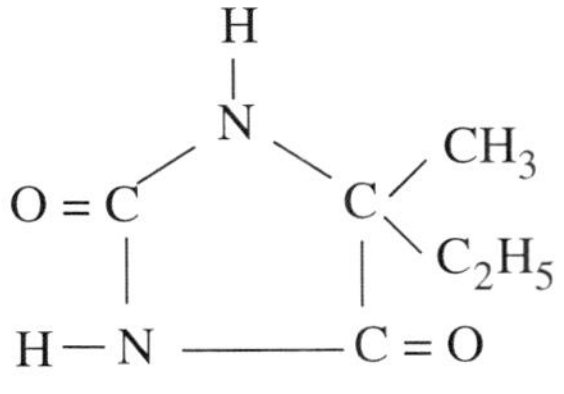

H
|
N — C(CH_3)(C_2H_5)
O = C |
| |
H—N ——— C = O

Solution: Molecular weight of the parent compound is 142. The fragment of m/e = 113 is formed because of the loss of a fragment of mass 29 (142 -113 = 29). This corresponds to an ethyl radical. This fragmentation is shown below.

Mol. Wt = 142 $\xrightarrow{-e}$ $M^+ = 142$ $\xrightarrow{-\dot{C}_2H_5}$ $(M - 29) = 113$

2) Example-2: Explain the formation of the abundant ions at m/e = 57 and m/e = 155 in the mass spectrum of the following compound having molecular weight of 170.

$(C_{12}H_{26})$ Mol wt = 170

$$H_3C-C(CH_3)_2-CH_2-C_7H_{15} \xrightarrow{-e} H_3C-\overset{+}{C}(CH_3)_2 \cdot CH_2-C_7H_{15} \longrightarrow H_3C-C^+(CH_3)_2 + \cdot CH_2-C_7H_{15}$$

m/e = 57

(tertiary carbocation)

$$H_3C-C(CH_3)_2-CH_2-C_7H_{15} \xrightarrow{-e} H_3C-\overset{\bullet +}{C}(CH_3)_2-CH_2-C_7H_{15} \longrightarrow H_3C-\overset{+}{C}(CH_3)-CH_2-C_7H_{15} + \cdot CH_3$$

m/e = 155 (tertiary carbocation)

(a) The fragment of m/e = 155 corresponds to the loss of mass equal to (170 -155 =15), i.e. the loss of $\cdot CH_3$ radical.

(b) The fragment of m/e = 57 corresponds to the loss of mass equal to (170 -57 = 113), i.e. the loss of $\cdot C_8H_{17}$ radical.

3) Example-3: The mass spectrum of 5-methyl-3-heptene has a molecular ion peak at m/e = 112. Explain the peaks at -

(a) m/e = 97 and

(b) m/e = 83

Solution:

(a) The fragment of m/e = 97 corresponds to the loss of mass equal to (112 -97 =15), i.e. the loss of $\cdot CH_3$ radical.

(b) The fragment of m/e = 83 corresponds to the loss of mass equal to (112 -83 = 29), i.e. the loss of $\cdot C_2H_5$ radical.

This fragmentation is shown below.

$$CH_3-CH_2-CH=CH-\underset{|}{\overset{CH_3}{CH}}-CH_2-CH_3 \xrightarrow{-e} CH_3-CH_2-\overset{+}{C}H-\overset{\bullet}{C}H-\overset{CH_3}{CH}-CH_2-CH_3$$

Mol. wt. = 112

$\downarrow -e$

$$CH_3-CH_2-\overset{+}{C}H-\overset{\bullet}{C}H-\overset{CH_3}{CH}-CH_2-CH_3 \qquad CH_3-CH_2-\overset{+}{C}H-\overset{\bullet}{C}H-\overset{\bullet}{\overset{CH_3}{CH}} + \overset{\bullet}{C}H_2-CH_3$$

$\downarrow -\overset{\bullet}{C}H_3$

$$CH_3-CH_2-\overset{+}{C}H \; CH=CH-CH_2-CH_3 \qquad CH_3-CH_2-\overset{+}{C}H \; CH=\overset{CH_3}{CH}$$

m/e = 97 m/e = 83

$$CH_3-CH_2-CH=CH-\overset{+}{C}H-CH_2-CH_3 \qquad CH_3-CH_2-CH=CH-\underset{+}{\overset{CH_3}{CH}}$$

4) Example-4: Are the following peaks indicated in the mass spectrum consistent with the structure –

(a) ethylbutyl ether; or

(b) methyl-n-pentyl ether

Justify your answer.

m/e = 102, 87, 73, 59, 45

Solution:

Ethylbutyl ether is – $CH_3—CH_2—O—CH_2—CH_2—CH_2—CH_3$

Methyl-n-pentyl ether is – $CH_3—O—CH_2—CH_2—CH_2—CH_2—CH_3$

(a) Molecular weight of both the compounds is 102.

(b) A fragment with m/e = 87 corresponds to the loss of mass equal to (102 – 87 = 15) units, which corresponds to the loss of a methyl ($\cdot CH_3$) radical.

(c) A fragment with m/e = 73 corresponds to the loss of mass equal to (102 –73 = 29) units, which corresponds to the loss of an ethyl ($\cdot C_2H_5$) radical.

(d) A fragment with m/e = 59 corresponds to the loss of mass equal to (102 – 59 = 43) units, which corresponds to the loss of a propyl ($\cdot C_3H_7$) radical.

(e) A fragment with m/e = 45 corresponds to the loss of mass equal to (102 – 45 = 57) units, which corresponds to the loss of a butyl ($\cdot C_4H_9$) radical.

This is shown by the following fragmentation pattern.

(A) Fragmentation in ethylbutyl ether

(i) Loss of methyl group

$$CH_3—CH_2—\ddot{\underset{\cdot\cdot}{O}}—CH_2—CH_2—CH_2—CH_3$$

Ethylbutyl ether (Mol. wt. = 102)

$$\downarrow -e$$

$$CH_3—CH_2—\overset{\bullet +}{\underset{\cdot\cdot}{O}}—CH_2—CH_2—CH_2—CH_3$$

M^+ ion (m/e = 102)

$$\downarrow$$

$$\dot{C}H_3 + \dot{C}H_2—\overset{\bullet +}{\underset{\cdot\cdot}{O}}—CH_2—CH_2—CH_2—CH_3$$

$$\downarrow$$

$$\dot{C}H_3 + CH_2=\overset{+}{\underset{\cdot\cdot}{O}}—CH_2—CH_2—CH_2—CH_3$$

(m/e = 102 -15 = 87)

(ii) Loss of ethyl group

$$CH_3-CH_2-\ddot{\underset{\cdot\cdot}{O}}-CH_2-CH_2-CH_2-CH_3$$

$\downarrow$ -e

$$CH_3-CH_2-\overset{\bullet +}{\underset{\cdot\cdot}{O}}-CH_2-CH_2-CH_2-CH_3$$

M^+ ion (m/e = 102)

$\downarrow$

$$CH_3-\dot{C}H_2 \;+\; {}^{+}\ddot{\underset{\cdot\cdot}{O}}-CH_2-CH_2-CH_2-CH_3$$

(m/e = 102 -29 = 73)

(iii) Loss of propyl group

$$CH_3-CH_2-\overset{\bullet +}{\underset{\cdot\cdot}{O}}-CH_2-CH_2-CH_2-CH_3$$

M^+ ion (m/e = 102)

$\downarrow$

$$CH_3-CH_2-\overset{\bullet +}{\underset{\cdot\cdot}{O}}-\dot{C}H_2 \;+\; \dot{C}H_2-CH_2-CH_3$$

$\downarrow$

$$CH_3-CH_2-\overset{+}{\underset{\cdot\cdot}{O}}=CH_2 \;+\; \dot{C}H_2-CH_2-CH_3$$

(m/e = 102 - 43 = 59)

(iv) Loss of butyl group

$$CH_3-CH_2-\overset{\bullet +}{\underset{\cdot\cdot}{O}}-CH_2-CH_2-CH_2-CH_3$$

M^+ ion (m/e = 102)

$\downarrow$

$$CH_3-CH_2-\ddot{\underset{\cdot\cdot}{O}}{}^{+} \;+\; \dot{C}H_2-CH_2-CH_2-CH_3$$

(m/e = 102 -57 = 45)

(B) Fragmentation in methyl-n-pentyl ether

$CH_3-\ddot{\underset{\cdot\cdot}{O}}-CH_2-CH_2-CH_2-CH_2-CH_3$

Methyl-n-pentyl ether (Mol. wt. = 102)

For methyl-n-pentyl ether, following peaks are obtained.

(a) peak corresponding to the M^+ ion (m/e = 102),
(b) peak corresponding to the loss of methyl radical ($\cdot CH_3$) (m/e = 102 -15 = 87),
(c) peak corresponding to the loss of butyl radical ($\cdot C_4H_9$) (m/e = 102 -57= 45),
(d) peak corresponding to the loss of pentyl radical ($\cdot C_5H_{11}$) (m/e = 102 -71=31), which is not obtained in the mass spectrum. This is shown below.

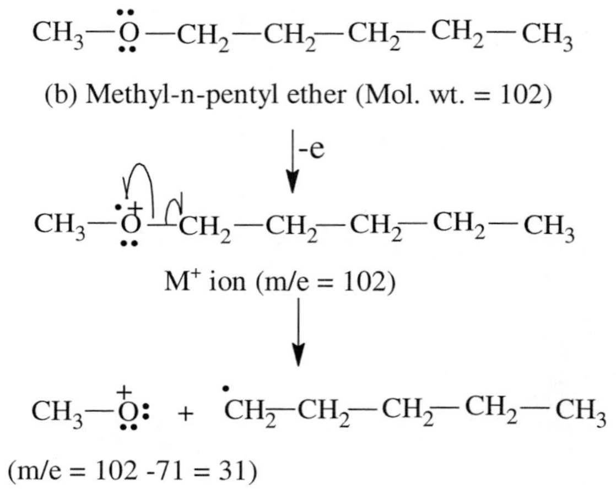

$CH_3-\ddot{\underset{\cdot\cdot}{O}}-CH_2-CH_2-CH_2-CH_2-CH_3$

(b) Methyl-n-pentyl ether (Mol. wt. = 102)

↓ -e

$CH_3-\overset{\cdot +}{\underset{\cdot\cdot}{O}}-CH_2-CH_2-CH_2-CH_2-CH_3$

M^+ ion (m/e = 102)

↓

$CH_3-\overset{+}{\underset{\cdot\cdot}{O}}: \; + \; \dot{C}H_2-CH_2-CH_2-CH_2-CH_3$

(m/e = 102 -71 = 31)

Similarly, this compound would not produce the peak corresponding to the loss of an ethyl radical and hence, would not show a peak at m/e = 73.

Hence, structure (a) of ethylbutyl ether is consistent with the spectral data and not the structure (b).

5) Example-5: The mass spectrum of heptyl chloride shows following peaks in its mass spectrum.

(a) m/e = 91 (100 %)
(b) m/e = 93 (35%)

Assign formulae to these fragments.

Solution:

(a) Heptyl chloride is $C_7H_{15}Cl$. This molecule can contain two isotopes of chlorine, viz., Cl^{35} and Cl^{37}.
(b) Its molecular weight is 134 or 136, depending on the presence of a particular isotope.
(c) The fragment with m/e = 91 corresponds to the loss in mass equal to (134 – 91 = 43).
(d) Mass loss of 43 units can be because of the propyl ($\cdot C_3H_7$) radical.
(e) Fragment with m/e = 93 (136 - 63) corresponds to the same loss in mass but it is produced by the compound with Cl^{37} isotope, i. e. it is an isotopic peak.

(f) Isotopic abundance for two isotopes of chlorine, Cl^{35}: Cl^{37} is in the ratio of 75.52: 24:47. Hence, the intensity of two peaks is in the ratio of 100 %: 35 %.

(g) Fractionation in heptyl chloride is shown as follows.

$CH_3—CH_2—CH_2—CH_2—CH_2—CH_2—CH_2—\ddot{Cl}:$

↓ -e

$CH_3—CH_2—CH_2—CH_2—CH_2—CH_2—CH_2—\overset{+}{\ddot{Cl}}$

↓

$CH_3—CH_2—\dot{C}H_2 + \dot{C}H_2—CH_2—CH_2—CH_2—\overset{+}{\ddot{Cl}}$

↓

$CH_3—CH_2—\dot{C}H_2$ + cyclic ($CH_2—CH_2—CH_2—CH_2—\ddot{Cl}^+$)

Cyclic chloronium ion

m/e = 91 for Cl^{35}

m/e = 93 for Cl^{37}

6) Example-6: The mass spectrum of methyl butyrate (Molecular weight = 102) contains peaks at m/e = 71 (55 %) and m/e = 43 (100 %). Suggest a mechanism to explain the formation of these ions.

Solution:

(a) Structure of methyl butyrate is $CH_3CH_2CH_2COOCH_3$. Its molecular weight is 102.

(b) The fragment F_1^+ at m/e = 71 is formed due to the loss of mass of (102 – 71 = 31) units.

(c) This would correspond to the loss of OCH_3 with mass equal to (16 + 15 = 31).

(d) The fragment F_2^+ at m/e = 43 is formed due to the loss of C=O, with mass equal to (12 + 16 = 28) from the fragment F_1^+. Mass of fragment F_1^+ is 71. Loss of carbon monoxide from it results in the formation of a fragment with mass equal to (71 – 28 = 43).

(e) These fragmentations are shown as below.

$$CH_3-CH_2-CH_2-\overset{\overset{\ddot{O}:}{||}}{C}-\ddot{O}CH_3$$

↓ -e

$$CH_3-CH_2-CH_2-\overset{\overset{\ddot{O}^{+\cdot}}{||}}{C}-\ddot{O}CH_3$$

M^+ ion, m/e = 102

↓

$$CH_3-CH_2-CH_2-\overset{\overset{\ddot{O}^{+\cdot}}{||}}{C}\cdot + \cdot\ddot{O}CH_3$$

↓

$$CH_3-CH_2-CH_2-\overset{\overset{\ddot{O}^{+}}{|||}}{C} + \cdot\ddot{O}CH_3$$

F_1^+, m/e = (102 - 31 = 71)

↓

$$CH_3-CH_2-CH_2-\overset{\overset{\ddot{O}:}{||}}{C}+ + \cdot\ddot{O}CH_3$$

↓

$$CH_3-CH_2-\overset{+}{C}H_2 + :C=\ddot{O}$$

F_2^+ , m/e = (71 - 28 = 43)

Since the positive charge is on the less electronegative carbon atom in fragment F_2^+, it is the most stable fragment and is obtained with 100 % intensity (a base peak). In fragment F_1^+, the positive charge is on more electronegative oxygen atom and hence, it is obtained with 55 % intensity.

7) Example-7: In the mass spectrum of 1-octanol (M = 130), an ion is observed at m/e = 84. This ion is formed by the elimination of water. Illustrate the cyclic transition state involved and also the loss of fragments during its fragmentation.

Solution:

(a) Fragmentation in1-octanol ($C_8H_{17}OH$) is shown below. Initially, a water molecule is lost by octanol, via the formation of a cyclic transition state.

(b) The fragment with m/e = 112 is formed by the loss of a water molecule corresponding to mass of 18.

(c) More stable fragment of m/e = 84 is formed by further elimination of an ethylene molecule corresponding to mass of 28.

-e

Cyclic transition state

$-H_2O$

m/e = (130 -18) =112

m/e = (112 -28) =84

Problems for practice:

1) Explain the formation of an ion at m/e = 68 in the mass spectrum of 1-methyl-1-cyclohexene.

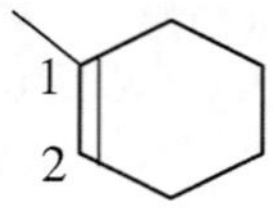

1
2

2) The mass spectrum of a compound contains a significant ion of m/e = 120. Which structure is most consistent with this data?

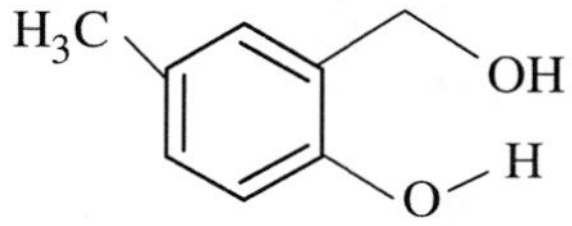

H_3C OH H O OR O CH_3 O H

(A) Mol. wt. = 138 (B) Mol. wt. = 138

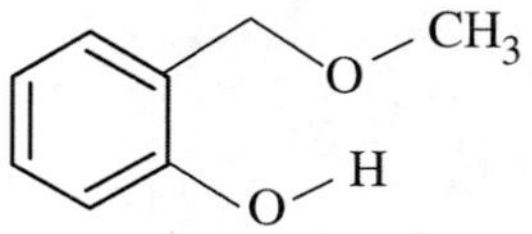

Answer: Structure A

3) In the mass spectrum of dimethyltetrahydrofuran (M = 100), ions are observed at –
(a) m/e =85 (67 %)
(b) m/e =56 (100 %)

Which isomer best fits this data?

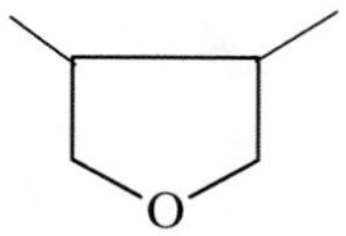

O O

(A) Mol. wt. = 100 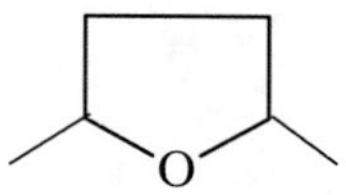 (B) Mol. wt. = 100

Answer: Structure B

MIXED PROBLEMS

Example-1: A compound having molecular weight 98 has following spectral data.

IR (cm^{-1}): 3429, 3385, 2900, 2210, 1660, 1620

^{1}H-NMR (δ ppm):

δ ppm	Multiplicity
2.14	t, 9.8 squares
3.40	t, 9.6 squares
4.03	s, 10 squares

Deduce the most probable structure of a compound.

Solution:

(a) Since there is no peak in the region corresponding to δ = 6-8 in the NMR spectrum of the compound, it is not an aromatic compound.

(b) Integration of all the peaks in the NMR spectrum is almost equal. Hence, the protons are in the ratio of 1:1:1. Hence, there are 3 protons or its multiple in the compound.

(c) Two triplets are recorded in the NMR spectrum. Hence, there is a possibility of a $- CH_2 - CH_2 -$ unit. Hence, the protons must be in the ratio of 2:2:2. On either side of this unit, the atoms which do not possess proton on them, should be present.

(d) A singlet at δ = 4.03 should also be produced by two protons. It may be because of the presence of an amino group.

(e) In the IR spectrum, the peaks at 3429 and 3385 cm^{-1} correspond to the symmetric and asymmetric N-H stretching vibrations of the primary amino group. The peak at 1620 cm^{-1} corresponds to N- H bending.

(f) The peak at 2210 cm^{-1} corresponds either to $C\equiv N$ or $C\equiv C$.

(g) The peak at 1660 cm^{-1} corresponds to C=O group.

Hence, the probable structure of a compound, which fits into the above data, is –

$$N\equiv C-CH_2-CH_2-\overset{\overset{\large O}{||}}{C}-NH_2$$

(Mol. formula: $C_4H_6N_2O$, Mol. wt. = 98)

Example-2: A compound of molecular weight 73 has the following spectral data.

Mass: m/e = 29, 44 (base peak), 57, 73.

^{1}H-NMR (δ ppm):

δ ppm	Multiplicity
1.15	t, 3H
2.25	q, 2H
6.4	s (broad, 2H), D_2O exchangeable

Deduce the most probable structure of a compound.

Solution:

(a) The NMR data suggests the presence of 7 protons in the compound.
(b) ^{1}H-NMR has one triplet and one quartet. This suggests the presence of CH_3-CH_2- unit.
(c) A broad singlet is produced because of the presence of two exchangeable protons of -NH_2 group.
(d) Thus, one CH_3-CH_2- unit and one -NH_2 group account for the weight corresponding to (15 + 14 + 16 = 45) units. This also accounts for all the 7 protons in the compound.
(e) Molecular weight of a compound is 73. Thus, a moiety having mass equal to (73-45 = 28) units remains to be accounted for. This can be achieved either by putting -CH_2-CH_2- unit or by C = O group or by putting $N \equiv N$ unit.
(f) The-CH_2-CH_2- unit cannot be put because the total number of protons getting recorded in ^{1}H-NMR spectrum is only 7 and all are accounted for.
(g)The structure obtained by putting C=O group, fits in the given data.

Hence, the most probable structure of a compound can be –

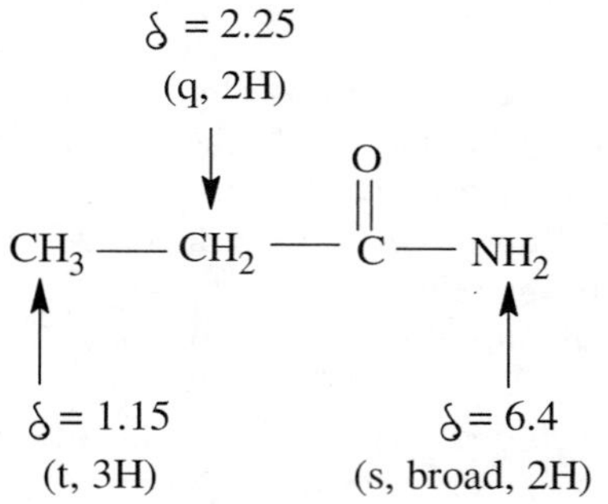

δ = 2.25 (q, 2H) → CH_2

$$CH_3 — CH_2 — C(=O) — NH_2$$

CH_3 ← δ = 1.15 (t, 3H)

NH_2 ← δ = 6.4 (s, broad, 2H)

The above structure also fits in the given mass spectral data. The mass spectrum of a compound can be explained by the following fragmentation pattern.

Fragmentation in mass spectrometry:

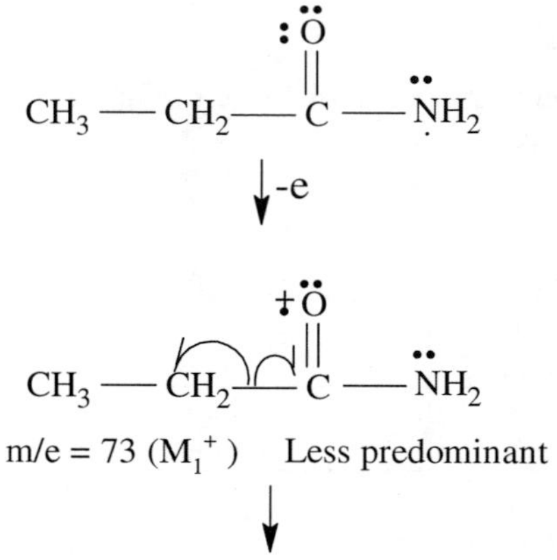

$$CH_3 — CH_2 — C(=\ddot{O}:) — \ddot{N}H_2$$

↓ -e

$$CH_3 — CH_2 — C(=\ddot{O}^{+\cdot}) — \ddot{N}H_2$$

m/e = 73 (M_1^+) Less predominant

↓

$$CH_3 - \dot{C}H_2 + \cdot C(=\overset{+}{O}) - NH_2$$

$$\downarrow$$

$$C^{+}(=O) - NH_2 \leftarrow C(\equiv \overset{+}{O}) - NH_2 \; (F_1^+)$$

m/e = 16 +12 + 14 +2 = 44

Less predominant

OR

$$CH_3 - CH_2 - C(=O) - NH_2$$

$$\downarrow -e$$

$$CH_3 - CH_2 - C(=O) - \overset{\cdot +}{N}H_2$$

m/e = 73 (M_2^+) More predominant

$$\downarrow$$

$$CH_3 - \dot{C}H_2 + \cdot C(=O) - \overset{\cdot +}{N}H_2$$

$$\downarrow$$

$$C^{+}(=O) - NH_2 \leftarrow C(=O) = \overset{+}{N}H_2 \; (F_2^+)$$

m/e = 16 +12 + 14 +2 = 44

More predominant

The peak at m/e = 73 is due to the formation of molecular ions (M_1^+) and (M_2^+). The molecular ion M_1^+ is less predominant, since the positive charge is present on the more electronegative oxygen atom. The peak corresponding to m/e = 44 is formed in two ways and it is the most intense peak or is the base peak. The fragment

F_1^{+} is less predominant, since the positive charge is present on the more electronegative oxygen atom.

The fragment with m/e = 29 corresponds to the formation of $CH_3CH_2^+$ ion as shown below.

$$CH_3-CH_2-\overset{\overset{+\ddot{O}:}{\parallel}}{C}-\ddot{N}H_2$$

m/e = 73 (M_1^+)

$$\downarrow$$

$$CH_3-CH_2-\overset{\overset{:\ddot{O}\cdot}{|}}{\underset{+}{C}}-\ddot{N}H_2$$

$$\downarrow$$

$$CH_3-\overset{+}{C}H_2 \;+\; :\overset{\overset{:\ddot{O}\cdot}{|}}{C}-\ddot{N}H_2$$

m/e = 29

$$\cdot\overset{\overset{:\ddot{O}}{\parallel}}{C}-\ddot{N}H_2$$

The fragment with m/e = 57 corresponds to the formation of $CH_3CH_2\ C\equiv O^+$ ion as shown below.

$$CH_3-CH_2-\overset{\overset{+\ddot{O}:}{\parallel}}{C}-\ddot{N}H_2$$

m/e = 73 (M_1^+)

$$\downarrow$$

$$CH_3-CH_2-\overset{\overset{+\ddot{O}:}{\parallel}}{C}\cdot \;+\; \cdot\ddot{N}H_2$$

$$\downarrow$$

$$CH_3-CH_2-\overset{\overset{\ddot{O}+}{\equiv}}{C}$$

m/e = 57

$$\downarrow$$

$$CH_3-CH_2-\overset{\overset{:\ddot{O}}{\parallel}}{\underset{+}{C}}$$

m/e = 57

Example-3: Deduce the structure of a compound of molecular weight 148 having following spectral data.

IR (cm^{-1}): 3010, 2701, 1662, 1627, 1521

^{1}H-NMR (δ ppm):

δ ppm	Multiplicity
9.8	s, 1H
7.3	m, 5H
6.1	s, 1H
5.9	s, 1H

Deduce the structure of a compound.

Solution:

(a) IR (cm^{-1}):

Frequency(cm^{-1})	Inference
3010	C – H str
2701	C – H str from aldehydic group
1662	C = O str
1627	C = N str or C = C str
1521	C = C str, aromatic

(b) ^{1}H-NMR (δ ppm):

δ ppm	Multiplicity
9.8 (s, 1H)	CHO, COOH, OH or NH group may be present
7.3 (m, 5H)	Monosubstituted phenyl ring may be present
6.1 (s, 1H)	-NH or –OH group may be present
5.9 (s, 1H)	-NH or –OH group may be present

(c) From the NMR data, the total number of protons in the molecule is 8.

(d) In the NMR spectrum, the peak at δ = 7.3 can be for a mono-substituted phenyl ring, which corresponds to C_6H_5 unit and accounts for the mass of (72 + 5 = 77) units.

(e) In the IR spectrum, the peak corresponding to 2701 cm^{-1} is because of C-H stretching from an aldehyde. The peak corresponding to 1662 cm^{-1} can be because of C=O stretching from an aldehyde. Hence, δ = 9.8 in NMR, confirms the presence of -CHO group in the molecule. It accounts for the mass of (12 + 1 + 16 = 29) units.

(f) Thus, the mass equal to (77 + 29 = 106) units is accounted for and the mass of (148 – 106 = 42) units and two more protons, remain to be accounted for.

(g) As per the NMR data, if two -NH groups are assumed to be present, then the mass of 30 units would be accounted for. Thus, the mass equal to (106 + 30 = 136) units is accounted for. Therefore, now, only the mass equal to (148 – 36) = 12 units, i.e. one more carbon atom, is required to be included in the structure.

Hence, the final structure can be –

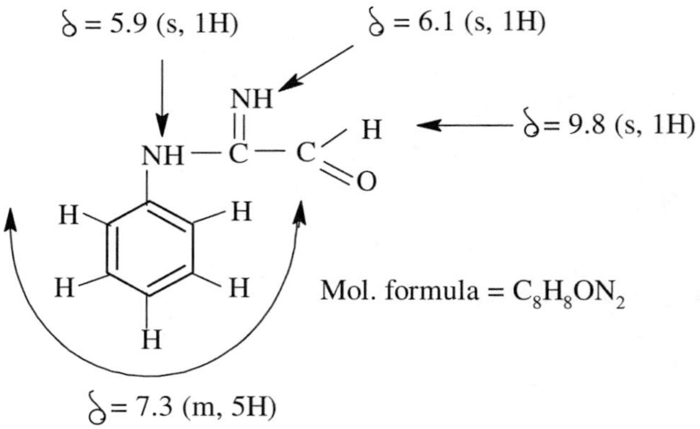

δ = 5.9 (s, 1H)

δ = 6.1 (s, 1H)

δ = 9.8 (s, 1H)

Mol. formula = $C_8H_8ON_2$

δ = 7.3 (m, 5H)

Example-4: A compound has following spectral characteristics. Deduce its structure.
Mass: 107 (M^+), 106 (100 %), 79, 78, 77
IR (cm^{-1}): 3410, 3305, 1610, 1508, 1452
^{1}H-NMR (δ ppm):

δ ppm	Multiplicity
7.3	m, 5H
3.8	s, 2H
5.9	s, 2H

Solution:

(a) From the NMR spectrum, the total number of protons in the molecule is 9.

(b) In the IR spectrum, peaks at 3410 and 3305 cm^{-1} suggest the presence of a primary amino group. The peak at δ = 5.9 in the NMR spectrum, corresponding to two protons, may be because of $-NH_2$ group.

(b) In the NMR spectrum, the peak at δ = 7.3 corresponding to 5 protons indicates the presence of a mono-substituted phenyl ring.

(c) One phenyl ring and one amino group account for the mass equal to C_6H_5 (72 + 5 = 77) and NH_2 (14+2 = 16), i.e. (77 + 16 = 93) units.

(d) The peak at m/e = 107 is the molecular ion peak. Hence, the molecular weight of the compound is 107.

(e) What remains to be accounted for is the mass equal to (107 – 93 = 14) units.

This can be fulfilled by introducing one CH_2 group, since two more protons at ä = 3.8 are also to be accounted for.

(f) Hence, the final structure can be –

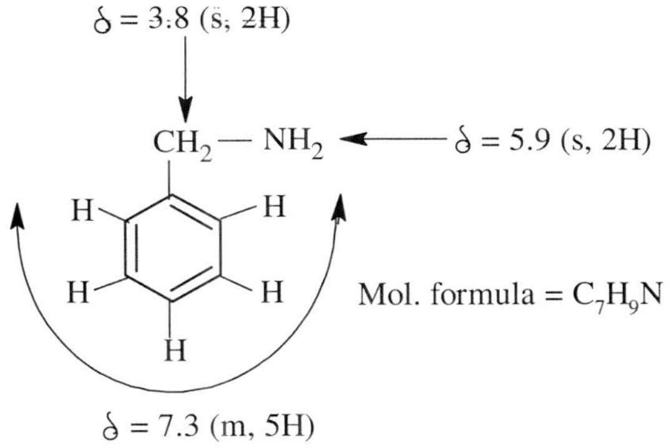

δ = 3.8 (s, 2H)

$CH_2 — NH_2$ ← δ = 5.9 (s, 2H)

δ = 7.3 (m, 5H)

Mol. formula = C_7H_9N

The fragmentation of this compound in the mass spectrum explains the peaks in its mass spectrum.

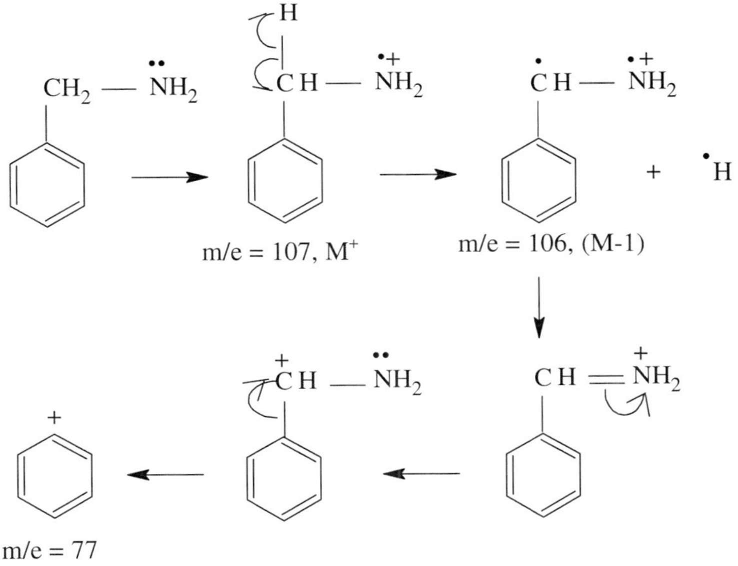

m/e = 107, M^+

m/e = 106, (M-1)

m/e = 77

Peaks at m/e = 78 and 79 are isotopic peaks.

Example-5: A compound has molecular weight of 99 and it exhibits the following spectral characteristics. Deduce its structure.

UV: No significant absorption

IR (cm^{-1}): 2910, 2235, 1470, 1400, 989

^1H-NMR (δ ppm):

δ ppm	Multiplicity
1.1	t, J = 6 Hz
2.7	t, J = 7 Hz
3.7	t, J = 7 Hz
4.7	q, J = 6 Hz

Solution:

(a) Protons with J = 6 Hz are coupled and hence, they are adjacent to each other.
(b) These protons produce a triplet and a quartet. Hence, they are from the CH_3-CH_2- unit.
(c) Similarly, protons with J = 7 Hz are coupled and hence, they are the neighboring protons. Both produce triplets and hence, they are from the -CH_2-CH_2- unit.
(d) These 2 units account for the mass of 29 (for CH_3-CH_2- unit) and 28 (for -CH_2- CH_2- unit). Both together account for the mass of (29 + 28 = 57) units.
(e) These two units should be separated by the group or atom which does not have proton on it.
(f) The peak at 2235 cm^{-1} in the IR spectrum, indicates the presence of –CN group, which accounts for the mass of (12 + 14) = 26 units.
(g) Thus, the total mass of (57 + 26) = 83 is accounted for.
(h) Hence, the mass to be accounted for is (99 – 83 = 16). This can be achieved by introducing one oxygen atom.

Hence, the final structure can be as follows.

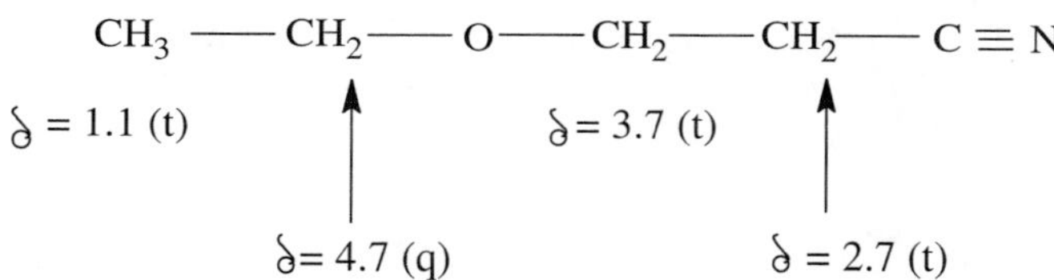

(Mol. formula = C_5H_9ON, Mol. wt. = 99).

Example-6: A compound having molecular weight 69 exhibits the following spectral characteristics. Deduce its structure.

UV: Above 210 nm
IR (cm^{-1}): 2941, 2857, 2273, 1460
^1H-NMR (ä ppm): 2.72 (septet, J = 6.7 Hz, 4.2 squares), 1.33 (doublet, J = 6.7 Hz, 25.8 squares)

Solution:

(a) From the NMR spectrum, the ratio of protons is 1:6.
(b) Protons with J = 6.7 Hz are coupled with each other and hence, they are the neighbors of each other.
(c) Septet at δ = 2.72 corresponding to one proton and a doublet at δ = 1.33 corresponding to six protons, indicate the presence of the following unit (an isopropyl group) in the molecule.

$$—CH\begin{matrix} CH_3 \\ CH_3 \end{matrix}$$

(d) This unit accounts for the mass of (13 + 15 + 15 = 43) units.
(e) The mass remains to be accounted for is (69 – 43 = 26) units.
(f) The peak in the IR spectrum at 2273 cm^{-1} indicates the presence of –CN group, which accounts for the mass of 26 units.

Hence, the probable structure of a compound can be –

$$N{\equiv}C{-}CH(CH_3)_2$$

Example-7: A compound having molecular weight 72 exhibits the following spectral characteristics. Deduce its structure.
UV: Above 274 nm
IR (cm^{-1}): 3011, 2817, 1658, 1425
^{1}H-NMR (δ ppm):

δ ppm	Multiplicity
2.48	quartet, J = 7.3 Hz, 12 squares
2.12	singlet, 17.6 squares
1.07	triplet, J =7.3 Hz, 18.2 squares

Solution:
(a) From the NMR spectrum, the ratio of protons is 2:3:3.
(b) Hence, the total number of protons can be 8 or its multiple.
(c) Protons with J = 7.3 Hz are coupled and hence, they are the neighbors of each other.
(d) Quartet at δ = 2.48 and a triplet at δ = 1.07, indicate the presence of an ethyl group (CH_3-CH_2) in the molecule. Thus, for a molecule containing 8 protons, 5 protons are accounted for.
(e) Singlet at δ = 2.12 corresponding to 3 protons can be because of CH_3 protons.
(f) Thus, the mass of one ethyl and one methyl unit, corresponding to (29 + 15 = 44) units, is accounted for.
(g) The mass of (72 – 44 = 28) units remains to be acccunted for. This can be achieved by putting C = O group in the structure, since the compound produces a peak at 1658 cm^{-1} in its IR spectrum.

Hence, the probable structure of a compound can be –

$$CH_3{-}CH_2{-}\overset{\overset{\displaystyle O}{||}}{C}{-}CH_3$$

Example-8: A compound with molecular formula, C_7H_9N exhibits the following spectral characteristics. Deduce its structure.
IR (cm^{-1}): 3341, 1610, 1525, 1451
^{1}H-NMR (δ ppm): 6.98 (m, 5H), 4.1 (s, 1H), 1.5 (s, 3H)

Solution:

(a) Total number of protons in the molecule is 9.

(b) Single peak at 3341 cm^{-1}in the IR spectrum indicates the presence of a secondary amino group. In the NMR spectrum, the peak at δ = 4.1, with integration corresponding to one proton, can be for an amino group (-NH).

(c) A singlet at δ = 1.5 corresponding to 3 protons, indicates the presence of a methyl group.

(d) In the NMR spectrum, the peak at δ = 6.98, corresponding to 5 protons, can be for a mono-substituted phenyl ring.

Hence, the probable structure of the molecule, which fits into the above spectral data is –

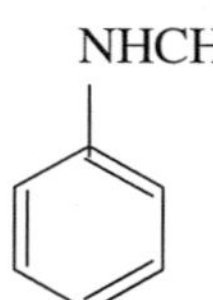

Problems for practice:

Answers to these problems are given at the end of three problems.

1. Molecular weight = 104

R (Cm^{-1}): 3325, 3125, 2857, 2695, 1675, 1449
^{1}H-NMR:

δ ppm	Multiplicity
10.95	s, 5.4 squares
4.13	s, 11.1 squares
3.66	q, 10.6 squares
1.27	t, 16.6 squares

2. Molecular weight = 99

IR (Cm^{-1}): 2910, 1470, 1400, 1000
^{1}H-NMR:

δ ppm	Multiplicity
4.7	q, J = 6 Hz
3.7	t, J = 7 Hz
2.7	t, J = 7 Hz
1.1	t, J = 6 Hz

3. Molecular weight = 82

IR (Cm^{-1}): 2900, 2210, 1120

^{1}H-NMR:

δ ppm	Multiplicity
4.03	s, 10 sq.
3.4	t, 9.6 sq.
2.14	t, 9.8 sq.

Answers to Mixed problems:

1. $H_3C - H_2C - O - CH_2 - O - CHO$

2. 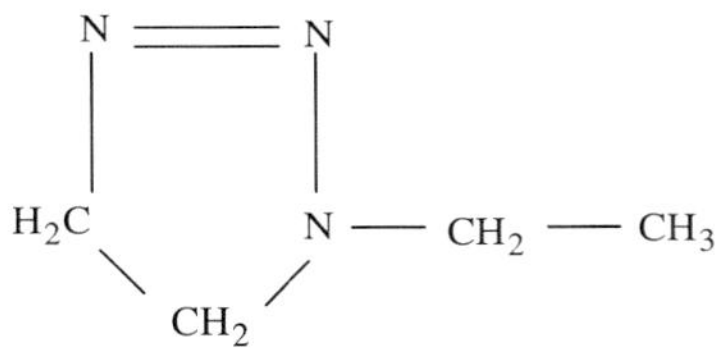 Five-membered ring: N = N, with N attached to H_2C and the other N bonded to $CH_2 - CH_3$; the ring is closed by a bridging CH_2 between H_2C and N-ethyl.

3. $N \equiv C - CH_2 - CH_2 - N = CH_2$

CHAPTER 18

UPKEEP AND MAINTENANCE OF ANALYTICAL INSTRUMENTS

Maintenance of an instrument is the process of maintaining or state of being maintained, i. e. the process of keeping/being kept in good condition by checking or repairing an instrument regularly. The best maintenance is the preventive maintenance, i. e. before an instrument gives trouble.

Upkeep of an instrument is the process of keeping an instrument in good condition.

The cost of the sophisticated analytical instruments is so high that proper precautions are necessary to keep them running for a longer period of time with high efficiency.

In order to maintain analytical instruments in good condition, regular preventive maintenance is required, i.e. the instruments are checked periodically for proper functioning to avoid the break down.

Some of the basic steps for upkeep and maintenance of instruments are mentioned below.

1. Keep analytical instruments preferably in a separate room, provided with a double door and which is dust free.
2. Provide temperature and moisture control in the instrument room. Humidity control is especially required for IR spectrometers, making use of beam splitters.
3. Provide a shock proof and sturdy platform for instruments.
4. Do not clutter the instrument room with unnecessary furniture.
5. Do not eat, drink or smoke in the instrument room.
6. Do not store chemicals in the instrument room
7. Do not expose instruments to harsh conditions like extreme temperature or corrosive vapor of chemicals.
8. Do not move instruments from one place to the other.
9. Do not spill any reagents on the instruments.
10. Prepare standard operating procedure (SOP) for all the instruments so that correct steps are followed by every operator.
11. Appoint one laboratory technician to take care of all the instruments regularly.
12. Calibrate the instruments from time to time.
13. Optimize the columns in HPLC and GC after regular intervals.
14. Do not leave electrodes open in air. Dip them in the appropriate solutions.
15. Rejuvenate electrodes whenever required.
16. Always use 'matched' pair of cuvettes for UV and fluorescence spectrometry. Do not handle the polished surface of cuvettes.
17. After the use, wash cuvettes with a suitable solvent and keep them dry.
18. Do not keep wet cuvettes in the instrument.
19. Make use of analytical grade (AR) reagents, whenever required.
20. Maintain a permanent log book for each instrument for the entry of an operator.
21. Keep foot-operated dust-bin in the instrument room.

INDEX